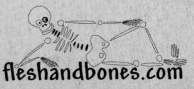

Self-assessment in Clinical Medicine

Dedicated to my wife Jayashree,
son Anoop and daughter Neena

For W. B. Saunders

Commissioning Editor: Ellen Green
Project Development Manager: Helen Leng
Project Manager: Nancy Arnott
Designer: Sarah Russell

Self-assessment in Clinical Medicine

Ragavendra R. Baliga
MB BS MD DNB FACC FRCP(Edin)

Clinical Assistant Professor of Medicine
Division of Cardiology
University Hospital
The University of Michigan
Ann Arbor, Michigan, USA

THIRD EDITION

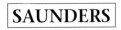

EDINBURGH   LONDON   NEW YORK   OXFORD   PHILADELPHIA   ST LOUIS   SYDNEY   TORONTO   2004

SAUNDERS
An imprint of Elsevier Limited

First edition 1994
Second edition 1999
Reprinted 2000, 2001, 2002
Third edition 2004
  Reprinted 2005

ISBN 0 7020 2666 2

British Library Cataloguing in Publication Data
A catalogue record for this book is available from
the British Library

Library of Congress Cataloging in Publication Data
A catalog record for this book is available from the
Library of Congress

Note
Medical knowledge is constantly changing.
Standard safety precautions must be followed, but
as new research and clinical experience broaden our
knowledge, changes in treatment and drug therapy
may become necessary as appropriate. Readers are
advised to check the most current product
information provided by the manufacturer of each
drug to be administered to verify the recommended
dose, the method and duration of administration,
and contraindications. It is the responsibility of the
practitioner, relying on experience and knowledge of
the patient, to determine dosages and the best
treatment for each individual patient. Neither the
publisher nor the author assumes any liability for
any injury and/or damage to persons or property
arising from this publication.

Cover image
Coloured MRI scan of whole human body (female)
Credit: Simon Fraser/Science Photo Library

Printed in China

Preface

Best of fives, extended matching questions (EMQs) and multiple choice questions (MCQs) are popular with examining bodies because they allow accurate ranking of examinees in a convenient manner. They are used for both undergraduate (MB BS, LRCP, PLAB, USMLE) and postgraduate (MRCP Part I and MRCGP) examinations in general internal medicine. Merely reading a medical text may not necessarily prepare students for such examinations. This book, which contains best of fives, EMQs and MCQs, derived from the 5th edition of Kumar and Clark's *Clinical Medicine*, should meet the needs of aspiring candidates. Limited explanations accompany the answers and candidates can refer to the main text for a better understanding of the material.

To make best use of the book I would recommend that the student reads the corresponding chapter in the original text before answering these questions. However, candidates using other texts should also find this book a useful revision guide. None of these questions have hidden meanings and are not meant to confuse the reader. To prepare for postgraduate examinations I recommend that the original textbook be read several times until the reader gets over 99% of the questions right.

Acknowledgements

I thank Professor Parveen Kumar and Dr. Michael Clark for allowing me to use *Clinical Medicine* 5E to derive the questions and answers.

I thank Prof. James Scott, FRCP, FRS for writing the Foreword.

I thank Thea Hulen-Picklesimer for taking on many of my responsibilities while I wrote this book, and Marsha Xedos for helping me to proofread this book.

I would like to thank Ellen Green, Commissioning Editor, and Helen Leng, Project Development Manager, at Elsevier. Finally I would like to thank Stephanie Pickering for painstakingly copyediting this book.

I dedicate this book to my wife Jayashree, my son Anoop and my daughter Neena for their support throughout the book's preparation.

Ragavendra R. Baliga
Ann Arbor, Michigan

Foreword

Best of fives, extended matching questions (EMQs) and multiple choice questions (MCQs) in general internal medicine are now an integral part of both undergraduate (MB BS and PLAB) and postgraduate (MRCP Part 1 and MRCGP) examinations.

Examining bodies use such questions to test more than factual recall; they are used to assess the understanding and application of essential facts. Simply reading a medical text will not prepare a candidate adequately for these examinations and to be well prepared the individual will have to solve several best of fives, EMQs and MCQs. These questions can also be used to determine areas of weakness and of expertise in general internal medicine. Although no bank of questions can be all-embracing, this book,

which contains over 900 best of fives, EMQs and MCQs, should be a valuable revision guide for aspiring students.

Prospective candidates, however, must be forewarned that merely solving these questions is not a satisfactory method of enhancing their medical knowledge. Sincere and dedicated students should use both this book and the clinical text on which it is based, Kumar and Clark's *Clinical Medicine*, as complementary approaches to enhance their understanding of clinical medicine.

Professor James Scott FRCP FRS
Imperial College of Science,
Technology and Medicine,
Hammersmith Hospital,
London

Contents

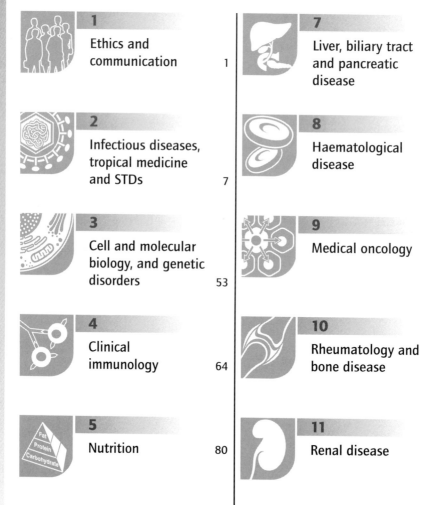

Ethics and communication

Q1.1

Which one of the following is the most common factor associated with failure of adherence to clinical advice following discharge from hospital?

A. No named doctor in charge of their care
B. No named nurse in charge of their care
C. Presence of pain most of the time
D. Being told on discharge when to resume normal activities
E. Scheduling of follow-up visits in outpatient clinics on discharge

Q1.2

Which one of the following qualities is seen in physicians who have never been subject to legal proceedings?

A. Normalizing ('Everyone feels that. Forget it!')
B. Jollying along ('Worse things happen at sea!')
C. Orientating patients to the process of the visit ('We are going to do this first, and then go on to do that.')
D. Passing the buck ('Nurse will tell you all about that.')
E. Switching the topic ('A headache? Tell me about your feet.')

Q1.3

'Patient-centred' communication improves the following

A. Incidence of acute urinary retention following surgery
B. Length of hospital stay following surgery
C. Blood pressure in hypertensives
D. Blood glucose control in diabetics
E. Pain following surgery

Q1.4

When a clinician learns about a patient complaint they should

A. Alter medical records to prevent lawsuit
B. Avoid offering a personal apology because this is an expression of guilt
C. Explain the reasons and circumstances behind the facts
D. Explain how things will improve
E. Avoid giving a written account, even though it is a clear account, because it could be used in a court of law later

Q1.5

When communicating with patients who are hard of hearing, the following are acceptable

A. Avoid speaking normally; mouth slowly
B. Put your face in a good light
C. Stay still and don't put things in your mouth

Ethics and communication

D. Trim moustaches and beards, avoid sunglasses, big earrings or background activity

E. Do not hesitate to say 'forget it' if the patient cannot follow you

Q1.6

1. Respect patients' privacy and dignity

2. Competence when making diagnoses and when giving or arranging treatment

3. Listen to patients and respect their views

4. Do not refuse or delay treatment because you believe that a patient's actions have contributed to his or her condition, or because you may be putting yourself at risk

5. An adequate assessment of the patient's condition and where necessary, an appropriate examination

6. Give patients the information they ask for or need about their condition, its treatment and prognosis

7. Provide or arrange investigations or treatments where necessary

8. Do not allow views about a patient's lifestyle, culture, beliefs, race, colour, sex, sexuality, age, social status or perceived economic worth to prejudice treatment

Select the best category for each of the above

A. The importance of protecting life and health

B. The importance of respect for autonomy

C. The importance of fairness and justice

Q1.7

1. Battery

2. Bolam test

3. Competent refusal

4. Negligence

5. Explicit consent

6. Implied consent

Select the best match for each of the above

A. Verbal or written consent

B. A doctor is not negligent if he has acted in accordance with the practice accepted as proper by a responsible body of medical men skilled in that particular case

C. Prima facie every adult has the right and capacity to decide whether or not he will accept medical treatment, even if a refusal may risk permanent injury to his health or even lead to premature death. Furthermore, it matters not whether the reasons for the refusal were rational or irrational, unknown or even non-existent. This is so notwithstanding the very strong public interest in preserving the life and health of all citizens

D. Patient accepts treatment without question, protest or any other physical sign that might be associated with rejection

E. To intentionally touch a competent person without their consent

F. Breach of professional duty to obtain adequate consent through not providing a reasonable amount of information about the risks of proposed treatment

Q1.8

1. Rhetorical leading question
2. Open screening question
3. Open question
4. Open directive question
5. Closed question
6. Reflecting question

Select the best question for each of the above categories

A. 'What has brought you to see me today?'
B. 'Is there anything else you want to tell me?'
C. 'How did the treatment for your headache go?'
D. 'Could you tell me a bit more about that?'
E. 'What date exactly did the headache start?'
F. 'The headache has got better on my treatment, hasn't it?'

Q1.9

1. The patient experiences being heard
2. The patient experiences being accepted
3. The patient experiences being seen
4. The clinician shows self-disclosure

Select the statement that best matches each of the above demonstrations of empathy

A. 'That last point made you look worried. Is there something more serious about that point you would like to tell me?'
B. 'I can tell you that most people in your circumstances get angry at some point, even with the people who have helped them.'
C. 'I'm a bit like you. Whenever I get heartburn I think it's a heart attack.'
D. 'I notice that you have talked about the death of your mother, but could I ask you to tell me something about how your brother died?'

Ethics and communication

A1.1

B

Problems identified as causing failure of adherence to clinical advice

In a random sample of 8303 patients from 66 hospitals in England and Wales (1994):

- 22% reported that no named doctor was in charge of their care
- 64% reported that no named nurse was in charge of their care
- 20% reported that they were in pain all or most of the time
- 62% were not told on discharge when to resume their normal activities

A1.2

C

Qualities leading to good relationships with patients

Primary care physicians who had never been sued:

- orientated patients to the process of the visit, e.g. introductory comments: 'We are going to do this first, and then go on to do that'
- used facilitative comments
- asked patients their opinion
- used active listening
- used humour and laughter
- conducted slightly longer visits (18 versus 15 minutes)

A1.3

A) T   B) T   C) T   D) T   E) T

Results from studies of communication and health outcomes

Condition	Outcome improved with better communication
Surgical operations	Shorter stay; less urinary retention and analgesia
Hypertension	Blood pressure control improved
Diabetes mellitus	Blood glucose control improved
Myocardial infarction	Rehabilitation improved, readmission rates reduced
Headache	Long-term symptom resolution

A1.4

A) F   B) F   C) T   D) T   E) F

When clinicians learn of a complaint they should: a) remain objective, not resentful or defensive – remember that there is a duty of care to the patient in this as every way; b) allow all the facts to speak through a clear account, verbal or written; c) explain the reasons and circumstances behind the facts; d) express regret (a personal apology is, as medical defence organizations emphasize, not an expression of guilt but a common courtesy, nor should it be wrapped up so carefully as to become a worthless token); e) explain how things will improve; f) remember that the patient is still a patient; g) leave all medical records strictly unaltered.

A1.5

A) F B) T C) T D) T E) F

Dos and don'ts of communicating with people who are deaf or hard of hearing (from RAD – Royal Association in Aid of Deaf People)

Smile and use eye contact
If you are stuck write it down
Speak normally, don't mouth slowly
Put your face in a good light
Stay still and don't put things in your mouth
Trim moustaches and beards, avoid sunglasses, big earrings or background activity
Never say 'forget it'

A1.6

1) B 2) A 3) B 4) C
5) A 6) B 7) A 8) C

General Medical Council, Good Medical Practice: 2–4

1. The importance of protecting life and health: a) 'an adequate assessment of the patient's condition … (and) … where necessary, an appropriate examination'; b) 'providing or arranging investigations or treatments where necessary'; c) 'competence when making diagnoses and when giving or arranging treatment'
2. The importance of respect for autonomy: a) 'listen to patients and respect their views'; b) 'respect patients' privacy and dignity'; c) 'give patients the information they ask for or need about their condition, its treatment and prognosis'
3. The importance of fairness and justice: a) '… (not allowing) … views about a patient's lifestyle, culture, beliefs, race, colour, sex, sexuality, age, social status, or perceived economic worth to prejudice … treatment'; b) '… (not refusing or delaying) treatment because you believe that patients' actions have contributed to their condition, or because you may be putting yourself at risk'

A1.7

1) E 2) B 3) C 4) F 5) A 6) D

Explicit consent may be either verbal or written, usually through the patient signing a consent form. Consent is explicit when it is given in relation to specific information about the proposed treatment. Consent may also be implied by the fact that the patient accepts treatment without question, protest or any other physical sign that might be associated with rejection. Clinicians may also be in breach of their professional duty to obtain adequate consent through not providing a reasonable amount of information about the *risks* of proposed treatment. It is unlawful intentionally to touch a competent person without their consent. To do so is battery. The Bolam test refers to the following judgement: 'A doctor is not negligent if he has acted in accordance with the practice accepted as proper by a responsible body of medical men skilled in that particular case'. Competent refusal refers to the following: 'Prima facie every adult has the right and capacity to decide whether or not he will accept medical treatment, even if a refusal may risk permanent injury to his health or even lead to premature death. Furthermore, it matters not whether the reasons for the refusal were rational or irrational, unknown or even non-existent. This is so notwithstanding the very strong public interest in preserving the life and health of all citizens.'

A1.8

1) F 2) B 3) A 4) C 5) E 6) D

Questioning style determines whether it is the clinician or the patient who talks more. The clinician will obtain more information by starting with open questions (e.g. 'What has brought you to see me today?'), then guiding the history by using closed questions (e.g. 'What date *exactly* did the headache start?') for further detail. If the clinician sits in complete silence, the patient will flounder and lose confidence. Eye contact or a smile show the patient that the clinician is listening attentively. Reflecting questions (e.g. 'Could you tell me a bit more about that?') allow the clinician to take up unexpected points as they arise or expand topics. As the history unfolds, detail can be brought into focus by using screening questions (e.g. 'Is there anything else you want to tell me?') and closed questions. Leading questions may be helpful but they should not end in the rhetorical 'isn't it?', or 'wouldn't it?' challenge (e.g. 'The headache has got better on my treatment, hasn't it?'), which makes the statement difficult to for the patient to discuss or contradict, even when it is completely wrong. This type of question is a major cause of misunderstanding. With certain patients (e.g. with organic brain disease or severe mental disease), clinicians require energy and imagination to make the best of the limited lines of communication. Open questions are often impossible for these patients; open directive questions (e.g. 'How did the treatment for your headache go?') have to be adjusted to the ability of each patient and non-verbal gestures used if necessary. Just as much ingenuity may be called upon to confirm the meaning of the responses. Third parties involved in the care of the patient can help. Much can be learned by watching a specialized speech therapist at work.

A1.9

1) D   2) B   3) A   4) C

Empathy has been described as 'imagination for others'. An empathic response is one which demonstrates a genuine interest in patients' experiences. This is a key skill in building the patient–clinician relationship and is highly therapeutic. Like other communication skills, it can be taught and learned and it cannot be counterfeited by a repertoire of routine mannerisms. Techniques which demonstrate empathy are:

- Seeing (e.g. 'That last point made you look worried. Is there something more serious about that point you would like to tell me?')
- Hearing (e.g. 'I notice that you have talked about the death of your mother but could I ask you to tell me something about how your brother died?')
- Accepting (e.g. 'I can tell you that most people in your circumstances get angry at some point, even with the people who have helped them')
- Using appropriate self-disclosure (e.g. 'I'm a bit like you. Whenever I get heartburn I think it's a heart attack')
- Acknowledging facial and bodily expressions, mode of dress and notable physical characteristics
- Avoiding physical barriers; sitting or standing at the same level as the patient without objects between
- Reflecting what the patient is feeling as they talk and what the patient sees as important and what the patient may be thinking
- Using the patient's own words and ideas
- Letting the patient correct any misunderstanding that arises
- Evaluating behaviour not judging the person.

Infectious diseases, tropical medicine and sexually transmitted diseases

Q2.1

A 45-year-old man has AIDS. Select from the organisms listed below the one most likely to cause a respiratory tract infection in this patient

A. *Escherichia coli*
B. *Klebsiella pneumoniae*
C. *Streptococcus pneumoniae*
D. *Pneumocystis carinii*
E. *Staphylococcus epidermidis*

Q2.2

A 38-year-old doctor receives chemotherapy for a malignant neoplasm, as a result of which she develops neutropenia. She is most likely to be susceptible to infection by which one of the following?

A. Respiratory syncytial virus
B. Cytomegalovirus
C. *Toxoplasma gondii*
D. *Pneumocystis carinii*
E. *Klebsiella pneumoniae*

Q2.3

A 43-year-old woman has a motorcycle accident. As a result of the trauma she requires a splenectomy. She is now most likely to be susceptible to infection by which one of the following?

A. *Toxoplasma gondii*
B. *Candida* spp.
C. *Aspergillus* spp.

D. *Strep. pneumoniae*
E. Herpes simplex

Q2.4

A 69-year-old man has chronic lymphatic leukaemia. He is most likely to be susceptible to infection by which one of the following?

A. Cytomegalovirus
B. *Aspergillus* spp.
C. *Candida* spp.
D. *Haemophilus influenzae*
E. *Mycobacterium avium-intracellulare*

Q2.5

An 18-year-old patient has streptococcal pharyngitis. Select the best antibiotic for treatment

A. Benzylpenicillin
B. Phenoxymethylpenicillin (penicillin V)
C. Ceftazidime
D. Tetracycline
E. Neomycin

Q2.6

A 14-year-old patient has meningococcal meningitis. Select the best antibiotic for treatment

A. Benzylpenicillin
B. Phenoxymethylpenicillin (penicillin V)
C. Ceftazidime
D. Tetracycline
E. Neomycin

Infectious diseases, tropical medicine and sexually transmitted diseases

Q2.7

A 14-year-old patient has a past history of rheumatic fever and requires prophylaxis. Select from the following antibiotics the one generally used for this purpose

A. Benzylpenicillin
B. Phenoxymethylpenicillin (penicillin V)
C. Ceftazidime
D. Tetracycline
E. Neomycin

Q2.8

A 23-year-old patient receiving chemotherapy for leukaemia has severe sepsis. Select the best antibiotic for treatment

A. Benzylpenicillin
B. Phenoxymethylpenicillin (penicillin V)
C. Ceftazidime
D. Tetracycline
E. Neomycin

Q2.9

A 23-year-old patient is diagnosed with syphilis. Select the best antibiotic for treatment

A. Benzylpenicillin
B. Phenoxymethylpenicillin (penicillin V)
C. Ceftazidime
D. Tetracycline
E. Neomycin

Q2.10

The infectious diseases specialist recommends, after reviewing blood culture results, that a 23-year-old man with septicaemia would benefit from a combination of intravenous benzylpenicillin and gentamicin. The nurse mixes both antibiotics in the same solution. The nurse's action results in

A. Increased potency of penicillin
B. Inactivation of penicillin
C. Inactivation of gentamicin
D. Increased potency of gentamicin
E. No interaction between the two antibiotics when in the same solution

Q2.11

A 52-year-old man has intra-abdominal sepsis. One day after blood cultures are drawn the microbiologist reports that the organism is an aerobic Gram-negative bacillus. The patient is allergic to aminoglycosides. Which one of the following antibiotics is the best option in combination therapy for this patient?

A. Tobramycin
B. Neomycin
C. Tetracycline
D. Aztreonam
E. Doxycycline

Q2.12

A 75-year-old patient is being treated with furosemide (frusemide) for her heart failure. She develops a fever and has positive blood cultures for which the infectious disease specialist starts a combination of antibiotics. Five days later she develops hearing difficulty. Which one of the following antibiotics is most likely to have contributed to her hearing difficulty?

A. Benzylpenicillin
B. Tetracyline
C. Doxycycline
D. Gentamicin
E. Cefuroxime

Q2.13

An 18-year-old patient develops acne. Select the best option for treating acne

A. Benzylpenicillin
B. Doxycycline
C. Aztreonam
D. Imipenem
E. Meropenem

Q2.14

The mother of a premature baby in a remote village in Bangladesh consults a village elder because her child has fever. He gives her an antibiotic for the child. Three days later the child has hypotension and is rushed to the hospital in the nearest town where the physician correctly diagnoses 'grey baby syndrome'. Which one of the following antibiotics is most likely to have caused this condition?

A. Tetracycline
B. Erythromycin
C. Ampicillin
D. Chloramphenicol
E. Co-trimoxazole

Q2.15

A 42-year-old man has hepatic amoebiasis. He is prescribed an antimicrobial agent. Three days later he has a beer in the local pub and soon suffers flushing, palpitations and dizziness. The most likely antimicrobial agent is

A. Vancomycin
B. Ketoconazole
C. Amphotericin B
D. Metronidazole
E. Griseofulvin

Q2.16

A 43-year-old patient with HIV on treatment develops red cell aplasia. The most likely aetiology is

A. Chronic HIV infection
B. Zidovudine therapy
C. Disseminated cytomegalovirus infection
D. Ganciclovir
E. Co-trimoxazole

Q2.17

A 23-year-old patient with AIDS develops increasing shortness of breath, fever, dry cough and malaise. Clinical examination reveals tachypnoea, tachycardia, cyanosis and signs of hypoxia. CD4 count is $100/mm^3$. On auscultation the lungs are clear. Chest X-ray is clear. First-line therapy is

A. Follow the patient regularly, perform serial X-rays and initiate therapy when there are clinical or X-ray changes
B. Systemic corticosteroids
C. Intravenous co-trimoxazole
D. Inhaled steroids
E. Inhaled pentamidine

Q2.18

A 39-year-old nurse with a prosthetic mitral valve has fever. Blood cultures reveal multiresistant *Staphylococcus aureus*. Select from the following the most useful in the management of this condition

A. Tetracycline
B. Bacitracin
C. Quinupristin with dalfopristin
D. Neosporin
E. Sulphonamides with trimethoprim

Infectious diseases, tropical medicine and sexually transmitted diseases

Q2.19

A 29-year-old patient with AIDS develops orbital pain, headache and decrease in visual acuity. He also complains of 'floaters' in his eyes. On examination he has a scotoma and the fundus reveals haemorrhages and exudates – the so-called 'pizza pie' appearance. The physician wishes to start therapy but notices that the patient has marked pancytopenia but his renal function is normal. Select the best treatment option

A. Intravenous ganciclovir
B. Intravenous foscarnet
C. Oral ganciclovir
D. Varicella zoster immunoglobulin
E. Intravenous co-trimoxazole

Q2.20

A 72-year-old man develops a skin rash along the back in the fifth intercostal space. The rash is preceded by severe pain along the fifth intercostal space. Select the best treatment for this condition

A. Griseofulvin
B. Topical steroids
C. Calamine lotion
D. Systemic steroids
E. Aciclovir

Q2.21

A 22-year-old heart transplant patient develops fever, cough and malaise. He has pneumonia, and tissue obtained at bronchoscopy shows typical intranuclear 'owl's eye' inclusions on histological staining and direct immunofluorescence. The treatment includes which one of the following?

A. Dapsone
B. Isoniazid
C. Steroids

D. Ganciclovir
E. Zoster immune globulin (ZIG)

Q2.22

A 29-year-old patient with HIV develops symptoms of diarrhoea and malabsorption. There is associated eosinophilia. He is found to have an overwhelming infection by a nematode. Which one of the following organisms is most likely to have caused this clinical picture?

A. *Trichuris trichiura*
B. *Necator americanus*
C. *Ancylostoma duodenale*
D. *Toxocara canis*
E. *Strongyloides stercoralis*

Q2.23

A 48-year-old patient with AIDS has dementia. Which of the following drugs is most likely to improve cognitive function without producing neuropathy?

A. Zalcitabine
B. Didanosine
C. Stavudine
D. Zidovudine
E. Aciclovir

Q2.24

A 28-year-old homosexual man develops plum-coloured plaques on his leg, on the tip of the nose, and around the mouth and palate. The most likely aetiological agent is

A. Herpes simplex-1
B. Human herpes virus type 6
C. Human herpes virus type 7
D. Human herpes virus type 8
E. Human parvovirus B19

Q2.25

A 29-year-old British businessman, 10 days after visiting the red light district in Bangkok, develops difficulty in passing urine and a purulent urethral discharge. The causative organism is most likely to be

A. Spirochaete
B. Gram-positive cocci in clusters
C. Gram-positive cocci in chains
D. Intracellular Gram-negative diplococci
E. Gram-positive diplococci

Q2.26

A 25-year-old pregnant woman develops vaginal discharge and postcoital bleeding. An endocervical swab reveals that the organism is *Chlamydia trachomatis*. The best option for treatment is

A. Benzylpenicillin
B. Oral penicillin
C. Doxycycline
D. Tetracycline
E. Erythromycin

Q2.27

Ten days after visiting a red light district a man notices an ulcer on his penis. On examination he has a painless, firm ulcer with painless inguinal lymphadenopathy. Dark-ground microscopy confirms the diagnosis. The most likely organism is

A. *Haemophilus ducreyi*
B. *Mycoplasma genitalium*
C. *Ureaplasma urealyticum*
D. *Treponema pallidum*
E. *Trichomonas vaginalis*

Q2.28

Ten days after visiting a red light district a man notices an ulcer on his penis. On examination he has a painless, firm ulcer with painless inguinal lymphadenopathy. Dark-ground microscopy confirms the diagnosis. This patient is known to be non-compliant. Select the best treatment option

A. Procaine benzylpenicillin 600 mg intramuscularly daily for 10 days
B. A single dose of benzathine penicillin G 2.4 g intravenously
C. Doxycycline 200 mg daily for 4 weeks
D. Erythromycin 500 mg four times daily is given orally for 2–4 weeks
E. A single dose of benzathine penicillin G 2.4 g intramuscularly

Q2.29

A 33-year-old man with multiple sexual partners develops multiple shallow, painful ulcers on the penis. Associated there is tender inguinal lymphadenopathy. On examination the lesions are still moist. The best treatment is

A. A single dose of azithromycin
B. A single dose of ceftriaxone
C. Famciclovir
D. Ciprofloxacin 500 mg twice daily for 3 days
E. Amantadine

Q2.30

A 49-year-old journalist returns to London from Africa. Soon afterwards he develops a high fever, headache, muscle aches, joint aches and a flushed face. Shortly after that he develops jaundice and hepatomegaly. Liver biopsy shows mid-zone necrosis and eosinophilic degeneration of hepatocytes. Which one of the following is typical of this condition?

Infectious diseases, tropical medicine and sexually transmitted diseases

A. Lewy bodies

B. Mallory bodies

C. Councilman bodies

D. Reed–Sternberg cells

E. Donovan bodies

Q2.31

A 49-year-old journalist returns to London from Africa. Soon afterwards he develops high fever, headache, muscle aches, joint aches and flushed face. Shortly after that he develops jaundice and hepatomegaly. Liver biopsy shows mid-zone necrosis, and eosinophilic degeneration of hepatocytes. Which one of the following could have prevented his condition?

A. MMR vaccine

B. Varicella zoster vaccine

C. Hepatitis A vaccine

D. Attenuated 17d chick embryo vaccine

E. Hepatitis B vaccine

Q2.32

An 8-year-old child in Pakistan develops malaise, fever, rhinorrhoea, cough and conjunctival suffusion. On examination she has small, greyish, irregular lesions surrounded by an erythematous base which are found in greatest numbers on the mucous membranes opposite the second molar tooth. In a day or two she is most likely to develop

A. Chickenpox

B. Erythema multiforme

C. A maculopapular rash that initially occurs on the face, particularly on the forehead and spreads to involve the rest of the body

D. Rubella

E. Influenza

Q2.33

A 33-year-old English architect is travelling through the Indian subcontinent when she develops intermittent diarrhoea, nausea and vomiting. Which one of the following tests confirms amoebic dysentery?

A. Presence of amoebic cysts in fresh stool

B. Motile trophozoites containing red blood cells in fresh stool

C. Sigmoidoscopy showing colonic ulcers

D. Barium enema showing ulcerative lesions in the colon

E. Presence of trophozoites in the bloodstream

Q2.34

A 22-year-old journalist returns to the UK after travelling from Eastern Europe. Soon after his return he develops anorexia, nausea and abdominal discomfort and bloating. As the weeks go by the stools become paler and he has characteristic steatorrhoea. Soon he begins to lose weight. The most likely cause for his symptoms is

A. *Wuchereria bancrofti*

B. *Brugia timori*

C. *Mansonella perstans*

D. *Loa loa*

E. *Giardia intestinalis*

Q2.35

A 28-year-old man living on the west coast of India develops fever, pain and tenderness in the scrotum. The scrotum is huge. He is seen by his physician who correctly diagnoses that he has recurrent epididymitis. The patient has an elevated eosinophil count. The most likely organism is

A. *Paragonimus westermani*
B. *Wuchereria bancrofti*
C. *Ascaris lumbricoides*
D. *Trichuris trichiura*
E. *Trichinella spiralis*

A. Epididymo-orchitis
B. CNS involvement
C. Pancreatitis
D. Hepatitis
E. Myocarditis

Q2.36

A 29-year-old man living in Yemen develops itching and redness of the eyes. Gradually his vision begins to deteriorate. On examination he has uveitis and secondary glaucoma. The Mazzotti reaction is positive. The most likely organism is

A. *Mansonella perstans*
B. *Dracunculus medinensis*
C. *Ascaris lumbricoides*
D. *Onchocerca volvulus*
E. *Enterobius vermicularis*

Q2.37

A 12-year-old child in India develops pain in the right lumbar region and has acute appendicitis. Biopsy specimen reveals several worms. The most likely organism to cause this picture is

A. *Dracunculus medinensis*
B. *Ascaris lumbricoides*
C. *Enterobius vermicularis*
D. *Trichuris trichiura*
E. *Loa loa*

Q2.38

A 12-year-old schoolboy in India develops fever, malaise, headache and loss of appetite. He has severe pain behind the left angle of the mandible. On examination the left ear lobe is elevated and he has tender enlargement behind the left angle of the mandible. He also has trismus. The most common extrasalivary manifestation of this condition is

Q2.39

Following a dog bite in rural India, a 12-year-old boy develops fever, malaise, headache, hallucinations and bizarre behaviour. He goes on to develop convulsions and respiratory paralysis, and succumbs to the illness 2 weeks later. Postmortem examination reveals Negri bodies in the cells of the hippocampus and cerebellum. The aetiological agent is

A. RNA retrovirus
B. A bullet-shaped virus that has spike-like structures arising from its surface containing glycoproteins
C. Hantavirus
D. Dengue virus
E. Japanese encephalitis

Q2.40

A 29-year-old Englishman presents with psychiatric disturbances and cerebellar signs. The most likely diagnosis is

A. Kuru
B. Gerstmann–Straussler–Scheinker disease
C. Classical Creutzfeldt–Jakob disease
D. Bovine spongiform encephalopathy
E. Ebola virus

Q2.41

A 5-year-old child develops malaise, fever, loss of appetite, runny nose and conjunctivitis. A week later he has paroxysms of coughing and a white cell count reveals that lymphocytes account

Infectious diseases, tropical medicine and sexually transmitted diseases

for over 90% of the total white blood cell count. The most likely organism is

A. *Corynebacterium diphtheriae*
B. *Bordetella pertussis*
C. *Streptococcus bovis*
D. *Mycoplasma pneumoniae*
E. *Chlamydia pneumoniae*

2.42

A 14-year-old schoolboy develops headache and vomiting. On examination he has neck stiffness. He then develops a purpuric rash. Prior to illness he has had close contact with his girlfriend. She has no symptoms and feels well. Which of the following is the best option for the management of his girlfriend?

A. Observation and treatment as soon as she develops symptoms
B. Intravenous benzylpenicillin
C. Oral rifampicin
D. Intramuscular benzathine penicillin
E. Tetracycline

2.43

Which one of the following is required to make a diagnosis of acute rheumatic fever using the revised Duckett Jones criteria?

A. Two major criteria will suffice
B. Two major criteria plus evidence of streptococcal infection
C. One major criterion plus two or more minor criteria
D. Three minor criteria
E. Elevated antistreptolysin O titre

2.44

A 14-year-old girl develops a sore throat. A throat swab confirms streptococcal infection. A few days later she develops fleeting joint pains beginning in the knees

followed by the ankles, elbows and wrists. She also develops mild fever and tachycardia out of proportion to her fever. In addition, she has a transient pink rash with slightly raised edges. Select the best option to prevent recurrent attacks of this condition

A. High dose salicylate therapy
B. Systemic corticosteroids
C. Single dose of benzathine penicillin
D. Oral phenoxymethylpenicillin daily until the age of 20 years or for 5 years after the latest attack
E. Oral phenoxymethylpenicillin daily for 1 week

2.45

A 29-year-old farmer develops mild fever followed by severe headache, malaise, anorexia and myalgia. He has hepatosplenomegaly. In the subsequent days he develops hepatic failure, renal failure, haemolytic anaemia and circulatory collapse. The aetiological agent is most likely to be

A. Gram-positive cocci in chains
B. Gram-positive cocci in clusters
C. Gram-negative cocci
D. Spirochaete
E. *Rickettsia*

2.46

A 19-year-old Mediterranean agricultural worker likes to drink raw milk. He develops malaise, headache, myalgia and night sweats. On examination he has hepatosplenomegaly. The most likely aetiological agent is

A. *Leptospira interrogans*
B. *Listeria monocytogenes*
C. *Brucella melitensis*
D. *Borrelia burgdorferi*
E. *Francisella tularensis*

Q2.47

A British nurse has been travelling through Central Africa for 2 months. She develops episodes of fever and can feel her lymph nodes. She is admitted to the hospital complaining of excessive sleepiness in the day, and headache. She is also confused. Lumbar puncture reveals increased protein and lymphocytes. Concentrated CSF specimens contain parasites. The best treatment is intravenous

A. Chloroquine
B. Quinine
C. Artesunate
D. Suramin
E. Sodium stibogluconate

Q2.48

A 14-year-old boy in South America is seen by a cardiologist. The cardiologist notes that this patient had fever 2 years ago which was treated with nifurtimox. Now he has dilated cardiomyopathy and the cardiologist believes that the patient's clinical features are due to a parasitic infection endemic to this part of the world. The best way to confirm the diagnosis is

A. Endomyocardial biopsy
B. Urine examination
C. Infection-free reduviid bugs are allowed to feed on the patient, and the insect gut is subsequently examined for parasites
D. CSF examination
E. Echocardiographic visualization of the parasite

Q2.49

A 25-year-old man in Africa has a 1-year history of low grade fever. On examination he has hepatosplenomegaly. Bone marrow aspirate reveals Donovan bodies. Select the best option for treatment

A. Chloroquine
B. Quinine
C. Artesunate
D. Suramin
E. Sodium stibogluconate

Q2.50

A 47-year-old man has saddle nose deformity with leonine facies. The ear lobes are thickened due to infiltration. Other abnormalities include glove and stocking anaesthesia, gynaecomastia, testicular atrophy, icthyosis, ulnar nerve palsy and loss of digits of the hands. Select the best treatment

A. Thalidomide
B. Combination therapy for 2 years with dapsone and 50 mg clofazimine daily, rifampicin and clofazimine 300 mg once a month
C. Combination therapy for 6 months consisting of rifampicin once a month and dapsone daily
D. Prednisolone 40 mg daily for 6 weeks
E. BCG vaccine

Q2.51

A 19-year-old student in India has a single hypopigmented patch on the arm that has no sensation. The edges are clearly demarcated and the cutaneous nerve leading to the patch is thickened. Another patch on the face is not anaesthetic. Select the best treatment

A. Thalidomide
B. Combination therapy for 2 years with dapsone and 50 mg clofazimine daily, rifampicin and clofazimine 300 mg once a month
C. Combination therapy for 6 months consisting of rifampicin once a month and dapsone daily

Infectious diseases, tropical medicine and sexually transmitted diseases

D. Prednisolone 40 mg daily for 6 weeks

E. BCG vaccine

Q2.52

A 22-year-old US postal worker in mid-2001 comes across a suspicious envelope while sorting mail. Microbiological examination confirms that it contains spores of *Bacillus anthracis*. He develops a non-productive cough and retrosternal discomfort. Select the best option for management

A. Observation until he develops systemic symptoms

B. Intravenous ciprofloxacin for 3 weeks followed by oral ciprofloxacin for a total of 60 days

C. Combination of gentamicin and vancomycin for 6 weeks

D. Dapsone and rifampicin in combination for 6 months

E. Streptomycin and isoniazid in combination for 18 months

Q2.53

A 29-year-old man in Bangladesh complains of profuse, watery stools which contain mucus. He has also vomited once. Examinaton of freshly-passed stools reveals rapidly motile organisms. Dark-field illumination reveals rapidly motile vibrios. The mainstay of treatment in this condition is

A. Oral tetracycline 500 mg four times daily for 3 weeks

B. Tetracycline 500 mg twice-daily for 3 days

C. Rehydration

D. Chloramphenicol

E. Ciprofloxacin

Q2.54

Following an epidemic of a febrile illness the local health authorities identify the vector as *Xenopsylla cheopis*, the causative organism as *Yersinia pestis* and the main reservoir as *Rattus rattus*. The best way to prevent further attacks is

A. Intramuscular streptomycin 1 g twice daily for 10 days for all contacts

B. Elimination of fleas before rodents

C. Elimination of rodents before fleas

D. Rifampicin for all contacts

E. Isoniazid to all contacts

Q2.55

Which one of the following malarial species is able to parasitize immature, young and old erythrocytes

A. *Plasmodium falciparum*

B. *Plasmodium malariae*

C. *Plasmodium vivax*

D. *Plasmodium ovale*

Q2.56

Blackwater fever is due to

A. Glomerulonephritis causing dark urine

B. Intravascular haemolysis of both parasitized and non-parasitized red cells

C. Intravascular haemolysis of parasitized red cells only

D. Disseminated intravascular coagulation

E. Sequestration of red cells in the spleen

Q2.57

A 12-year-old boy develops glomerulonephritis and nephrotic syndrome following a malarial infection. The most likely species is

Infectious diseases, tropical medicine and sexually transmitted diseases

A. *Plasmodium falciparum*
B. *Plasmodium malariae*
C. *Plasmodium vivax*
D. *Plasmodium ovale*

Q2.58

A 6-year-old child is admitted with high fever, confusion and convulsions. Examination of a blood smear confirms malaria. The most likely species is

A. *Plasmodium falciparum*
B. *Plasmodium malariae*
C. *Plasmodium vivax*
D. *Plasmodium ovale*

Q2.59

A 14-year-old boy living in a region where malaria is endemic presents with severe fatigue. He is anaemic and has massive splenomegaly. This condition is associated with elevated levels of

A. IgA
B. IgG
C. IgE
D. IgM
E. IgD

Q2.60

A 29-year-old diabetic patient has a tooth extracted in the lower jaw, following which healing is slow. He has little pain. There is no lymphadenopathy. Sinuses and tracts develop with discharge of 'sulphur granules'. The best antimicrobial is

A. Ketoconazole
B. Nystatin
C. Amphotericin B
D. Intravenous penicillin
E. Gentamicin

Q2.61

A 67-year-old farmer from the Mississippi river valley has a chronic cough and weight loss. Chest X-ray reveals pulmonary cavities, infiltrates and fibrous streaking from the periphery towards the hilum. Investigation excludes all acid-fast bacilli as the aetiological agent. The best antimicrobial agent for this condition is

A. Isoniazid
B. Rifampicin
C. Amphotericin B
D. Ethambutol
E. Combination of isoniazid and rifampicin

Q2.62

A 38-year-old patient who is an orthotopic heart transplant recipient develops cough and fever. Chest X-ray reveals consolidation and microbiological examination of bronchial washings reveals *Aspergillus fumigatus*. The best management is

A. Intravenous benzylpenicillin
B. Tetracycline
C. Oral ketoconazole
D. Intravenous amphotericin B
E. Prolonged course of oral sulphonamides

Q2.63

A 22-year-old AIDS patient develops headache and fever. CSF examination reveals a yeast-like fungus, *Cryptococcus neoformans*. The best treatment is

A. Intravenous amphotericin B
B. Intravenous benzylpenicillin
C. Nystatin
D. Itraconazole
E. Pentamidine

Infectious diseases, tropical medicine and sexually transmitted diseases

Q2.64

A 31-year-old insulin-dependent diabetic patient is admitted in ketoacidosis. She complains of nasal stuffiness and facial pain. Examination of the nasal turbinates reveals blackish discoloration. The most likely diagnosis is

A. Cryptococcosis
B. Coccidioidomycosis
C. Blastomycosis
D. Invasive zygomycosis
E. Mycetoma

Q2.65

1. A 21-year-old woman with a previous history of rheumatic fever
2. A 55-year-old patient with a prosthetic heart valve before a dental procedure
3. A 23-year-old medical student who has had a splenectomy
4. A 16-year-old schoolgirl who is exposed to a friend with meningococcal meningitis
5. A 23-year-old man who has been in close contact with a friend diagnosed with *H. influenzae* type b
6. A 23-year-old nurse exposed to a patient with tuberculosis. A year before exposure, during annual employee screening, she was found to be tuberculin negative

Select the best option for antibiotic chemoprophylaxis for each of the above

A. Oral isoniazid 5 mg/kg daily for 6–12 months
B. Rifampicin 100 mg daily for 4 days
C. Rifampicin 600 mg twice-daily for 2 days
D. Phenoxymethylpenicillin 500 mg 12-hourly
E. Oral amoxicillin 3 g 1 hour before procedure
F. Phenoxymethylpenicillin 250 mg twice-daily

Q2.66

1. *Borrelia burgdorferi*
2. *Yersinia pestis*
3. *Toxoplasma gondii*
4. *Cryptosporidium parvum*
5. *Echinococcus granulosus*

Select the animal reservoir for each of the above pathogens

A. Cats and other mammals
B. Cattle
C. Dogs
D. Deer
E. Rodents

Q2.67

1. Anthrax
2. Lyme disease
3. Plague
4. Yellow fever
5. Cutaneous larva migrans

Select the mode of transmission for each of the above infections

A. Flea bite
B. Mosquito bite
C. Tick bite
D. Penetration of skin by larvae
E. Contact; ingestion and inhalation

Q2.68

1. Block bacterial cell wall mucopeptide formation by binding to and inactivating peptidases involved in the final stages of cell wall assembly and division
2. Interrupt bacterial protein synthesis by inhibiting ribosomal function (messenger and transfer RNA)
3. Competes with messenger RNA for ribosomal binding. It also inhibits peptidyl transferase

4. Block thymidine and purine synthesis by inhibiting microbial folic acid synthesis

5. Inhibits bacterial DNA synthesis by inhibiting topoisomerase IV and DNA gyrase

Select the best match for each of the above

A. Sulphonamides
B. Ciprofloxacin
C. Chloramphenicol
D. Ceftazidime
E. Gentamicin

Q2.69

1. A 35-year-old heart transplant recipient with systemic aspergillosis

2. An 18-year-old army recruit with ringworm

3. A traveller with pulmonary histoplasmosis of moderate severity

4. A 54-year-old patient with fungal nail infection

5. A 45-year-old patient with cryptococcal meningitis who is allergic to amphotericin B

Select the best treatment for each of the above

A. Griseofulvin
B. Fluconazole
C. Clotrimazole
D. Amphotericin B
E. Ketoconazole

Q2.70

1. Aciclovir
2. Interferon-alpha
3. Foscarnet
4. Zanamivir
5. Ribavirin

Select the mechanism of action for each of the above

A. Acyclic nucleoside analogue that acts as terminator of herpesvirus DNA synthesis

B. Pyrophosphate analogue which inhibits viral DNA polymerases

C. Inhibits the neuraminidase of influenza A and B

D. Synthetic purine nucleoside derivative which interfaces with 5′-capping of messenger RNA, and is active against several RNA viruses

E. Renders uninfected cells resistant to infection with the same – or in some circumstances different – viruses

Q2.71

1. A 17-year-old boy has moderate watery diarrhoea. The causative organism produces these symptoms by effacement of intestinal mucosa

2. A 16-year-old girl has dysentery

3. An 18-year-old army recruit develops profuse watery diarrhoea. The diarrhoea is due to secretion of fluid without mucosal drainage

4. A 21-year-old man develops vomiting and variable diarrhoea. The diarrhoea is due to paralysis of the autonomic nervous system

5. A 45-year-old woman develops bloody diarrhoea. There is damage to the intestinal mucosa

Select the best match for each of the above

A. Enterohaemorrhagic E. coli (EHEC)
B. Staphylococcus aureus producing enterotoxin B
C. Enterotoxigenic E. coli (ETEC)
D. Enteroinvasive E. coli (EIEC)
E. Enteropathogenic E. coli (EPEC)

Infectious diseases, tropical medicine and sexually transmitted diseases

Q2.72

1. A 23-year-old pregnant woman's blood cultures grow *Listeria monocytogenes*

2. A 22-year-old woman develops acute Q fever but has no complications

3. A 24-year-old deer hunter develops erythema chronicum migrans accompanied by fever, headache, myalgia, arthralgia and lymphadenopathy. He then develops meningoencephalitis. Despite treatment he develops chronic and persistent neurological disease

4. A 33-year-old abattoir worker develops an ulceroglandular lesion followed by tender, suppurative lymphadenopathy. Blood cultures reveal *Francisella tularensis*

5. A 53-year-old farmer in Malta develops brucellosis.

Select the best therapeutic option for each of the above

A. Combination of ampicillin and gentamicin
B. Combination of doxycycline and rifampicin for 6 weeks
C. Doxycycline alone
D. Intravenous benzylpenicillin
E. Streptomycin or gentamicin

Q2.73

1. A 23-year-old student in India has a single hypopigmented patch on the arm that has no sensation. The edges are clearly demarcated and the cutaneous nerve leading to the patch is thickened. Another patch on the face is not anaesthetic

2. A 42-year-old man has several small patches with numerous satellite lesions around the larger ones. The peripheral nerves (but not the cutaneous nerves) are thickened and there is deformity of the hands and feet

3. A 29-year-old man has numerous macules, papules and plaques of varying size and form. He has typical punched-out skin lesions with loss of sensation in the centre. There is widespread involvement of the nerves and deformity of the limbs

4. A 47-year-old woman has a large number of asymmetrical skin lesions which are strongly positive for acid-fast bacilli. The skin between the lesions is normal and negative for acid-fast bacilli

5. A 37-year-old man has saddle nose deformity with leonine facies. The ear lobes are thickened due to infiltration. Other abnormalities include glove and stocking anaesthesia, gynaecomastia, testicular atrophy, icthyosis, ulnar nerve palsy and loss of digits of the hands

Select the best match for each of the above

A. Borderline leprosy
B. Lepromatous leprosy
C. Tuberculoid leprosy
D. Borderline tuberculoid leprosy
E. Borderline lepromatous leprosy

Q2.74

1. A 22-year-old refugee in Ethiopia develops fever, headache and a measles-like rash. He subsequently develops hepatosplenomegaly and pneumonia before he recovers. The vector is the human body louse and man is the reservoir

2. A 33-year-old man develops a mild fever and recovers from it. The vector is the rat flea and the reservoir is rodents

3. A 42-year-old man is bitten by the larval trombiculid mite. An eschar is seen at the site of the bite. The patient develops a mild febrile illness. The trombiculid mite is both vector and reservoir

4. A 23-year-old outdoor enthusiast is camping in the Rocky Mountains in the USA where he is bitten by a hard tick. An eschar develops at the site of the bite and there is regional lymph node enlargement. The reservoir is rodents

5. A 33-year-old man develps a mild febrile illness and maculopapular rash following the bite of a mite. The vector is rodents

Select the causative organism in each of the above

A. *Rickettsia rickettsii*
B. *Rickettsia akari*
C. *Rickettsia tsutsugamushi*
D. *Rickettsia typhi*
E. *Rickettsia prowazekii*

Q2.75

The malarial parasite multiplies in the hepatocytes as merozoites. After a few days the infected hepatocytes rupture releasing the merozoites into the blood where they are rapidly taken up by erythrocytes. A few parasites remain dormant in the liver as hypnozoites (which can subsequently reactivate to cause relapsing infection)

A. *Plasmodium falciparum*
B. *Plasmodium malariae*
C. *Plasmodium vivax*
D. *Plasmodium ovale*

Q2.76

A 29-year-old British doctor is planning to travel to the tropics where there is significant resistance of malaria to chloroquine. The following regimens are recommended for prophylaxis

A. Chloroquine 300 mg weekly
B. Mefloquine 250 mg weekly
C. Doxycycline 100 mg daily
D. Malarone 4 tablets daily
E. Proguanil 200 mg daily

Q2.77

1. A 25-year-old Central African farmer develops painless haematuria towards the end of micturition

2. A 25-year-old Central African farmer develops hepatitis followed by progressive periportal fibrosis, leading to portal hypertension, oesophageal varices and splenomegaly. Hepatocellular function is well preserved

3. A 45-year-old man eats inadequately cooked shellfish and develops fever, cough and mild haemoptysis. Sputum contains eggs of the causative organism

4. A 45-year-old woodcutter eats the undercooked meat of a bear he has killed. Following this he develops fever, oedema and myalgia. There is associated eosinophilia and serological tests confirm the causative organism

5. A 14-year-old boy who loves dogs presents with fever and urticaria. He has eosinophilia. He also complains of difficulty in seeing objects and has granulomatous ocular swellings mimicking retinoblastoma

6. A 29-year-old Chinese farmer eats raw fish. Thereafter, he has repeated attacks of cholangitis. Stool microscopy reveals the eggs of the causative organism

Infectious diseases, tropical medicine and sexually transmitted diseases

7. A 43-year-old Chinese farmer who enjoys eating pork presents with convulsions. CT of the head reveals cysts in the brain

8. A 43-year-old Australian sheep farmer uses dogs to control his livestock. He presents with pain in the right hypochondrium and fever. He has eosinophilia. Ultrasound of the liver reveals a large solitary cyst in the liver

9. A 23-year-old Japanese man enjoys eating raw fish. He develops a parasitic infestation with megaloblastic anaemia. The parasite utilizes most of the vitamin B_{12} resulting in this blood picture

Select the most likely organism for each of the above

A. *Trichinella spiralis*
B. *Paragonimus westermani*
C. *Clonorchis sinesis*
D. *Diphyllobothrium latum*
E. *Echinococcus granulosus*
F. *Taenia solium*
G. *Taenia saginata*
H. *Schistosoma mansoni*
I. *Schistosoma haematobium*
J. *Toxocara canis*

Q2.78

A 35-year-old patient with pneumococcal pneumonia develops resistance to antibiotic treatment.

1. Single point change of the nucleotide sequence of bacterial DNA

2. Incorporation of donor's naked DNA into recipient bacterium's chromosomal DNA

3. Transfer of DNA via a bacteriophage (virus) which is then incorporated into recipient bacterium's chromosomal DNA

4. Transfer of extrachromosomal DNA (a plasmid) from one bacterium to another during direct contact

Which term best describes each of the above mechanisms?

A. Mitosis
B. Conjugation
C. Transduction
D. Transformation
E. Mutation

Q2.79

An 88-year-old woman has pneumonia. Blood cultures reveal *Staphylococcus aureus*. The following metabolic changes occur in this condition

A. Diversion of synthesis away from albumin towards acute-phase reactants
B. Increased immunoglobulin production
C. Marked decreases in nitrogen losses
D. Metabolic acidosis
E. Respiratory acidosis

Q2.80

A 29-year-old nurse with HIV and bluish red nodules on the forehead has a CD4 count of $300/mm^3$, rapidly falling. The following drug combinations will eradicate HIV

A. Stavudine+didanosine+efavirenz
B. Stavudine+lamivudine+nevirapine
C. Zidovudine+didanosine+indinavir
D. Zodovudine+lamivudine+indinavir+ ritonavir
E. Zidovudine+zalcitabine+nelfinavir

Q2.81

A 28-year-old man has genital herpes. He may develop the following complications

A. Keratitis
B. Acute encephalitis
C. Erythema multiforme
D. Acute myocardial infarction
E. Uraemia

Q2.82

An 11-year-old girl develops malaise, fever and a skin rash. The skin rash rapidly progresses from macules to papules to vesicles to pustules in a few hours. The rash is present on the face, scalp and trunk and to a lesser extent on the extremities. Eventually the pustules crust and heal without scarring. Complications of this condition include

A. Kuru
B. Pneumonitis
C. Acute truncal cerebellar ataxia
D. Multiorgan involvement
E. Shingles

Q2.83

A 19-year-old nursing student develops fever, headache, malaise and sore throat. Her general practitioner prescribes ampicillin following which she develops a macular rash. On examination her posterior cervical lymph nodes are palpable and her spleen is just felt. The aetiological agent of this condition is also responsible for

A. Rosacea
B. Oral hairy leucoplakia in AIDS
C. Burkitt's lymphoma
D. Nasopharyngeal carcinoma
E. Immunoblastic lymphoma of AIDS

Q2.84

A 4-year-old boy in Bangladesh develops weakness of his left leg. This is preceded by fever, sore throat and muscle aches, particularly in the lower back. On examination he has weakness of the muscles of the left leg but no sensory loss. Late complications of this condition include

A. Guillain–Barré syndrome
B. Aspiration pneumonia
C. Myocarditis
D. Paralytic ileus
E. Urinary calculi

Q2.85

A 28-year-old farmer in India, following an accident on his farm, develops a wound on his foot. A week later he has general malaise, rapidly followed by trismus. Within 72 hours he develops painful reflex spasms. The following statements regarding his management are correct

A. The wound should be cleaned but not debrided since the latter hastens the toxin's effects on the central nervous system
B. Human tetanus immunoglobulin when given intramuscularly will neutralize the circulating toxin
C. Human tetanus antitoxin should be given with intramuscular injection of tetanus toxoid
D. Benzodiazepines should not be used to control spasm since they suppress the respiratory system
E. The patient should be nursed in an isolated, quiet, well-ventilated room
F. Intravenous metronidazole should be administered

Infectious diseases, tropical medicine and sexually transmitted diseases

Q2.86

A 28-year-old British doctor travels to India. On his return he has fever, diarrhoea, headache and abdominal pain. On examination he has a maculopapular rash, 'rose red spots' on his abdomen, and hepatosplenomegaly. He has associated leucopenia. The complications of this condition include

A. Meningitis
B. Lobar pneumonia
C. Osteomyelitis
D. Intestinal perforation
E. Intestinal haemorrhage

Q2.87

A 28-year-old chef at an Indian restaurant in London is found to be the source of a *Salmonella typhi* outbreak. He himself is asymptomatic. Ultrasound of the abdomen reveals that he has a thick-walled gall bladder with calculi. Prevention of future outbreaks of this condition is best done by

A. Laparoscopic cholecystectomy
B. Laparotomy and cholecystectomy
C. Endoscopic retrograde cholangiopancreatography and administration of chloramphenicol directly into the gall bladder
D. Intravenous chloramphenicol
E. Combination of gentamicin and vancomycin

Q2.88

A 23-year-old journalist who is in the first trimester of her pregnancy develops vaginal discharge, dysuria and intermenstrual bleeding. Microscopy of an endocervical specimen reveals intracellular, Gram-negative cocci. Complications of this condition include

A. Abscesses of Bartholin's glands
B. Fitz-Hugh–Curtis syndrome
C. Infertility
D. Rectal infection
E. Ophthalmia neonatorum

Q2.89

A 29-year-old farmer in East Asia, who is accustomed to walking barefoot, develops epigastric pain and peptic ulcer-like symptoms. Investigations reveal a microcytic anaemia and low serum ferritin levels. The following are likely to have caused this clinical picture

A. *Enterobius vermicularis*
B. *Ascaris lumbricoides*
C. *Ancylostoma duodenale*
D. *Necator americanus*
E. *Trichinella spiralis*

Q2.90

Two months after intercourse, a 22-year-old homosexual man develops fever, arthralgia, myalgia and lymphadenopathy. The illness lasts for 3 weeks. Laboratory abnormalities which are typically seen in this condition include

A. Lymphocytosis
B. Thrombocytosis
C. Raised liver enzymes
D. Markedly elevated CD4 lymphocytes
E. Markedly depleted CD8 lymphocytes

Q2.91

Drugs which are nephrotoxic used in the treatment of HIV include

A. Foscarnet
B. Amphotericin B
C. Pentamidine
D. Sulfadiazine
E. Indinavir

Q2.92

A 22-year-old woman develops malaise and fever in the first trimester of pregnancy. She has mild conjunctivitis. The suboccipital, posterior auricular and posterior cervical lymph nodes are palpable. Four days later she develops a rash which appears on the forehead and then spreads to involve the trunk and limbs. The rash is pinkish-red, macular and discrete. The rash fades by the second day and is gone by the third day. Complications of this condition include

A. Thrombocytopenia
B. Encephalitis
C. Patent ductus arteriosus in the newborn
D. Ventricular septal defect in the fetus
E. Microcephaly of the child

Q2.93

A 22-year-old woman develops malaise and fever late in the third trimester of pregnancy. She has mild conjunctivitis. The suboccipital, posterior auricular and posterior cervical lymph nodes are palpable. Four days later she develops a rash which appears on the forehead and then spreads to involve the trunk and limbs. The rash is pinkish-red, macular and discrete. The rash fades by the second day and is gone by the third day. Complications of this condition include

A. Congenital rubella syndrome
B. Expanded rubella syndrome
C. Patent ductus arteriosus in the newborn
D. Ventricular septal defect in the fetus
E. Microcephaly of the child

Q2.94

A 12-month-old child in Pakistan develops malaise, fever, rhinorrhoea, cough and conjunctival suffusion. On examination she has small, greyish, irregular lesions surrounded by an erythematous base. These are found in greatest numbers on the mucous membranes opposite the second molar tooth. She develops a maculopapular rash. Complications of this condition include

A. Bacterial pneumonia
B. Bronchitis
C. Otitis media
D. Gastroenteritis
E. Subacute sclerosing panencephalitis

Q2.95

A 4-year-old child develops malaise, fever, loss of appetite, runny nose and conjunctivitis. A week later he has paroxysms of coughing and a white cell count reveals that lymphocytes account for over 90% of the total white blood cell count. Complications of this condition include

A. Pneumonia
B. Cerebral anoxia and convulsions
C. Rectal prolapse
D. Inguinal hernia
E. Bronchiectasis

Infectious diseases, tropical medicine and sexually transmitted diseases

Q2.96

A 29-year-old pregnant woman has fever, and palpable lymph nodes in the neck. She has several cats in her house and she acknowledges that at times it is unhygienic. The Sabin–Feldman dye test is positive. As a consequence of her clinical condition the fetus is predisposed to

A. Microcephaly
B. Hydrocephalus
C. Encephalitis
D. Mental retardation
E. Choroidoretinitis

Q2.97

An 8-year-old child presents with fever and sore throat. On the second day she develops a rash on the neck. The rash initially blanches on pressure but rapidly becomes punctate, erythematous and generalized. It is prominent in the flexures but absent on the face, palms and soles. The tongue has a white coating, through which prominent bright red papillae can be seen – the strawberry tongue. Complications of this condition include

A. Otitis media
B. Rheumatic fever
C. Glomerulonephritis
D. Retropharyngeal abscess
E. Peritonsillar abscess

Q2.98

An 8-year-old child in Sri Lanka develops fever and a sore throat. On examination the tonsils and pharynx are markedly inflamed. There is a membrane covering the tonsils which is firmly adherent to the underlying tissue. The lymph nodes are enlarged and tender, producing the so-called 'bull-neck'. The following statements about the management of this condition are correct

A. The patient should be isolated
B. Bed rest should be avoided
C. Antibiotics have no role since this condition is due to a toxin
D. Antitoxin therapy is the only specific treatment
E. This condition can be prevented by active immunization in childhood

A2.1

D

Deficiency	Causes	Organisms
Cellular immune defects	HIV infection Lymphoma Bone marrow transplant Congenital syndromes	Respiratory syncytial virus Cytomegalovirus Epstein–Barr virus Herpes simplex and zoster *Salmonella* spp. *Mycobacterium* spp. (esp. *M. avium-intracellulare*) *Cryptococcus neoformans* *Candida* spp. *Cryptosporidium parvum* *Pneumocystis carinii* *Toxoplasma gondii*

A2.2

E

Deficiency	Causes	Organisms
Neutropenia	Chemotherapy Bone marrow transplant Immunosuppressant drugs	*Escherichia coli* *Klebsiella pneumoniae* *Staphylococcus aureus* *Staph. epidermidis* *Aspergillus* spp. *Candida* spp.

A2.3

D

Deficiency	Causes	Organisms
Splenectomy	Surgery Trauma	*Strep. pneumoniae* *Neisseria meningitidis* *Haemophilus influenzae* Malaria

A2.4

D

Deficiency	Causes	Organisms
Humoral immune deficiencies	Congenital syndromes Chronic lymphocytic leukaemia Corticosteroids	*Haemophilus influenzae* *Strep. pneumoniae* Enteroviruses

Infectious diseases, tropical medicine and sexually transmitted diseases

A2.5

B

See answer to question 2.7.

A2.6

A

See answer to question 2.7.

A2.7

B

Phenoxymethylpenicillin (penicillin V) is an oral preparation that is used chiefly to treat streptococcal pharyngitis and as prophylaxis against rheumatic fever. Benzylpenicillin can only be given parenterally and is often the drug of choice for serious infections, notably infective endocarditis, meningococcal, streptococcal and gonococcal infections, clostridial infections (tetanus, gas gangrene), actinomycosis, anthrax, and spirochaetal infections (syphilis, yaws). Tetracyclines are active against Gram-positive and Gram-negative bacteria but their use is now limited, partly owing to increasing bacterial resistance. A tetracycline is used for the treatment of acne and rosacea. Tetracyclines are also active against *Vibrio. cholerae*, *Rickettsia* spp., *Mycoplasma* spp., *Coxiella burnetii*, *Chlamydia* spp. and *Brucella* spp. They were formerly used widely in lower respiratory tract infection, but resistance is now common among *Strep. pneumoniae*. The cephalosporins have an advantage over the penicillins in that they are resistant to staphylococcal penicillinases (but are still inactive against methicillin-resistant staphylococci) and have a broader range of activity that includes both Gram-negative and Gram-positive organisms, but excludes enterococci and anaerobic bacteria.

Ceftazidime and cefpirome are active against *Pseudomonas aeruginosa*. These potent broad-spectrum antibiotics are useful for the treatment of serious systemic infections, particularly when the precise nature of the infection is unknown. They are commonly used for serious sepsis in postoperative and immunocompromised patients, particularly during cytotoxic chemotherapy of leukaemia and other malignancies. Neomycin is an aminoglycoside that is used only for the topical treatment of eye and skin infections and in the management of portosystemic encephalopathy. Even though it is poorly absorbed, prolonged oral administration can produce ototoxicity.

A2.8

C

Cephalosporins are commonly used for serious sepsis in postoperative and immunocompromised patients, particularly during cytotoxic chemotherapy of leukaemia and other malignancies.

A2.9

A

Benzylpenicillin can only be given parenterally and is often the drug of choice for serious infections, notably infective endocarditis, meningococcal, streptococcal and gonococcal infections, clostridial infections (tetanus, gas gangrene), actinomycosis, anthrax, and spirochaetal infections (syphilis, yaws).

A2.10

C

Penicillins inactivate aminoglycosides when mixed in the same solution.

A2.11

D

Aztreonam's spectrum of activity is limited to aerobic Gram-negative bacilli. With the exception of urinary tract infections, aztreonam should be used in combination with metronidazole (for anaerobes) and an agent active against Gram-positive cocci (a penicillin or erythromycin). It is a useful alternative to aminoglycosides in combination therapy, largely for the treatment of intra-abdominal sepsis.

A2.12

D

When gentamicin is used with some diuretics, ototoxicity may occur.

A2.13

B

Tetracyclines are active against Gram-positive and Gram-negative bacteria but their use is now limited, partly owing to increasing bacterial resistance. A tetracycline is used for the treatment of acne and rosacea.

A2.14

D

Chloramphenicol should not be given to premature infants or neonates because of their inability to conjugate and excrete this drug; high blood levels lead to circulatory collapse and the often fatal 'grey baby syndrome'.

A2.15

D

Metronidazole is of major importance in the treatment of anaerobic bacterial infections, particularly those due to *Bacteroides* spp. It is also used prophylactically in colonic surgery. It may be given orally, by suppository (well absorbed and cheap) or intravenously (very expensive). It is also the treatment of choice for amoebiasis, giardiasis and infection with *Trichomonas vaginalis*. It can produce a disulfiram-like reaction with ethanol and enhance the anticoagulant effect of warfarin.

A2.16

B

Anaemia, neutropenia and thrombocytopenia are all common in advanced HIV infection. Pancytopenia occurs because of underlying opportunistic infection or malignancies, in particular *Mycobacterium avium-intracellulare*, disseminated cytomegalovirus and lymphoma. Myelotoxic drugs include zidovudine (megaloblastic anaemia, red cell aplasia, neutropenia), ganciclovir (neutropenia), systemic chemotherapy (pancytopenia) and co-trimoxazole (agranulocytosis).

A2.17

C

In *Pneumocystis carinii* infection fine crackles are heard on auscultation, although in mild cases there may be no auscultatory abnormality. In early infection the chest X-ray is normal but the typical appearances are of bilateral perihilar interstitial infiltrates, which can progress to confluent alveolar shadows

Infectious diseases, tropical medicine and sexually transmitted diseases

throughout the lungs. Treatment should be instituted as early as possible. First-line therapy is with intravenous co-trimoxazole (100 mg/kg per day sulfamethoxazole and 20 mg/kg per day trimethoprim in divided doses) for 21 days.

A2.18

C

The streptogramin antibiotics quinupristin with dalfopristin, effective against Gram-positive bacteria including methicillin-resistant *Staphylococcus aureus* (MRSA), should be reserved for multiresistant organisms.

A2.19

B

Cytomegalovirus (CMV) retinitis tends to occur once the CD4 count is below 100 and is found in up to 30% of AIDS cases. Presenting features depend on the area of retina involved (loss of vision being most common with macular involvement) and include floaters, loss of visual acuity, field loss and scotomata, orbital pain and headache. Examination of the fundus reveals haemorrhages and exudates, which follow the vasculature of the retina (so-called 'pizza pie' appearance). Treatment for CMV should be started as soon as possible with either ganciclovir (10 mg/kg daily) or foscarnet (60 mg/kg 8-hourly) given intravenously. The decision about which drug to use is based on the overall condition of the patient and concurrent medication, because a major side-effect of ganciclovir is myelosuppression and foscarnet is nephrotoxic. Treatment doses should be continued for at least 3 weeks or until the retinitis is quiescent.

A2.20

E

Shingles (herpes zoster) is treated with aciclovir and the duration of lesion formation and time to healing can be reduced by early treatment. Aciclovir, valaciclovir and famciclovir have all been shown to reduce the burden of zoster-associated pain when treatment is given at the acute phase. Shingles involving the ophthalmic division of the trigeminal nerve has an associated incidence of acute and chronic ophthalmic complications of 50%. Early treatment with aciclovir reduces this to 20% or less. All immunocompromised individuals should be given aciclovir at the onset of shingles.

A2.21

D

In the immunosuppressed, ganciclovir (5 mg/kg daily for 14–21 days) reduces retinitis and gastrointestinal damage and can eliminate cytomegalovirus (CMV) from blood, urine and respiratory secretions. It is less effective against pneumonitis. In patients with continuing immunocompromise, particularly AIDS, maintenance therapy may be necessary. Drug resistance has been reported in AIDS patients and transplant recipients and bone marrow toxicity is common. No antiviral drugs are currently available for routine treatment of CMV in neonates and the toxicity of ganciclovir prohibits its use in most cases. Two other drugs, foscarnet and cidofovir, are currently in use for the treatment of CMV infection. Both are nephrotoxic and, as with ganciclovir, their use should be restricted to those with severe disease.

A2.22

E

Strongyloides stercoralis is a small (2 mm long) worm which lives in the small intestine. In patients who are immunosuppressed (e.g. by corticosteroid therapy or intercurrent illness) filariform larvae may penetrate directly through the bowel wall in huge numbers, causing an overwhelming and usually fatal generalized infection (the strongyloidiasis hyperinfestation syndrome). This condition is often complicated by septicaemia due to bowel organisms.

A2.23

D

Zidovudine has a beneficial effect on HIV neurological disease, with startling improvement in cognitive function in many patients with AIDS dementia complex (ADC). It may also have a neuroprotective role. Zalcitabine, didanosine and stavudine produce a similar neuropathy as a major toxic side-effect and must be used with caution in patients with HIV neuropathy.

A2.24

D

Human herpes virus 8, first described in 1994, is strongly associated with the aetiology of classical and AIDS-related Kaposi's syndrome. Antibody prevalence is high in those with tumours but relatively low in the general population of most industrialized countries. High rates of infection (>50% population) have been described in central and southern Africa

and this matches the geographic distribution of Kaposi's sarcoma before the era of AIDS. HHV-8 can be sexually transmitted among homosexual men, through heterosexual sex and through exposure to blood from needle sharing. It is thought that salivary transmission may be the predominant route in Africa. HHV-8 RNA transcripts have been detected in Kaposi's sarcoma cells and in circulating mononuclear cells from patients with the tumour.

A2.25

D

Neisseria gonorrhoeae is a Gram-negative intracellular diplococcus, which infects epithelium particularly of the urogenital tract, rectum, pharynx and conjunctivae. Humans are the only host and the organism is spread by intimate physical contact. The incubation period is 2–14 days with most symptoms occurring between days 2 and 5. In men the most common symptom is one of anterior urethritis causing dysuria and/or urethral discharge.

A2.26

E

Tetracyclines or macrolide antibiotics are most commonly used to treat *Chlamydia*. Doxycycline 100 mg 12-hourly for 7 days or azithromycin 1 g as a single dose are both effective for uncomplicated infection. Tetracyclines are contraindicated in pregnancy. Other effective regimens include erythromycin 500 mg four times daily.

Infectious diseases, tropical medicine and sexually transmitted diseases

A2.27

D

In primary syphilis, between 10 and 90 days (mean 21 days) after exposure to the pathogen a papule develops at the site of inoculation. This ulcerates to become a painless, firm chancre. There is usually painless regional lymphadenopathy in association. *Treponema pallidum* is not amenable to *in vitro* culture – the most sensitive and specific method is identification by dark-ground microscopy.

A2.28

E

Early syphilis (primary or secondary) should be treated with long-acting penicillin such as procaine benzylpenicillin (e.g. Jenacillin A which also contains benzylpenicillin) 600 mg intramuscularly daily for 10 days. For late-stage syphilis, particularly when there is cardiovascular or neurological involvement, the treatment course should be extended for a further week. For patients sensitive to penicillin, either doxycycline 200 mg daily or erythromycin 500 mg four times daily is given orally for 2–4 weeks depending on the stage of the infection. Non-compliant patients can be treated with a single dose of benzathine penicillin G 2.4 g intramuscularly. Benzathine penicillin is never administered intravenously.

A2.29

C

Famciclovir and valaciclovir are useful in primary genital herpes if patients are seen while lesions are still moist.

A2.30

C

In yellow fever the pathology of the liver shows mid-zone necrosis, and eosinophilic degeneration of hepatocytes (Councilman bodies).

A2.31

D

Yellow fever is an internationally notifiable disease. It is easily prevented using the attenuated 17d chick embryo vaccine. Vaccination is not recommended for children under 9 months and immunosuppressed patients unless there are compelling reasons. For the purposes of international certification, immunization is valid for 10 years, but protection lasts much longer than this and probably for life. The WHO Expanded Programme of Immunization includes yellow fever vaccination in endemic areas.

A2.32

C

Typical measles has two stages:

- The pre-eruptive and catarrhal stage. This is the stage of viraemia and viral dissemination. Malaise, fever, rhinorrhoea, cough, conjunctival suffusion and the pathognomonic Koplik's spots are present during this stage. Koplik's spots are small, greyish, irregular lesions surrounded by an erythematous base and are found in greatest numbers on the mucous membrane opposite the second molar tooth. They occur a day or two before the onset of the rash.

- The eruptive or exanthematous stage. This is characterized by the presence of a maculopapular rash that initially occurs on the face, chiefly the forehead, and then spreads rapidly to involve the rest of the body. At first the rash is discrete but later it may become confluent and patchy, especially on the face and neck. It fades in about 1 week and leaves behind a brownish discoloration.

A2.33

B

The most important human disease due to amoebae is amoebiasis, which is caused by *Entamoeba histolytica*. The organism formerly known as *E. histolytica* is now known to consist of two distinct species: *E. histolytica*, which is pathogenic, and *E. dispar*, which is non-pathogenic. Cysts of the two species are identical, but can be distinguished by molecular techniques after culture of the trophozoite. *E. histolytica* can be distinguished from all amoebae except *E. dispar*, and from other intestinal protozoa, by microscopic appearance. Microscopic examination of fresh stool or colonic exudate obtained at sigmoidoscopy is the simplest way of diagnosing colonic amoebic infection. To confirm the diagnosis motile trophozoites containing red blood cells must be identified: the presence of amoebic cysts alone does not imply disease. Sigmoidoscopy and barium enema examination may show colonic ulceration but are rarely diagnostic.

A2.34

E

Giardia intestinalis is a flagellate that is found world-wide. It causes small intestinal disease, with diarrhoea and malabsorption. Prevalence is high throughout the tropics, and it is the most common parasitic infection in travellers returning to the UK. In certain parts of Europe, and in some rural areas of North America, large water-borne epidemics have been reported.

A2.35

B

The clinical picture of filariasis depends on the individual immune response, which in turn may depend on factors such as age at first exposure. In endemic areas many people have asymptomatic infection. Sometimes early infection is marked by bouts of fever accompanied by pain, tenderness and erythema along the course of affected lymphatics. Involvement of the spermatic cord and epididymis are common in Bancroftian filariasis. These acute attacks subside spontaneously in a few days, but usually recur. Recurrent episodes cause intermittent lymphatic obstruction, which in time can become fibrotic and irreversible. Obstructed lymphatics may rupture, causing cellulitis and further fibrosis; there may also be chylous pleural effusions and ascites. Over time there is progressive enlargement, coarsening, and fissuring of the skin, leading to the classical appearances of elephantiasis. The limbs or scrotum may become hugely swollen.

Infectious diseases, tropical medicine and sexually transmitted diseases

A2.36

D

Onchocerciasis (river blindness) is found in well-defined areas of West and East Africa, Yemen, and parts of Central and South America. It is the result of infection with *Onchocerca volvulus*. Infection is transmitted by day-biting flies of the genus *Simulium*: principally *S. damnosum* in West Africa, *S. neavei* in East Africa, and *S. metallicum* in America. Onchocerciasis is a major cause of morbidity in parts of West Africa, where the whole adult population may be affected and blindness rates exceed 10%. Live microfilariae cause relatively little harm, but dead parasites may cause severe allergic reactions, with hyaline necrosis and loss of tissue collagen and elastin. In the eye a similar process causes conjunctivitis, sclerosing keratitis, uveitis, and secondary glaucoma. Choroidoretinitis is also occasionally seen. In order to identify parasites, skin snips taken from the iliac crest or shoulder are placed in saline under a cover slip. After 4 hours, microscopy will show microfilariae wriggling free on the slide. If this is negative a 50 mg dose of diethylcarbamazine (DEC) can be given: this will provoke an allergic rash in the majority of patients (the Mazzotti reaction).

A2.37

B

Infection with *Ascaris lumbricoides* (roundworm) is usually asymptomatic, although heavy infections are associated with nausea, vomiting, abdominal discomfort and anorexia. Worms can sometimes obstruct the small intestine, the most common site being at the ileocaecal valve. They may also occasionally invade the appendix, causing acute appendicitis, or the bile duct, resulting in biliary obstruction and suppurative cholangitis. Larvae in the lung may produce pulmonary eosinophilia. Heavy infection in children, especially those who are already malnourished, may have significant effects on nutrition and development. Serious morbidity and mortality are rare in ascariasis, but the huge number of people infected means that on a global basis roundworm infection causes a significant burden of disease, especially in children.

A2.38

B

CNS involvement is the most common extrasalivary-gland manifestation of mumps. Clinical meningitis occurs in 5% of all infected patients, and 30% of patients with CNS involvement have no evidence of parotid gland involvement. Epididymo-orchitis develops in about one-third of patients who develop mumps after puberty. Bilateral testicular involvement results in sterility in only a small percentage of these patients. Pancreatitis, oophoritis, myocarditis, mastitis, hepatitis and polyarthritis may also occur.

A2.39

B

Rabies is a major problem in some countries, and established infection is invariably fatal. The rabies virus is bullet-shaped and has spike-like structures arising from its surface containing glycoproteins that cause the host to produce neutralizing, haemagglutination-inhibiting antibodies. The virus has a marked affinity for nervous tissue and the salivary glands. It exists in two major epidemiological settings. a) Urban rabies is most frequently transmitted to humans through rabid dogs and, less frequently, cats. b) Sylvan (wild) rabies is maintained in the wild by a host of animal reservoirs such as foxes, skunks, jackals, mongooses and bats.

A2.40

D

The human prion diseases are Creutzfeldt–Jakob disease (CJD), including the classical sporadic, familial, iatrogenic and variant forms of the disease Gerstmann–Straussler–Scheinker syndrome, fatal familial insomnia, and kuru. Creutzfeldt–Jakob disease usually occurs sporadically at an annual rate of one per million of the population. In the UK, knowledge that large numbers of cattle with the prion disease bovine spongiform encephalopathy (BSE) had gone into the human food chain led to enhanced surveillance for emergence of the disease in humans. The evidence is now convincing, based on transmission studies in mice and on glycosylation patterns of prion proteins, that this has occurred and, to date, there have been 79 confirmed and suspected cases of variant CJD (human BSE) in the UK. In contrast to classical CJD, which presents with dementia at a mean age of onset of 60 years, variant CJD presents with psychiatric and cerebellar signs at a mean age of onset of 29 years. Gerstmann–Straussler–Scheinker syndrome and fatal familial insomnia are rare prion diseases usually occurring in families with a positive history. The pattern of inheritance is as an autosomal dominant with some degree of variable penetrance. Kuru was described and characterized in the Fore highlanders in north-eastern New Guinea. Transmission was associated with ritualistic cannibalism of deceased relatives. With the cessation of cannibalism by 1960, the disease has gradually diminished and recent cases had all been exposed to the agent before 1960.

A2.41

B

Pertussis occurs world-wide. Humans are both the natural hosts and reservoirs of infection. The disease is caused by *Bordetella pertussis* which is a Gram-negative coccobacillus. *B. parapertussis* and *B. bronchiseptica* produce milder infections. Malaise, anorexia, mucoid rhinorrhoea and conjunctivitis are present. The paroxysmal stage, so called because of the characteristic paroxysms of coughing, begins about a week later. Paroxysms with the classic inspiratory whoop are seen only in younger individuals in whom the lumen of the respiratory tract is compromised by mucus secretion and mucosal oedema.

A2.42

C

For close contacts of a case of meningococcal disease, household and 'kissing' contacts should be given prophylaxis with oral rifampicin or ciprofloxacin (the latter should not be given to children) to eradicate the bacteria from the nasopharynx. In the case of group C disease, contacts should be offered immunization.

Infectious diseases, tropical medicine and sexually transmitted diseases

A2.43

B

Evidence of streptococcal infection is required to make diagnosis of acute rheumatic fever in addition to two or more major criteria or one major plus two or more minor criteria. Evidence of streptococcal infection includes a positive throat culture for group A streptococci, elevated antistreptolysin O titre or other streptococcal antibodies, or a history of recent scarlet fever.

A2.44

D

Recurrences of rheumatic fever are most common when persistent cardiac damage is present, and are prevented by the continued administration of oral phenoxymethylpenicillin 250 mg daily or by monthly injections of 916 mg of benzathine penicillin until the age of 20 years or for 5 years after the latest attack. A sulphonamide (e.g. sulfadiazine) may be used if the patient is allergic to penicillin. Any streptococcal infection that does develop should be treated very promptly.

A2.45

D

The diagnosis of leptospirosis is usually a clinical one. Leptospires can be cultured from blood or CSF during the first week of illness, but culture requires special media and may take several weeks. In England and Wales only 20–30 cases of leptospirosis are diagnosed every year (although many mild infections probably go undiagnosed), and it remains largely an occupational disease of farmers, vets and others who work with animals. In some parts of the world (e.g. Hawaii, where the annual incidence is about 130/100 000), it is associated with a variety of recreational activities which bring people into closer contact with rodents. Weil, in 1886, described a severe illness consisting of jaundice, haemorrhage and renal impairment caused by L. icterohaemorrhagiae, but fortunately 90–95% of infections are subclinical or cause only a mild fever.

A2.46

C

Brucellosis (Malta fever, undulant fever) is a zoonosis and has a world-wide distribution, although it has been virtually eliminated from cattle in the UK. The highest incidence is in the Mediterranean countries, the Middle East and the tropics; there are about 500 000 new cases diagnosed per year. Spread is usually by the ingestion of raw milk from infected cattle or goats, although occupational exposure is also common.

A2.47

D

Sleeping sickness is caused by trypanosomes transmitted to humans by the bite of the tsetse fly (genus Glossina). It is endemic in a belt across sub-Saharan Africa, extending to about 14°N and 20°S; this marks the natural range of the tsetse fly. Two subspecies of trypanosome cause human sleeping sickness: Trypanosoma brucei gambiense ('Gambian sleeping sickness'), and T. b. rhodesiense ('Rhodesian sleeping sickness'). Gambian sleeping sickness is found from Uganda in Central Africa, west to Senegal and south as far as Angola. The treatment of sleeping sickness has remained largely unchanged for more than 40 years, although there have been recent developments in the management of *T. b. gambiense* infection. In both forms, treatment is usually effective if given before the onset of CNS involvement, but much less so in neurological disease. The drug of choice in early trypanosomiasis is suramin, given intravenously at a dose of 20 mg/kg at 5- to 7-day intervals up to a total dose of 5 g. Severe reactions are relatively common, and a test dose of 100 mg is usually given prior to this regimen. Intramuscular pentamidine is effective against *T. b. gambiense* only: a number of different regimens are in use. A single dose of suramin should be given to patients with parasitaemia prior to lumbar puncture, to avoid inoculation into the CSF.

A2.48

C

In chronic Chagas' disease, parasites of *Trypanosoma cruzi* may be detected by xenodiagnosis: infection-free reduviid bugs are allowed to feed on the patient, and the insect gut subsequently examined for parasites. Serological tests can also detect both acute and chronic Chagas' disease.

A2.49

E

The most widely used drugs for visceral leishmaniasis are the pentavalent antimony salts (e.g. sodium stibogluconate, which contains 100 mg of antimony per mL), given intravenously or intramuscularly at a dose of 20 mg of antimony per kg for 21 days. Resistance to antimony salts is increasing, and relapses may occur following treatment. The drug of choice where resources permit is intravenous amphotericin B (preferably given in the liposomal form).

A2.50

B

This patient has lepromatous leprosy. The treatment is as shown in the table.

Recommended treatment regimens for leprosy in adults
Multibacillary leprosy (LL, BL, BB)
Rifampicin 600 mg once-monthly, supervised
Clofazimine 300 mg once-monthly, supervised
Clofazimine 50 mg daily, self-administered
Dapsone 100 mg daily, self-administered
Treatment continued for 2 years
Paucibacillary leprosy (BT, TT)
Rifampicin 600 mg once-monthly, supervised
Dapsone 100 mg daily, self-administered
Treatment continued for 6 months

LL, lepromatous; BL, borderline lepromatous; BB, borderline; BT, borderline tuberculoid; TT, tuberculoid

A2.51

C

This patient has tuberculoid leprosy. The treatment is as shown in the table accompanying Answer 2.50, above.

A2.52

B

Penicillin or ciprofloxacin are the best treatments for anthrax. In mild cutaneous infections, oral therapy for 2 weeks is adequate. In more severe infections high doses of intravenous antibiotics are needed, along with appropriate supportive care.

Infectious diseases, tropical medicine and sexually transmitted diseases

A2.53

C

Cholera is caused by the curved, flagellated Gram-negative bacillus, *Vibrio cholerae*. The mainstay of treatment is rehydration, and with appropriate and effective rehydration therapy mortality has decreased to less than 1%. Oral rehydration is usually adequate, but intravenous therapy is occasionally required. Antibiotics such as tetracycline 500 mg four times daily for 3 days help to eradicate the infection, decrease stool output, and shorten the duration of the illness. Drug resistance is becoming an increasing problem, and ciprofloxacin is now used more frequently.

A2.54

B

Plague is caused by *Yersinia pestis*, a Gram-negative bacillus. The main reservoirs are woodland rodents, which transmit infection to domestic rats (*Rattus rattus*). The usual vector is the rat flea, *Xenopsylla cheopis*. These fleas bite humans when there is a sudden decline in the rat population. Prevention of plague is largely dependent on the control of the flea population. Outhouses, or huts, should be sprayed with insecticides that are effective against the local flea. During epidemics rodents should not be killed until the fleas are under control, as the fleas will leave dead rodents to bite humans. Tetracycline 500 mg four times daily or sulphonamides 2–4 g daily for 7 days are effective chemoprophylactic agents. A partially effective formalin-killed vaccine is available for use by travellers to plague-endemic areas.

A2.55

A

In malaria, the parasites multiply inside the red cells, changing from merozoite, to trophozoite, to schizont, and finally appearing as 8–24 new merozoites. The erythrocyte ruptures, releasing the merozoites to infect further cells. Each cycle of this process, which is called erythrocytic schizogeny, takes about 48 hours in *P. falciparum*, *P. vivax* and *P. ovale*, and about 72 hours in *P. malariae*. *P. vivax* and *P. ovale* mainly attack reticulocytes and young erythrocytes, while *P. malariae* tends to attack older cells; *P. falciparum* will parasitize any stage of erythrocyte.

A2.56

B

Blackwater fever is due to widespread intravascular haemolysis, affecting both parasitized and unparasitized red cells, giving rise to dark urine.

A2.57

B

In children, *P. malariae* infection is associated with glomerulonephritis and nephrotic syndrome.

A2.58

A

Cerebral malaria is one of the features of severe falciparum malaria. It is marked by diminished consciousness, confusion, and convulsions, often progressing to coma and death. Untreated it is universally fatal.

A2.59

D

Hyperreactive malarial splenomegaly (tropical splenomegaly syndrome, TSS) is seen in older children and adults in areas where malaria is hyperendemic. It is associated with an exaggerated immune response to repeated malaria infections, and is characterized by anaemia, massive splenomegaly, and elevated IgM levels. Malaria parasites are scanty or absent. TSS usually responds to prolonged treatment with prophylactic antimalarial drugs.

A2.60

D

Cervicofacial actinomycosis usually occurs following dental infection or extraction. It is often indolent and slowly progressive, associated with little pain, and results in induration and localized swelling of the lower part of the mandible. Lymphadenopathy is uncommon. Occasionally acute inflammation occurs. Sinuses and tracts develop with discharge of 'sulphur' granules. *Actinomyces* spp. are Gram-positive branching higher bacteria which are normal mouth and intestine commensals; they are particularly associated with poor mouth hygiene. Treatment of actinomycosis often involves surgery as well as antibiotics: penicillin is the drug of choice. Intravenous penicillin 2.4 g 4-hourly is given for 4–6 weeks, followed by oral penicillin for some weeks after clinical resolution. Tetracyclines are also effective.

A2.61

C

Histoplasmosis occurs world-wide and is commonly seen in Ohio and the Mississippi river valley regions where over 80% of the population have been subclinically exposed. Transmission is mainly by inhalation of the spores. Chronic pulmonary histoplasmosis is clinically indistinguishable from pulmonary tuberculosis. It is usually seen in white males over the age of 50 years. Radiologically, pulmonary cavities, infiltrates and characteristic fibrous streaking from the periphery towards the hilum are seen. Only symptomatic acute pulmonary histoplasmosis, chronic histoplasmosis and acute disseminated histoplasmosis require therapy. Ketoconazole or itraconazole are indicated for moderate disease. Severe infection is treated with intravenous amphotericin B to a total dose of 1.5 g. Patients with AIDS usually require treatment with parenteral amphotericin B. Surgical excision of histoplasmomas (pulmonary granuloma due to *H. capsulatum*) or chronic cavitatory lung lesions and release of adhesions following mediastinitis is often required.

A2.62

D

Invasive aspergillosis occurs in immunosuppressed patients and presents as acute pneumonia, meningitis or an intracerebral abscess, lytic bone lesions, and granulomatous lesions in the liver; less commonly endocarditis, paranasal *Aspergillus* granuloma or keratitis may occur. Urgent treatment with intravenous amphotericin B is required.

A2.63

A

Cryptococcosis is caused by a yeast-like fungus, *Cryptococcus neoformans*. Amphotericin B (0.3–0.5 mg/kg daily i.v.) alone or in combination with flucytosine (100–200 mg/kg daily) has reduced the mortality of this once universally fatal condition. Therapy should be continued for 3 months if meningitis is present. Fluconazole has greater CSF penetration and is used when toxicity is encountered with amphotericin B and flucytosine and as maintenance therapy in immunocompromised patients, especially those with HIV. Itraconazole does not penetrate the blood–brain barrier.

A2.64

D

Invasive zygomycosis (mucormycosis) is rare and is caused by several fungi, including *Mucor* spp., *Rhizopus* spp. and *Absidia* spp. It occurs in severely ill patients. The hallmark of the disease is vascular invasion with marked haemorrhagic necrosis. Rhinocerebral mucormycosis is the most common form. Nasal stuffiness, facial pain and oedema, and necrotic, black nasal turbinates are characteristic. It is rare and is mainly seen in diabetics with ketoacidosis.

A2.65

1) F   2) E   3) D   4) C   5) B   6) A

Antibiotic chemoprophylaxis (see British National Formulary)		
Clinical problem	Aim	Drug regimen
Rheumatic fever	To prevent recurrence and further cardiac damage	Phenoxymethylpenicillin 250 mg twice-daily, or sulfadiazine 1g when penicillin-allergic
Infective endocarditis	To prevent infection on abnormal, prosthetic or homograft heart valves, patent ductus or septal defect (see 'special'-risk patients)	*Dental/upper respiratory tract procedures (LA)* Oral amoxicillin 3 g 1 hour before procedure For penicillin-allergic individuals, clindamycin 600 mg 1 hour before procedure Chlorhexidine mouthwash may also be used
		Dental under GA At induction: i.v. amoxicillin 1 g Six hours later: oral amoxicillin 500 mg
		'Special'-risk patients only (prosthetic valves and/or previous endocarditis):
		Gastrointestinal, obstetric or gynaecological, dental (GA) and genitourinary procedures: At induction: i.v. amoxicillin 1 g i.v. gentamicin 120 mg Six hours after procedure, amoxicillin 500 mg (vancomycin for penicillin-allergic patient)
Splenectomy/spleen malfunction	To prevent serious pneumococcal sepsis	Phenoxymethylpenicillin 500 mg 12-hourly
Meningitis: Due to meningococci	To prevent infection in close contacts	Adults: rifampicin 600 mg twice daily for 2 days Children < 1 month: 5 mg/kg Children > 1 month: 10 mg/kg
Due to *H. influenzae* type b	To reduce nasopharyngeal carriage and prevent infection in close contacts	Adults: rifampicin 100 mg daily for 4 days Children: 20 mg/kg
Tuberculosis	To prevent infection in exposed (close contacts) tuberculin-negative individuals, infants of infected mothers and immunosuppressed patients	Oral isoniazid 5 mg/kg daily for 6–12 months

Infectious diseases, tropical medicine and sexually transmitted diseases

A2.66

1) D 2) E 3) A 4) B 5) C

Zoonotic infections	
Pathogen	Animal reservoir
Prion protein	Cattle
Arenavirus	Multimammate rat
Flavivirus	Pigs
Rhabdovirus	Dog and other mammals
Flavivirus	Primates
E. coli 0157	Cattle, chickens
S. enteritidis and others	Chickens, cattle
C. jejuni	Various
L. icterohaemorrhagiae and others	Rodents
B. abortus	Cattle
B. melitensis	Sheep
B. anthracis	Cattle, sheep
B. burgdorferi	Deer
B. henselae	Cats
Y. pestis	Rodents
Various Rickettsia spp.	Various
C. psittaci	Psittacine birds
T. gondii	Cats and other mammals
C. parvum	Cattle
E. granulosus	Dogs
A. caninum	Dogs

A2.67

1) E 2) C 3) A 4) B 5) D

Zoonotic infections	
Disease	Mode of transmission
Prions	
nvCJD	Ingestion (CNS tissue)
Viruses	
Lassa fever	Direct contact
Japanese encephalitis	Mosquito bite
Rabies	Saliva, faeces (bats)
Yellow fever	Mosquito bite
Bacteria	
Gastrococci	Ingestion (meat)
Salmonellosis	Ingestion (meat, eggs)
Campylobacter	Ingestion (meat, milk, water)
Leptospirosis	Ingestion (urine)
Brucellosis	Contact; ingestion of milk/cheese
Anthrax	Contact; ingestion
Lyme disease	Tick bite
Cat scratch fever	Flea bite
Plague	Flea bite
Typhus	Arthropod bite
Psittacosis	Aerosol
Others	
Toxoplasmosis	Ingestion (meat, faeces)
Cryptosporidiosis	Ingestion (faeces)
Hydatid disease	Ingestion (faeces)
Cutaneous larva migrans	Penetration of skin by larvae

nvCJD, new variant Creutzfeldt–Jakob disease

A2.68

1) D 2) E 3) C 4) A 5) B

β-lactams (penicillins, cephalosporins and monobactams) block bacterial cell wall mucopeptide formation by binding to and inactivating specific penicillin-binding proteins (PBPs), which are peptidases involved in the final stages of cell wall assembly and division. Aminoglycosides interrupt bacterial protein synthesis by inhibiting ribosomal function (messenger and transfer RNA). Chloramphenicol competes with messenger RNA for ribosomal binding. It also inhibits peptidyl transferase. Sulphonamides block thymidine and purine synthesis by inhibiting microbial folic acid synthesis. The quinolone group of bactericidal drugs such as ciprofloxacin, norfloxacin, ofloxacin and levofloxacin, inhibit bacterial DNA synthesis by inhibiting topoisomerase IV and DNA gyrase, the enzyme responsible for maintaining the superhelical twists in DNA.

A2.69

1) D   2) C   3) E   4) A   5) B

Amphotericin B is used intravenously in severe systemic fungal infections. Clotrimazole is used topically for the treatment of ringworm and cutaneous and genital candidiasis. Ketoconazole is effective in candidiasis and deep mycoses including histoplasmosis and blastomycosis but not in aspergillosis and cryptococcosis. Fluconazole is noted for its ability to enter CSF and is used for candidiasis and for the treatment of central nervous system (CNS) infection with *Cryptococcus neoformans*. Griseofulvin, a naturally occurring antifungal, is widely used for the treatment of more extensive superficial mycoses and onychomycosis. Only symptomatic acute pulmonary histoplasmosis, chronic histoplasmosis and acute disseminated histoplasmosis require therapy. Ketoconazole or itraconazole are indicated for moderate disease. Severe infection is treated with intravenous amphotericin B to a total dose of 1.5 g. Patients with AIDS usually require treatment with parenteral amphotericin B. Surgical excision of histoplasmomas (pulmonary granuloma due to *H. capsulatum*) or chronic cavitatory lung lesions and release of adhesions following mediastinitis is often required.

A2.70

1) A   2) E   3) B   4) C   5) D

Aciclovir is an acyclic nucleoside analogue that acts as a chain terminator of herpesvirus DNA synthesis. This drug is converted to aciclovir monophosphate by a virus-encoded thymidine kinase produced by alpha herpesviruses, herpes simplex types 1 and 2 and varicella zoster virus. Foscarnet (sodium phosphonoformate) is a simple pyrophosphate analogue which inhibits viral DNA polymerases. It is active against herpesviruses. Two drugs that inhibit the action of the neuraminidase of influenza A and B have been introduced. Zanamivir is administered by inhalation and oseltamivir is an oral preparation. Both have been shown to be effective in reducing the duration of illness in influenza. Ribavirin, a synthetic purine nucleoside derivative which interfaces with 5'-capping of messenger RNA, is active against several RNA viruses. It is administered by a small-particle aerosol generator (SPAG) to infants with acute respiratory syncytial virus (RSV) infection. Interferons are stimulated by a number of factors, including viral nucleic acid, and render uninfected cells resistant to infection with the same – or in some circumstances different – viruses. They have been synthesized commercially either by culture of lymphoblastoid cells or by recombinant DNA technology and are licensed for therapeutic use. Currently, infection with hepatitis viruses B and C (and certain malignancies) are treated with regular injections of α-interferon.

Infectious diseases, tropical medicine and sexually transmitted diseases

A2.71

1) E   2) D   3) C   4) B   5) A

Pathogenic mechanisms of bacterial gastroenteritis

Pathogenesis	Mode of action	Clinical presentation	Examples
Mucosal adherence	Effacement of intestinal mucosa	Moderate watery diarrhoea	Enteropathogenic *E. coli* (EPEC)
Mucosal invasion	Penetration and destruction of mucosa	Dysentery	*Shigella* spp. *Campylobacter* spp. Enteroinvasive *E. coli* (EIEC)
Toxin production			
Enterotoxin	Fluid secretion without mucosal damage	Profuse watery diarrhoea	*Vibrio cholerae* *Salmonella* spp. *Campylobacter* spp. Enterotoxigenic *E. coli* (ETEC)
Neurotoxin	Paralysis of autonomic nervous system	Variable diarrhoea and vomiting	*Bacillus cereus* *Staphylococcus aureus* producing enterotoxin B
Cytotoxin	Damage to mucosa	Bloody diarrhoea	*Salmonella* spp. *Campylobacter* spp. Enterohaemorrhagic *E. coli* (EHEC)

A2.72

1) A   2) C   3) D   4) E   5) B

In pregnant women listeria causes a flu-like illness, but infection of the fetus can lead to septic abortion, premature labour and stillbirth. Early treatment of listeria in pregnancy may prevent this, but the overall fetal loss rate is about 50%. The treatment of choice for adult listeriosis is ampicillin plus gentamicin. Q fever is a zoonosis caused by the rickettsia-like organism *Coxiella burnetii*. Treatment with doxycycline 200 mg daily reduces the duration of the acute illness, but it is not known whether this correlates with eradication of the organism. For chronic Q fever, including endocarditis, doxycycline is often combined with rifampicin or clindamycin. Lyme disease, caused by the spirochaete *Borrelia burgdorferi*, is a zoonosis of deer and other wild mammals. Infection is transmitted from animal to man by ixodid ticks, and is most likely to occur in rural wooded areas in spring and early summer. Amoxicillin or doxycycline given early in the course of the disease shortens the duration of the illness in approximately 50% of patients. Late disease should be treated with 2–4 weeks of intravenous benzylpenicillin or ceftriaxone. Tularaemia should be treated with streptomycin or gentamicin. Brucellosis is treated with a combination of doxycycline 200 mg daily and rifampicin 600–900 mg daily for 6 weeks, but relapses occur.

A2.73

1) C   2) D   3) A   4) E   5) B

In tuberculoid leprosy (TT) the characteristic, usually single, skin lesion is a hypopigmented, anaesthetic patch with thickened, clearly demarcated edges, central healing, and atrophy. The face, gluteal region and extremities are most commonly affected. The nerve leading to the hypopigmented patch, and the regional nerve trunk, are often thickened and tender. Unlike other parts of the body, a tuberculoid patch on the face is not anaesthetic. Nerve involvement leads to marked muscle atrophy. Tuberculoid lesions are known to heal spontaneously. Borderline tuberculoid (BT) leprosy resembles TT but skin lesions are usually more numerous, smaller, and may be present as small 'satellite' lesions around larger ones. Peripheral but not cutaneous nerves are thickened, leading to deformity of hands and feet. In borderline (BB) leprosy skin lesions are numerous, varying in size and form (macules, papules, plaques). The annular, rimmed lesion with punched-out, hypopigmented anaesthetic centre is characteristic. There is widespread nerve involvement and limb deformity. In borderline lepromatous (BL) leprosy there are a large number of florid asymmetrical skin lesions of variable form, which are strongly positive for acid-fast bacilli. Skin between the lesions is normal and often negative for bacilli. In lepromatous leprosy (LL), although practically every organ can be involved, the changes in the skin are the earliest and most obvious manifestation. Peripheral oedema and rhinitis are the earliest symptoms. The skin lesions predominantly occur on the face, the gluteal region and the upper and lower limbs. They may be macules, papules, nodules or plaques: of these, the macule is the first to appear. Infiltration is most noticeable in the ear lobes. Thinning of the lateral margins of the eyebrows is characteristic. The mucous membranes are frequently involved, resulting in nasal stuffiness, laryngitis and hoarseness of the voice. Nasal septal perforation with collapse of the nasal cartilages produces a saddle-nose deformity. With progression of the disease, the typical leonine facies due to infiltration of the skin becomes apparent. Glove and stocking anaesthesia, gynaecomastia, testicular atrophy, ichthyosis and nerve palsies (facial, ulnar, median and radial) develop late in the disease. Neurotrophic atrophy affecting the phalanges leads to the gradual disappearance of fingers. Nerve involvement is less pronounced than in TT.

Infectious diseases, tropical medicine and sexually transmitted diseases

2.74

1) E 2) D 3) C 4) A 5) B

Infections caused by rickettsiae			
Disease	Organism	Reservoir	Vector
Typhus fever group			
Epidemic typhus	*Rickettsia prowazekii*	Man	Human body louse
Endemic (murine) typhus	*R. typhi*	Rodents	Rat flea
Scrub typhus	*R. tsutsugamushi*	Trombiculid mite	Trombiculid mite
Spotted fever group			
African tick typhus	*R. conorii, R. africae*	Various mammals	Hard tick
Fièvre boutonneuse	*R. conorii*	Rodents, dog	Hard tick
Rocky Mountain spotted fever	*R. rickettsii*	Rodents	Hard tick
Rickettsial pox	*R. akari*	Rodents	Mite

2.75

A) F B) F C) T D) T

The sporozoites are inoculated into a new human host, and those which are not destroyed by the immune response are rapidly taken up by the liver. Here they multiply inside hepatocytes as merozoites: this is pre-erythrocytic (or hepatic) sporogeny. After a few days the infected hepatocytes rupture, releasing merozoites into the blood from where they are rapidly taken up by erythrocytes. In the case of *P. vivax* and *P. ovale*, a few parasites remain dormant in the liver as hypnozoites. These may reactivate at any time subsequently, causing relapsing infection.

2.76

A) F B) T C) T D) T E) F

Malaria prophylaxis for adult travellers		
Area visited	Prophylactic regimen	Alternatives
No chloroquine resistance	Chloroquine 300 mg weekly	Proguanil 200 mg daily
Limited chloroquine resistance	Chloroquine 300 mg weekly *plus* Proguanil 200 mg daily *or* Mefloquine 250 mg weekly	Chloroquine 300 mg weekly *plus* Maloprim 1 tablet weekly
Significant chloroquine resistance	Mefloquine 250 mg weekly	Doxycycline 100 mg daily *or* Malarone 4 tablets daily

A2.77

1) I 2) H 3) B 4) A 5) J 6) C
7) F 8) E 9) D

The normal hosts of *Trichinella spiralis*, the cause of trichinosis, include pigs, bears and warthogs. Man is infected by eating undercooked meat from these animals. Ingested larvae mature in the small intestine, where adults release new larvae which penetrate the bowel wall and migrate through the tissues. Eventually these larvae encyst in striated muscle. Light infections are usually asymptomatic. Heavier loads of worms produce gastrointestinal symptoms as the adults establish themselves in the small intestine, followed by systemic symptoms as the larvae invade. The latter include fever, oedema, and myalgia. Massive infection may occasionally be fatal, but usually the symptoms subside once the larvae encyst. Eggs of the dog roundworm, *Toxocara canis*, are occasionally ingested by humans, especially children. The eggs hatch and the larvae penetrate the small intestinal wall and enter the mesenteric circulation, but are then unable to complete their life cycle in a 'foreign' host. In most cases infection is asymptomatic, and the larvae die without causing serious problems. In heavy infections there may be generalized symptoms (fever and urticaria) and eosinophilia, as well as focal signs related to the migration of the parasites. Pulmonary involvement may cause bronchospasm and chest X-ray changes. Ocular infection may produce a granulomatous swelling mimicking a retinoblastoma, while cardiac or neurological involvement may occasionally be fatal. The earliest symptom of *Schistosoma haematobium* infection (bilharzia) is usually painless terminal haematuria. As bladder inflammation progresses there is increased urinary frequency and groin pain. Obstructive uropathy develops, leading to hydronephrosis, renal failure, and recurrent urinary infection. There is a strong association between chronic urinary schistosomiasis and squamous cell bladder carcinoma. *Schistosoma mansoni* usually affects the large bowel. Early disease produces superficial mucosal changes, accompanied by blood-stained diarrhoea. Later the mucosal damage becomes more marked, with the formation of rectal polyps, deeper ulceration, and eventually fibrosis and stricture formation. Ectopic eggs are carried to the liver, where they cause an intense granulomatous response. Hepatitis is followed by progressive periportal fibrosis, leading to portal hypertension, oesophageal varices and splenomegaly. Hepatocellular function is usually well preserved. Over 20 million people are infected with lung flukes of the genus *Paragonimus*. The adult worms (of which the major species is *P. westermani*) live in the lungs, producing eggs which are expectorated or swallowed and passed in the faeces. Humans and other mammalian hosts become infected after consuming uncooked shellfish. The common clinical features are fever, cough and mild haemoptysis. In heavy infections the disease may progress, sometimes mimicking pneumonia or pulmonary tuberculosis. The diagnosis is made by detection of ova on sputum or stool microscopy. Serological tests are also available. The human liver flukes, *Clonorchis sinensis*, *Opisthorchis felineus*, and *O. viverrini*, are almost entirely confined to east and South East Asia, where they infect more than 20 million people. Infection is often asymptomatic, but may be associated with cholangitis and biliary carcinoma. *Taenia solium*, the pork tapeworm, is generally smaller than *T. saginata*, although it can still reach 6 metres in length. It is particularly common in South America, South Africa, China, and parts of South East Asia. As with *T. saginata* infection is usually asymptomatic. Man can act as both primary and intermediate host for *T. solium*. The latter situation arises when eggs are ingested, or possibly when they are regurgitated from the small intestine to the stomach. Larvae are liberated, penetrate the intestinal wall, and are carried to various parts of the body where they develop into cysticerci. These are cysts, 0.5–1 cm in diameter, containing the scolex of a new adult worm. Common sites for cysticerci include subcutaneous tissue, skeletal muscle and brain. Cysts in the brain can cause a variety of problems including epilepsy, personality change, hydrocephalus and focal neurological signs. Infection with the fish tapeworm, *Diphyllobothrium latum*, is common in northern Europe and Japan, owing to the consumption of raw fish. The adult worm reaches a length of several metres, but like the other tapeworms usually causes no symptoms. A megaloblastic anaemia (due to competitive utilization of B_{12} by the parasite) may occur. Hydatid disease occurs when humans become an intermediate host of the dog tapeworm, *Echinococcus granulosus*. The adult worm lives in the gut of domestic and wild canines, and the larval stages are usually found in sheep, cattle and camels. Man may become infected either from direct contact with dogs, or from food or water contaminated with dog faeces. It is common in Australia, Argentina, the Middle East and parts of East Africa; small foci of infection are still found in North Wales and rural Scotland. Symptoms depend mainly on the site of the cyst. The liver is the most common organ affected (60%), followed by the lung (20%), kidneys (3%), brain (1%) and bone (1%). The symptoms are those of a slowly growing benign tumour. Pressure on the bile ducts may cause jaundice. Rupture into the abdominal cavity, pleural cavity or biliary tree may occur. In the latter situation, intermittent jaundice, abdominal pain and fever associated with eosinophilia result.

A2.78

1) E   2) D   3) C   4) B

The development or acquisition of resistance to an antibiotic by bacteria invariably involves either a mutation at a single point in a gene or transfer of genetic material from another organism. Larger fragments of DNA may be introduced into a bacterium either by transfer of 'naked' DNA or via a bacteriophage (a virus) DNA vector. Both the former (transformation) and the latter (transduction) are dependent on integration of this new DNA into the recipient chromosomal DNA. This requires a high degree of homology between the donor and recipient chromosomal DNA. Finally, antibiotic resistance can be transferred from one bacterium to another by conjugation, when extrachromosomal DNA (a plasmid) containing the resistance factor (R factor) is passed from one cell into another during direct contact. Transfer of such R factor plasmids can occur between unrelated bacterial strains and involve large amounts of DNA and often codes for multiple antibiotic resistance. Transformation is probably the least clinically relevant mechanism, whereas transduction and R factor transfer are usually responsible for the sudden emergence of multiple antibiotic resistance in a single bacterium. Increasing resistance to many antibiotics has developed.

A2.79

A) T   B) T   C) F   D) T   E) T

During acute infection, three major changes occur in protein metabolism. a) There is a diversion of synthesis away from somatic and circulating proteins such as albumin towards acute-phase proteins. b) Protein synthesis is also directed towards immunoglobulin production and there is increased production of lymphocytes, neutrophils and other phagocytic cells. c) There is a marked increase in nitrogen losses due to tissue breakdown, which may reach 10–15 g per day. Acid–base balance disturbance is common. Causes include respiratory alkalosis following tachypnoea related to fever, respiratory acidosis and hypoxaemia associated with pneumonia, and metabolic acidosis associated with septicaemia.

A2.80

A) F   B) F   C) F   D) F   E) F

None of the current drug combinations can eradicate HIV. Plasma RNA levels rise when therapy is stopped. Studies suggest that even in patients in whom viral replication is suppressed below the limits of detection for prolonged periods, viral replication is ongoing.

A2.81

A) T   B) T   C) T   D) F   E) F

Complications of HSV-1 infection include transfer to the eye (dendritic ulceration, keratitis), acute encephalitis, skin infections such as herpetic whitlow, and erythema multiforme.

A2.82

A) F   B) T   C) T   D) T   E) T

The child has chickenpox which is due to varicella zoster virus. Important complications of chickenpox include pneumonia, which generally begins 1–6 days after the skin eruption, and bacterial superinfection of skin lesions. Pneumonia is more common in adults than in children and cigarette smokers are at particular risk. Pulmonary symptoms are usually more striking than the physical findings, although a chest radiograph usually shows diffuse changes throughout both lung fields. CNS involvement occurs in about 1 per 1000 cases and most commonly presents as an acute truncal cerebellar ataxia. The immunocompromised are susceptible to disseminated infection with multiorgan involvement. Varicella zoster virus (VZV) produces two distinct diseases, varicella (chickenpox) and herpes zoster (shingles). Shingles never occurs as a primary infection but results from reactivation of latent VZV from the dorsal root and/or cranial nerve ganglia.

A2.83

A) F   B) T   C) T   D) T   E) T

This patient has infectious mononucleosis (glandular fever) which is caused by the Epstein–Barr virus (EBV). EBV is also the cause of oral hairy leucoplakia in AIDS patients and is the major aetiological agent responsible for Burkitt's lymphoma, nasopharyngeal carcinoma, post-transplant lymphoma and the immunoblastic lymphoma of AIDS patients. Different levels of expression of EBV latency genes occur in the various clinical conditions caused by the virus.

Infectious diseases, tropical medicine and sexually transmitted diseases

A2.84

A) F B) T C) T D) T E) T

Aspiration pneumonia, myocarditis, paralytic ileus and urinary calculi are late complications of poliomyelitis. The diagnosis of polio is a clinical one. Distinction from Guillain–Barré syndrome is easily made by the absence of sensory involvement and the asymmetrical nature of the paralysis in poliomyelitis.

A2.85

A) F B) T C) T D) F E) T
F) T

When tetanus is suspected any wound must be cleaned and debrided if necessary, to remove the source of toxin. Human tetanus antitoxin 250 units should be given along with an intramuscular injection of tetanus toxoid. If the patient is already protected a single booster dose of the toxoid is given; otherwise the full three-dose course of adsorbed vaccine is given. Patients are nursed in a quiet, isolated, well-ventilated, darkened room. Benzodiazepines are used to control spasm and sedate the patient; if the airway is compromised intubation and mechanical ventilation may be necessary. Antibiotics and antitoxin should be administered, even in the absence of an obvious wound. Intravenous metronidazole is the drug of choice, although penicillin is also effective. Human tetanus immunoglobulin (HTIG) 500 IU should be given by intramuscular injection to neutralize any circulating toxin.

A2.86

A) T B) T C) T D) T E) T

This patient has enteric fever due to *Salmonella typhi*. Without treatment (and occasionally even after treatment) serious complications can arise, usually in the third week of illness. These include meningitis, lobar pneumonia, osteomyelitis, intestinal perforation and intestinal haemorrhage.

A2.87

A) F B) F C) F D) F E) F

Prolonged antibiotic therapy may eliminate the carrier state of *Salmonella typhi*, but in the presence of gall bladder disease it is rarely effective. Cholecystectomy is not usually justified on clinical or public health grounds.

A2.88

A) T B) T C) T D) T E) T

In women the primary site of infection for gonorrhoea is usually the endocervical canal. Symptoms include an increased or altered vaginal discharge, pelvic pain due to ascending infection, dysuria, and intermenstrual bleeding. Complications include Bartholin's abscesses and in rare cases a perihepatitis (Fitz-Hugh–Curtis syndrome) can develop. On a global basis gonorrhoea is one of the most common causes of female infertility. Rectal infection, due to local spread, occurs in women and is usually asymptomatic, as is pharyngeal infection. Conjunctival infection is seen in neonates born to infected mothers and is one cause of ophthalmia neonatorum.

A2.89

A) F B) F C) T D) T E) F

Hookworm infections, caused by the human hookworms *Ancylostoma duodenale* and *Necator americanus*, are found world-wide. They are relatively rare in developed countries, but very common in areas with poor sanitation and hygiene: overall about 25% of the world's population are affected. Hookworm infection is a major contributing factor to anaemia in the tropics. *A. duodenale* is found mainly in East Asia, North Africa and the Mediterranean, while *N. americanus* is the predominant species in South and Central America, South East Asia and sub-Saharan Africa. Light infections, especially in a well-nourished person, are often asymptomatic. Heavier worm loads may be associated with epigastric pain and nausea, resembling peptic ulcer disease. Chronic heavy infection, particularly on a background of malnourishment, may cause iron deficiency anaemia. Blood loss has been estimated at about 0.15 mL/worm/day for *A. duodenale*, and 0.03 mL/worm/day for *N. americanus*.

A2.90

A) F B) F C) T D) F E) F

Laboratory abnormalities seen in a primary illness of HIV include lymphopenia with atypical reactive lymphocytes noted on blood film, thrombocytopenia and raised liver enzymes. CD4 lymphocytes may be markedly depleted and the CD4:CD8 ratio reversed. Antibodies to HIV may be absent during this early stage of infection although the level of circulating viral RNA is high and p24 core protein may be detectable.

A2.91

A) T B) T C) T D) T E) T

Many nephrotoxic drugs are used in the management of HIV-associated pathology, particularly foscarnet, amphotericin B, pentamidine, sulfadiazine and indinavir.

A2.92

A) T B) T C) T D) T E) T

Complications of rubella include superadded pulmonary bacterial infection, arthralgia, haemorrhagic manifestations due to thrombocytopenia, encephalitis and the congenital rubella syndrome. Rubella affects the fetuses of up to 80% of all women who contract the infection during the first trimester of pregnancy. Congenital rubella syndrome is characterized by the presence of fetal cardiac malformations, especially patent ductus arteriosus and ventricular septal defect, eye lesions (especially cataracts), microcephaly, mental retardation and deafness. The expanded rubella syndrome consists of the manifestations of the congenital rubella syndrome plus other effects including hepatosplenomegaly, myocarditis, interstitial pneumonia and metaphyseal bone lesions.

A2.93

A) F B) F C) F D) F E) F

The incidence of congenital abnormalities of the fetus due to maternal rubella diminishes in the second trimester and no ill-effects result from infection in the third trimester.

Infectious diseases, tropical medicine and sexually transmitted diseases

A2.94

A) T   B) T   C) T   D) T   E) T

Although measles is a relatively mild disease in the healthy child, it carries a high mortality in the malnourished and in those who have other diseases. Complications are common in such individuals and include bacterial pneumonia, bronchitis, otitis media and gastroenteritis. Less commonly, myocarditis, hepatitis and encephalomyelitis may occur. In those who are malnourished or those with defective cell-mediated immunity, the classical maculopapular rash may not develop and widespread desquamation may occur. The virus also causes the rare condition, subacute sclerosing panencephalitis, which may follow measles infection occurring early in life (<18 months of age). Persistence of the virus with reactivation prior to puberty results in accumulation of virus in the brain, progressive mental deterioration and a fatal outcome.

A2.95

A) T   B) T   C) T   D) T   E) T

Complications of whooping cough (pertussis) include pneumonia, atelectasis, rectal prolapse and inguinal hernia. Cerebral anoxia may occur, especially in younger children, resulting in convulsions. Bronchiectasis is a rare sequel.

A2.96

A) T   B) T   C) T   D) T   E) T

Congenital toxoplasmosis may be asymptomatic, but can produce serious disease. Clinical manifestations include microcephaly, hydrocephalus, encephalitis, convulsions and mental retardation. Choroidoretinitis is common; occasionally this may be the only feature.

A2.97

A) T   B) T   C) T   D) T   E) T

Scarlet fever may be complicated by peritonsillar or retropharyngeal abscesses and otitis media. Non-suppurative complications include acute glomerulonephritis and rheumatic fever.

A2.98

A) T   B) F   C) F   D) T   E) T

The patient with diphtheria should be isolated and bed rest is advised. Antitoxin therapy is the only specific treatment. It must be given promptly to prevent further fixation of toxin to tissue receptors, since fixed toxin is not neutralized by antitoxin. Antibiotics should be administered concurrently to eliminate the organisms and thereby remove the source of toxin production. Benzylpenicillin 1.2 g four times daily is given for 1 week. Diphtheria is prevented by active immunization in childhood.

Cell and molecular biology and genetic disorders

3

Q3.1

Normally, old cellular proteins are mopped up by a small cofactor molecule called ubiquitin. This acts as a signal for destruction. Which one of the following conditions is associated with the accumulation of ubiquinated proteins that are resistant to ubiquitin-mediated proteolysis?

A. Pneumonia
B. Acute myocardial infarction
C. Hypertension
D. Liver failure
E. Alzheimer's disease

Q3.2

Pinocytosis of low-density lipoprotein receptors results in surface clumping and internal accumulation of

A. DNA
B. RNA
C. Clathrin
D. Histone
E. Desmosomes

Q3.3

1. LH receptor
2. Epidermal growth factor receptor
3. T-cell receptor
4. TGF-β receptor
5. CD45 receptor
6. Platelet-derived growth factor receptor
7. Atrial natriuretic peptide receptor

Select the best match for each of the above

A. Receptor linked onto the outer membrane leaflet of the cell membrane by a glycan phosphatidylinositol anchor
B. Serpentine receptor with seven transmembrane domains
C. Transmembrane with large extra- and intracellular domain
D. Guanylyl cyclase-linked receptor
E. Tyrosine kinase receptor
F. Tyrosine phosphatase receptor
G. Serine/threonine kinase receptor

Q3.4

1. Zellweger's syndrome
2. Rhizomelic dwarfism
3. Synthesis of protein peptide chain
4. Maturation of primary processed peptides into functional proteins
5. Osteoclast remodelling of bone
6. Enzymes of the Krebs cycle
7. Proteins of the *bcl2–bax* family

Select the site of function or dysfunction for each of the above

A. Endoplasmic reticulum
B. Golgi apparatus
C. Lysozomes
D. Peroxisomes
E. Outer membrane of mitochondria
F. Inner matrix of mitochondria

53

Cell and molecular biology and genetic disorders

Q3.5

1. Colchicine
2. Vinblastine
3. Keratin intermediate fibres
4. Vimentin
5. Dynein

Select the best match for each of the above

A. Responsible for beating of cilia
B. Disrupts the microtubule assembly
C. Found in epithelial cells only
D. Found in mesothelial cells only

Q3.6

1. Mutations of claudin-16
2. Autoantibodies against desmoglein-3
3. Autoantibodies against desmoglein-1
4. Mutant connexons
5. Changes in cadherin expression
6. Defective integrin expression
7. Selectins

Select the best match for each of the above

A. Bernard–Soulier syndrome
B. Metastatic potential of tumours
C. Leucocyte rolling
D. X-linked form of Charcot–Marie–Tooth disease
E. Pemphigus foliaceus
F. Pemphigus vulgaris
G. Gitelman's syndrome

Q3.7

1. Transcription of proteins necessary for DNA replication
2. Genome replication
3. Preparation phase for separating diploid chromosomes into two daughter cells
4. Mitosis
5. Resting or quiescent

Select the best match for each of the above

A. G0
B. G1
C. G2
D. S
E. M

Q3.8

1. Portion of the DNA that contains the codes for a polypeptide sequence
2. AT-rich promoter site on eukaryotic genes
3. Chain of adenine nucleotides
4. Inverted guanidine nucleotide on 5′ end of mRNA
5. Initiation of translation begins with this codon
6. Stop codon

Select the best match for each of the above

A. AUG (methionine)
B. UAG
C. Gene
D. TATA box
E. CAP
F. Poly A

Q3.9

1. Steroid receptor
2. cAMP response element binding protein (CREB protein)
3. c-*jun* cell replication oncogene
4. *myc* oncogene
5. *mad* oncogene

Select the best DNA-binding proteins for each of the above

A. Helix–loop–helix
B. Helix–turn–helix
C. Zinc finger
D. Leucine zipper

Q3.10

1. Technique used for blotting RNA fragments on to membranes

2. Used to separate very long pieces of DNA (hundreds of kilobases)

3. Allows visualization of individual DNA fragments

4. Amplifies minute amounts of DNA over a million times within a few hours

5. Allows identification of the exact nucleotide sequence of a piece of DNA

Select the best match for each of the above

A. DNA sequencing
B. Polymerase chain reaction
C. Southern blotting
D. Pulsed-field gel electrophoresis
E. Northern blotting

Q3.11

1. A 23-year-old man with infertility, decreased crown–pubis:pubis–heel ratio, eunuchoid features, testicular atrophy and learning difficulties

2. An infant with absent iris and Wilms' tumour of the kidney

3. A 21-year-old man with bilateral loss of central vision and cardiac arrhythmias. He has a family history of blindness

4. A 22-year-old man has wasting of the small muscles of the hand and of the muscles of the calves of the leg which stop abruptly giving an inverted champagne bottle appearance. There is stocking distribution sensory loss, and nerve conduction studies in the lower limbs indicate demyelination

5. An 18-year-old girl who is 4 ft 11 in tall, has a webbed neck, cubitus valgus, primary amenorrhoea, infantilism and normal IQ

Select the best match for each of the above

A. The chromosome fails to separate during meiosis so that the cells have only an X chromosome and no Y chromosome

B. Point mutation of a mitochondrial chromosome

C. Duplication of a part of a chromosome

D. Deletion of a part of an arm of a chromosome

E. The chromosome fails to separate during meiosis so that the cells have two copies of the X chromosome and one copy of the Y chromosome

Q3.12

1. A 12-year-old boy has difficulty in getting up from a squatting position. On examination he has weakness of the proximal muscles of the lower limbs with hypertrophy of the calf

2. A 23-year-old man has a family history of chronic renal failure and is on long-term haemodialysis. Ultrasound of the kidneys reveals several cysts

3. A 23-year-old black woman presents with abdominal pain following an infection. She has anaemia, and investigation reveals markedly decreased haptoglobin levels

4. An 8-year-old boy has pectus carinatum and bowing of the legs which does not respond to vitamin D therapy

5. A 42-year-old man is bald and has difficulty kicking a ball. He has difficulty releasing your hand after a handshake. He has an expressionless face. Other features include diabetes, testicular atrophy and cataracts

Cell and molecular biology and genetic disorders

Select the best match for each of the above

A. Point mutation resulting in change in one codon from GAG to GTG on the globin gene
B. The three nucleotides GCT are repeated about 35 times on the mutated allele with an expanded 3′UTR region
C. One of the two copies of the autosomes has a mutation and the protein produced by the normal form of the gene cannot compensate
D. The X-chromosome has a mutation
E. Deletion of the large sequences in the dystrophin gene

Q3.13

1. Lod score of +3
2. Used to isolate genes whose protein products are not known but whose existence can be inferred from a disease phenotype
3. Requires a working knowledge of biochemistry of the disease
4. Over-expression of *bcl2*
5. Hardy–Weinberg equilibrium
6. Trinucleotide repeats expand within the disease gene with each generation and somatic expansion with cellular replication is observed

Select the best match for each of the above

A. Functional cloning
B. Positional cloning
C. Anticipation
D. Polycythaemia vera
E. Evidence of linkage
F. Suggests that the chance of having trinucleotide repeats is increased
G. Describes the outcome of random mating within the population

Q3.14

Examination of a newborn child reveals that the bridge of the nose is collapsed, there are epicanthic folds and low-set ears. Examination of the eye reveals Brushfield spots and the hands show a simian crease. Correct statements about this condition include

A. Most children with this condition are born to women above the age of 35
B. Most individuals with this condition have a high IQ
C. There is a strong association between this condition and the development of acute childhood leukaemia
D. This condition is associated with low maternal α-fetoprotein in the second trimester
E. Most patients with this condition will develop Alzheimer-like neuronal degeneration after the age of 40 years

Q3.15

Apoptosis is important in

A. The rapid growth of cancer cells
B. Wound healing
C. Embryogenesis
D. Autodestruction of the endometrium in menstruation
E. Chemotherapy of tumours

Q3.16

The geneticist wants to examine chromosomes in actively dividing cells. The following cells can be used

A. Lymphocytes in peripheral blood
B. Amniotic fluid
C. Chorionic villus sampling
D. Bone marrow
E. Skin

Q3.17

Telomeres

A. Contain genes
B. Contain the sites where the replication of chromosomes occur
C. Are extremely short in progeria
D. Are shorter in stem cells than in their terminally differentiated daughters
E. Contain enzymes called telomerases which are usually inactivated in cancers

Cell and molecular biology and genetic disorders

A3.1

E

Old cellular proteins are mopped up by a small cofactor molecule called ubiquitin, which interacts with these worn proteins via their exposed (hydrophobic) lysine residues. The ubiquitin acts as a signal for destruction, and a complex containing more than five ubiquitin molecules is rapidly degraded by a large proteolytic multienzyme array termed 26S proteasome. The failure to remove worn proteins can result in the development of chronic debilitating disorders. Alzheimer and Pick's dementias are associated with the accumulation of ubiquinated proteins (prion-like proteins), which are resistant to ubiquitin-mediated proteolysis.

A3.2

C

Pinocytosis is a much smaller-scale model of phagocytosis and is continually occurring in all cells. In contrast to phagocytosis, receptors for smaller molecular complexes such as low-density lipoprotein (LDL) result in surface clumping and the internal accumulation of a protein called clathrin. Clathrin-coated pits pinch inwards as clathrin-coated vesicles. Clathrin prevents fusion of lysosomes, and thus its removal will result in lysosomal fusion and degradation of the contents. Maintenance of a clathrin coat can result in transcellular transit of the contents and their exocytosis at another side of the plasma membrane, i.e. apical-to-basal surface transcytosis.

A3.3

1) B   2) C   3) A   4) G   5) F
6) E   7) D

Structurally, these plasma membrane receptors can be: a) serpentine (seven transmembrane domains, e.g. the luteinizing hormone (LH) receptor); b) transmembrane with large extra- and intracellular domains (e.g. the epidermal growth factor (EGF) receptor); c) transmembrane with a large extracellular domain only; d) entirely linked onto the outer membrane leaflet by a lipid moiety known as a GPI (glycan phosphatidylinositol) anchor (e.g. T-cell receptor). Enzyme-linked surface receptors usually have a single transmembrane-spanning region, and a cytoplasmic domain that has intrinsic enzyme activity or will bind and activate other membrane-bound or cytoplasmic enzyme complexes. Four classes of enzymes have been designated. a) Guanylyl cyclase-linked receptors (e.g. the atrial natriuretic peptide receptor) produce cyclic GMP. This in turn activates a cGMP-dependent kinase (G-kinase), which binds to and phosphorylates serine and threonine residues of specific secondary messengers. b) Tyrosine kinase receptors (e.g. the platelet-derived growth factor (PDGF) receptor) either specifically phosphorylate kinases on a small set of intracellular signalling proteins, or associate with proteins that have tyrosine kinase activity. c) Tyrosine phosphatase receptors (e.g. CD45) remove phosphates from tyrosine residues of specific intracellular signalling proteins. d) Serine/threonine kinase receptors (e.g. the transforming growth factor-beta (TGF-β) receptor) phosphorylate specific serine and threonine residues of intracellular signalling proteins.

A3.4

1) D   2) D   3) A   4) B   5) C
6) F   7) E

The endoplasmic reticulum (ER) is involved in the processing of proteins: the ribosomes translate mRNA into a primary sequence of amino acids of a protein peptide chain. This chain is synthesized into the ER where it is first folded and modified into mature peptides. The primary processed peptides of the ER are exported to the Golgi apparatus for maturation into functional proteins (e.g. glycosylation of proteins which are to be excreted occurs here) before packaging into secretory granules and cellular vesicles that bud off the end. Lysosomal action is crucial to the function of macrophages and polymorphs in killing and digesting infective agents, tissue remodelling during development and osteoclast remodelling of bone. The inability of the peroxisomes to function correctly can lead to rare metabolic disorders such as Zellweger's syndrome and rhizomelic dwarfism. Proteins of the *bcl2–bax* family are incorporated in this outer membrane and can release mitochondrial enzymes that trigger apoptosis. The inner matrix of mitochondria contains the enzymes of the Krebs cycle that generate the substrates of both the electron transport chain ($FADH_2$ and NADH) and central metabolism (e.g. succinyl CoA, α-oxoglutarate, oxaloacetate).

A3.5

1) B   2) B   3) C   4) D   5) A

Dynein is responsible for the beating of cilia. Drugs that disrupt the microtubule assembly (e.g. colchicine and vinblastine) affect the positioning and morphology of the organelles. The intermediate filament fibre proteins are specific to the embryonic lineage of the cell concerned, for example keratin intermediate fibres are only found in epithelial cells, while vimentin is only found in mesothelial (fibroblastic) cells.

A3.6

1) G   2) F   3) E   4) D   5) B
6) A   7) C

The kidney displays a differential expression of claudin proteins. Mutations of claudin-16 (which is only expressed in the thick ascending limb of the loop of Henle, where magnesium is reabsorbed) are responsible for some forms of Gitelman's syndrome – a rare inherited hypomagnesaemia characterized by massive urinary magnesium loss, hypercalciuria and seizures at an early age. In blistering dermatological disorders autoantibodies cause damage by attacking tight junction desmosomal proteins such as desmoglein-3 in pemphigus vulgaris and desmoglein-1 in pemphigus foliaceus. Connexons are made up of six subunits surrounding a channel and their isoforms in tissues are encoded by different genes. Mutant connexons can cause disorders such as the X-linked form of Charcot–Marie–Tooth disease. Changes in cadherin expression are often associated with tumour metastatic potential. Defective integrins are associated with many immunological and clotting disorders such as Bernard–Soulier syndrome and Glanzmann's thrombasthenia. All three selectins play a part in leucocyte rolling.

Cell and molecular biology and genetic disorders

A3.7

1) B   2) D   3) C   4) E   5) A

Regulation of the cell cycle is complex. Cells in the quiescent G0 phase (G, gap) of the cycle are stimulated by the receptor-mediated actions of growth factors (e.g. EGF, epithelial growth factor; PDGF, platelet-derived growth factor; IGF, insulin growth factor) via intracellular second messengers. Stimuli are transmitted to the nucleus where they activate transcription factors and lead to the initiation of DNA synthesis, followed by mitosis and cell division. Cell cycling is modified by the cyclin family of proteins that activate or deactivate proteins involved in DNA replication by phosphorylation (via kinases and phosphatase domains). Thus from G0 the cell moves on to G1 (gap 1) when the chromosomes are prepared for replication. This is followed by the synthetic (S) phase, when the 46 chromosomes are duplicated into chromatids, followed by another gap phase (G2), which eventually leads to mitosis (M).

A3.8

1) C   2) D   3) F   4) E   5) A   6) B

A gene is a portion of DNA that contains the codes for a polypeptide sequence. Eukaryotic genes have two AT-rich promoter sites. The first, the TATA box, is located about 25 bp upstream of (or before) the transcription start site, while the second, the CAAT box, is 75 bp upstream of the start site. The initial or primary mRNA is a complete copy of one strand of DNA and therefore contains both introns and exons. While still in the nucleus, the mRNA undergoes post-transcriptional modification whereby the 5′ and 3′ ends are protected by the addition of an inverted guanidine nucleotide (CAP) and a chain of adenine nucleotides (Poly A). Translation begins when the triplet AUG (methionine) is encountered. All proteins start with methionine but this is often lost as the leading sequence of amino acids of the native peptides are removed during protein folding and post-translational modification into a mature protein. Similarly the Poly A tail is not translated (3′ untranslated region) and is preceded by a stop codon, UAA, UAG or UGA.

A3.9

1) C   2) B   3) D   4) A   5) A

Examples of DNA-binding proteins	
Class of DNA-binding protein	Examples
Helix–turn–helix	CREB (cAMP response element binding protein)
Zinc finger	Steroid and thyroid hormone receptors Retinoic acid and vitamin D receptors bc16 oncogene product (lymphoma) WT1 oncogene product (Wilms' tumour) GATA-1 erythrocyte differentiation and Hb expression factor
Leucine zippers	c-jun cell replication oncogene c-fos cell replication oncogene
Helix–loop–helix	myc oncogene mad oncogene max oncogene

A3.10

1) E   2) D   3) C   4) B   5) A

Southern blotting allows the visualization of individual DNA fragments. A similar technique for blotting RNA fragments (which are not cut by restriction enzymes, but which are blotted as full-length mRNAs) on to membranes is called Northern blotting, and one for blotting proteins is called Western blotting. Minute amounts of DNA can be amplified over a million times within a few hours using polymerase chain reaction. Pulsed-field gel electrophoresis (PFGE) can be used to separate very long pieces of DNA (hundreds of kilobases) which have been cut by restriction enzymes that cut at rare sites in the genome. In this technique, DNA molecules are subjected to two perpendicular electric fields that are switched on alternately. The DNA molecules are separated on the basis of molecular size, and this technique can be used for long-range mapping of the genome to detect major deletions and rearrangements.

A3.11

1) E   2) D   3) B   4) C   5) A

In addition to the 23 pairs of chromosomes in the nucleus of every diploid cell, the mitochondria in the cytoplasm of the cell also have their own chromosomes. Sex-chromosome trisomies (e.g. Klinefelter's syndrome, XXY) are relatively common. The sex-chromosome monosomy in which the individual has an X chromosome only and no second X or Y chromosome is known as Turner's syndrome and is estimated to occur in 1 in 2500 live-born girls. Aniridia–Wilms syndrome is characterized by deletion of part of the short arm of chromosome 11.

A form of the neuropathy, Charcot–Marie–Tooth disease, is due to a small duplication of a region of chromosome 17. Leber's hereditary optic neuropathy (LHON) is the commonest cause of blindness in young men, with bilateral loss of central vision and cardiac arrhythmias, and is an example of a mitochondrial disease caused by a point mutation in one gene.

A3.12

1) E   2) C   3) A   4) D   5) B

Point mutation is the simplest type of change and involves the substitution of one nucleotide for another, so changing the codon in a coding sequence. In sickle cell disease a mutation within the globin gene changes one codon from GAG to GTG, so that instead of glutamic acid, valine is incorporated into the polypeptide chain, which radically alters its properties. Insertion or deletion of one or more bases is a more serious change, as it results in the alteration of the rest of the following sequence to give a frame-shift mutation. For example, some large deletions in the dystrophin gene remove coding sequences and this results in Duchenne muscular dystrophy. Each diploid cell contains two copies of all the autosomes. An autosomal dominant disorder occurs when one of the two copies has a mutation and the protein produced by the normal form of the gene cannot compensate, e.g. adult polycystic kidney disease. Genes carried on the X chromosome are said to be 'X-linked', and can be dominant or recessive in the same way as autosomal genes. As females have two X chromosomes they will be unaffected carriers of X-linked recessive diseases. However, since males have just one X chromosome, any deleterious mutation in an X-linked gene will manifest

Cell and molecular biology and genetic disorders

itself because no second copy of the gene is present. X-linked dominant disorders are rare. Vitamin D-resistant rickets is the best-known example. In the gene responsible for myotonic dystrophy, the mutated allele was found to have an expanded 3'UTR region in which three nucleotides, GCT, were repeated up to 35 times.

A3.13

1) E   2) B   3) A   4) D   5) G   6) C

Functional cloning requires a working knowledge of the biochemistry of the disease such that the defective protein/enzyme has previously been characterized in some way. Positional cloning is used to isolate genes whose protein products are not known, but whose existence can be inferred from a disease phenotype. The likelihood of recombination between the marker under study and the disease allele must be taken into account. This measure of likelihood is known as the 'lod score' (the logarithm of the odds) and is a measure of the statistical significance of the observed co-segregation of the marker and the disease gene, compared with what would be expected by chance alone. By convention a lod score of +3 is taken to be definite evidence of linkage because this indicates 1000 to 1 odds that the co-segregation of the DNA marker and the disease did not occur by chance alone. The expression of the *bcl2* protein is protective against apoptosis and heightens the threshold to which a cell will respond to a signal to undergo apoptosis. Thus, over-expression of *bcl2* is a component of oncogenesis for some tumours and proliferative states (e.g. polycythaemia vera). An unusual phenomenon observed by geneticists studying myotonic dystrophy and

Huntington's chorea in the early 1900s was termed 'anticipation'. Trinucleotide repeats such as CTG (myotonic dystrophy) and CAG (Huntington's chorea) expand within the disease gene with each generation, and somatic expansion with cellular replication is also observed. The Hardy–Weinberg equilibrium is a concept based on a mathematical equation that describes the outcome of random mating within populations. It states that 'in the absence of mutation, non-random mating, selection, and genetic drift, the genetic constitution of the population remains the same from one generation to the next'.

A3.14

A) F   B) F   C) T   D) F   E) T

Most Down's individuals have an IQ of between 20 and 80; 61% will require surgery for congenital heart, gastrointestinal and ophthalmic defects; there is a strong association with the development of acute childhood leukaemia; and 60–70% will develop Alzheimer-like neuronal degeneration after the age of 40 years. Although women over 35 are at higher risk, they account for only 7% of pregnancies. In fact, 70–80% of all Down's children are born to women under this age. Maternal serum is widely used in the second trimester (15–22 weeks) for screening for neural tube defects and aneuploid fetuses. High levels of maternal serum fetoprotein are associated with neural tube defects and some other fetal abnormalities. Altered levels of maternal serum α-fetoprotein, unconjugated estriol and human chorionic gonadotrophin (hCG) are associated with aneuploid pregnancies, in particular trisomy 21 (Down's syndrome).

A3.15

A) F   B) T   C) T   D) T   E) T

Chemotherapy employs systemically administered drugs that directly damage cellular DNA (and RNA). It kills cells by promoting apoptosis and sometimes frank necrosis. Apoptosis is essential for many life processes from tissue structure formation in embryogenesis and wound healing to normal metabolic processes such as autodestruction of the thickened endometrium to cause menstruation in a non-conception cycle. In oncology it has become clear that chemotherapy and radiotherapy regimens only work if they can trigger the tumour cells' own apoptotic pathways. Failure to do so in resistant tumours can result in the accumulation of further genetic damage to the surviving cells.

A3.16

A) T   B) T   C) T   D) T   E) T

Chromosomes can only be seen easily in actively dividing cells. Typically, lymphocytes from the peripheral blood are stimulated to divide and are processed to allow the chromosomes to be examined. Cells from other tissues can also be used – for example amniotic fluid, placental cells from chorionic villus sampling, bone marrow and skin.

A3.17

A) F   B) F   C) T   D) F   E) F

The ends of chromosomes, telomeres, do not contain genes but many repeats of a hexameric sequence TTAGGG. Replication of linear chromosomes starts at coding sites (origins of replication) within the main body of chromosomes and not at the two extreme ends. Stem cells have longer telomeres than their terminally differentiated daughters. However, germ cells replicate without shortening of their telomeres. This is because they express an enzyme called telomerase, which protects against telomere shortening by acting as a template primer at the extreme ends of the chromosomes. Most somatic cells (unlike germ and embryonic cells) switch off the activity of telomerase after birth and die as a result of apoptosis. Many cancer cells, however, reactivate telomerase, contributing to their immortality. Conversely, cells from patients with progeria (premature ageing syndrome) have extremely short telomeres.

4 Clinical immunology

Q4.1

When neutrophils arrive at the site of inflammation, attracted by chemoattractants they roll along the blood-vessel wall. Their progress is halted by

A. L-selectin
B. $\beta 5\alpha$ integrins
C. $\beta 6\alpha$ integrins
D. $\beta 8\alpha$ integrins
E. $\beta 7\alpha 4$/LPAM-1 integrins

Q4.2

The main factor that affects the erythrocyte sedimentation rate (ESR) reading is

A. C-reactive protein
B. Serum amyloid P protein
C. Complement components
D. Fibrinogen
E. Ferritin

Q4.3

The presence of antigen-specific IgM in a newborn infant suggests that

A. The mother is infected and has passed on immunity to the child *in utero*
B. The mother was infected by the child
C. The child developed an intrauterine infection
D. The child had intrauterine IgA deficiency and it is compensating by increasing IgM

E. The child is normal because all normal children are protected by the maternal transfer of IgM

Q4.4

A 45-year-old man is receiving a kidney from his wife. Which one of the following statements is correct?

A. The possibility of two different individuals having the same combination of HLA molecules is very remote
B. Usually there is considerable overlap between HLA type of the donor and the recipient, and therefore the organ graft will almost always be recognized as self and will not be rejected by the immune system of the host
C. The identification of the set of HLA antigens in the tissues of a given individual always requires specific antisera and mixed lymphocyte culture (MLC) for typing
D. Polymerase chain reaction is a crude method of identification of the set of HLA antigens in the tissues of a given individual
E. There is very little inter-racial variation in HLA antigens.

Q4.5

A 43-year-old man has a neutrophil count of 0.5×10^9/L secondary to leukaemia. He is most susceptible to infection by

A. Pneumococcus
B. Measles virus
C. Mycoplasma infection
D. *Aspergillus fumigatus*
E. Meninogococcus

Q4.6

A 53-year-old man has a neutrophil count of 0.5×10^9/L secondary to zidovudine therapy. However, his monocyte count is normal. In comparison to a patient with a markedly reduced monocyte count and neutropenia, this patient is

A. Less susceptible to infection
B. More susceptible to infection when exposed to a single organism
C. Equally susceptible to infection
D. More susceptible to bacterial infection rather than viral infection
E. More susceptible to viral infections rather than bacterial

Q4.7

A 14-year-old boy has a history of mucocutaneous sepsis in the mouth and perianal areas. Past history includes delayed separation of the umbilical stump. The most likely cause is

A. Opsonin defects
B. C1 esterase inhibitor deficiency
C. Defect in neutrophil function
D. Cell-mediated immunodeficiency
E. Lytic complement pathway defects

Q4.8

A 23-year-old asthmatic is on corticosteroids. The main effect of corticosteroids on neutrophils is to

A. Decrease neutrophil count
B. Impair leucocyte–endothelial adhesion
C. Enhance phagosome–lysozyme fusion

D. Impair production of oxygen radicals
E. Promote catalase activity

Q4.9

A 23-year-old man with HIV is treated with antiretroviral therapy. As a result he shows a marked improvement in CD4 cell numbers within 6 weeks. This is mainly due to

A. Regeneration of cells showing the naive phenotype
B. Antigen-specific response
C. Redistribution of lymphocytes from the tissues
D. Lymphopenia
E. Increase in neutrophil count

Q4.10

1. Initiation of inflammatory responses by the release of pro-inflammatory mediators such as histamine, leukotrienes and platelet-activating factor

2. Physiological function is parasite control

3. Cells which bear high-affinity IgE receptors (CD23) which rapidly absorb any local IgE

4. Cells which have receptors for the Fc portion of antibody molecules (FcR) and complement (CR)

5. Cells which kill microbes via reducing oxygen by a cytochrome-dependent NADH oxidase

Select the best match for each of the above

A. Neutrophil
B. Mast cell
C. Natural killer cell
D. Eosinophil
E. Lymphocyte

Clinical immunology

Q4.11

1. Antigen–antibody immune complex
2. Apoptotic cells
3. C-reactive protein bound to ligand
4. Bacterial endotoxin
5. Fungal cell wall
6. Tumour cells
7. Microbes with terminal sugar groups that are similar in structure to C1q and without the activation of antibody

For each of the above triggers select the best pathway

A. Alternative complement pathway
B. Classical pathway
C. Mannose-binding lectin (MBL) pathway

Q4.12

1. Interferon-α
2. Interferon-β
3. Gamma-interferon
4. Mannose-binding lectin
5. Heat-shock protein
6. Nuclear factor kappa B
7. TREM-1
8. Toll-4 receptor

Select the best match for each of the above

A. Act as molecular chaperones, preserving the cell's protein structure
B. Initiates complement activity inducing opsonization
C. Treatment of chronic hepatitis B and C infections
D. Reduces the relapse rate of multiple sclerosis
E. Used in the treatment of chronic granulomatous disease
F. Signalling receptor that initiates nuclear factor kappa B induction
G. Associates with DAP-12 to trigger secretion of pro-inflammatory cytokines
H. A pivotal transcription factor in chronic inflammatory disease

Q4.13

1. Cells that recognize tiny fragments of virus or tumour antigen that are expressed on the surface of affected cells and are able to destroy the cell and pathogen within it
2. Cells that are unable to destroy pathogens or cells directly, but through cytokine production are able to activate macrophages to kill organisms within them and further activate cytotoxic T cells
3. In response to antigen challenge and usually under T-cell help, these cells divide and are activated to become plasma cells which secrete large amounts of antibody
4. Cells that recognize abnormal cells in two ways. Firstly, they bear immunoglobulin receptors (FcR) and bind antibody-coated targets leading to antibody-dependent cellular cytotoxicity (ADCC). Secondly, they have surface receptors for MHC class I
5. Mucosa-associated lymphoid tissue (MALT)

Select the best match for each of the above

A. Natural killer cells
B. Peyer's patches
C. B cells
D. These cells usually CD4 positive
E. These cells usually bear CD8

Q4.14

1. This antibody is confined mainly to the intravascular pool
2. Patients who lack this antibody suffer recurrent and even life-threatening infections
3. Localized antigen exposure results in an increased response to this antibody widely in the mucosa-associated lymphoid tissue resulting in generalized mucosal immunity which is important for vaccination
4. Levels are high in conditions with B-cell activation such as systemic lupus erythematosus, AIDS and Hodgkin's disease
5. Important in the pathogenesis of type I hypersensitivity (atopic or allergic disease)

Select the best match for each of the above

A. IgD
B. IgM
C. IgG
D. IgA
E. IgE

Q4.15

1. HLA-A antigen
2. HLA-B antigen
3. HLA-C antigen
4. HLA D-antigen
5. HLA-DR antigen

Select the best match for each of the above

A. Constitutively expressed only on professional antigen-presenting cells (B cells, monocytes/macrophages, Langerhans' cells, dendritic cells) and activated T cells
B. Expressed on all cell types except erythrocytes and trophoblasts

Q4.16

1. Defect in phagocytes
2. B cell defects
3. T cell deficiencies
4. Common T and B cell deficiencies
5. Complement deficiency

Select the best match for each of the above

A. Mannan-binding lectin deficiency
B. Hypersplenism
C. Splenectomy
D. Ciclosporin treatment
E. Epstein–Barr virus-associated immunodeficiency

Q4.17

1. Burns patients
2. Smokers
3. Cystic fibrosis patients
4. Patients with urinary obstruction
5. Indwelling venous catheters and other foreign bodies

Select the best option for opportunist organisms in each of the above situations

A. Gram-negative infections
B. Staphylococcal and candidal infections
C. Staphylococcal and *Pseudomonas* infections
D. *Pseudomonas* infections
E. *Haemophilus influenzae* and pneumococcal infections

Q4.18

1. A 33-year-old woman with lupus nephritis
2. A 22-year-old man with extrinsic asthma
3. A 34-year-old patient with Addison's disease
4. A 33-year-old patient with Goodpasture's syndrome

Clinical immunology

5. A 65-year-old patient with pulmonary tuberculosis

6. A 1-month-old with hyperthyroidism

Select the type of hypersensitivity reaction mediating each of the above

A. Type I or immediate hypersensitivity
B. Type II or cytotoxic
C. Type III or immune complex mediated
D. Type IV or delayed hypersensitivity
E. Type V or due to stimulating antibody

Q4.19

1. Dressler's syndrome in which patients with myocardial infarction develop acute pericarditis secondary to the production of antimyocardial antibodies

2. The association of Coxsackie virus infection with the development of insulin-dependent diabetes

3. Quinine-induced thrombocytopenia

4. Methyldopa-induced haemagglutination

5. Production of anticardiac antibodies (antimyosin) after streptococcal infection leading to rheumatic fever

Select the mechanism for each of the above

A. There are some autoantigens to which the developing immune system is not usually exposed because these antigens are 'hidden' within the cells or tissues. Therefore clonal deletion of self-reactive cells does not occur. Normally these self-antigens remain hidden, so no autoimmune disease develops. If, however, the tissue is damaged by trauma, infection or tumour, the antigens may be released and evoke an autoimmune response

B. T cell bypass, which is a mechanism by which T cells are tricked into providing help to autoreactive B cells rather than suppressing them. For this to occur the self-antigen needs to be attached to a foreign antigen that is recognized by the T cell. T-cell activation will occur with the production of cytokines such as IL-4. If an autoreactive B cell has also bound the self-antigen it will then receive the signals to proliferate and produce autoantibody

C. Molecular mimicry which occurs when an organism has a similar antigenic structure to self-molecules. The infection generates antigen-specific T cells and antibodies that cross-react with host tissues and cause autoimmune disease

D. T cells regulate any autoreactive T and B cells that have survived clonal deletion. It is hypothesized that dysregulation of T-cell function could therefore lead to loss of control and the development of autoimmune disease

Q4.20

Neutrophils arrive at the site of inflammation, attracted by chemoattractants. The main chemoattractants for neutrophils in vivo are

A. N-formyl-methionyl-leucylphenylalanine (FMLP)
B. Leukotriene B_4
C. Interleukin-8
D. Complement C5a
E. Laminin

Q4.21

Neutrophils arrive at the site of inflammation, attracted by chemoattractants. These substances cause migration of neutrophils by the following mechanisms

A. Downregulation of neutrophil adhesion molecule L-selectin
B. Decrease in vascular endothelial cell expression of adhesion molecule E-selectin
C. Increase in vascular endothelial cell expression of adhesion molecule ICAM-1
D. Stimulation of neutrophil chemotaxis
E. Upregulation of vitronectin receptor

Q4.22

A 33-year-old patient is undergoing elective splenectomy. The following vaccines are recommended before this type of surgery

A. BCG vaccination
B. Measles vaccination
C. Pneumococcal vaccination
D. Meningococcal vaccination
E. Hib vaccination

Q4.23

A 22-year-old man with HIV has a low CD4 count. The mechanisms of CD4 loss/dysfunction in HIV include

A. Direct cytopathic effects of HIV
B. Lysis of infected cells by HIV-specific cytotoxic T cells
C. Cytotoxic T-cell-mediated lysis of uninfected CD4+ T cells that have bound gp120 to the CD4 molecule
D. Molecular mimicry between gp120/160 and MHC class I inducing autoimmune destruction
E. Immunosuppressive effects of soluble HIV proteins on uninfected cells

Q4.24

A 45-year-old man is on high-dose corticosteroid therapy. As a result he has impaired cell-mediated immunity, in particular T cell–macrophage cooperation. As a result he is susceptible to the following infections

A. *Pneumocystis carinii* infection
B. Tuberculosis
C. Cytomegalovirus infection
D. Candidiasis
E. Non-typhi *Salmonella* septicaemia

Clinical immunology

A4.1

A

Neutrophils, like most of the cells involved in immune responses, are not static within a particular tissue but are mobile cells. Neutrophils travel within the blood, either flowing freely as part of the circulating pool or rolling along the vascular endothelium as the marginating pool. Neutrophils arrive at the site of the inflammation, attracted by chemoattractants which upregulate L-selectin. The neutrophils roll along the blood-vessel wall and their progress is halted by L-selectin on their surface binding to a carbohydrate structure, e.g. sialyl-Lewis^x, an adhesion molecule. On activation, the L-selectin is replaced by another cell surface adhesion molecule, e.g. integrin which binds to E-selectin.

A4.2

D

Interleukin-6 induces the liver to synthesize large amounts of the acute-phase reactants, particularly complement components, C-reactive protein (CRP), mannan-binding lectin and fibrinogen. Many of these are important opsonins. CRP and fibrinogen (the factor which affects the ESR reading) are measured diagnostically to monitor infection and inflammatory conditions.

A4.3

C

IgM does not cross the placenta, and is not normally produced in the child until after birth. Therefore, if present in the newborn infant, antigen-specific IgM is a good marker for intrauterine infection

A4.4

A

The possibility of two different individuals having the same combination of HLA molecules is very remote. It is this particular aspect of the immune system that presents problems for organ transplantation. Unless the HLA type of the donor and the recipient are virtually identical, the organ graft will be recognized as non-self and rejected by the immune system of the host. Thus donors and recipients have to be tissue typed to find the best-matched organ or bone marrow. This involves the identification of the set of HLA antigens in the tissues of a given individual. In the past, specific antisera and mixed lymphocyte culture (MLC) were used for typing, although the polymerase chain reaction is now becoming the method of choice. There is a wide inter-racial variation in HLA antigens.

A4.5

D

Immune defects and some opportunist organisms
Neutropenia and defective neutrophil function
Staphylococcus aureus
Staphylococcus epidermidis
Escherichia coli
Klebsiella pneumoniae
Proteus mirabilis
Pseudomonas aeruginosa
Serratia marcescens
Bacteroides spp.
Aspergillus fumigatus
Candida spp. (systemic)
Mucor spp.

A4.6

A

The risk of infection rises steeply once the neutrophil count falls below 0.5×10^9/litre, regardless of cause. The risk is less if the monocyte count is preserved, as these cells can serve as a back-up phagocyte population. (In cyclical neutropenia, monocytes usually have cycles of opposite phase, which is probably why serious infections are uncommon.)

A4.7

C

Defects of neutrophil function (some of which also affect monocyte/macrophage function) interfere with migration into the tissues through vascular endothelium, locomotion in tissues, phagocytosis or intracellular killing. Mucocutaneous sepsis in the mouth and perianal areas is common and local infections often lead to chronic abscess formation in the tissues or draining lymph nodes. Granulomas may be seen, because of failure of neutrophils to degrade microbes effectively. Systemic spread is less common than with neutropenia. Congenital causes may first present with infection or delayed separation of the umbilical stump.

A4.8

B

The main effect of corticosteroids on neutrophils is to impair leucocyte–endothelial adhesion. This reduces the marginated pool of leucocytes and impairs their attachment to endothelium at the site of tissue injury or infection. Corticosteroids thus prevent neutrophils reaching the tissues. The corollary of reduced margination is a rise in the neutrophil count; this can be deceptive if its significance is not appreciated.

A4.9

C

Antiretroviral therapy, using combinations of drugs against the reverse transcriptase and protease enzymes, has proved effective in controlling HIV replication. On these regimes, many patients show a marked improvement in CD4 cell numbers within a matter of 4–8 weeks, mainly due to redistribution of lymphocytes from the tissues. Functional improvement with regeneration of T cells showing the naive phenotype, and antigen-specific responses (immune reconstitution) takes about 6 months.

Clinical immunology

A4.10

1) B   2) D   3) B   4) A   5) A

Neutrophils can only ingest particles smaller than themselves and are therefore mainly active against extracellular infections, particularly bacteria and some fungi, protecting the blood and viscera from these types of organisms. Once the neutrophils have been recruited, phagocytosis (ingestion) and intracellular killing of microbes begins. Ingestion and killing of organisms is much more effective if the particle is first coated or opsonized ('made ready to eat') with specific antibody and complement. This is because neutrophils have receptors for the Fc portion of antibody molecules (FcR), and complement (CR). In developed countries eosinophilia is most commonly associated with allergic disease, but their physiological function is in parasite control. Basophils are morphologically similar to mast cells but are found in very small numbers in the blood. These cells also bear high-affinity IgE receptors FcεR1 (CD23) which rapidly absorb any local IgE and also participate in immediate-type hypersensitivity reactions. The main function of mast cells appears to be in the initiation of inflammatory responses (increased vascular permeability, bronchoconstriction) by the release (following degranulation) of pro-inflammatory mediators such as histamine, leukotrienes and platelet-activating factor (PAF).

A4.11

1) B   2) B   3) B   4) A   5) A
6) A   7) C

The complement pathways are triggered by different factors:
a) Classical pathway by antigen–antibody immune complexes, apoptotic cells, C-reactive protein bound to ligand and certain viruses and bacteria.
b) Alternative pathway by bacterial endotoxin, fungal cell walls, viruses and tumour cells. The pathways converge in the activation of C3 (by the formation of either classical or alternative C3 convertase). This leads into a final common pathway with the assembly of components C5–C9 to form the membrane attack complex (MAC) which assembles into a 'doughnut-like' transmembrane channel leading to cell lysis by osmotic shock.
c) Mannose-binding lectin (MBL) pathway by microbes with terminal mannose groups. MBL has a similar structure to C1q and activates through the classical pathway without the requirement for antibody.

A4.12

1) C   2) D   3) E   4) B   5) A
6) H   7) G   8) F

Interferon (IFN)-α is used in the treatment of chronic hepatitis B and C infections as well as in some forms of leukaemia. IFN-β reduces the relapse rate in multiple sclerosis. Gamma-interferon is used therapeutically in the congenital neutrophil defect (chronic granulomatous disease), in patients with defects in IFN-γ production or receptor expression, and in the adjunct therapy of some infections (leishmaniasis, atypical mycobacterial disease). Pattern recognition receptors include: a) mannose-binding lectin, which initiates complement activity inducing opsonization; b) endocytic pattern recognition receptors, which act by enhancing antigen presentation on macrophages, by recognizing micro-organisms with mannose-rich carbohydrates on their surface or by binding to bacterial cell walls and scavenging bacteria from the circulation – all lead to phagocytosis; and c) signalling receptors that initiate nuclear factor kappa B induction (e.g. toll-like receptor TLR-4) and immune response genes leading to cell activation. NFκB (nuclear factor kappa B) is a pivotal transcription factor in chronic inflammatory diseases. It is stimulated by, for example, cytokines, protein C activators and viruses and itself regulates various proteins (e.g. pro-inflammatory cytokines, chemokines, adhesion molecules, inflammatory enzymes and receptors). Heat-shock proteins are a family of highly conserved proteins which act as immunodominant antigens in many infections. They act as molecular chaperones, housekeeping proteins within cells, preserving the cell's protein structure. They are similar in configuration to antigens found on certain microorganisms and may induce autoimmunity through molecular mimicry.

'perforins'; granzymes are injected through these pores and cause the induction of apoptosis. As normal host cells are MHC class I positive, the 'death pathway' is inhibited by the NK cell binding to this receptor. However, tumour cells and viruses often cause downregulation of class I and thus it leaves them open to NK cell attack. Cytotoxic T cells recognize tiny fragments of virus or tumour antigen that are expressed on the surface of affected cells and are able to destroy the cell and pathogen within it. Helper T cells are unable to destroy pathogens or cells directly, but through cytokine production are able to activate macrophages to kill organisms within them and further activate cytotoxic T cells. Lymphoid tissue is frequently found distributed in mucosal surfaces in non-encapsulated patches. This is termed mucosa-associated lymphoid tissue (MALT), consisting of gut-associated lymphoid tissue (GALT, mainly Peyer's patches), bronchus-associated lymphoid tissue (BALT, found in the lobes of the lungs along the main bronchi) and skin-associated lymphoid tissue (SALT).

A4.13

1) E   2) D   3) C   4) A   5) B

Natural killer (NK) cells recognize abnormal cells in two ways. Firstly, they bear immunoglobulin receptors (FcR) and bind antibody-coated targets leading to antibody-dependent cellular cytotoxicity (ADCC). Secondly, they have surface receptors for major histocompatibility complex (MHC) class I. If these MHC receptors are not bound on interaction with a cell, the NK cell is programmed to lyse this target cell. It does this by making holes in its cell membrane by secreting

A4.14

1) B   2) C   3) D   4) A   5) E

IgM antibody is confined mainly to the intravascular pool. IgG appears to be the most important antibody in resistance to infection, as patients who are lacking in IgG suffer with recurrent, even life-threatening bacterial infections. Those with isolated IgA or IgM deficiency have much less severe problems. For IgA responses, localized antigen exposure gives rise to generalized mucosal immunity, which is of importance in vaccination. This is because after encountering antigen, IgA precursor B cells in the mucosal lymphoid follicles journey to regional lymph nodes. After clonal expansion the cells return to the systemic circulation via the thoracic duct and circulate to settle widely in the mucosa-associated lymphoid tissue, not just the area where antigen exposure occurred. IgD is present on the surface of B lymphocytes, and may have an immunoregulatory role. Levels are high in conditions with B-cell activation such as systemic lupus erythematosus (SLE), AIDS and Hodgkin's disease. IgE is a monomer that is normally present in very low levels in serum, as most is membrane-bound to the high-affinity receptors on mast cells and basophils. Its main physiological role is its antinematode activity, but its most common clinical relevance is in the pathogenesis of type 1 hypersensitivity (atopic or allergic) disease.

1) B   2) B   3) B   4) A   5) A

Class I (HLA-A, -B and -C) antigens are expressed on all cell types except erythrocytes and trophoblasts. Striated muscle cells and liver parenchymal cells are normally negative but become strongly positive in inflammatory reactions. Class I molecules interact with CD8 T cells during antigen presentation and therefore are involved in driving mainly cytotoxic reactions. Class II antigens (HLA-D and -DR) are constitutively expressed only on professional antigen-presenting cells (B cells, monocytes/macrophages, Langerhans' cells, dendritic cells) and activated T cells. Other cells do not normally express this antigen but may be induced to do so in the presence of gamma-interferon at sites of inflammation and can then become antigen-presenting cells. Class II antigens link with CD4 molecules during antigen presentation and the reaction induced by cells bearing this molecule is therefore of the helper type.

A4.16

1) B   2) C   3) D   4) E   5) A

Congenital and acquired immunodeficiencies

Congenital	Acquired
Phagocytes	
Congenital neutropenia	Neutropenia due to myelosuppression
Cyclical neutropenia	Hypersplenism
Leucocyte adhesion defects	Autoimmune neutropenia
Hyper-IgE syndrome	Corticosteroid therapy
Shwachman's syndrome	Diabetes mellitus
Chronic granulomatous disease	Hypophosphataemia
Other intrinsic killing defects	Myeloid leukaemias
Storage diseases	Influenza
Chediak–Higashi syndrome	
Complement deficiency	
C3, Clq, I, H deficiencies	
C5, 6, 7, 8, 9 deficiencies	
Mannan-binding lectin deficiency	
Complement-dependent opsonization defects	
Antibody deficiency (B cell defects)	
X-linked hypogammaglobulinaemia	Myeloma, lymphoma
Common variable immunodeficiency	Splenectomy
IgA ($\pm$IgG$_2$) deficiency	Congenital rubella
Specific antibody deficiencies	
T cell deficiencies	AIDS
DiGeorge anomaly	Measles
IL-2 deficiency	Corticosteroid therapy
Signal transduction defect	Ciclosporin, tacrolimus
Combined T and B cell immunodeficiencies	
Severe combined immunodeficiency:	
Adenosine deaminase deficiency	Protein–calorie malnutrition
Purine nucleoside phosphorylase deficiency	Immunodeficiency of prematurity
Non-expression of MHC class II	
Reticular dysgenesis	
Wiskott–Aldrich syndrome	
Ataxia telangiectasia	
EBV-associated immunodeficiency	

A4.17

1) C   2) E   3) D   4) A   5) B

Examples of opportunist organisms in the setting of non-immunological innate defence defects include: staphylococci and *Pseudomonas* in burns patients; *Haemophilus influenzae* and pneumococci in smokers; *Pseudomonas* in cystic fibrosis patients; Gram-negative infections where there is urinary obstruction; staphylococcal and candidal infections with indwelling venous catheters and other foreign bodies; *Candida* and pathogenic *Escherichia coli* following elimination of gut flora after antibiotic therapy.

A4.18

1) C 2) A 3) B 4) B 5) D 6) E

Hypersensitivity reactions

	I (immediate)	II (cytotoxic)	III (immune complex)	IV (delayed)	V (stimulating/ blocking)*
Antigens	Pollens, moulds, mites, drugs, food and parasites	Cell surface or tissue bound	Exogenous (viruses, bacteria, fungi, parasites) Autoantigens	Cell/tissue bound	Cell surface receptors
Mediators	IgE and mast cells	IgG, IgM and complement	IgG, IgM, IgA and complement	TD, Tc, activated macrophages and lymphokines	IgG
Diagnostic tests	Skin-prick tests: weal and flare Specific IgE in serum	Coombs' test Indirect immuno-fluorescence (antibodies) Red cell agglutination Precipitating antibodies ELISA	Immune complexes	Skin test: erythema induration (e.g. tuberculin test)	Indirect immuno-fluorescence
Time taken for reaction to develop	5–10 min	6–36 hours	4–12 hours	48–72 hours	Variable
Immuno-pathology	Oedema, vasodilation, mast cell degranulation, eosinophils	Antibody-mediated damage to target cells	Acute inflammatory reaction, neutrophils. vasculitis	Perivascular inflammation, mononuclear cells, fibrin Granulomas Caseation and necrosis in TB	Hypertrophy or normal
Diseases and conditions produced	Asthma (extrinsic) Urticaria/ oedema Allergic rhinitis Anaphylaxis	Autoimmune haemolytic anaemia Transfusion reactions Haemolytic disease of newborn Goodpasture's syndrome Addisonian pernicious anaemia Myasthenia gravis	Autoimmune (e.g. SLE, glomerulo-nephritis, rheumatoid arthritis) Low-grade persistent infections (e.g. viral hepatitis) Disease caused by environmental antigens (e.g. farmer's lung)	Pulmonary TB Contact dermatitis Graft-versus-host disease Insect bites Leprosy	Neonatal hyperthyroidism Graves' disease Myasthenia gravis
Treatment	Antigen avoidance Antihistamines Corticosteroids (usually topical) Sodium cromoglicate Adrenaline (epinephrine) or life-threatening conditions	Exchange transfusion Plasmapheresis Immuno-suppressives/ cytotoxics	Corticosteroids Immuno-suppressives Plasmapheresis	Immunosuppressives Corticosteroids Removal of antigen	Treatment of individual disease

*Type V hypersensitivity may also be classified with type II reactions
RAST, radioallergosorbent test; SLE, systemic lupus erythematosus; TB, tuberculosis; Tc, T cytotoxic; TD, T delayed hypersensitivity

A4.19

1) A   2) A   3) B   4) B   5) C

There are several mechanisms proposed to account for loss of self-tolerance.

a) Immune dysregulation: T cells regulate any autoreactive T and B cells that have survived clonal deletion. It is hypothesized that dysregulation of T-cell function could therefore lead to loss of control and the development of autoimmune disease. This is backed up by the observation that immunodeficiency diseases such as hypogammaglobulinaemia and HIV infection are commonly associated with autoimmune phenomena. However, most patients with autoimmune disease do not have obvious immune deficiency.

b) Tissue damage: there are some autoantigens to which the developing immune system is not usually exposed because these antigens are 'hidden' within the cells or tissues. Therefore clonal deletion of self-reactive cells does not occur. Normally these self-antigens remain hidden, so no autoimmune disease develops. If, however, the tissue is damaged by trauma, infection or tumour, the antigens may be released and evoke an autoimmune response. Examples of this in clinical practice are Dressler's syndrome in which patients with myocardial infarction develop acute pericarditis secondary to the production of antimyocardial antibodies, or the association of Coxsackie virus infection with the development of insulin-dependent diabetes. The presence of inflammatory cytokines at the site of injury may enhance the expression of costimulatory molecules on local antigen-presenting cells and increase the likelihood of an autoreactive T-cell

response still further. This hypothesis may be supported by the observation that patients given alpha-interferon (which upregulates class I expression) develop thyroid autoantibodies on therapy.

c) T-cell bypass: this is a mechanism by which T cells are tricked into providing help to autoreactive B cells rather than suppressing them. For this to occur the self-antigen needs to be attached to a foreign antigen that is recognized by the T cell. T-cell activation will occur with the production of cytokines such as IL-4. If an autoreactive B cell has also bound the self-antigen it will then receive the signals to proliferate and produce autoantibody. There are several examples of this in drug-induced autoimmune responses. Quinine binds to platelets, creating a foreign epitope for T cells and inducing autoreactive B cells to make antiplatelet antibodies with sometimes fatal thrombocytopenia developing. Methyldopa or infection with mycoplasma causes changes in red cell epitopes to induce a similar autoantibody response to red cells with haemagglutination or lysis.

d) Molecular mimicry: this occurs when an organism has a similar antigenic structure to self-molecules. The infection generates antigen-specific T cells and antibodies that cross-react with host tissues and cause autoimmune disease. Examples where there is known cross-reaction between an infective agent and host antigen are in the production of anticardiac antibodies (antimyosin) after streptococcal infection leading to rheumatic fever, between klebsiella and HLA-B27 in ankylosing spondylitis, and Coxsackie and glutamic acid

Clinical immunology

decarboxylase in insulin-dependent diabetes. The development of autoimmune disease can be viewed as either a loss of tolerogenic signals to lymphocytes, or an increase in immunogenic signals. The underlying mechanism appears to be the activation of lymphocytes by different pathways.

A4.20

A) T   B) T   C) T   D) T   E) F

The main chemoattractants for neutrophils in vivo are N-formyl-methionyl-leucylphenylalanine (FMLP) from bacterial cell walls, which in turn causes the release of another chemoattractant, leukotriene B_4 (LTB_4) from tissue mast cells; the chemokine (chemoattractant cytokine) interleukin-8 (from macrophages); and C5a from the activation of complement.

A4.21

A) F   B) F   C) T   D) T   E) F

Chemoattractants cause migration of neutrophils by three mechanisms: a) upregulation of neutrophil adhesion molecules, L-selectin and the integrin LFA-1 (leucocyte function antigen), which increases the stickiness of the cells; b) increase in vascular endothelial cell expression of the adhesion molecules E-selectin and ICAM-1 which causes increased stickiness of the endothelium. The selectin expression causes the circulating neutrophil to be tethered and roll along the endothelium slowly (margination), whereas the reaction between the integrins LFA-1 and ICAM-1

is much stronger, causing the cells to stop moving. c) Stimulation of neutrophil chemotaxis (directed movement along the chemoattractant gradient towards the stimulus).

A4.22

A) F   B) F   C) T   D) T   E) T

Splenectomy causes impairment of defence against capsulated bacteria, especially pneumococcus, partly because T-independent antibody responses are largely made in the spleen and partly because of its role as part of the fixed reticuloendothelial system. Hyposplenism associated with severe sickle cell disease is responsible for the increased risk of infection in such patients. Pneumococcal, meningococcal and Hib vaccination before elective splenectomy and the use of penicillin prophylaxis can largely eliminate risk of serious infection.

A4.23

A) T   B) T   C) T   D) T   E) T

Mechanism of CD4 loss/dysfunction in HIV infection

Direct cytopathic effects of HIV
Lysis of infected cells by HIV-specific cytotoxic T cells
Tc-mediated lysis of uninfected CD4+ T cells that have bound gp120 to the CD4 molecule
Immunosuppressive effects of soluble HIV proteins on uninfected cells, e.g. gp120 envelope protein leading to decreased proliferation
Molecular mimicry between gp120/160 and MHC class I inducing autoimmune destruction
Signal transduction defects and induction of programmed cell death (apoptosis) by unknown mechanisms

A4.24

A) T **B)** T **C)** T **D)** T **E)** T

Corticosteroid therapy interferes with cell-mediated immunity, in particular T cell–macrophage cooperation. This is due to effects on T-cell traffic and impairment of macrophage responses to cytokines, together with impaired antigen presentation. Mucocutaneous candidiasis, *Pneumocystis carinii* pneumonia, cytomegalovirus infection, mycobacterial infection, *Nocardia*, non-typhi *Salmonella* septicaemia and cryptococcosis are some of the very many infections seen with prolonged high-dose steroid therapy.

Nutrition

Q5.1

In the basal state, energy demands are highest for which one of the following?

A. Skeletal muscle
B. Brain
C. Heart
D. Abdominal viscera
E. Lungs

Q5.2

An 11-year-old boy in Africa has been complaining of difficulty seeing at night. On examination he has corneal thickening. Correct treatment is with which one of the following?

A. Vitamin B
B. Vitamin K
C. Vitamin D
D. Vitamin E
E. Vitamin A

Q5.3

A 37-year-old woman has diarrhoea. She also complains of a painful tongue and recurrent mouth infections. On examination her tongue is red, and raw. She has chronic thickening, dryness and pigmentation of the skin in sun-exposed areas – Casal's necklace. Which one of the following is the best option for treatment?

A. Pyridoxine therapy
B. Thiamine
C. Riboflavin therapy
D. Nicotinamide
E. Ascorbic acid

Q5.4

A young doctor wants to prevent haemorrhagic disease of the newborn. Which one of the following vitamins must be given prophylactically?

A. Vitamin B
B. Vitamin K
C. Vitamin D
D. Vitamin E
E. Vitamin A

Q5.5

In southern Thailand a mother brings in her 3-month-old breast-fed baby with a history of anorexia and some degree of aphonia. On examination the baby has tachycardia and tachypnoea. Treatment includes

A. Intravenous vitamin A
B. Vitamin K
C. Vitamin B_1
D. Vitamin C
E. Vitamin B_6

Q5.6

1. The mother of a 3-year-old girl in Bangladesh brings her child to the doctor with a history of frequent diarrhoea. The child is emaciated, with muscle wasting and loss of body fat. The hair is thin and dry. The child is not apathetic or anorexic. There is no peripheral oedema

2. A 2-year-old boy in a Romanian orphanage is being examined by the Red Cross doctor. The child is apathetic and lethargic. He has severe anorexia. The hair is dry and sparse with a reddish hue. There is generalized oedema and thickening and pigmentation of the skin. Examination of the abdomen reveals hepatomegaly with ascites. Serum albumin is 15 g/L

3. An 11-year-old boy from Nigeria has been complaining of difficulty with his vision at night. The conjunctiva are dry and thickened. White plaques – Bitot's spots – are found on the conjunctiva

4. A 28-year-old Scottish woman who has been ingesting vitamins and health foods complains of hair loss, double vision and headaches. Liver function tests are abnormal

5. A 35-year-old housewife in Thailand eats mainly polished rice. She initially had heaviness and stiffness of the legs, followed by weakness, numbness and pins and needles. The ankle jerk reflexes are lost and eventually all the signs of polyneuropathy are found

6. A 45-year-old woman with primary biliary cirrhosis complains of fatty stools. Her INR is markedly elevated

7. Gross ataxia in a child with abetalipoproteinaemia

Select the best match for each of the above

A. Dry beriberi
B. Vitamin E deficiency
C. Vitamin K deficiency
D. Marasmus
E. Kwashiorkor
F. Vitamin A deficiency
G. Vitamin A excess

Q5.7

1. A 47-year-old alcoholic male who lives on the streets has ophthalmoplegia, nystagmus and ataxia. He also has dementia

2. A 22-year-old volunteer is deprived of this vitamin as a part of a nutrition study. She develops fissuring at the corners of the mouth, red inflamed tongue and seborrhoeic dermatitis involving the vulva

3. A 45-year-old Nigerian farmer virtually eats maize only. Sun-exposed areas of the skin have cracks, with ulceration. He complains of a painful, red tongue, glossitis and diarrhoea. On examination he has dementia

4. A 43-year-old patient with TB being treated with isoniazid develops polyneuropathy

5. A 64-year-old Asian woman who eats rice and chapatis complains of muscle pain and fatigue. She has swollen, spongy gums, anaemia and spontaneous haemorrhage. Examination of the skin shows perifollicular haemorrhage

Select the best match for each of the above

A. Vitamin C deficiency
B. Niacin deficiency
C. Riboflavin deficiency
D. Vitamin B_6 deficiency
E. Wernicke–Korsakoff syndrome

Nutrition

Q5.8

1. Vitamin A
2. Vitamin K
3. Vitamin E
4. Niacin
5. Riboflavin
6. Vitamin C
7. Thiamine

Select the best match for each of the above

A. Found in green leafy vegetables, dairy products, rape seed and soya bean oils
B. Vegetables and seed oils, including soya bean, saffron, sunflower, cereals and nuts, are the main sources. Animal products are poor sources of the vitamin
C. It is found in many foodstuffs, including cereals, grains, beans, nuts, as well as pork and duck
D. Widely distributed throughout all plant and animal cells. Good sources are dairy products, offal and leafy vegetables. It is not destroyed appreciably by cooking, but is destroyed by sunlight
E. It is found in many foodstuffs, including plants, meat (particularly offal) and fish. It is lost by removing bran from cereals but is added to processed cereals and white bread in many countries
F. The richest food source is liver, but it is also found in milk, butter, cheese, egg yolks and fish oils
G. It is present in all fresh fruit and vegetables. Unfortunately, it is easily leached out of vegetables when they are placed in water and it is also oxidized during cooking, or by exposure to copper or alkalis. Potatoes are a good source as many people eat a lot of them, but the vitamin is lost during storage

Q5.9

1. Vitamin A
2. Vitamin E
3. Niacin
4. Riboflavin
5. Vitamin C
6. Thiamine pyrophosphate
7. Vitamin B_6
8. Vitamin K

Select the best match for each of the above

A. It is an essential cofactor in carbohydrate metabolism. It is involved in the oxidative decarboxylation of acetyl CoA in mitochondria
B. It is a flavoprotein that is a cofactor for many oxidative reactions in the cell
C. This is the generic name for two chemical forms. Both act as hydrogen acceptors in many oxidative reactions, and in their reduced forms act as hydrogen donors in reductive reactions
D. It is a cofactor in the metabolism of many amino acids
E. It is a simple sugar and a powerful reducing agent, its main role being to control the redox potential within cells. It is involved in the hydroxylation of proline to hydroxyproline, which is necessary for the formation of collagen
F. It is a cofactor for the post-translational carboxylation of specific protein-bound glutamate residues in γ-carboxyglutamate (Gla). Gla residues bind calcium ions to phospholipid templates, and this action on factors II, VII, IX and X, and on proteins C and S, is necessary for coagulation to take place
G. One form of this protein is found in the opsin proteins in the rods (rhodopsin) and cones (iodopsin) of the retina

H. The biological activity of this vitamin results principally from its antioxidant properties. In biological membranes it contributes to membrane stability

Q5.10

1. Menkes' kinky hair disease
2. Keshan cardiomyopathy
3. Acrodermatitis enteropathica
4. Endemic goitre
5. Pitting and discoloration of the teeth
6. Anorexia, weakness, osteoporosis
7. Growth retardation, skeletal abnormalities, and glucose intolerance

Select the best match for each of the above

A. Phosphate deficiency
B. Selenium deficiency
C. Manganese deficiency
D. Iodine deficiency
E. Fluorosis
F. Zinc deficiency
G. Copper deficiency

Q5.11

The physiologist wishes to measure the total energy expenditure of a group of normal volunteers. The following methods are used to measure total energy expenditure

A. Gallium scanning
B. Thallium uptake
C. Double-labelled water technique
D. CO_2 production by isotopic dilution
E. Protein uptake

Q5.12

A 19-year-old college student has a body mass index of 34. This is a feature of the following conditions

A. Protein–energy malnutrition
B. Laurence–Moon–Biedl syndrome
C. Cushing's syndrome
D. Stein–Leventhal syndrome
E. Prader–Willi syndrome

Q5.13

A 29-year-old man has a blood pressure of 160/90 mmHg, heart rate of 67 beats/min, temperature of 37.1°C, oxygen saturation of 95% on room air and body mass index of 42. Correct statements include

A. The leptin mRNA in subcutaneous adipose tissue is usually substantially lower than in control individuals whose body mass index is 20
B. Plasma leptin levels are usually very low
C. Basal metabolic rate is lower than in lean subjects
D. There is an increased risk of early death mainly from diabetes, coronary heart disease and cerebrovascular disease
E. Tend to expend less energy during physical activity than control individuals whose body mass index is 20

Q5.14

A 45-year-old lawyer whose initial body weight is 100 kg makes a determined effort to lose weight. He loses 15 kg. Potential benefits from his weight loss include

A. A fall in total mortality risk
B. A fall in risk of diabetes-related death
C. A fall in risk of obesity-related cancer death

Nutrition

D. Reduces the risk of developing diabetes
E. Results in a fall in both systolic and diastolic blood pressure

A. Stroke
B. Fluid and electrolyte disturbances
C. Pneumothorax
D. Liver dysfunction
E. Sepsis

Q5.15

Correct statements about food intake in obesity include

A. All obese people eat more than they need
B. Not all obese people eat more than the average person
C. Obese patients eat more than they admit to eating
D. The increase in obesity in social class 5 is due to increased protein intake
E. The long-term overall success rate of losing weight by reducing calorie intake is close to 70%

Q5.16

1. Phentermine

2. Sibutramine

3. Orlistat

Select the mechanism of action of each of the above

A. Stimulates dopamine receptors
B. Acts on serotoninergic and noradrenergic pathways
C. Acts on noradrenergic pathways
D. Stimulates pancreatic and gastric lipases
E. Inhibits pancreatic and gastric lipases

Q5.17

A 75-year-old man in the ICU has been advised that he will require parenteral nutrition via a central venous catheter using the infraclavicular approach. His daughter would like to know the possible complications of his treatment. The following are recognized complications

Q5.18

A 42-year-old businessman drinks 160 g ethanol per day. The potential long-term physical effects of this intake of alcohol include

A. Protects against heart disease
B. Macrocytosis
C. Hyperuricaemia
D. Carcinoma of the oesophagus
E. Thrombocytopenia

Q5.19

1. A raised concentration of this sulphur-containing amino acid, derived from methionine, is an independent risk factor for vascular disease

2. The synthesis of haem in haemoglobin requires this amino acid

3. The synthesis of melanin requires this amino acid

4. Quantitatively the most important amino acid in the circulation which is important for inter-organ exchange

5. The synthesis of glutathione, which is a part of the defence system against free radicals, requires this amino acid

Select the best amino acid for each of the above statements

A. Glycine
B. Homocysteine
C. Tyrosine
D. Glutamine
E. Myristic acid

Q5.20

Deficiency of vitamin K occurs in the newborn owing to

A. Interference by vitamin C
B. Poor placental transfer of vitamin K
C. Little vitamin K in breast milk
D. No hepatic stores of menaquinone (no intestinal bacteria in the neonate)
E. Interference by vitamin D

Q5.21

The 38-year-old TV presenter who is a strong believer in alternative medicine asks her general practitioner whether a dietary supply of the following fatty acids is essential

A. Eicosapentaenoic acid
B. Docosahexaenoic acid
C. Lauric acid
D. Linoleic acid
E. α-Linolenic acid

Q5.22

The ingestion of sufficient fat to provide about 45% of dietary energy can result in

A. Breast cancer
B. Colon cancer
C. Prostate cancer
D. Type 1 diabetes
E. Cardiovascular disease

Q5.23

1. Saturated fatty acids

2. n-6 fatty acids

3. n-3 fatty acids

4. *Trans* fatty acids

Select the best dietary source for each of the above

A. Margarine
B. Fish oils
C. Vegetable oils and other plant foods
D. Mainly animal fat

Q5.24

The owner of a weight-reduction clinic wants to clarify with her general practitioner the current UK recommendations for fat intake. The following statements are accurate

A. *Cis*-polyunsaturated fat intake should provide at least 20% of dietary energy
B. Saturated fatty acids should provide approximately 10% of dietary energy
C. *Cis*-monosaturated fatty acids should provide approximately 20% of dietary energy
D. Total fat intake should be no more than 35% of total dietary energy
E. Polyunsaturated fatty acids should be derived mainly from n-6 and n-3 polyunsaturated fatty acids

Q5.25

The 67-year-old patient with intracerebral haemorrhage has been on parenteral nutrition with glucose and protein only. This patient has an increased ratio of triene (n-9) to tetraene (n-6) in plasma acids. The patient is likely to develop

A. Dermatitis
B. Alopecia
C. Anaemia
D. Thrombocytopenia
E. Acute myocardial infarction

Nutrition

Q5.26

Non-starch polysaccharides (NSPs) which are digested by gut enzymes include

A. Cellulose
B. Hemicelluloses
C. Pectins
D. Gums
E. Lignins

Q5.27

The following common conditions are associated with protein–energy malnutrition

A. Sepsis
B. Dementia
C. Malignancy
D. Anorexia nervosa
E. Depression

Q5.28

A 45-year-old woman has diarrhoea. She also complains of a painful tongue and recurrent mouth infections. On examination she has a red, raw tongue. Sun-exposed areas of her skin show pigmentation. There is chronic thickening, dryness and pigmentation on the dorsal surfaces of the hands. The lesions are symmetrical. This may occur in the following circumstances

A. Isoniazid therapy
B. Hartnup's disease
C. Carcinoid syndrome
D. Phaeochromocytoma
E. Addison's disease

A5.1

D

In the basal state, energy demands for resting muscle are 20% of the total energy required, abdominal viscera 35–40%, brain 20% and heart 10%. There can be more than a 50-fold increase in muscle energy demands during exercise.

A5.2

E

Vitamin A deficiency and xerophthalmia is the major cause of blindness in young children in Africa despite intensive preventative programmes. Impaired adaptation followed by night blindness is the first effect. There is dryness and thickening of the conjunctiva and the cornea (xerophthalmia occurs as a result of keratinization). Bitot's spots – white plaques of keratinized epithelial cells – are found on the conjunctiva of young children with vitamin A deficiency. These spots can, however, be seen without vitamin A deficiency, possibly caused by exposure. Corneal softening, ulceration and dissolution (keratomalacia) eventually occur; superimposed infection is a frequent accompaniment and both lead to blindness.

A5.3

D

In endemic areas the treatment of pellagra is based on the clinical features, remembering that other vitamin deficiencies can produce similar changes (e.g. angular stomatitis). Nicotinamide (approximately 300 mg daily by mouth) with a maintenance dose of 50 mg daily is given with dramatic improvement in the skin and diarrhoea. Mostly, however, vitamin B complex is given, as other deficiencies are often present.

A5.4

B

Vitamin K deficiency leads to a haemorrhagic disease of the newborn which can be prevented by prophylactic vitamin K. However, in the UK there is no agreement on whether prophylactic therapy is necessary.

A5.5

C

Infantile beriberi occurs, usually acutely, in breast-fed babies at approximately 3 months of age. The mothers show no signs of thiamin deficiency but presumably their body stores are virtually nil. The infant becomes anorexic, develops oedema and has some degree of aphonia. Tachycardia and tachypnoea develop and, unless treatment is instituted, death occurs quickly.

A5.6

1) D   2) E   3) F   4) G   5) A   6) C   7) B

Marasmus is the type of severe protein energy malnutrition (PEM) seen most commonly. A child looks emaciated, there is obvious muscle wasting and loss of body fat. There is no oedema. The hair is thin and dry. The child is not so apathetic or anorexic as with kwashiorkor. Diarrhoea is frequently present and signs of infection must be looked for carefully. Kwashiorkor shows the child to be apathetic and lethargic with severe anorexia. There is generalized oedema with skin pigmentation and thickening. The hair is dry, sparse and may become reddish or yellow in colour. The abdomen is distended owing to hepatomegaly and/or ascites. The serum albumin is always low.

Nutrition

Vitamin A deficiency and xerophthalmia is the major cause of blindness in young children. There is dryness and thickening of the conjunctiva and the cornea (xerophthalmia occurs as a result of keratinization). Bitot's spots – white plaques of keratinized epithelial cells – are found on the conjunctiva of young children with vitamin A deficiency. With high intakes of vitamin A, chronic ingestion of retinol can cause liver and bone damage, hair loss, double vision, vomiting, headaches and other abnormalities.

When bile flow into the intestine is interrupted, malabsorption of vitamin K occurs as no bile salts are available to facilitate absorption and the prothrombin time increases. In patients with chronic cholestasis (e.g. primary biliary cirrhosis) oral therapy using a water-soluble preparation, menadiol sodium phosphate 10 mg daily, is used.

Vitamin E deficiency is seen only in children with abetalipoproteinaemia and in patients on long-term parenteral nutrition. The severe neurological deficit (gross ataxia) can be prevented by vitamin E injection.

Thiamine deficiency is seen as beriberi where the only food consumed is polished rice. Dry beriberi usually presents insidiously with a symmetrical polyneuropathy. The initial symptoms are heaviness and stiffness of the legs, followed by weakness, numbness, and pins and needles. The ankle jerk reflexes are lost and eventually all the signs of polyneuropathy that may involve the trunk and arms are found.

A5.7

1) E   2) C   3) B   4) D   5) A

Thiamine deficiency also presents with polyneuropathy or with the Wernicke–Korsakoff syndrome. This syndrome, which consists of dementia, ataxia, varying ophthalmoplegia and nystagmus, presents acutely and should be suspected in all heavy drinkers. If treated promptly it is reversible; if left it becomes irreversible. It is a major cause of dementia in the USA.

Riboflavin is widely distributed throughout all plant and animal cells. There is no definite deficiency, although many communities have low dietary intakes. Studies in volunteers taking a low riboflavin diet have produced angular stomatitis or cheilosis (fissuring at the corners of the mouth), a red, inflamed tongue and seborrhoeic dermatitis, particularly involving the face (around the nose) and the scrotum or vulva.

Pellagra is found in people who eat virtually only maize, for example in parts of Africa. The classical features are of dermatitis, diarrhoea and dementia. Although this is an easily remembered triad, not all are always present and the mental changes are not a true dementia.

Vitamin C deficiency is seen mainly in infants fed boiled milk and in the elderly and single people who cannot be bothered to eat vegetables. In the UK it is also seen in Asians eating only rice and chapatis, and in food faddists.

A5.8

1) F   2) A   3) B   4) E   5) D
6) G   7) C

A5.9

1) G   2) H   3) C   4) B   5) E
6) A   7) D   8) F

Vitamin A has several metabolic roles. a) Retinaldehyde in its *cis* form is found in the opsin proteins in the rods (rhodopsin) and cones (iodopsin) of the retina. Light causes retinaldehyde to change to its *trans* isomer, and this leads to changes in membrane potentials that are transmitted to the brain. b) Retinol and retinoic acid are involved in the control of cell proliferation and differentiation. c) Retinyl phosphate is a cofactor in the synthesis of most glycoproteins containing mannose.

Vitamin K is a cofactor necessary for the production not only of blood clotting factors but also for proteins necessary in the formation of bone. Vitamin K is a cofactor for the post-translational carboxylation of specific protein-bound glutamate residues in γ-carboxyglutamate (Gla). Gla residues bind calcium ions to phospholipid templates, and this action on factors II, VII, IX and X, and on proteins C and S, is necessary for coagulation to take place. Bone osteoblasts contain three vitamin K dependent proteins, osteocalcin, matrix Gla protein and protein S, which have a role in bone matrix formation. Osteocalcin contains three Gla residues which bind tightly to the hydroxyapatite matrix depending on the degree of carboxylation; this leads to bone mineralization.

The biological activity of vitamin E results principally from its antioxidant properties. In biological membranes it contributes to membrane stability. It protects cellular structures against damage from a number of highly reactive oxygen species, including hydrogen peroxide, superoxide and other oxygen radicals. Vitamin E may also affect cell proliferation and growth.

Thiamine diphosphate, often called thiamine pyrophosphate (TPP), is an essential cofactor, particularly in carbohydrate metabolism. TPP is involved in the oxidative decarboxylation of acetyl CoA in mitochondria. In the Krebs cycle, TPP is the key enzyme for the decarboxylation of α-ketoglutarate to succinyl CoA. TPP is also the cofactor for transketolase, a key enzyme in the hexose monophosphate shunt.

Riboflavin is a flavoprotein that is a cofactor for many oxidative reactions in the cell.

Niacin is the generic name for the two chemical forms, nicotinic acid and nicotinamide, the latter being found in the two pyridine nucleotides, nicotinamide adenine dinucleotide (NAD) and nicotinamide adenine dinucleotide phosphate (NADP). Both act as hydrogen acceptors in many oxidative reactions, and in their reduced forms (NADH and NADPH) act as hydrogen donors in reductive reactions. Many oxidative steps in the production of energy require NAD, and NADP is equally necessary in the hexose monophosphate shunt for the generation of NADPH, which is necessary for fatty-acid synthesis.

A5.10

1) G   2) B   3) F   4) D   5) E
6) A   7) C

1. Menkes' kinky hair syndrome is a rare condition caused by malabsorption of copper. Infants with this sex-linked recessive abnormality develop growth failure, mental retardation, bone lesions and brittle hair.

2. Deficiency of selenium is rare except in areas of China where Keshan disease, a selenium-responsive cardiomyopathy, occurs. Selenium deficiency may also cause a skeletal myopathy.

Nutrition

3. Acrodermatitis enteropathica is an inherited disorder caused by malabsorption of zinc. Infants develop growth retardation, severe diarrhoea, hair loss and associated *Candida* and bacterial infections.

4. Many mountainous areas throughout the world lack iodine in the soil, and so iodine deficiency, which impairs brain development, is a World Health Organization priority. Endemic goitre occurs in remote areas where the daily intake is below 70 µg, and in those parts of the world 1–5% of babies are born with cretinism.

5. Excessive fluoride intake in areas where the water fluoride level is above 3 mg/L can result in fluorosis, in which there is infiltration into the enamel of the teeth, producing pitting and discoloration.

6. Dietary deficiency of phosphates has not been described. Patients taking large amounts of aluminium hydroxide can however, develop phosphate deficiency owing to binding in the gut lumen. It can also be seen in total parenteral nutrition. Symptoms include anorexia, weakness and osteoporosis.

7. Manganese deficiency causes growth retardation, skeletal abnormalities and glucose intolerance.

A5.11

A) F   B) F   C) T   D) T   E) F

Daily energy expenditure is the sum of the basal metabolic rate (BMR), the thermic effect of food eaten, occupational activities and non-occupational activities. Total energy expenditure can be measured using a double-labelled water technique. Water containing the stable isotopes ^2H and ^{18}O is given orally. As energy is expended carbon dioxide and water are produced.

An alternative tracer technique for measuring total energy expenditure is to estimate CO_2 production by isotopic dilution.

A5.12

A) F   B) T   C) T   D) T   E) T

Conditions in which obesity is an associated feature
Genetic syndromes associated with hypogonadism (e.g. Prader–Willi syndrome, Laurence–Moon–Biedl syndrome)
Hypothyroidism
Cushing's syndrome
Stein–Leventhal syndrome
Drug-induced (e.g. corticosteroids)
Hypothalamic damage (e.g. due to trauma, tumour)

A5.13

A) F   B) F   C) F   D) T   E) F

In massively obese subjects, leptin mRNA in subcutaneous adipose tissue is 80% higher than in controls. Plasma levels of leptin are also very high, correlating with the body mass index (BMI). Basal metabolic rate (BMR) in obese subjects is higher than in lean subjects, which is not surprising since obesity is associated with an increase in lean body mass. Obese patients tend to expend more energy during physical activity as they have a larger mass to move. On the other hand, many obese patients decrease their amount of physical activity. Obese patients are at risk of early death, mainly from diabetes, coronary heart disease and cerebrovascular disease.

A5.14

A) T B) T C) T D) T E) T

Potential benefits that may result from the loss of 10 kg in patients who are initially 100 kg and suffer from co-morbidities

Mortality	20–25% fall in total mortality 30–40% fall in diabetes-related deaths 40–50% fall in obesity-related cancer deaths
Blood pressure	Fall of about 10 mmHg (systolic and diastolic)
Diabetes	Reduces risk of developing diabetes by >50% Fall of 30–50% in fasting glucose Fall of 15% in HbA$_{1c}$
Lipids	Fall of 10% in total cholesterol Fall of 15% in LDL Fall of 30% in triacylglycerol Increase of 8% in HDL cholesterol

A5.15

A) T B) T C) T D) F E) F

Not all obese people eat more than the average person, but all obviously eat more than they need. It is relatively easy for most people to lose the first few kilograms, but long-term success in moderate obesity is poor, with an overall success rate of no more than 10%. The increase in obesity in social class 5 can usually be related to the type of food consumed (i.e. food containing sugar and fat). It has been shown that obese patients eat more than they admit to eating, and over the years a very small daily excess can lead to a large accumulation of fat.

A5.16

1) C 2) B 3) E

In obesity drugs can be used in the short term (up to 3 months) as an adjunct to the dietary regimen, but they do not substitute for strict dieting.

Centrally acting drugs:

- drugs acting on the noradrenergic pathways, e.g. phentermine, which has minor stimulant properties, and produces its main effects by suppressing appetite

- drugs acting on both serotoninergic and noradrenergic pathways, e.g. sibutramine.

Peripherally acting drugs. Orlistat is an inhibitor of pancreatic and gastric lipases. It reduces dietary fat absorption and aids weight loss. Weight regain occurs after the drug is stopped. It has been used continuously in a large-scale trial for up to 2 years. Patients may complain of diarrhoea during treatment and constipation after treatment.

A5.17

A) F B) T C) T D) T E) T

Complications of intravenous parenteral nutrition include catheter-related, metabolic (e.g. hyperglycaemia – insulin therapy is usually necessary), fluid and electrolyte disturbances, hypercalcaemia and liver dysfunction. Complications of catheter placement include central vein thrombosis, pneumothorax and embolism, but the major problem is catheter-related sepsis. Organisms, mainly staphylococci, enter along the side of the catheter, leading to bacteraemia. Sepsis can be prevented by careful and sterile placement of the catheter, by not removing the dressing over the catheter entry site, and by not giving other substances (e.g. blood products, antibiotics) via the central vein catheter. Sepsis should be suspected if the patient develops fever and leucocytosis. In two-thirds of cases, organisms can be grown from the catheter tip. Treatment involves removal of the catheter and appropriate systemic antibiotics.

Nutrition

A5.18

A) F   B) T   C) T   D) T   E) T

Physical effects of excess alcohol consumption

Central nervous system
Epilepsy
Wernicke–Korsakoff syndrome
Polyneuropathy

Muscles
Acute or chronic myopathy

Cardiovascular system
Cardiomyopathy
Beriberi heart disease
Cardiac arrhythmias
Hypertension

Metabolism
Hyperuricaemia (gout)
Hyperlipidaemia
Hypoglycaemia
Obesity

Endocrine system
Pseudo-Cushing's syndrome

Respiratory system
Chest infections

Gastrointestinal system
Acute gastritis
Carcinoma of the oesophagus or large bowel
Pancreatic disease
Liver disease

Haemopoiesis
Macrocytosis (due to direct toxic effect on bone marrow or folate deficiency)
Thrombocytopenia
Leucopenia

Bone
Osteoporosis
Osteomalacia

A5.19

1) B   2) A   3) C   4) D   5) A

Of all the amino acids, glutamine is quantitatively the most important one in the circulation and involved in inter-organ exchange. Alanine is also an important amino acid released from muscle; it is deaminated and converted into pyruvic acid before entering the citric acid cycle. Homocysteine is a sulphur-containing amino acid which is derived from methionine in the diet. A raised plasma concentration is an independent risk factor for vascular disease. Amino acids may be utilized to synthesize products other than protein or urea. For example: haem requires glycine; melanin and thyroid hormones require tyrosine; nucleic acid bases require glutamine, aspartate and glycine; and glutathione, which is part of the defence system against free radicals, requires glutamate, cysteine and glycine.

A5.20

A) F   B) T   C) T   D) T   E) F

Deficiency of vitamin K occurs in the newborn owing to:

- poor placental transfer of vitamin K
- little vitamin K in breast milk
- no hepatic stores of menaquinone (no intestinal bacteria in the neonate).

A5.21

A) F B) F C) F D) T E) T

The essential fatty acids (EFAs) are linoleic and α-linolenic acid, both of which are precursors of prostaglandins. Eicosapentaenoic and docosahexaenoic are physiologically important, but can be made to a limited extent in the tissues from linoleic and linolenic and thus a dietary supply is not essential.

A5.22

A) T B) T C) T D) F E) T

A high fat intake has been implicated in the causation of cardiovascular disease, cancer (e.g. breast, colon and prostate), obesity and type 2 diabetes.

A5.23

1) D   2) C   3) B   4) A

Dietary sources of fatty acids	
Type of acid	Sources
Saturated fatty acids	Mainly animal fat
n-6 fatty acids	Vegetable oils and other plant foods
n-3 fatty acids	Vegetable foods, rapeseed oil, fish oils
Trans fatty acids	Hydrogenated fat or oils, often in margarine

A5.24

A) F B) T C) F D) T E) T

The current recommendations for fat intake for the UK are as follows: a) saturated fatty acids should provide approximately 10% of the dietary energy; b) cis-monounsaturated acids (mainly oleic acid) should continue to provide approximately 12% of the dietary energy; c) cis-polyunsaturated acids should provide 6% of dietary energy, and are derived from n-6 and n-3 polyunsaturated fatty acids; d) total fat intake should be no more than 35% of the total dietary energy, and restriction to 30% is desirable.

A5.25

A) T B) T C) T D) T E) F

Essential fatty acid deficiency may accompany protein energy malnutrition (PEM), but it has been clearly defined as a clinical entity only in patients on long-term parenteral nutrition given glucose, protein and no fat. Alopecia, thrombocytopenia, anaemia and a dermatitis occur within weeks with an increased ratio of triene (n-9) to tetraene (n-6) in plasma fatty acids.

A5.26

A) F B) F C) F D) F E) F

Dietary fibre, which is largely non-starch polysaccharide (NSP) (entirely NSP according to some authorities), is often removed in the processing of food. This leaves highly refined carbohydrates such as sucrose which contribute to the development of dental caries and obesity. Lignin is included in dietary fibre in some classification systems, but it is not a polysaccharide. It is only a minor component of the human diet. The principal classes of NSP are cellulose, hemicelluloses, pectins and gums. None of these is digested by gut enzymes. However, NSP is partly broken down in the gastrointestinal tract, mainly by colonic bacteria, producing gas and volatile fatty acids, e.g. butyrate.

Nutrition

A5.27

A) T   B) T   C) T   D) T   E) T

Common conditions associated with protein–energy malnutrition

Sepsis	Psychological: anorexia
Trauma	nervosa, depression
Surgery, particularly	Dementia
of GI tract with	Malignancy
complications	Metabolic disease: renal
GI disease,	failure
particularly involving	Any very ill patient
the small bowel	

A5.28

A) T   B) T   C) T   D) T   E) F

Pellagra may also occur in the following circumstances:

- Isoniazid therapy can lead to a deficiency of vitamin B$_6$, which is needed for the synthesis of nicotinamide from tryptophan – vitamin B$_6$ is now given concomitantly with isoniazid

- In Hartnup's disease, a rare inborn error in which basic amino acids, including tryptophan, are not absorbed by the gut. There is also loss of this amino acid in the urine

- In generalized malabsorption (rare)

- In alcohol-dependent patients who do not eat

- In very low protein diets given for renal disease or taken as a food fad

- In the carcinoid syndrome and phaeochromocytomas, tryptophan metabolism is diverted away from the formation of nicotinamide to form amines

Gastrointestinal disease 6

Q 6.1

A 42-year-old patient has a 25-year history of extensive ulcerative colitis. She would like to know the risk of cancer for herself and her sister who has long-standing Crohn's disease. Which one of the following statements is correct?

A. Her risk of cancer is lower than that of her sister who has Crohn's disease
B. The cumulative risk of cancer is more than double the risk she had 5 years ago
C. The risk of cancer decreases each year after 10 years of ulcerative colitis
D. Colonoscopy with biopsy done every year after 10 years of ulcerative colitis is recommended because several clinical trials have demonstrated that this reduces mortality
E. Her sister should undergo colonoscopy with biopsy done every year after 10 years of Crohn's colitis. This is recommended because several clinical trials have demonstrated that it reduces mortality

Q 6.2

A 45-year-old woman presents with steatorrhoea, abdominal discomfort, bloating and weight loss. On examination she has mouth ulcers and angular stomatitis. Her symptoms improve with the removal of wheat, rye and barley from the diet. Which one of the following is the investigation of first choice?

A. Anti-reticulin antibodies
B. Jejunal biopsy
C. A small bowel follow-through
D. Endomysial (EMA) and tissue transglutaminase (tTG) antibodies (IgA)
E. Anti-gliadin antibodies

Q 6.3

A 45-year-old woman presents with steatorrhoea, abdominal discomfort, bloating and weight loss. On examination she has mouth ulcers and angular stomatitis. Her symptoms improve with the removal of wheat, rye and barley from the diet. She also develops a blistering subepidermal eruption of the skin. The skin condition is most likely to respond to which one of the following?

A. Tetracycline
B. Amoxicillin
C. Dapsone
D. Isoniazid
E. Erythromycin

Q 6.4

A 38-year-old man living in a village in Bangladesh has diarrhoea of 8 months' duration. The onset was sudden. Associated symptoms are abdominal discomfort and loss of weight. Which one of the following medications is indicated in this condition?

A. Prednisolone
B. Methotrexate

Gastrointestinal disease

C. Tetracycline
D. Ciclosporin
E. Mycophenolate

Q6.5

A 45-year-old woman presents with steatorrhoea, abdominal discomfort, bloating and weight loss. On examination she has mouth ulcers and angular stomatitis. Her symptoms improve with the removal of wheat, rye and barley from the diet. Which one of the following complications is most likely to occur, even with a long-term gluten-free diet?

A. Infertility
B. Polyneuropathy
C. Depression
D. Osteoporosis
E. Osteomalacia

Q6.6

A 32-year-old hospital doctor presents with an 8-month history of intermittent bleeding per rectum. He has no family history of colon cancer. Select the best option from the following list

A. Barium enema must be performed to exclude ischaemic colitis
B. Colonoscopy is mandatory to exclude colorectal cancer
C. Per rectal examination and sigmoidoscopy are adequate
D. Given his age, angiography for angiodysplasia must be performed
E. Proctoscopy is useful to screen for colorectal cancer

Q6.7

An 18-year-old student had dental caries. She has a sweet tooth and consumes a lot of sweets. Which one of the following is the organism most likely to cause dental caries?

A. Herpesvirus 8
B. Epstein–Barr virus
C. *Streptococcus bovis*
D. *Streptococcus mutans*
E. *Streptococcus viridans*

Q6.8

A 47-year-old HIV-infected homosexual man has white vertical corrugations on the lateral borders of the tongue. Immunostaining is most likely to show which one of the following?

A. Herpesvirus 8
B. Epstein–Barr virus
C. *Streptococcus bovis*
D. *Streptococcus mutans*
E. *Streptococcus viridans*

Q6.9

A 37-year-old HIV-infected homosexual man has a reddish-purple macule on the palate. This lesion is associated with which one of the following?

A. Herpesvirus 8
B. Epstein–Barr virus
C. *Streptococcus bovis*
D. *Streptococcus mutans*
E. *Streptococcus viridans*

Q6.10

A 48-year-old man complains of constipation, painful abdomen and faeculent vomiting. Which one of the following is most likely to cause this presentation?

A. Gastric outlet obstruction
B. Gastroparesis
C. Hypercalcaemia
D. Gastrocolic fistula
E. Increased intracranial pressure

Q6.11

A 38-year-old Bangladeshi woman complains of fever, weight loss and abdominal distension. On examination she has a distended abdomen with shifting dullness. Ascitic fluid examination reveals a protein concentration of 30 g/L. No tubercle bacilli are isolated. The most likely diagnosis is which one of the following?

A. Congestive heart failure
B. Tuberculous peritonitis
C. Retroperitoneal fibrosis
D. Polyserositis
E. Primary mesothelioma

Q6.12

A 45-year-old woman with a long-standing history of peptic ulcer complains of repeated bouts of projectile vomiting. The most likely cause for her symptom is which one of the following?

A. Psychogenic
B. Gastric outlet obstruction
C. Gastrocolic fistula
D. Pregnancy
E. Low intestinal obstruction

Q6.13

A 28-year-old swimming coach complains of a 2-year history of persistent pain in the right hypochondrium. There is no weight loss and the patient has been able to continue her job without much interference. Which of the following is the most likely cause?

A. Gall bladder disease
B. Biliary tract disease
C. Chronic appendicitis
D. Functional bowel disease
E. Gastric carcinoma

Q6.14

A 58-year-old woman has gastro-oesophageal reflux disease. Which one of the following mechanisms has been implicated in this disease?

A. Increased lower oesophageal sphincter relaxation
B. Decreased oesophageal mucosal sensitivity
C. Increased oesophageal clearance of acid
D. Increased gastric emptying
E. Low resting lower oesphageal sphincter tone

Q6.15

A 45-year-old woman with prolonged QT interval has gastro-oesophageal reflux disease (GORD). Which one of the following medications should be avoided in this patient?

A. Alginate-containing antacids
B. Magnesium trisilicate
C. Aluminium hydroxide
D. Omeprazole
E. Cisapride

Q6.16

A 67-year-old man has gastro-oesophageal reflux disease (GORD). He develops diarrhoea. Which one of the following drugs is most likely to cause this symptom?

A. Alginate-containing antacids
B. Magnesium trisilicate
C. Aluminium hydroxide
D. Omeprazole
E. Lansoprazole

Gastrointestinal disease

Q6.17

A 68-year-old man has gastro-oesophageal reflux disease (GORD). He develops reflux symptoms every week. Which one of the following statements applies to this patient?

A. He is unlikely to develop peptic stricture

B. He is more likely to develop Mallory–Weiss syndrome

C. He is less likely to develop squamous cell carcinoma of the oesophagus

D. He is more likely to develop a duodenal ulcer

E. He is eight times more likely to develop adenocarcinoma than an asymptomatic individual

Q6.18

A 67-year-old retired mechanic complains of a 2-year history of pain in the right iliac fossa. The pain is persistent and unrelated to food. There is no weight loss. Which one of the following is the most likely cause for his symptoms?

A. Chronic appendicitis

B. Functional bowel disease

C. Proctalgia

D. Acute diverticulitis

E. Gall bladder disease

Q6.19

A 75-year-old woman complains of difficulty in swallowing. She feels both liquid and solid foods get 'stuck'. Select the best barium contrast study for this patient

A. Barium meal

B. Barium swallow

C. Small bowel follow-through

D. Small bowel enema

E. Barium enema

Q6.20

A 26-year-old woman has a 3-month history of frequent episodes of vomiting occurring on at least three separate days in a week. She does not have any features to suggest eating disorder, rumination or major psychiatric disease. Her vomiting is not self-induced or brought on by medication. She does not have any abnormalities in the gut, central nervous system or metabolic disease to explain the recurrent vomiting. Which one of the following is the most likely diagnosis?

A. Globus

B. Functional dyspepsia

C. Aerophagia

D. Functional vomiting

E. Rumination syndrome

Q6.21

A 29-year-old software engineer has a 4-month history of epigastric pain and vomiting. Select the best barium contrast study for this patient

A. Barium meal

B. Barium swallow

C. Small bowel follow-through

D. Small bowel enema

E. Barium enema

Q6.22

A 42-year-old accountant has a 3-month history of diarrhoea and epigastric pain. Select the best barium contrast study for this patient

A. Barium meal

B. Barium swallow

C. Small bowel follow-through

D. Double-contrast barium meal

E. Barium enema

Q6.23

A 32-year-old Caucasian woman has chronic diarrhoea with blood and mucus, accompanied by lower abdominal discomfort. She has about 8 stools per day. Albumin is 29 g/L, haemoglobin is 9 g/dL and ESR is 60 mm/1 h. A colonoscopy reveals left-sided proctocolitis. Biopsy shows a chronic inflammatory cell infiltrate in the lamina propria. Crypt abscesses and goblet cell depletion are seen. Select the best medication for this patient

A. Oral aminosalicylates only
B. Parenteral aminosalicylates
C. Oral aminosalicylates with prednisolone 20 mg enema
D. Oral aminosalicylates with oral prednisolone
E. Oral sulfapyridine

Q6.24

A 22-year-old woman has a 6-week history of altered bowel habit and pain in the left hypochondrium. There is blood and mucus in the stools. Select the best barium contrast study for this patient

A. Barium meal
B. Barium swallow
C. Small bowel follow-through
D. Double-contrast barium meal
E. Barium enema

Q6.25

A 39-year-old man complains of abdominal pain. He points at the epigastrium to localize the site of pain. The pain usually comes on at night and is worse when he is hungry. Sometimes nausea accompanies the pain and is somewhat relieved by antacids. Clinical examination is unremarkable; he has mild tenderness in the epigastrium. The quick and easy way of confirming the diagnosis is which one of the following?

A. Immunoassay of the stool
B. ^{13}C Urea breath test
C. Barium swallow
D. Upper GI endoscopy and rapid urease test
E. Upper GI endoscopy and histology

Q6.26

1. A 68-year-old obese patient complains of oesophageal reflux
2. A 29-year-old woman is suspected to have Meckel's diverticulum with gastric mucosa
3. The gastroenterologist wishes to determine the extent of inflammation in a 22-year-old patient with inflammatory bowel disease
4. A 65-year-old patient is suspected to have gastrointestinal loss of blood
5. A 32-year-old patient has protein-losing enteropathy and the extent of the albumin loss needs to be determined
6. A 55-year-old is suspected to have malabsorption due to excessive bile salts in the colon
7. A 48-year-old is suspected to have malabsorption due to bacterial overgrowth
8. A 68-year-old is suspected to have a neuroendocrine tumour

Select the best investigation for each of the above

A. Radiolabelled octreotide and whole-body scanning
B. [^{99}mTc]-technetium-sulphur colloid incorporated into food
C. [^{99}mTc]-pertechnetate
D. [^{99}mTc]-hexamethylpropylene amine oxime labelled white cells
E. Administering $^{51}CrCl_3$ intravenously
F. Whole body scanning and counting the

activity in the faeces following oral ^{75}Se-homochoyl taurine (SeHCAT)

G. Measuring $^{14}CO_2$ in the breath following oral ^{14}C-glycocholic acid

H. ^{57}Co-B$_{12}$

I. Administering ^{51}Cr red cells and measuring radioactivity in faeces

___

6.27

1. A 28-year-old woman has a long history of intermittent dysphagia for both liquids and solids. Occasionally food gets stuck but she has learned to overcome this by drinking large quantities. She has lost 3 lb in weight since the onset of symptoms

2. A 42-year-old patient complains of retrosternal chest pain and dysphagia. Barium swallow shows 'corkscrew' oesophagus

3. An 87-year-old patient complains of dysphagia. Barium swallow shows prominent indentation or 'bar'

4. 42-year-old patient complains of dysphagia on swallowing a large bolus of bread. The barium swallow reveals an oesophagus well distended with barium. The barium-coated bread will lodge at the narrowing

5. A 58-year-old patient complains of dysphagia which is progressive and unrelenting. Initially the patient had difficulty only in swallowing solids but more recently he also has dysphagia for liquids. He has lost weight and complains of anorexia

Select the correct diagnosis for each of the above

A. Carcinoma of the oesophagus
B. Achalasia
C. Diffuse oesophageal spasm
D. Cricopharyngeal dysfunction
E. Schatzki ring

6.28

1. A 56-year-old man has a long history of dyspepsia. He now has no pain but complains of projectile vomiting. The vomitus has a huge volume and contains particles of food eaten the day before

2. A 69-year-old man has new onset dyspepsia. The pain is relieved by food and antacids. He also has nausea, dysphagia and weight loss. There is a palpable gastric mass

3. A 64-year-old patient has past history of peptic ulcer successfully treated several years ago with gastrectomy. He now has nausea, distension, sweating, fainting and palpitations

4. A 38-year-old complains of epigastric pain and oedema. Investigations reveal hypochlorhydria and hypoalbuminaemia. Endoscopy reveals giant gastric folds. Histology of gastric mucosa shows hyperplasia of gastric pits, atrophy of glands and an increase in overall mucosal thickness

5. A 28-year-old patient complains of epigastric pain. Investigations reveal achlorhydria, and pernicious anaemia

Select the best match for each of the above

A. Ménétrier's disease
B. Autoimmune gastritis
C. Gastric carcinoma
D. Dumping syndrome
E. Pyloric stenosis

___

6.29

1. Colestyramine

2. Orlistat

3. Thyrotoxicosis

4. Diabetes mellitus

5. Hypogammaglobulinaemia

Select the best match for each of the above

A. Causes steatorrhoea owing to secondary infestation with *Giardia intestinalis*
B. Diarrhoea occurs owing to increased gastric emptying and increased intestinal motility
C. Diarrhoea, malabsorption and steatorrhoea may occur owing to bacterial overgrowth from stasis
D. Binds bile salts and produces steatorrhoea
E. Inhibits gastric pancreatic lipase resulting in diarrhoea and steatorrhoea

Q6.30

1. A 42-year-old man presents with steatorrhoea, abdominal pain, fever and weight loss. Histologically the small bowel shows stunted villi and contains diagnostic periodic acid-Schiff (PAS)-positive macrophages. Electron microscopy shows bacilli within the macrophages

2. A 47-year-old man has diarrhoea and steatorrhoea. Aspiration of the upper jejunum reveals the presence of *Escherichia coli* and/or *Bacteroides*, both in concentrations greater than 10^6/mL. The patient wants to avoid surgery

3. A 28-year-old woman from the Punjab presents with diarrhoea, abdominal pain, fever, anorexia and weight loss. On examination a mass is palpable in the right iliac fossa. X-ray shows infiltration of the upper lobe and the sputum contains acid-fast bacilli

4. 78-year-old man complains of bluish-red flushing of the face and neck. He also has abdominal pain and recurrent watery diarrhoea. On examination there is pulmonary stenosis. Examination of the abdomen reveals hepatomegaly

5. A 39-year-old patient has a family history of gastrointestinal polyps. There is pigmentation around the mouth, hands and feet. Colonoscopy shows multiple polyps in the small bowel

Select the best match for each of the above

A. The gene responsible is *LKB1*
B. Octreotide may inhibit tumour growth
C. Rotating course of antibiotics such as metronidazole and tetracycline or ciprofloxacin
D. Treatment is rifampicin, isoniazid and pyrazinamide for 1 year
E. Patient has a dramatic response to antibiotic therapy with trimethoprim/sulfamethoxazole

Q6.31

1. A 25-year-old woman presents with chronic watery diarrhoea. Colonoscopy reveals normal mucosa. Histopathology reveals a chronic inflammatory infiltrate in the lamina propria, with deformed crypt architecture, and goblet cell depletion with crypt abscesses

2. A 27-year-old man presents with chronic watery diarrhoea. Colonoscopy reveals that the mucosa is normal. Histopathology reveals surface epithelial injury, prominent lymphocytic infiltrate in the surface epithelium and increased lamina propria mononuclear cells

3. A 41-year-old woman presents with chronic watery diarrhoea. Colonoscopy reveals that the mucosa is normal. Histopathology reveals a thickened subepithelial collagen layer adjacent to the basal membrane with increased infiltration of the lamina propria, with lymphocytes and plasma cells and surface epithelial cell damage

Gastrointestinal disease

Select the best match for each of the above

A. Associated with high prevalence of antibiotic use
B. Microscopic ulcerative colitis
C. Associated with primary biliary cirrhosis
D. Associated with myocardial infarction
E. Associated with dilated cardiomyopathy

Q6.32

An 82-year-old man presents with a history of passing fewer than two stools per week for 2 months. He rarely experiences a call to stool. He undergoes marker studies of colonic transit. Capsules containing 21 radio-opaque shapes are swallowed by him on days 1, 2 and 3 and an abdominal X-ray is obtained 120 hours after his first capsule. On the X-ray it is noted that there are more than 12 shapes from the third capsule. Correct statements about this patient's condition include

A. The diagnosis is best confirmed by performing evacuation proctography
B. His clinical picture suggests the presence of an anterior rectocele
C. The main focus of his treatment should be directed to decreasing the fibre in his diet
D. The use of enemas is contraindicated because of his advanced age
E. Loperamide should be prescribed in advanced stages

Q6.33

1. A 7-year-old boy has a long-standing history of constipation. Investigation reveals that a short segment of the rectum is dilated. A rectal biopsy on frozen section reveals an elevated staining for acetylcholinesterase. Manometric studies reveal a failure of relaxation of the internal sphincter

2. A 56-year-old man presents with intermittent left iliac fossa pain and an erratic bowel habit. Clinical examination is unremarkable. His blood count reveals polymorphonuclear leucocytosis and elevated ESR. Spiral CT of the lower abdomen reveals thickening of the colonic wall, pericolic abscess and diverticula in the sigmoid colon

3. A 78-year-old woman presents with sudden onset abdominal pain with the passage of bright red blood in the stools and some loose stools. The abdomen is distended and tender. A straight abdominal X-ray reveals thumb printing at the site of splenic flexure

4. A 65-year-old man has abdominal pain and diarrhoea. X-ray of the abdomen reveals multiple gas-filled cysts in the sub-mucosa of the colon

5. A 38-year-old nurse has chronic diarrhoea. The diarrhoea is of high volume, and serum potassium is 3.2 mEq/L. Sigmoidoscopy shows pigmented mucosa, and rectal biopsy shows pigment-laden macrophages

Select the best match for each of the above

A. Hirschsprung's disease
B. Outpatient treatment with cephalosporin and metronidazole
C. Ischaemic colitis
D. Oxygen therapy
E. Purgative abuse

Q6.34

A 47-year-old alcoholic and diabetic with end-stage renal disease and heart failure due to coronary artery disease complains of vomiting. The following explain his symptoms

A. Uraemia
B. Diabetic ketoacidosis
C. Serum digoxin levels of 3 ng/ml
D. Inferior myocardial infarction
E. Alcohol excess

Q6.35

A 67-year-old woman presents with rapidly progressive abdominal distension and pain. X-ray shows a gas-filled large bowel. The patient's symptoms respond to intravenous neostigmine therapy. This syndrome can complicate the following clinical situations

A. Intra-abdominal sepsis
B. Pneumonia
C. Parkinson's disease
D. Malnutrition
E. Use of opiates following orthopaedic surgery

Q6.36

A 25-year-old alcoholic with diabetic nephropathy complains of early-morning vomiting. The most likely causes of early-morning vomiting are

A. Haematochezia
B. Uraemia
C. Alcohol excess
D. Pregnancy
E. Anorexia

Q6.37

Mouth ulcers are a feature of the following systemic disorders

A. Crohn's disease
B. Ulcerative colitis
C. Behçet's disease
D. Neutropenia
E. Reiter's disease

Q6.38

In the dermatology department the doctor recognizes licheniform eruptions in the mouth. He believes that drugs cause this condition. The following drugs are reported to cause this condition

A. Antimalarials
B. Gold salts
C. Methyldopa
D. Tolbutamide
E. Penicillamine

Q6.39

A medical student recognizes gingival hyperplasia in a 45-year-old patient who has had cardiac transplantation and a history of epilepsy and hypertension. The following medications are likely to cause fibrous gingival hyperplasia

A. Aciclovir
B. Mycophenolate mofetil
C. Ciclosporin
D. Nifedipine
E. Phenytoin

Q6.40

A 67-year-old woman complains of a dry mouth. The following can cause a dry mouth

A. Radiotherapy
B. Sjögren's syndrome
C. Tricyclic antidepressants
D. Clonidine
E. Antihistamines

Gastrointestinal disease

Q6.41

A 35-year-old woman complains of difficulty in swallowing. Causes of this symptom include

A. Goitre
B. Enlarged left atrium
C. Scleroderma
D. Bulbar palsy
E. Myasthenia gravis

Q6.42

A 28-year-old man complains of painful swallowing without difficulty. Causes of this symptom include

A. Achalasia
B. Diffuse oesophageal spasm
C. Oesophageal webs
D. Candidiasis
E. Herpes simplex

Q6.43

Correct statements about the normal stomach and duodenum include

A. The lower third of the stomach contains parietal cells
B. The antrum contains G cells which secrete gastrin
C. The duodenal mucosa lacks Brunner's glands
D. Somatostatin is produced by specialized antral cells
E. Recent evidence suggests that absorption is a major function of the stomach

Q6.44

Risk factors for adenocarcinoma of the oesophagus include

A. Heavy alcohol intake
B. Plummer–Vinson syndrome
C. Tylosis
D. Diet deficient in vitamins
E. Coeliac disease

Q6.45

A 67-year-old patient is diagnosed as having squamous cell carcinoma of the oesophagus. The following statements are correct

A. Squamous cell carcinoma is more common in females
B. Radiotherapy provides the best chance for cure
C. These tumours arise from Barrett's oesophagus
D. Most patients present with stage 3 disease
E. To confirm the diagnosis endoscopy is almost always preceded by barium swallow to prevent risks of perforation

Q6.46

A 39-year-old man complains of abdominal pain. He points at the epigastrium to localize the site of pain. The pain usually comes on at night and is worse when he is hungry. Sometimes nausea accompanies the pain and it is somewhat relieved by antacids. Clinical examination is unremarkable; he has mild tenderness in the epigastrium. The ^{13}C urea breath test confirms the diagnosis of *Helicobacter pylori* infection. Medications which have been used in the treatment of this condition include

A. Beta-blockers
B. Proton-pump inhibitors
C. Metronidazole
D. Clarithromycin
E. Bismuth chelate
F. Amoxicillin
G. H$_2$-receptor blockers
H. Sodium–potassium pump inhibitors

Q6.47

A 58-year-old patient with severe rheumatoid arthritis and pain gets relief of symptoms with NSAIDs. The patient develops ulcer dyspepsia. Stopping NSAIDs is not possible because of the pain. The following are options

A. Use an NSAID with low GI side-effects at lowest dose possible
B. Gastrectomy
C. Use of proton-pump inhibitor or misoprostol as prophylactic therapy
D. COX-2 therapy
E. Steroid therapy

Q6.48

A 67-year-old man presents with black tarry stools for 2 days. The following statements are correct

A. As little as 10 mL of blood is adequate to produce this symptom
B. It can occur with bleeding from any lesion proximal to the sigmoid colon
C. The passage of black tarry stools is known as haematemesis
D. This symptom is unlikely to be due to chronic peptic ulceration
E. The black colour of the stools is due to partially digested blood

Q6.49

A 74-year-old woman with chronic rheumatoid arthritis who is on ibuprofen and the normal therapeutic dose of prednisolone presents with haematemesis. She is also on warfarin for atrial fibrillation. The night before admission she was at a party and admits to having had several alcoholic drinks. On examination she has stigmata of chronic liver disease but no splenomegaly. The following statements are correct

A. NSAIDs can produce GI haemorrhage from both duodenal and gastric ulcers
B. It is well recognized that normal therapeutic doses of corticosteroids result in severe upper GI haemorrhage
C. Warfarin *per se* causes acute GI haemorrhage
D. Alcohol *per se* can cause upper GI haemorrhage
E. The absence of splenomegaly rules out oesophageal varices

Q6.50

A 53-year-old man presents with haematemesis and melaena. On examination the patient has pallor, cold nose, a heart rate of 120 beats/minute and systolic blood pressure of 90 mmHg. The patient's haemoglobin is 11 mg/dL. The patient continues to have brisk bleeding. The following statements about management of this patient are correct

A. Central venous access is not necessary in this patient
B. Blood substitutes are preferred to whole blood in this patient
C. Pulse rate and venous pressure are crude guides to monitor transfusion rates
D. Haemoglobin is an excellent indicator of the need to transfuse whole blood
E. Blood volume must be restored rapidly in this patient

Q6.51

A 47-year-old woman presents with haematemesis and hypotension on a Friday evening. Her blood volume is restored rapidly and her symptoms abate. Correct statements about management include

A. Endoscopy can be delayed until Monday
B. Endoscopy detects the cause of bleeding in less than 10% of cases

Gastrointestinal disease

C. On endoscopy in the presence of a peptic ulcer the presence of an organized blood clot suggests that the patient is unlikely to re-bleed
D. At first endoscopy all bleeding ulcers should be injected with adrenaline (epinephrine) and a sclerosant
E. Intravenous omeprazole has been shown to substantially reduce re-bleeding rates

Q6.52

An 82-year-old woman presents with haematemesis and melaena. The following statements about mortality due to GI haemorrhage are correct

A. H_2-receptor antagonists reduce the mortality rate
B. Proton-pump inhibitors reduce the mortality rate
C. The injection of adrenaline (epinephrine) and a sclerosant at first endoscopy reduces the mortality rate
D. Recurrent haemorrhage has an increased mortality
E. Melaena is usually more hazardous than haematemesis

Q6.53

Following ingestion of a meal the nutrients are absorbed. The following statements about absorption are correct

A. Vitamin B_{12} is absorbed in the terminal ileum
B. Glucose is absorbed by simple diffusion
C. Dietary starch is broken down to monosaccharides before absorption
D. Dietary protein is broken down to oligopeptides and amino acids before absorption
E. Emulsification of fat predominantly occurs in the stomach
F. Bile salts are absorbed in the jejunum

Q6.54

The gut of the normal adult has contractile patterns. The following statements regarding these patterns are correct

A. During fasting migrating motor complexes occur in a cyclical fashion
B. Phase III migrating motor complexes are associated with decreased gastric, intestinal and biliary secretions
C. Phase I migrating motor complexes propel food towards the colon
D. After a meal the pattern of the migrating motor complex is disrupted
E. Irregular contractions after feeding have a mixing function

Q6.55

A 45-year-old woman presents with steatorrhoea, abdominal discomfort, bloating and weight loss. On examination she has mouth ulcers and angular stomatitis. Her symptoms improve with the removal of wheat, rye and barley from her diet. The following statements about this condition are correct

A. It is common in black Africans
B. About 70% of first-degree relatives have this condition
C. α-Gliadin is the main damaging peptide in gluten
D. Histology of the small intestine shows an absence of villi and crypt hyperplasia with chronic inflammatory cells in the lamina propri
E. It may occur at any age

6.56

A 45-year-old woman presents with steatorrhoea, abdominal discomfort, bloating and weight loss. On examination she has mouth ulcers and angular stomatitis. Her symptoms improve with the removal of wheat, rye and barley from her diet. Complications of this condition include

A. Osteoporosis
B. Infertility
C. Polyneuropathy
D. Depression
E. Osteomalacia

6.57

A 45-year-old woman presents with steatorrhoea, abdominal discomfort, bloating and weight loss. On examination she has mouth ulcers and angular stomatitis. Her symptoms improve with the removal of wheat, rye and barley from her diet. The following conditions are associated with this patient's condition

A. Atopy
B. Epilepsy
C. IgM deficiency
D. Primary biliary cirrhosis
E. Diabetes

6.58

A 57-year-old man undergoes resection of the terminal ileum. The following statements about complications are correct

A. Removal of the ileocaecal valve decreases the incidence of diarrhoea
B. Serum vitamin B_{12} is low
C. There is a decrease in the formation of renal oxalate stones
D. Increased loss of bile salts decreases the formation of gallstones

E. Glucagon-like peptide 2 (GLP-2) is increased following intestinal resection

6.59

A 55-year-old presents with microcytic anaemia. Colonoscopy reveals four sessile polyps which are ~3 cm in diameter. The following statements are correct

A. The risk of malignancy is low
B. Colonoscopic removal of the polyps with surveillance substantially reduces the incidence of colon cancer
C. This patient should have surveillance colonoscopy every 10 years after polypectomy
D. These clinical features are typical of Peutz–Jegher's syndrome
E. Most colorectal cancers develop from sporadic polyps

6.60

An 18-year-old man has a family history of polyposis. Colonoscopy reveals several hundreds to thousands of colorectal adenomas. The following statements about this condition are correct

A. It usually arises from mutations of the *APC* gene
B. Prophylactic colectomy should be offered before the age of 20 years
C. The average age of developing colorectal cancer is 25 years
D. Congenital hypertrophy of the retinal pigment epithelium is a recognized feature
E. Tracing and screening of relatives is essential after the age of 20 years

Gastrointestinal disease

6.61

The gastroenterologist diagnoses hereditary non-polyposis colorectal cancer in his patient. The following statements are correct

A. Familial adenomatous polyposis is a component of this condition
B. Three or more cases of colorectal cancers occur in a minimum of two generations
C. One affected individual must be a first-degree relative of the other two (or more) cases
D. Endometrial cancer is a feature of this condition
E. Mutations in *hMLH1* and *hMSH2* genes account for over 95% of cases

6.62

A 42-year-old physician has change in bowel habit, passing mucus per rectum, anorexia and weight loss. The following statements about his condition are correct

A. Colonoscopy is the gold standard for diagnosis
B. Even though 80% of patients undergo surgery, fewer than half survive more than 5 years
C. Long-term survival is only likely when the lesion is completely removed
D. High levels of microsatellite instability have a less favourable outlook
E. Adjuvant postoperative chemotherapy does not improve disease-free survival once the lymph nodes are involved

6.63

A 27-year-old patient has a history of chronic diarrhoea. SeHCAT shows that a <5% retention of the radiolabelled bile acid analogue occurs at 7 days. This condition is associated with

A. Ileal resection
B. Colchicine
C. Biguanides
D. Cystic fibrosis
E. Diabetic diarrhoea

6.64

1. A 29-year-old woman has a 3-month history of abdominal discomfort relieved with defecation. Increased frequency of stool is the predominant symptom
2. A 32-year-old woman has a 3-month history of abdominal discomfort relieved with defecation. Constipation is the predominant symptom
3. A 48-year-old man has epigastric and back pain. The pain is accompanied by vomiting. Serum amylase levels are more than five times normal
4. A 23-year-old man has pain around the navel. The pain is of sudden onset and radiates around the right iliac fossa. He has nausea, vomiting and diarrhoea. On palpation he has tenderness in the right iliac fossa. Serum amylase is about three times normal before it starts falling
5. A 33-year-old woman presents with acute right hypochondrial pain, fever and mildly abnormal liver biochemistry

Select the best match for each of the above

A. Fitz-Hugh–Curtis syndrome
B. Acute pancreatitis
C. Acute appendicitis
D. Hydroxytryptamine ($5HT_3$) receptor antagonist
E. $5HT_4$-receptor agonist
F. Crigler–Najjar syndrome
G. Zieve's syndrome

Q6.65

A 27-year-old nurse has long-standing ulcerative colitis. She requires prednisolone of 60 mg/day to keep her colitis in remission. After discussion with her gastroenterologist and surgeon she opts for surgical management of her condition. The following statements regarding her surgical options are correct

A. Ileorectal anastomosis is used to avoid permanent ileostomy
B. With ileo-anal anastomosis, continence is rarely achieved
C. There is a reduced incidence of pouchitis when ileo-anal anastomosis is performed in patients who also have primary sclerosing cholangitis
D. With ileo-anal anastomosis the stapling of the ileal pouch to the lower rectal mucosa usually results in night-time incontinence
E. With ileal pouch–distal rectal anastomosis the stapling of the ileal pouch to the lower rectal mucosa substantially reduces the risk of cancer in the residual diseased mucosa

Q6.66

A 27-year-old woman with active inflammatory bowel disease (IBD) wishes to conceive. The following statements regarding pregnancy in IBD are correct

A. Fertility is unaffected in active disease
B. Patients with active disease are twice as likely to have spontaneous abortion than those with inactive disease
C. The risk of exacerbation of IBD is increased in pregnancy
D. Aminosalicylates, steroids and azathioprine are unsafe at the time of conception
E. Aminosalicylates, steroids and azathioprine are unsafe during pregnancy

Q6.67

A 21-year-old patient with distal inflammatory proctitis due to ulcerative colitis wishes to know the prognosis. The following statements are correct

A. About two-thirds of patients will develop more proximal colitis
B. A third of patients will develop total colitis
C. Most patients will only have a single attack and the remaining minority will have a relapsing course
D. Two-thirds of patients will undergo colectomy within 10 years of diagnosis
E. About two-thirds of patients undergoing colectomy will require a second operation

Q6.68

A 27-year-old Caucasian woman has chronic diarrhoea with blood and mucus, accompanied by lower abdominal discomfort. Biopsy obtained during sigmoidoscopy shows a chronic inflammatory cell infiltrate in the lamina propria. Crypt abscesses and goblet cell depletion are seen. The following statements about her condition are correct

A. It is unlikely she will have first-degree relatives with a similar diagnosis
B. It is more likely to be present in smokers
C. It usually affects the gastrointestinal tract from the mouth to the anus
D. On histology typically there is transmural inflammation
E. Enteric fistulae, e.g. to bladder or vagina, occur in 20–40% of cases

Gastrointestinal disease

Q6.69

A 21-year-old Scottish woman has an 8-month history of intermittent diarrhoea, abdominal pain and weight loss. On examination she has aphthous ulcers of the mouth. Abdominal examination reveals a tender mass in the right iliac fossa. Per rectal examination reveals oedematous anal tags, and perianal abscesses. Biopsy reveals an increase in chronic inflammatory cells and lymphoid hyperplasia. Non-caseating epithelioid cell granulomas are present. The following statements about medical management of her condition are correct

A. Loperamide is not indicated for control of diarrhoea
B. Steroids have been shown to be effective in severe attacks of this condition
C. Enteral nutrition is contraindicated in this condition
D. Mycophenolate mofetil is effective in maintaining remission
E. Infliximab is contraindicated in this condition

Q6.70

A 32-year-old Caucasian woman has chronic diarrhoea with blood and mucus, accompanied by lower abdominal discomfort. Biopsy obtained during sigmoidoscopy shows a chronic inflammatory cell infiltrate in the lamina propria. Crypt abscesses and goblet cell depletion are seen. The following suggest a severe attack

A. Five stools per day with blood
B. Temperature of 38°C
C. Heart rate of 98 beats per minute
D. ESR of 50 mm per hour
E. Haemoglobin 9 g/dL
F. Albumin 32 g/L

A6.1

B

Patients with extensive ulcerative colitis of more than 10 years' duration are at an increased risk of developing colorectal cancer (cumulative risk 5% after 20 years, 12% at 25 years). Although patients with Crohn's colitis are also at risk, this is lower than with ulcerative colitis. Many centres recommend that colonoscopy and multiple biopsies should be undertaken at 1–2-year intervals in patients with extensive ulcerative colitis of more than 10 years' duration and those with evidence of high-grade dysplasia should undergo colectomy. There is, however, no supportive evidence for this strategy. There is insufficient evidence to support the use of a surveillance programme in patients with Crohn's colitis.

A6.2

D

Endomysial (EMA) and tissue transglutaminase (tTG) antibodies have a high sensitivity and specificity for the diagnosis of untreated coeliac disease and can also be used as screening tests. They are now the investigation of first choice. In the presence of a typical clinical picture and the presence of these antibodies, a confirmatory jejunal biopsy may not always be required.

A6.3

C

Dermatitis herpetiformis is an uncommon blistering subepidermal eruption of the skin associated with a gluten-sensitive enteropathy. Rarely there may be gross malabsorption, but usually the jejunal morphological abnormalities are not as severe as in coeliac disease. The skin condition responds to dapsone but both the gut and the skin will improve on a gluten-free diet.

A6.4

C

Tropical sprue is endemic in most of Asia, some Caribbean islands, Puerto Rico and parts of South America. Epidemics occur, lasting up to 2 years, and in some areas repeated epidemics occur at varying intervals of up to 10 years. Most patients require an antibiotic (usually tetracycline 1 g daily) to ensure a complete recovery; it may be necessary to give this for up to 6 months.

A6.5

D

Osteoporosis is common in coeliac disease and occurs even in patients on long-term gluten-free diets. Rare complications include tetany, osteomalacia, or gross malnutrition with peripheral oedema.

A6.6

C

Isolated episodes of rectal bleeding in the young (<45 years) only require rectal examination and sigmoidoscopy. Colorectal cancer is rare in this age group without a strong family history.

A6.7

D

Streptococcus mutans is the main bacterial cause of dental caries in man. These bacteria are cariogenic only in the presence of dietary sugar.

Gastrointestinal disease

A6.8

B

Oral hairy leucoplakia is almost pathognomonic of HIV infection and may be an early sign. It is more common in HIV-infected homosexual men than in any other high-risk group. It is characterized by white vertical corrugations on the lateral borders of the tongue and immunostaining shows Epstein–Barr virus. Treatment is rarely necessary.

A6.9

A

Kaposi's sarcoma presents as a red, purple or blue macule or nodule, most commonly on the palate. It is diagnostic of AIDS. The lesion is associated with herpesvirus 8.

A6.10

D

Faeculent vomit suggests low intestinal obstruction or the presence of a gastrocolic fistula.

A6.11

B

Three subgroups of abdominal TB can be identified: wet, dry and fibrous. a) In patients with the wet type, ascitic fluid should be examined for protein concentration (>20 g/L) and tubercle bacilli (rarely found). b) In the dry form, patients present with subacute intestinal obstruction which is due to tuberculous small bowel adhesions. c) In the fibrous form, patients present with abdominal pain, distension and ill-defined irregular tender abdominal masses. The diagnosis of peritoneal TB can be supported by findings on ultrasound or CT screening (mesenteric

thickening and lymph node enlargement). A histological diagnosis is not always required before instituting treatment.

A6.12

B

Projectile vomiting is due to gastric outflow obstruction.

A6.13

D

Right hypochondrial pain is usually from the gall bladder or biliary tract. Hepatic congestion (e.g. in hepatitis) and sometimes peptic ulcer can present with pain in the right hypochondrium. Chronic, often persistent, pain in the right hypochondrium is a frequent symptom in healthy females suffering from functional bowel disease. This chronic pain is not due to gall bladder disease.

A6.14

E

The following mechanisms have been implicated in gastro-oesophageal reflux disease (GORD). a) Transient lower oesophageal sphincter (LOS) relaxations. b) Low resting LOS tone which fails to increase when the patient is lying flat, as occurs normally. c) The LOS tone fails to increase when intra-abdominal pressure is increased by tight clothing or pregnancy. d) There is increased oesophageal mucosal sensitivity to acid. e) There is reduced oesophageal clearance of acid because of poor oesophageal peristalsis. The reduced acid clearance is exacerbated with a hiatus hernia owing to trapping of acid within the hernial sac. f) A large hiatus hernia can impair the 'pinchcock' mechanism of the crural diaphragm. g) Delayed gastric emptying occurs, which may increase the chance of reflux. h) Prolonged episodes of gastro-oesophageal reflux which occur at night and postprandially.

A6.15

E

Cisapride increases the QT_c interval and has been withdrawn because of the risk of arrhythmias.

A6.16

B

Simple antacids magnesium trisilicate and aluminium hydroxide are readily available and are often used initially by patients. The former tends to cause diarrhoea while the latter causes constipation.

A6.17

E

Patients with weekly reflux symptoms are nearly eight times more likely to develop adenocarcinoma compared with those without symptoms. The greater the frequency, severity and duration of reflux symptoms, the greater the risk.

A6.18

B

Acute pain in the left iliac fossa is usually colonic in origin (e.g. acute diverticulitis). Chronic pain is most commonly associated with functional bowel disease. In females, lower abdominal pain occurs in a number of gynaecological disorders and the differentiation from GI disease is often difficult. Persistent pain in the right iliac fossa over a long period is not due to chronic appendicitis. Proctalgia is a severe pain deep in the rectum that comes on suddenly but lasts only for a short time. It is not due to organic disease.

A6.19

B

In a barium swallow, the oesophagus is visualized as barium is swallowed in the upright and prone positions. Motility abnormalities as well as anatomical lesions can then be observed. Reflux of barium from the stomach into the oesophagus is demonstrated with the patient tipped head down. The severity of this reflux can be gauged by administering an effervescent tablet and asking the patient to drink water (water siphon test). Swallowing bread with the barium (to add bulk) is sometimes useful in a case of dysphagia.

A6.20

D

Functional vomiting is a rare condition in clinical practice but often extensive investigation is required before reaching a diagnosis. Clinically, functional vomiting is characterized by: a) frequent episodes of vomiting, occurring on at least three separate days in a week; b) absence of criteria for an eating disorder, rumination or major psychiatric disease; c) absence of self-induced and medication-induced vomiting; d) absence of abnormalities in the gut or central nervous system and metabolic disease to explain the recurrent vomiting.

A6.21

A

Double-contrast barium meal is performed to examine the stomach and duodenum. A small amount of barium is given together

Gastrointestinal disease

with effervescent granules or tablets to produce carbon dioxide so that a double contrast between air and barium is obtained. This technique has a high accuracy rate when performed carefully but many prefer gastroscopy to examine the stomach.

A6.22

C

Small bowel follow-through is used to examine the small bowel and ideally should be performed separately from a barium meal as a different technique is employed. Barium is swallowed and allowed to pass into the small intestine through the jejunum and into the ileum. This technique is the only way of demonstrating the gross anatomy of the small intestine. Specific views of the terminal ileum are routinely obtained using compression to separate the loops.

A6.23

D

In left-sided proctocolitis oral aminosalicylates plus local rectal steroid preparations may be effective but in moderate to severe attacks oral prednisolone will be required.

A6.24

E

In barium enema, patients are given a low-fibre diet for 3 days and the colon is thoroughly cleansed with oral laxative preparations. Barium and air are insufflated via a rectal catheter and double-contrast views obtained of the entire colon. Rectal examination and sigmoidoscopy should precede this examination. An 'instant' barium enema involving no bowel preparation is used in colitis.

A6.25

B

Helicobacter pylori is causally associated with duodenal ulcer (DU) disease: in patients with DU 95% are infected with H. pylori and cure of the infection stops duodenal ulcer recurrence. The precise mechanism of how duodenal ulceration occurs is unclear as only 15% of patients infected with H. pylori (approximately 50–60% of the adult population world-wide) develop duodenal ulcers. ^{13}C Urea breath test is a quick and easy way of detecting the presence of H. pylori and is used as a screening test. The measurement of $^{13}CO_2$ in the breath, after ingestion of ^{13}C urea, requires a mass spectrometer, which is expensive, but the test is very sensitive (98%) and specific (95%).

A6.26

1) B   2) C   3) D   4) I   5) E   6) F
7) G   8) A

Radionuclides are used in the diagnosis of gastrointestinal disease, to a varying degree, depending on local enthusiasm and expertise. Indications are: a) to demonstrate oesophageal reflux using [^{99m}Tc] technetium–sulphur colloid; b) to determine the rate of gastric emptying using [^{99m}Tc] technetium–sulphur colloid; c) to demonstrate a Meckel's diverticulum using [^{99m}Tc] pertechnetate, which has an affinity for gastric mucosa; d) to show the extent of inflammation and the presence of any inflammatory collections in inflammatory bowel disease using ^{99m}Tc HMPAO (hexamethylpropylene amine oxime) labelled white cells. Isotopes can also be used: a) to assess gastrointestinal loss of red cells by giving ^{51}Cr red cells and measuring radioactivity in the faeces, or by labelling red cells with ^{99m}Tc and scanning the abdomen, e.g. Meckel's diverticulum; b) to assess albumin loss in the stools in protein-losing enteropathy by giving ^{51}CrCl$_3$ intravenously; c) to assess bile salt malabsorption by whole-body scanning and counting the activity in the faeces following oral ^{75}Se-homochoyl taurine (SeHCAT); d) to detect bacterial overgrowth by measuring ^{14}CO$_2$ in the breath following ^{14}C glycocholic acid orally; e) to detect neuroendocrine tumours using radiolabelled octreotide and whole-body scanning; f) to assess B$_{12}$ malabsorption using ^{57}Co-B$_{12}$.

A6.27

1) B **2)** C **3)** D **4)** E **5)** A

Carcinoma of the oesophagus occurs mainly in those aged 60–70 years, although it is now occurring in younger age groups. Dysphagia is the most common single symptom and is progressive and unrelenting. Initially there is difficulty in swallowing solids, but eventually dysphagia for liquids also occurs. Benign strictures, on the other hand, initially produce intermittent dysphagia. Impaction of food causes pain, but more persistent pain implies infiltration. Achalasia is a disease characterized by aperistalsis in the body of the oesophagus and failure of relaxation of the lower oesophageal sphincter on initiation of swallowing. Patients usually have a long history of intermittent dysphagia for both liquids and solids. Regurgitation of food from the dilated oesophagus may be induced by the patient or may occur spontaneously, particularly at night, and aspiration pneumonia may result. Occasionally food gets stuck but patients often learn to overcome this by drinking large quantities, thereby increasing the head of pressure in the oesophagus and forcing the food through. Severe retrosternal chest pain occurs particularly in younger patients with vigorous non-peristaltic contraction of the oesophagus. The dysphagia in these patients can be mild and the pain misdiagnosed as cardiac in origin. Weight loss is usually not marked. Diffuse oesophageal spasm is a severe form of abnormal oesophageal motility that can sometimes produce retrosternal chest pain and dysphagia. It can accompany gastro-oesophageal reflux disease (GORD). Swallowing is accompanied by bizarre and marked contractions of the oesophagus without propagation of the waves. On barium swallow the appearance may be that of a 'corkscrew'. However, changes in oesophageal motility are not infrequent, particularly in patients over the age of 60 years (presbyoesophagus). In cricopharyngeal dysfunction there is poor relaxation of the cricopharyneal muscle during swallowing so that a prominent indentation or 'bar' is seen on a barium swallow. It occurs in the elderly. Dysphagia is treated with dilation but surgical myotomy may be necessary. Schatzki ring is a narrowing of the lower end of the oesophagus due to a ridge of mucosa or a fibrous membrane. The ring may be asymptomatic, but it can very occasionally produce dysphagia after swallowing a large bolus of bread or meat. A barium swallow (with the oesophagus well distended with barium) often shows the narrowing; barium-coated bread will lodge at the narrowing.

Gastrointestinal disease

A6.28

1) E   2) C   3) D   4) A   5) B

Autoimmune gastritis affects the fundus and body of the stomach (pangastritis), leading to atrophic gastritis with loss of parietal cells. This leads to achlorhydria and intrinsic factor deficiency causing pernicious anaemia. Autoantibodies to gastric parietal cells and intrinsic factor are found in the serum. Ménétrier's disease is a rare condition consisting of giant gastric folds, mainly in the fundus and the body of the stomach. Histologically there is hyperplasia of the gastric pits, atrophy of glands and an increase overall of mucosal thickness. Hypochlorhydria is usually present.The patient may complain of epigastric pain and occasionally peripheral oedema may occur because of hypoalbuminaemia resulting from protein loss through the gastric mucosa. Dumping syndrome is the term used to describe a number of upper abdominal symptoms (e.g. nausea and distension associated with sweating, faintness and palpitations) that occur in patients following gastrectomy or gastroenterostomy. It is due to 'dumping' of food into the jejunum, which is followed by rapid fluid dilution of the high osmotic load. A number of patients have mild symptoms of dumping but learn to cope with them. The most common symptom of carcinoma of the stomach is epigastric pain, which is indistinguishable from the pain of peptic ulcer disease, both being relieved by food and antacids. The pain can vary in intensity, but may be constant and severe. Most patients with carcinoma of the stomach have advanced disease at the time of presentation, and also have nausea, anorexia and weight loss. Vomiting is frequent and can be severe if the tumour is near the pylorus. Dysphagia can occur with tumours involving the fundus. Gross haematemesis is unusual,

but anaemia from occult blood loss is frequent. The main symptom of pyloric stenosis is vomiting, usually without pain as the characteristic ulcer pain has abated owing to healing. Vomiting is projectile and huge in volume, and the vomitus contains particles of yesterday's food. On examination of the abdomen the patient may have a succussion splash.

A6.29

1) D   2) E   3) B   4) C   5) A

Drugs that bind bile salts (e.g. colestyramine) and some antibiotics (e.g. neomycin) produce steatorrhoea. Orlistat, used in obesity, inhibits gastric and pancreatic lipase, reducing fat absorption. Side-effects include diarrhoea and steatorrhoea. Diarrhoea, rarely with steatorrhoea, occurs in thyrotoxicosis owing to increased gastric emptying and increased motility. In some patients with diabetes mellitus, diarrhoea, malabsorption and steatorrhoea occur, sometimes owing to bacterial overgrowth from stasis. Hypogammaglobulinaemia, which is seen in a number of conditions including lymphoid nodular hyperplasia, causes steatorrhoea owing either to an abnormal jejunal mucosa or to secondary infestation with *Giardia intestinalis*.

A6.30

1) E   2) C   3) D   4) B   5) A

In Whipple's disease a dramatic improvement occurs with antibiotic therapy, which should include an antibiotic that crosses the blood–brain barrier (e.g. trimethoprim/sulfamethoxazole) for 6 months. Peutz–Jeghers syndrome consists of mucocutaneous pigmentation (circumoral, hands and feet) and gastrointestinal polyps and has an autosomal dominant inheritance. The gene *LKB1* responsible for Peutz–Jeghers is a serine protein kinase and can be used for genetic analysis. In carcinoid syndrome, octreotide and lanreotide are octapeptide somatostatin analogues that have been shown to inhibit the release of many gut hormones. They alleviate the flushing and diarrhoea and can control a carcinoid crisis. In bacterial overgrowth, if possible, the underlying lesion should be corrected (e.g. a stricture should be resected). With multiple diverticula, grossly dilated bowel or in Crohn's disease, this may not be possible and rotating courses of antibiotics are necessary, such as metronidazole and tetracycline, or ciprofloxacin. Drug treatment for intestinal TB is similar to that for pulmonary TB – rifampicin, isoniazid and pyrazinamid – but treatment should last 1 year.

A6.31

1) B   2) A   3) C

Patients with microscopic inflammatory colitis present with chronic or fluctuating watery diarrhoea. Although the macroscopic features on colonoscopy are normal, the histopathological findings on biopsy are abnormal. There are three distinct forms of microscopic inflammatory colitis: a) microscopic ulcerative colitis; b) microscopic lymphocytic colitis; c) microscopic collagenous colitis. In microscopic ulcerative colitis, there is a chronic inflammatory cell infiltrate in the lamina propria, with deformed crypt architecture, and goblet cell depletion with or without crypt abscesses. Treatment is as for ulcerative colitis although many patients respond to treatment with aminosalicylates alone. In microscopic lymphocytic colitis there is surface epithelial injury, prominent lymphocytic

infiltration in the surface epithelium and increased lamina propria mononuclear cells. It affects males and females equally and is associated with a high prevalence of antibiotic use. In microscopic collagenous colitis there is a thickened subepithelial collagen layer (>10 μm) adjacent to the basal membrane with increased infiltration of the lamina propria with lymphocytes and plasma cells and surface epithelial cell damage. It is predominantly a disorder of middle-aged or elderly women, and is associated with a variety of autoimmune disorders (arthritis, thyroid disease, CREST syndrome and primary biliary cirrhosis).

A6.32

A) F   B) F   C) F   D) F   E) F

This patient has slow-transit constipation. The severity of slow-transit constipation can be assessed by undertaking a simple abdominal X-ray and in more problematical cases by undertaking marker studies of colonic transit. Capsules containing 21 radio-opaque shapes are swallowed on days 1, 2 and 3 and an abdominal X-ray obtained 120 hours after ingestion of the first capsule. Each capsule contains shapes of different configuration and the presence of more than 4 shapes from the first capsule, 6 from the second and 12 from the third denotes moderate to severe slow transit. The common causes of 'obstructive' disorders of defecation include the presence of an anterior rectocele whereby a weakness of the rectovaginal septum results in protuberances of the anterior wall of the rectum with trapping of stool if the diameter is >3 cm. In patients with slow-transit constipation the main focus should be directed to increasing the fibre content of the diet in conjunction with increasing fluid intake. The use of enemas should be restricted to the management of elderly, infirm and immobile patients and those with neurological disorders. Loperamide is used to treat diarrhoea, not constipation.

A6.33

1) A   2) B   3) C   4) D   5) E

In Hirschsprung's disease, which presents in the first years of life, an aganglionic segment of the rectum gives rise to constipation and subacute obstruction. Occasionally Hirschsprung's disease affects only a short segment of the rectum and can be missed in childhood. A preliminary rectal biopsy is performed and stained with special stains for ganglion cells in the submucosal plexus. In doubtful cases full-thickness biopsy, under anaesthesia, should be obtained. A frozen section is stained for acetylcholinesterase, which is elevated in Hirschsprung's disease. Manometric studies show failure of relaxation of the internal sphincter, which is diagnostic of Hirschsprung's disease. This disease can be successfully treated surgically. Acute diverticulitis most commonly affects diverticula in the sigmoid colon. It presents with severe pain in the left iliac fossa, often accompanied by fever and constipation. These symptoms and signs are similar to appendicitis but on the left side. On examination the patient is often febrile with a tachycardia. Abdominal examination shows tenderness, guarding and rigidity on the left side of the abdomen. A palpable tender mass is sometimes felt in the left iliac fossa. Spiral CT of the lower abdomen will show colonic wall thickening, diverticula and often pericolic collections and abscesses. There is usually a streaky increased density extending into the immediate pericolic fat with thickening of the pelvic fascial planes. These findings are diagnostic of acute diverticular disease and differ from malignant disease. Acute attacks can be treated on an outpatient basis using a cephalosporin and metronidazole. Patients who are more ill will require admission for bowel rest, intravenous fluids and antibiotic therapy (e.g. gentamicin, or a cephalosporin) and metronidazole. Pneumatosis cystoides intestinalis is a rare condition in which multiple gas-filled cysts are found in the submucosa of the intestine, chiefly the colon. The cause is unknown but many cases are associated with chronic bronchitis and some with peptic ulceration. Patients are usually asymptomatic, but abdominal pain and diarrhoea do occur and occasionally the cysts rupture to produce a pneumoperitoneum. This condition is diagnosed on X-ray of the abdomen, barium enema or sigmoidoscopy when cysts are seen. Treatment is often unnecessary but continuous oxygen therapy will help to disperse the largely nitrogen-containing cysts. Metronidazole may help. Occlusion of branches of the superior mesenteric (SMA) or inferior mesenteric arteries (IMA), often in the older age group, commonly presents with sudden onset of abdominal pain and the passage of bright red blood per rectum, with or without diarrhoea. There may be signs of shock and there may be evidence of underlying cardiovascular disease. The majority of cases affect the splenic flexure and left colon. This condition has also been described in women taking the contraceptive pill and in patients with thrombophilia and small- or medium-vessel vasculitis. On examination the abdomen is distended and tender. A straight abdominal X-ray often shows thumb printing (a characteristic sign of ischaemic disease) at the site of the splenic flexure. Purgative abuse is most commonly seen in females who surreptitiously take high-dose laxatives and are often extensively investigated for chronic diarrhoea. The diarrhoea is usually of high volume (1 litre daily) and patients may have a low serum potassium. Sigmoidoscopy may show pigmented mucosa, a condition known as melanosis coli. Histologically the rectal biopsy shows pigment-laden macrophages in patients taking an anthraquinone purgative (e.g. senna). Melanosis coli is also seen in people regularly taking purgatives in normal doses.

A6.34

A) T   B) T   C) T   D) T   E) T

Causes of vomiting	
Any gastrointestinal disease	Drugs, e.g.
Acute infections, e.g.	digoxin toxicity
influenza	opiates
pertussis	chemotherapy
Central nervous disease, e.g.	immunotherapy
raised intracranial pressure	Reflex, e.g.
meningitis	severe pain:
vestibular disturbances	myocardial
migraine	infarction
Metabolic causes, e.g.	Psychogenic
uraemia	Pregnancy
diabetes: ketoacidosis	Alcohol excess
or gastroparesis	
hypercalcaemia	

A6.35

A) T   B) T   C) T   D) T   E) T

It is now recognized that a clinical picture mimicking mechanical obstruction may develop in patients who do not have a mechanical cause. Colonic pseudo-obstruction is the commonest form. In more than 80% of cases it complicates other clinical conditions, for example:
a) intra-abdominal trauma, pelvic, spinal and femoral fractures; b) postoperatively

(abdominal, pelvic, cardiothoracic, orthopaedic, neurosurgical); c) intra-abdominal sepsis; d) pneumonia; e) metabolic (e.g. electrolyte disturbances, malnutrition, diabetes mellitus, Parkinson's disease); f) drugs – opiates (particularly after orthopaedic surgery), antidepressants, antiparkinsonian drugs.

A6.36

A) F   B) T   C) T   D) T   E) F

Early-morning vomiting is seen in pregnancy, alcohol dependence and some metabolic disorders (e.g. uraemia). Haematochezia means blood in the stools.

A6.37

A) T   B) T   C) T   D) T   E) T

Oral ulceration is seen in gastrointestinal disorders, such as Crohn's disease, ulcerative colitis and coeliac disease in approximately 10–20% of cases. Other diseases associated with oral ulceration include lupus erythematosus (systemic and discoid), Behçet's disease, neutropenia and immunodeficiency disorders. In Reiter's disease, ulceration occurs in approximately 25–30% of patients.

A6.38

A) T   B) T   C) T   D) T   E) T

Certain drugs can cause oral lichenoid eruptions. They include antimalarials, methyldopa, tolbutamide, penicillamine and gold salts.

A6.39

A) F   B) F   C) T   D) T   E) T

Fibrous gingival hyperplasia is a result of hereditary gingival fibromatosis or

Gastrointestinal disease

associated with drugs (e.g. phenytoin, ciclosporin, nifedipine). Inflammatory swellings are seen in pregnancy, gingivitis and scurvy.

A6.40

A) T B) T C) T D) T E) T

Xerostomia (dry mouth) can result from:

- Sjögren's syndrome

- Drugs (e.g. anticholinergic, antiparkinsonian, antihistamines, lithium, monoamine oxidase inhibitors, tricyclic and related antidepressants, and clonidine)

- Radiotherapy

- Psychogenic causes

- Dehydration, shock and renal failure

A6.41

A) T B) T C) T D) T E) T

Causes of dysphagia

Disease of mouth and tongue (e.g. tonsillitis)	Extrinsic pressure: Mediastinal glands
Neuromuscular disorders:	Goitre
Pharyngeal disorders	Enlarged left
Bulbar palsy (e.g.	atrium
motor neurone disease)	Intrinsic lesion:
Myasthenia gravis	Foreign body
Oesophageal motility	Stricture
disorders:	benign –
Achalasia	peptic, corrosive
Scleroderma	malignant –
Diffuse oesophageal	carcinoma
spasm	Lower oesophageal
Presbyoesophagus	rings
Diabetes mellitus	Oesophageal web
Chagas' disease	Pharyngeal pouch

A6.42

A) F B) F C) F D) T E) T

Painful swallowing without real difficulty is a symptom of candidiasis and herpes simplex infection. Both these conditions are seen in AIDS patients. Ingestion of tablets such as bisphosphonates and potassium (slow release) will produce local ulceration if they lodge in the gullet when swallowed lying down and without water.

A6.43

A) F B) T C) F D) T E) F

The upper two-thirds of the stomach contains parietal cells, which secrete hydrochloric acid, and chief cells, which secrete pepsinogen (which initiates proteolysis). The antrum contains mucus-secreting and G cells, which secrete gastrin. Somatostatin is also produced by specialized antral cells (D cells). The duodenal mucosa contains Brunner's glands, which secrete alkaline mucus. Absorption in the stomach is of only minimal importance.

A6.44

A) F B) F C) F D) F E) F

Risk factors for cancer of the oesophagus

Squamous cell carcinoma	Adenocarcinoma
Tobacco smoking	Long-standing
Heavy alcohol intake	GORD
Plummer–Vinson syndrome	Barrett's oesophagus
Achalasia	Tobacco smoking
Coeliac disease	
Tylosis*	
Diet deficient in vitamins; high dietary carotenoids and vitamin C possibly decrease the risk	

* Tylosis is an autosomal dominant condition with hyperkeratosis of the palms and soles

A6.45

A) F   B) F   C) F   D) T   E) F

Squamous cell carcinoma (SCC) of the oesophagus is more common in men. Many gastroenterologists like to go directly to oesophagoscopy which provides histological or cytological proof of the carcinoma; 90% of oesophageal carcinomas can be confirmed with this technique. Barium swallow is also a very sensitive technique and is useful in the younger patient with dysphagia where the differential diagnosis is of a motility disorder. Most patients present with stage 3 disease. Surgery provides the best chance of a cure and should be used only when staging has shown that the tumour has not infiltrated outside the oesophageal wall. Surgery in this group shows an 80% 5-year survival rate if the postoperative pathology confirms the staging. Radiotherapy is used, with limited success, for squamous carcinoma of the upper and middle third of the oesophagus with a 20% 5-year survival for stage 3 disease. Oesophagitis and stricture formation occur. Adenocarcinoma is less radiosensitive.

A6.46

A) F   B) T   C) T   D) T   E) T
F) T   G) T   H) F

Currently favoured regimens are triple therapy with a proton-pump inhibitor (PPI) along with two antibiotics for 1 week. For example: a) omeprazole 20 mg twice daily + metronidazole 400 mg twice daily and clarithromycin 500 mg twice daily; b) omeprazole 20 mg twice daily + clarithromycin 500 mg twice daily and amoxicillin 1 g twice daily. Resistance to amoxicillin has not yet been demonstrated. Tripotassium dicitratobismuthate (bismuth chelate) binds to the ulcer crater and stimulates prostaglandin secretion. It is effective against *H. pylori* and is used in some eradication therapies with two antibiotics. It blackens the tongue and stools. In some regimens, H_2-receptor antagonists, e.g. ranitidine or ranitidine bismuth citrate, are included instead of a PPI.

A6.47

A) T   B) F   C) T   D) T   E) F

In many patients with severe arthritis, stopping NSAIDs may not be possible. Use: a) an NSAID with low GI side-effects at lowest dose possible; b) prophylactic therapy, e.g. proton-pump inhibitor (PPI) or misoprostol for all high-risk patients (i.e. over 65 years), those with a peptic ulcer history, particularly with complications, and patients on therapy with corticosteroids or anticoagulants; c) COX-2 therapy.

A6.48

A) F   B) F   C) F   D) F   E) T

Haematemesis is the vomiting of blood from a lesion proximal to the distal duodenum. Melaena is the passage of black tarry stools; the black colour is due to altered blood – 50 mL or more is required to produce this. Melaena can occur with bleeding from any lesion from areas proximal to and including the caecum. Following a massive bleed from the upper GI tract, unaltered blood (owing to rapid transit) can appear per rectum, but this is rare. The colour of the blood appearing per rectum is dependent not only on the site of bleeding but also on the time of transit in the gut. Chronic peptic ulceration still accounts for approximately half of all cases of upper GI haemorrhage.

Gastrointestinal disease

A6.49

A) T B) F C) T D) F E) F

Aspirin (even 75 mg a day) and other NSAIDs can produce gastric lesions. These agents are also responsible for GI haemorrhage from both duodenal and gastric ulcers, particularly in the elderly. Remember, these drugs are available over the counter and careful questioning is necessary. Corticosteroids in the usual therapeutic doses probably have no influence on GI haemorrhage. Anticoagulants do not cause acute GI haemorrhage *per se* but bleeding from any cause is greater if the patient is anticoagulated. Splenomegaly suggests portal hypertension but its absence does not rule out oesophageal varices. Alcohol in high concentration damages the gastric mucosal barrier and is associated with acute gastric mucosal erosions and subepithelial haemorrhage which can lead to upper GI bleeding.

A6.50

A) F B) F C) T D) F E) T

In upper GI haemorrhage, the major principle is to rapidly restore the blood volume to normal. This can be best achieved by transfusion of whole blood via one or more large-bore intravenous cannulae. It may be necessary to give a blood substitute initially to a severely shocked patient or to a patient with blood compatibility problems. The rate of blood transfusion must be monitored carefully to avoid overtransfusion and consequent heart failure. The pulse rate and venous pressure are the best guides to transfusion rates. All patients with organ failure and requiring blood transfusion as well as patients with severe hypotension should have a central venous pressure line. Anaemia does not develop immediately as haemodilution has not taken place, and therefore the haemoglobin level is a poor indicator of the need to transfuse. If the level is low (less than 10 g/dL) and the patient has either bled recently or is actively bleeding, transfusion may be necessary.

A6.51

A) F B) F C) F D) T E) T

Endoscopy should be performed within 24 hours in most patients. Early endoscopy helps to make a diagnosis and to make decisions regarding discharge from hospital, particularly in patients with minor bleeds and under 60 years of age. Urgent endoscopy (i.e. after resuscitation) should be performed in patients with shock, suspected liver disease or with continued bleeding. Endoscopy can detect the cause of the haemorrhage in 80% or more of cases. In patients with a peptic ulcer, if the stigmata of a recent bleed are seen (i.e. a spurting artery, active oozing, fresh or organized blood clot or black spots) the patient is more likely to re-bleed. At first endoscopy all bleeding ulcers should be either injected with adrenaline (epinephrine) and a sclerosant or the vessel coagulated either with a heater probe or with laser therapy. In one study intravenous omeprazole substantially reduced the re-bleeding rate in this group and should be given.

A6.52

A) F B) F C) F D) T E) F

All bleeding ulcers should be either injected with adrenaline (epinephrine) and a sclerosant or the vessel coagulated either with a heater probe or with laser therapy. These methods reduce the incidence of re-bleeding, although they do not significantly improve mortality as re-bleeding still occurs in 20% within 72 hours. There is little evidence that H_2-receptor antagonists or proton-pump inhibitors (PPIs) affect the mortality rate of GI haemorrhage, but PPIs are usually given to patients with ulcers because of their longer-term benefits. Below the age of 60 years mortality from GI bleeding is small, <0.1%, but above the age of 80 the mortality is greater than 20%. Patients with recurrent haemorrhage have an increased mortality. Melaena is usually less hazardous than haematemesis.

stimulates the release of enterokinase, which activates trypsinogen to trypsin, and this in turn activates the other proenzymes, chymotrypsin and elastase. These enzymes break down protein into oligopeptides. Some di- and tripeptides are absorbed intact by a carrier-mediated process, while the remainder are broken down into free amino acids by peptidases on the microvillus membranes of the cell, prior to absorption in a similar way to disaccharides. These amino acids are transported into the cell by a variety of carrier systems.

A6.53

A) T B) F C) T D) T E) T F) F

Nutrients can be absorbed throughout the small intestine, with the exception of vitamin B_{12} and bile salts, which have specific receptors in the terminal ileum. Glucose enters the enterocyte on the luminal side via a sodium-dependent carrier molecule (sodium/glucose cotransporter I, SGLTI) and leaves on the serosal side via a sodium-independent carrier (Glut-2) that is found in the basolateral membrane. The breakdown products of starch digestion, together with sucrose and lactose, are hydrolysed on the brush border membrane by their appropriate oligo- and disaccharidases to form the monosaccharides glucose, galactose and fructose. These monosaccharides are transported into the cells. Dietary fat consists mainly of triglycerides with some cholesterol and fat-soluble vitamins. Emulsification of fat occurs in the stomach and is followed by hydrolysis of triglycerides in the duodenum by pancreatic lipase to yield fatty acids and monoglycerides. Dietary protein is digested by pancreatic enzymes prior to absorption. These proteolytic enzymes are secreted by the pancreas as proenzymes and transformed to active enzymes in the lumen. The presence of protein in the lumen

A6.54

A) T B) F C) F D) T E) T

The contractile patterns of the small intestinal muscular layers are primarily determined by integrated neural circuits within the gut wall – the enteric nervous system. During fasting, a distally migrating sequence of motor events termed the migrating motor complexes (MMC) occurs in a cyclical fashion. The MMC consists of a period of motor quiescence (phase I) followed by a period of irregular contractile activity (phase II), culminating in a short (5–10 minutes) burst of regular phasic contractions (phase III). In the duodenum, phase III is associated with increased gastric, pancreatic and biliary secretions. The role of the MMC is unclear, but the strong phase III contractions propel secretions, residual food and desquamated cells towards the colon, acting as an 'intestinal housekeeper'. After a meal, the MMC pattern is disrupted and replaced by irregular contractions. This seemingly chaotic-fed pattern lasts typically for 2–5 hours, depending on the size and nutrient content of the meal. The irregular contractions of the fed pattern have a mixing function, moving intraluminal contents to and fro, aiding the digestive process.

Gastrointestinal disease

A6.55

A) F B) F C) T D) T E) T

Coeliac disease is a condition in which there is an inflammation of the jejunal mucosa that improves when the patient is treated with a gluten-free diet and relapses when gluten is reintroduced. Gluten is contained in the cereals wheat, rye and barley. Coeliac disease can present at any age. It occurs throughout the world, but is rare in black Africans. There is an increased incidence of coeliac disease within families but the exact mode of inheritance is unknown; 10–15% of first-degree relatives will have the condition, although it may be asymptomatic. Gluten is a high-molecular-weight, heterogeneous compound that can be fractionated to produce α-, β-, γ- and ω-gliadin peptides. α-Gliadin is the main damaging peptide to the small intestinal mucosa although the other peptides are also 'toxic'. The exact mechanism of how the damage is produced is still not understood.

A6.56

A) T B) T C) T D) T E) T

Infertility and neuropsychiatric symptoms of anxiety and depression may occur in coeliac disease. Osteoporosis is common. Rare complications include tetany, osteomalacia, or gross malnutrition with peripheral oedema. Neurological symptoms such as paraesthesia, muscle weakness or a polyneuropathy occur.

A6.57

A) T B) T C) F D) T E) T

In coeliac disease there is an increased incidence of atopy and autoimmune disease, including thyroid disease, insulin-dependent diabetes, primary biliary cirrhosis and Sjögren's syndrome. Other associated diseases include inflammatory bowel disease, chronic liver disease, fibrosing allergic alveolitis and epilepsy. IgA deficiency is more common than in the general population.

A6.58

A) F B) T C) F D) F E) F

The following occur in ileal resection. a) Bile salts and fatty acids enter the colon and cause malabsorption of water and electrolytes leading to diarrhoea. b) Increased bile salt synthesis can compensate for loss of approximately one-third of the bile salts in the faeces. Greater loss than this results in decreased micellar formation and steatorrhoea, and lithogenic bile and gallstone formation. c) Increased oxalate absorption is caused by the presence of bile salts in the colon. This gives rise to renal oxalate stones. d) There is a low serum B_{12} and macrocytosis. e) Glucagon-like peptide 2 (GLP-2) is low following ileal resection. GLP-2 is a specific growth hormone for the enterocyte and this deficiency may explain the lack of adaptation with an ileal resection.

A6.59

A) F B) T C) F D) F E) T

Port-mortem studies have shown the incidence of adenomas to be 30–40% in western populations, and more than 70% of colorectal cancers develop from sporadic adenomatous polyps. Polyps rarely produce symptoms and most are diagnosed on X-ray or on colonoscopy performed for other reasons. Large polyps may bleed intermittently and cause anaemia. The National Polyp Study conducted in the USA showed that colonoscopic polypectomy with surveillance reduced colorectal cancer incidence by 76–90%. Current recommendations, based on this study, suggest that surveillance colonoscopy intervals of around 6 years after polypectomy are appropriate.

A 6.60

A) T   B) T   C) F   D) T   E) F

Familial adenomatous polyposis (FAP) arises from germline mutations of the *APC* gene located on chromosome 5q and is inherited in an autosomal dominant fashion. The mean age of adenoma development is 16 years, whereas the average age for developing colorectal cancer is 39 years. Tracing and screening of relatives is essential (usually after 12 years of age) and affected individuals should be offered a prophylactic colectomy, often before the age of 20. Extraintestinal lesions include osteomas, epidermoid cysts and desmoid tumours. Congenital hypertrophy of the retinal pigment epithelium (CHRPE) occurs in many families with FAP.

A 6.61

A) F   B) T   C) T   D) T   E) T

Hereditary non-polyposis colorectal cancer (HNPCC) arises from germline mutations in any one of five mismatch repair (MMR) genes. Mutations in two of these, *hMLH1* and *hMSH2*, account for >95% of HNPCC families. Mutations in these genes lead to microsatellite instability in the tumours of affected individuals. Modified Amsterdam Criteria for hereditary non-polyposis colorectal cancer include: a) three or more cases of colorectal cancer in a minimum of two generations; b) one affected individual must be a first-degree relative of the other two (or more) cases; c) one case must be diagnosed at age <50; d) colorectal cancer can be replaced by endometrial or small bowel cancer; e) familial adenomatous polyposis should be excluded.

A 6.62

A) T   B) T   C) T   D) F   E) F

Patients aged more than 35–40 years presenting with new large bowel symptoms should be investigated. The alarm symptoms suggestive of colorectal cancer include: change in bowel habit, rectal bleeding, anorexia and weight loss, faecal incontinence, tenesmus and passing mucus per rectum. Colonoscopy is the gold standard for investigation and allows biopsies and polypectomies to obtain specimens for histological examination. About 80% of patients with colorectal cancer undergo surgery though fewer than half survive more than 5 years. Long-term survival is only likely when the cancer is completely removed. Adjuvant postoperative chemotherapy will improve disease-free survival and overall survival in TNM stage III (Dukes' C) colon cancer. Cancers with high levels of microsatellite instability may have a more favourable outlook.

A 6.63

A) T   B) T   C) T   D) T   E) T

Causes of bile acid malabsorption

Ileal resection
Ileal disease, e.g. active or inactive Crohn's disease
Idiopathic or primary bile acid malabsorption (structurally normal ileum)
Postinfective gastroenteritis
Associated with:
    Post-cholecystectomy diarrhoea
    Diabetic diarrhoea
    Post-vagotomy diarrhoea
    Chronic pancreatitis
    Cystic fibrosis
    Coeliac disease
    Microscopic inflammatory colitis
    Drugs (e.g. colchicine, biguanides)

Bile acid malabsorption is an underdiagnosed cause of chronic diarrhoea.

Gastrointestinal disease

A6.64

1) D   2) E   3) B   4) C   5) A

Therapies for irritable bowel syndrome (IBS) include hydroxytryptamine ($5HT_3$)-receptor antagonists for diarrhoea-predominant IBS and $5HT_4$-receptor agonists for constipation-predominant IBS. In the acute abdomen, high levels of serum amylase (more than five times normal) indicate acute pancreatitis. Raised levels below this can occur in any acute abdomen and should not be considered diagnostic of pancreatitis. In acute appendicitis most patients present with abdominal pain; in many it starts vaguely in the centre of the abdomen, becoming localized to the right iliac fossa in the first few hours. Nausea, vomiting and occasional diarrhoea can occur. Because of the motile position of the appendix, symptoms and signs are variable. Examination of the abdomen reveals tenderness in the right iliac fossa, with guarding due to the localized peritonitis. In the Fitz-Hugh–Curtis syndrome the chlamydia infection tracks up the right paracolic gutter to cause a perihepatitis. Patients can present with acute right hypochondrial pain, fever and mildly abnormal liver biochemistry.

A6.65

A) T   B) F   C) F   D) F   E) F

In acute disease, subtotal colectomy with end ileostomy and preservation of the rectum is the operation of choice. At a later date a number of surgical options are available. These include proctectomy with a permanent ileostomy. To avoid a permanent ileostomy, ileorectal anastomosis can be performed. With an ileo-anal anastomosis, a pouch of ileum is formed that acts as a reservoir. The pouch is anastomosed to the anus at the dentate line following endoanal excision of the mucosa of the distal rectum and anal canal. Continence is usually achieved. The incidence of 'pouchitis' is twice as high in patients with primary sclerosing cholangitis. In the hopes of improving night-time continence some surgeons advocate stapling the reservoir to the lower rectal or upper anal mucosa (ileal pouch–distal rectal anastomosis). The disadvantage of this technique is the cancer risk associated with the residual diseased mucosa.

A6.66

A) F   B) T   C) F   D) F   E) F

Women with inactive inflammatory bowel disease (IBD) have normal fertility. Fertility, however, may be reduced in those with active disease, and patients with active disease are twice as likely to suffer spontaneous abortion than those with inactive disease. Although the risk of an exacerbation of IBD is not increased in pregnancy, when exacerbations occur they do so most commonly in the first trimester and during the immediate postpartum period. Aminosalicylates, steroids and azathioprine are safe at the time of conception and during pregnancy.

A6.67

A) F   B) F   C) F   D) F   E) T

A third of patients with distal inflammatory proctitis due to ulcerative colitis will develop more proximal disease, with 5–10% developing total colitis. A third of patients with ulcerative colitis will have a single attack and the others will have a relapsing course. A third of patients with ulcerative colitis will undergo colectomy within 20 years of diagnosis. About 60–70% will require a second operation.

A6.68

A) F   B) F   C) F   D) F   E) F

Ulcerative colitis (UC) is more common among relatives of patients than in the general population; 6–10% of patients affected with UC have one or more relatives with the disease. The risk of UC in first-degree relatives of a Crohn's disease (CD) patient is eight times higher than in the general population. There is an increased risk of UC in non- or ex-smokers and nicotine has been shown to be an effective treatment in UC. Ulcerative colitis can affect the rectum alone (proctitis), can extend proximally to involve the sigmoid and descending colon (left-sided colitis), or may involve the whole colon (total colitis). In a few of these patients there is also inflammation of the distal terminal ileum (backwash ileitis). In Crohn's disease the inflammation extends through all layers (transmural) of the bowel, whereas in ulcerative colitis a superficial inflammation is seen. Enteric fistulae, e.g. to bladder or vagina, occur in 20–40% of cases of Crohn's disease, equally divided between internal and external fistulae; the latter usually occurring after surgery.

A6.69

A) F   B) T   C) F   D) T   E) F

The aim of management is to induce and then maintain a remission. Patients with mild symptoms may require only symptomatic treatment. Diarrhoea can be controlled with loperamide, codeine phosphate or diphenoxylate. Corticosteroids are commonly used to induce remission in moderate and severe attacks of Crohn's disease. Enteral nutrition is an underutilized means of inducing remission in moderate and severe attacks of Crohn's disease, and efficacy is independent of nutritional status. Mycophenolate mofetil, which suppresses the proliferation of T and B lymphocytes, is also effective in maintaining remission. Biological treatments directed against specific inflammatory mediators, e.g. anti-TNFα antibody (infliximab), are being used. A single infusion of this has been shown to be effective in producing clinical improvement in up to 60% of patients with steroid-resistant disease, and in those responding to the initial infusion, a further four doses at 8-weekly intervals had maintained remission in 50% of patients by 8 weeks after the final infusion.

A6.70

A) F   B) T   C) T   D) T   E) T   F) F

Definition of a severe attack of ulcerative colitis	
Stool frequency	>6 stools per day with blood
Fever	>37.5°C
Tachycardia	>90 per minute
ESR	>30 mm per hour
Anaemia	Haemoglobin <10 g/dL
Albumin	<30 g/L

7

Liver, biliary tract and pancreatic disease

Q7.1

A 49-year-old patient with cirrhosis presents with melaena. Urgent upper GI endoscopy does not reveal varices or peptic ulceration. There is chronic gastric congestion, punctate erythema and gastric erosions. Which one of the following is the most likely source of the bleeding?

A. Variceal haemorrhage
B. Rectal polyps
C. Portal hypertensive gastropathy
D. Mallory–Weiss syndrome
E. Duodenal ulcer

Q7.2

A patient presents with jaundice, vomiting and abdominal pain in the last trimester of pregnancy. Investigations reveal hepatocellular damage, hyperuricaemia and thrombocytopenia. CT scanning of the liver shows low density. Liver biopsy is most likely to show which one of the following?

A. Macronodular cirrhosis
B. Micronodular cirrhosis
C. Centrilobular necrosis
D. Microvesicles of fat in liver cells with little necrosis
E. Subcapsular haematoma

Q7.3

A 51-year-old woman with ischaemic heart disease and primary biliary cirrhosis presents with haematemesis. Which one of the following is the best choice to stop bleeding from oesophageal varices?

A. Propranolol
B. Terlipressin infusion
C. Somatostatin infusion
D. Balloon tamponade
E. Acute variceal sclerotherapy and banding

Q7.4

A 48-year-old alcoholic with ascites presents with clinical deterioration of her general condition. On examination she is afebrile and there is no tenderness. Ascitic fluid cell count reveals 400 cell/mm^3. Which one of the following statements is correct?

A. Since the patient is afebrile she needs no treatment but should be observed in hospital
B. There is sufficient evidence to start antibiotic treatment with a third-generation cephalosporin
C. The clinical picture is an absolute contraindication for liver transplantation
D. The prognosis is excellent
E. Prednisolone should be injected into the ascitic fluid

Q7.5

A 42-year-old alcoholic with cirrhosis is being diuresed vigorously. Urine output falls, blood urea nitrogen (BUN) increases and urine sodium is low. Select the most likely finding on renal biopsy

A. The glomeruli are damaged
B. The collecting tubules are damaged
C. Tubular function is intact
D. Renal artery stenosis
E. Loop of Henle is damaged

Q7.6

A 45-year-old woman presents with itching and jaundice. Which of the following is the investigation of first choice?

A. Plain X-ray abdomen
B. Ultrasound of the abdomen
C. Cholecystogram
D. ^{99m}Tc-iodide scan
E. CT of abdomen
F. Magnetic resonance imaging of the abdomen

Q7.7

A 42-year-old patient undergoes liver biopsy. Two days after the biopsy she develops biliary colic, jaundice and melaena. Which of the following is the most likely diagnosis?

A. Hepatitis A
B. Hepatitis B
C. Haemobilia
D. Intraperitoneal bleeding
E. Glycogen storage disease

Q7.8

A 42-year-old woman drinks one large whisky a day. She now presents with jaundice and itching. On examination she has xanthomas in the palmar creases and above the eyes. Which of the following is the most likely diagnosis?

A. Haemochromatosis
B. Primary biliary cirrhosis
C. Hepatitis A
D. Hepatitis B
E. Wilson's disease

Q7.9

A 42-year-old woman with primary biliary cirrhosis is referred to liver transplantation. Which one of the following makes it most likely that she will be considered for transplantation?

A. Albumin 45 g/L, bilirubin 25 μmol/L and absence of ascites
B. Albumin 45 g/L, bilirubin 50 μmol/L and absence of ascites
C. Albumin 35 g/L, bilirubin 90 μmol/L and absence of ascites
D. Albumin 28 g/L, bilirubin 111 μmol/L and presence of ascites
E. Albumin 33 g/L, bilirubin 25 μmol/L and absence of ascites

Q7.10

A 17-year-old nursing student is brought in confused and disoriented. She was seen to be active and normal the day before. On examination she has jaundice with signs of hepatic encephalopathy. Investigations reveal hyperbilirubinaemia and high serum aminotransferases. Paracetamol overdose is confirmed. Which one of the following suggests the need for liver transplantation?

Liver, biliary tract and pancreatic disease

A. Arterial pH >7.3
B. Serum creatinine >300 μmol/L, PT >100 s, Grade IV hepatic encephalopathy
C. Serum creatinine >300 μmol/L, PT >50 s, Grade II hepatic encephalopathy
D. Interval from onset of jaundice to encephalopathy >7 days
E. Serum creatinine >300 μmol/L, PT >5 s, Grade III hepatic encephalopathy

Q7.11

1. A 49-year-old woman with primary biliary cirrhosis

2. A 42-year-old woman with autoimmune hepatitis

3. A 67-year-old man with hepatocellular carcinoma

4. A 25-year-old man with Wilson's disease

5. A 45-year-old male non-smoker with emphysema and cirrhosis

6. A 57-year-old man with haemochromatosis

7. A 29-year-old woman with sclerosing cholangitis

Among the following blood tests, select the best option for each of the above

A. α-Fetoprotein
B. Serum ferritin
C. α_1-Antitrypsin
D. Antinuclear, smooth muscle (actin), liver/kidney microsomal antibody
E. Antinuclear cytoplasmic antibodies
F. Serum caeruloplasmin
G. Antimitochondrial antibodies

Q7.12

1. A 29-year-old hypertensive is on medication for the control of blood pressure. Serum bilirubin is 102 μmol/L, the level of unconjugated bilirubin is raised, serum transferases, alkaline phosphatase and albumin are normal. Serum haptoglobins are low

2. A 22-year-old man is asymptomatic and on routine annual check his serum bilirubin is 6 mg/dL (102 μmol/L) and the unconjugated bilirubin level rises on fasting. All other liver biochemistry is normal and there are no signs of liver disease. Reticulocyte count is normal. There is a family history of jaundice

3. An 18-year-old man presents with jaundice with elevated unconjugated bilirubin. Liver histology is normal. Mutation of the gene for UDP-glucoronosyl transferase has been demonstrated in this condition

4. A 28-year-old woman presents with jaundice. She has conjugated bilirubinaemia and liver biopsy shows melanin deposition

5. A 31-year-old woman presents with recurrent attacks of jaundice, severe itching, steatorrhoea and weight loss. The patient has conjugated bilirubinaemia and serum γ-GT is normal. The gene responsible has been mapped to the FICI locus

Which of the following best matches each of the above?

A. Recurrent familial intrahepatic cholestasis or benign recurrent intrahepatic cholestasis
B. Dubin–Johnson syndrome
C. Crigler–Najjar syndrome
D. Gilbert's syndrome
E. Methyldopa treatment

Q7.13

1. A 25-year-old man presents with fever. He has mild jaundice and minor abnormalities of liver biochemistry. Peripheral blood shows atypical lymphocytes. Five days later he undergoes liver biopsy which shows that the sinusoids and portal tracts are infiltrated with large mononuclear cells but the liver architecture is preserved. A Paul–Bunnell test is positive

2. A 27-year-old kidney transplant recipient presents with acute hepatitis. The offending virus is isolated in the urine. The liver biopsy shows intranuclear inclusions and giant cells

3. A 42-year-old businessman who travels frequently presents with jaundice. Liver biopsy shows hepatic necrosis. The viral infection he has is carried by the mosquito *Aedes aegypti*

4. A 32-year-old heart transplant recipient presents with acute hepatitis. He has cold sores around his lips. Aminotransferases are massively elevated. Liver biopsy shows extensive necrosis. Aciclovir is used to treat this patient's infection

5. A 25-year-old man presents with fever. He has mild jaundice and minor abnormalities of liver biochemistry. A Paul–Bunnell test is negative. The Sabin–Feldman dye test is positive

Select the best match for each of the above

A. Toxoplasmosis
B. Cytomegalovirus
C. Herpes simplex
D. Yellow fever
E. Infectious mononucleosis

Q7.14

1. A 44-year-old man with chronic hepatitis B and decompensated liver disease

2. A 23-year-old man with chronic hepatitis on histology with HCV RNA in the serum and elevated aminotransferases for 6 months

3. A 33-year-old patient with chronic liver disease who is HBsAg-positive and also has anti-delta antibody. Reverse polymerase chain reaction (PCR) reveals HDV RNA in the serum

4. An 18-year-old woman who has had jaundice and elevated aminotransferases which have not improved with time. Anti-liver/kidney (anti-LKM1) antibodies are present. Liver biopsy shows chronic hepatitis

5. A 25-year-old patient with chronic hepatitis. Liver biopsy shows the changes of chronic hepatitis. Plasma cell infiltration is seen. Serum IgG is twice normal. Antinuclear and anti-smooth muscle antibodies are detected

Select the best match for each of the above

A. Treatment is with alpha-interferon only since there are few data regarding the use of lamivudine
B. Interferon should not be routinely used but the patient could be treated with lamivudine
C. Combination therapy with alpha-interferon and ribavirin
D. Combination therapy with prednisolone and azathioprine
E. Treatment with aspirin only

Liver, biliary tract and pancreatic disease

Q7.15

1. A 22-year-old woman with schizophrenia is started on chlorpromazine. She develops jaundice and elevated liver enzymes

2. A 16-year-old nursing student takes an overdose of paracetamol

3. A 44-year-old olympic runner has been ingesting anabolic steroids

4. A 29-year-old woman with menorrhagia is being treated with ferrous sulphate

5. A 67-year-old patient with rheumatoid arthritis is being treated with methotrexate

Select the best match for each of the above

A. Zone 1 necrosis of liver
B. Zone 3 necrosis of liver
C. Pelioses hepatitis
D. Liver fibrosis
E. Hepatocanalicular cholestasis

Q7.16

1. A 42-year-old patient presents with variceal haemorrhage. Liver histology shows mild portal fibrosis

2. A 29-year-old farmer from Egypt presents with melaena. On examination the patient has ascites. Liver biopsy shows extensive pipe-stem fibrosis

3. A 45-year-old woman presents with abdominal distension. On examination she has mild jaundice. The liver is enlarged and the caudate lobe of the liver is palpable. The hepatojugular reflex is negative and the spleen is palpable

4. A 17-year-old patient presents with recurrent attacks of fever, abdominal pain and Gram-negative septicaemia. Jaundice and portal hypertension are absent. Endoscopic retrograde cholangiopancreatography (ERCP) shows saccular dilatation of intrahepatic ducts

5. 45-year-old man presents with loss of appetite and weight loss. On examination there is deep jaundice, hepatomegaly, splenomegaly and ascites. Liver biopsy shows fatty change, infiltration by polymorphonuclear leucocytes and hepatocyte necrosis mainly in zone 3. The patient has dense cytoplasmic inclusions called Mallory bodies and giant mitochondria. In addition he has micronodular cirrhosis.

Select the best match for each of the above

A. Caroli's disease
B. Alcoholic liver disease
C. Schistosomiasis
D. Non-cirrhotic portal fibrosis
E. Budd–Chiari syndrome
F. Wilson's disease
G. Primary biliary cirrhosis
H. Amoebic liver disease
I. Malaria

Q7.17

A 43-year-old woman complains of pruritus. On examination she has hepatomegaly but no jaundice. Blood tests reveal a raised serum alkaline phosphatase and autoantibodies. Pigmented xanthelasma are seen on the eyelids. The following statements about this condition are correct

A. The presence of antimitochondrial antibodies in high titre correlates with the severity of the condition
B. The presence of antimitochondrial antibodies in high titre correlates with the histological picture of this condition
C. Serum antimitochondrial antibodies are found in almost all patients with this condition

D. The antigen to M2 antibody is specific to this condition
E. Ursodeoxycholic acid improves long-term prognosis
F. Given her clinical picture, it is likely that this patient will die of liver failure in 5 years unless transplanted
G. Keratoconjunctivitis sicca occurs in over two-thirds of cases

Q7.18

A 39-year-old newly diagnosed diabetic complains of shortness of breath. On examination he has hepatomegaly, skin pigmentation and hypogonadism. Echocardiography reveals cardiomegaly. The following statements about his condition are correct

A. Most patients with this condition are homozygous for the Cys 282 Tyr mutation
B. There is an increase in total iron binding capacity
C. The most likely diagnosis is Wilson's disease
D. Venesection prolongs life in this condition
E. Liver biochemistry is often normal even with established cirrhosis
F. The risk of malignancy remains despite venesection
G. Serum ferritin is used as a screeing test to detect early and asymptomatic disease in all first-degree relatives
H. Diabetes, testicular atrophy and chondrocalcinosis disappear with venesection

Q7.19

An 18-year-old man presents to the neurologist with tremor, dysarthria and involuntary movements. On examination the patient has signs of chronic liver disease and a greenish brown pigment at the corneoscleral junction. The following statements are correct

A. The diagnosis is hereditary haemochromatosis
B. This condition is an autosomal dominant disorder
C. The basic problem is a failure of biliary excretion of iron
D. In most patients serum caeruloplasmin is elevated
E. Liver biopsy varies from chronic hepatitis to macronodular cirrhosis
F. The patient requires lifetime therapy with penicillamine
G. Liver transplantation is contraindicated in this condition

Q7.20

A 45-year-old alcoholic patient has severe liver disease. The following processes may be affected

A. Degradation of amino acids
B. Glucose homeostasis
C. Synthesis of albumin
D. Synthesis of gamma globulins
E. Coagulation cascade

Liver, biliary tract and pancreatic disease

Q7.21

A 29-year-old man has dyslipidaemia. The following statements are correct

A. Triglycerides can be of dietary origin but most are synthesized in the liver
B. Cholesterol is mainly of dietary origin but is also formed in the liver
C. Hepatic lipase removes triglyceride from intermediate-density lipoproteins to produce low-density lipoproteins
D. The liver synthesizes very-low-density lipoproteins
E. Lecithin–cholesterol acyltransferase catalyses the conversion of free cholesterol to cholesterol ester

Q7.22

In the liver the multidrug resistance protein mediates the transport of

A. Sodium
B. Water
C. Bilirubin diglucoronide
D. Glucuronidated bile acids
E. Sulphated bile acids

Q7.23

Bile acids

A. Are synthesized in hepatocytes from cholesterol
B. Are conjugated with glycine
C. Are converted into secondary bile acids by intestinal bacteria
D. Undergo enterohepatic circulation
E. Act as detergents; their main function is lipid solubilization

Q7.24

A 27-year-old student nurse has jaundice. She obtaines information about bilirubin metabolism on the internet. The following statements are accurate

A. Bilirubin is produced mainly from the breakdown of myoglobin
B. Normally the body does not produce any bilirubin
C. The enzyme uridine diphosphoglucurosyl transferase catalyses the formation of bilirubin monoglucuronide
D. Conjugated bilirubin is water-soluble
E. Conjugated bilirubin is absorbed in the small intestine
F. Urobilinogen is formed in the intestine
G. When hepatic excretion of conjugated bilirubin is impaired, a small amount of conjugated bilirubin is found strongly bound to serum albumin

Q7.25

A 42-year-old woman with alcoholic cirrhosis presents with anorexia, nausea and vomiting. Her liver function tests show a prolonged International Normalized Ratio (INR), serum albumin of 20 mg/dL, mildly elevated aminotransferases and alkaline phosphatase. The following statements about liver function tests are correct

A. Aspartate aminotransferase is more specific to liver disease than alanine aminotransferase
B. A raised serum alkaline phosphatase in cholestasis helps to differentiate between intrahepatic liver disease and disease from an extahepatic cause
C. In liver disease the globulin fraction is depressed
D. A falling serum albumin is a bad prognostic sign

E. An elevated prothrombin time despite vitamin K therapy excludes liver disease

Q7.26

A second-year medical student on examination of the hands of a patient correctly detects palmar erythema. This occurs in the following conditions

A. Cardiogenic shock
B. Pregnancy
C. Thyrotoxicosis
D. Rheumatoid arthritis
E. Severe acute liver disease

Q7.27

A 15-year-old schoolboy living in India presents with nausea, anorexia and distaste for his favourite foods. On examination the liver is moderately enlarged and the spleen is just palpable. Complete blood count reveals leucopenia with relative lymphocytosis. Serum bilirubin is elevated but serum alkaline phosphatase is only minimally elevated. Aspartate aminotransferase and alanine aminotransferase are both raised. The following statements are correct

A. The virus causing this hepatitis is a DNA virus
B. This condition has a carrier state
C. The incubation period is less than 3 weeks
D. Spread of infection is by the faeco-oral route
E. Chronic liver disease is a common feature

Q7.28

A 15-year-old schoolboy living in India presents with nausea, anorexia and distaste for his favourite foods. On examination the liver is moderately enlarged and the spleen is just palpable. Complete blood count reveals leucopenia with relative lymphocytosis. Serum bilirubin is elevated but serum alkaline phosphatase is only minimally elevated. Aspartate aminotransferase and alanine aminotransferase are both raised. Extra-hepatic complications of this condition include

A. Arthritis
B. Vasculitis
C. Myocarditis
D. Renal failure
E. Osteomyelitis

Q7.29

A 22-year-old woman living in the Middle East presents with nausea and anorexia and is passing dark-coloured urine. The patient also has a maculopapular rash and polyarthritis of the small joints during the prodromal period. On examination the liver is moderately enlarged and the patient is jaundiced. Serum bilirubin is elevated but serum alkaline phosphatase is only minimally elevated. Aspartate aminotransferase and alanin aminotransferase are both raised. HbeAg is elevated. The following statements are correct

A. HBeAg is more useful than HBV DNA in detecting infectivity
B. The spread of this condition is through the faeco-oral route
C. Liver cancer is a well-recognized feature of this condition

Liver, biliary tract and pancreatic disease

D. Active immunization of this condition is with a recombinant yeast vaccine produced by the insertion of a plasmid containing the gene of HbsAg into a yeast
E. A carrier state has been described in this condition

A. Elevated serum aminotransferases
B. INR >3.0
C. Respiratory acidosis
D. Serum creatinine >300 µmol/L
E. Hypotension after resuscitation with fluid

Q7.30

A 42-year-old man who is a former intravenous drug abuser has routine blood tests which reveal a raised alanine transferase. ELISA-3 assay incorporating antigens NS3, NS4 and NS5 regions of the offending hepatitis virus is positive. The following statements are correct

A. Sexual transmission plays a major role in the transmission of this viral agent
B. There is a higher incidence of diabetes in this condition
C. The virus is transmitted by blood and blood products
D. Interferon is useful when administered early in acute cases
E. Cirrhosis develops in about 20–30% of patients within 10–30 years

Q7.31

A 17-year-old nursing student is brought in confused and disoriented. She was seen to be active and normal the day before. On examination she has jaundice with signs of hepatic encephalopathy. Neurological examination reveals spasticity and plantar responses are flexor. Investigations reveal hyperbilirubinaemia and high serum aminotransferases. Transfer criteria to specialized units for patients with liver injury include

Q7.32

A 33-year-old woman, 3 months after the delivery of her daughter, develops colicky pain in the right upper quadrant area. The following statements are correct

A. An abdominal ultrasound is the single most useful investigation for the diagnosis of gallstone-related disease
B. Cholecystectomy is the treatment of choice for virtually all patients with symptomatic gall bladder stones
C. Chenodeoxycholic acid should be used for almost pure cholesterol stones with a diameter of less than 10 mm
D. Simvastatin is contraindicated in patients who are on ursodeoxycholic acid for dissolution of gallstones
E. Fragmentation of stones with extracorporeal shock wave lithotripsy tends to occur when the stones are greater than 10 mm in diameter

Q7.33

A 34-year-old woman presents with colicky abdominal pain and fever. On examination she has icterus and tenderness in the right upper quadrant. The following statements are correct

A. The presence of fever indicates biliary sepsis
B. A bilirubin concentration >200 µmol/L reflects complete bile duct obstruction
C. The initial imaging technique of choice is abdominal ultrasound

D. Even a mild elevation of serum amylase indicates pancreatitis
E. CT with i.v. contrast is of limited use in obese patients
F. Although endoscopic retrograde cholangiography is useful in diagnosis it has no role in the treatment of this condition

Q7.34

A 40-year-old man with a history of inflammatory bowel disease presents with a history of fluctuating pruritus, jaundice and cholangitis. The following statements about this condition are correct

A. The cholangiogram characteristically shows both intra- and extrahepatic bile duct strictures
B. Liver histology shows inflammation of the intrahepatic biliary radicals with considerable associated scar tissue classically described as being onion skin in appearance
C. This condition ultimately leads to cirrhosis
D. Cholangiocarcinoma occurs in about four-fifths of patients with this condition
E. The only proven treatment is liver transplantation

Q7.35

A 56-year-old woman presents with epigastric pain often accompanied by nausea and vomiting of 8 hours duration. Physical examination reveals some tenderness in the upper abdominal region and periumbilical bruising. The white cell count is 17×10^9/L, blood glucose 8 mmol/L, serum urea 20 mmol/L, serum albumin 28 g/L, serum aminotransferase 300 U/L, serum calcium 1.8 mmol/L,

serum LDH 700 U/L and P_aO_2 7 kPa. The following statements about this condition are correct

A. Morphine derivatives are the drugs of choice for pain control
B. A three-fold elevation of the serum amylase within 24 hours of the onset of pain is an extremely sensitive test
C. An erect chest X-ray is mandatory in this patient
D. Endoscopic retrograde cholangiopancreatography is the investigation of choice for diagnosis
E. The prognosis in this patient is excellent

Q7.36

A 48-year-old alcoholic man presents with epigastric pain radiating to the back. He has had several such episodes in the past 18 months during which he has had anorexia. In addition the patient has steatorrhoea and severe weight loss. The following statements regarding this condition are correct

A. Serum amylase and lipase levels have considerable diagnostic value in this condition
B. Faecal elastase levels will be abnormal in a majority of patients with moderate to severe pancreatic disease
C. Magnetic resonance cholangiopancreatography has largely replaced endoscopic retrograde cholangiopancreatography for confirming the diagnosis
D. Tricyclic antidepressants should not be used for the management of chronic pain
E. The most common structural complication of chronic pancreatitis is a pancreatic pseudocyst

Liver, biliary tract and pancreatic disease

Q7.37

A 65-year-old woman presents with abdominal pain, anorexia and weight loss. The pain is dull in character with radiation to the back. There is partial relief of pain on sitting forward. The gall bladder is palpable. The patient has associated polyarthritis and skin nodules. The following statements about this condition are correct

A. Contrast enhanced spiral CT is an essential part of assessment prior to surgical resection
B. Percutaneous needle biopsy is essential before surgery
C. The CA19.9 levels are highly sensitive
D. The CA242 levels are high false-positive compared to CA19.9 levels
E. The 5-year survival rate for this condition is close to 50%
F. In the majority of the cases the management is palliative

Q7.38

A 42-year-old patient has had hepatitis for 8 months. The following statements are correct

A. Cell infiltrates comprising lymphyocytes and plasma cells are typically absent in the portal tracts
B. The degree of hepatitis and inflammation is used for staging the hepatitis
C. The severity of fibrosis or cirrhosis is used for grading the hepatitis
D. 'Piecemeal necrosis' is preferred to 'interface hepatitis' to describe the loss of definition of the portal/periportal limiting plate
E. The chronic nature of this patient's hepatitis excludes viral aetiology

Q7.39

A 42-year-old man is diagnosed with cirrhosis. The following statements are correct

A. Over a period of 10 years about a fifth of such patients develop gastro-oesophageal varices
B. About two-thirds of patients with varices will bleed from them
C. With advanced therapeutic techniques the mortality from variceal haemorrhage is less than 1%
D. Bleeding is less likely to occur with large varices with red signs on the varices
E. In a patient with melaena upper GI endoscopy is not required to confirm the diagnosis of varices since there is clinical evidence of bleeding

Q7.40

A 49-year-old woman with cirrhosis is readmitted with haematemesis. She had a similar episode a week ago when her varices were injected with a sclerosing agent and banded. The following statements are correct

A. Only a small minority of patients rebleed within 10 days
B. Transjugular intrahepatic portocaval shunt (TIPS) is used because it has been shown to improve portal hypertension in the long term
C. Oesophageal transection and ligation of feeding vessels is the most common surgical technique used when other measures fail
D. Acute portosystemic shunt surgery is infrequently performed because it produces significant hepatic encephalopathy
E. TIPS is used in cases where bleeding cannot be stopped only after ten sessions of endoscopic therapy within 5 days

Q7.41

A 59-year-old man with alcoholic cirrhosis presents with a rapidly developing history of weight loss, anorexia, fever, ache in the right hypochondrium and ascites. On examination he has an enlarged, irregular, tender liver. The following statements are correct

A. The risk of this condition in HCV is as high or higher than in HBV
B. Serum α-fetoprotein is normal in at least a third of patients
C. Ultrasound may show a filling defect in 90% of cases
D. Chemotherapy and radiotherapy prolong survival
E. Survival is seldom more than 6 months

Q7.42

A 42-year-old man has ascites due to cirrhosis. The pathogenesis of ascites is due to

A. Increased plasma oncotic pressure due to changes in serum albumin
B. Increased splanchnic production of lymph and transudation of fluid into the peritoneal cavity due to portal hypertension
C. Sodium and water retention which occur as a result of peripheral arterial vasodilatation and consequent reduction in effective blood volume
D. Passage of pleural fluid from pleural effusion through congenital defects in the diaphragm
E. Secondary hypoaldosteronism

Q7.43

A 29-year-old woman has ascites due to cirrhosis. Her serum sodium is 140 mEq/L, K 4.5 mEq/L and creatinine is 240 μmol/L. The following statements are correct

A. An ascitic protein of 5 g/L below the serum albumin level suggests that it is a transudate
B. The diuresis due to bed rest in practice is the most helpful method of reducing abdominal distension
C. Fluid restriction is the cornerstone in the management of this condition
D. Aldosterone 100 mg/day is the diuretic of choice in this patient
E. The maximum rate at which ascitic fluid can be mobilized is 1.5 L in 24 hours

Q7.44

A 58-year-old patient with ascites and cirrhosis presents wtih a history of nausea, vomiting and weakness. She is irritable and disorientated. The patient is unable to draw a five-pointed star. The following statements are correct

A. Ammonia-induced alteration of brain neurotransmitter balance – especially at the astrocyte–neurone interface – is the leading concept of causation for this condition
B. Constipation can precipitate this condition
C. EEG shows an increase in frequency of α-waves
D. Transjugular intrahepatic portocaval shunt (TIPS) is used to treat this condition
E. Immediate management of this condition includes evacuation of the bowels and sterilizing the bowel

Liver, biliary tract and pancreatic disease

Q7.45

A patient with advanced cirrhosis and ascites is treated aggresively with diuretics. As a consequence the patient develops renal failure and urine output is low. The following statements regarding this condition are correct

A. Tubular function (the ability to concentrate urine) is intact
B. Urine sodium is high
C. Liver transplantation is contraindicated
D. Terlipressin improves overall prognosis
E. Eicosanoids have been implicated in the pathogenesis

Q7.46

The following patients risk developing cholesterol gallstones

A. A 45-year-old woman with nine children
B. A 52-year-old man with a body mass index (BMI) of 40
C. A 29-year-old acromegalic patient being treated with octreotide
D. A 49-year-old hunter who eats a diet high in animal fat
E. A 54-year-old woman with cirrhosis

Q7.47

A 51-year-old smoker has emphysema and cirrhosis. Serum α_1-antitrypsin is 60% of the normal level. The following statements about this condition are correct

A. This patient most likely has the PiZZ phenotype of the condition
B. This deficiency is inherited as an autosomal recessive trait

C. The main role of the protein associated with this condition is to to inhibit the proteolytic enzyme, neutrophil elastase
D. Patients should be advised to stop smoking
E. α_1-Antitrypsin constitutes 90% of the serum α_1-globulin seen on electrophoresis

Q7.48

A 43-year-old man is diagnosed with chronic hepatitis B. The following statements regarding his condition are correct

A. Clinical relapse is associated with seroconversion of HBeAg to anti-HBe
B. Clinical relapse is associated with seroconversion of anti-HBe to HBeAg
C. Patients with HBsAg, HBeAg and HBV DNA in the serum with abnormal serum aminotransferases and chronic hepatitis on liver biopsy should not be treated because liver changes are irreversible
D. The main aim of treatment is to eliminate HBeAg and HBV DNA from the serum
E. Pegylated interferon should be avoided because it causes elevation of transaminases
F. In patients in whom HBeAg disappears, remission is usually sustained
G. If this patient had no HBeAg his response to treatment with interferon would be significantly superior to that of a patient with HBeAg
H. Overall, the response rate with disappearance of HBeAg is close to 90%

A7.1

C

Endoscopy should be performed to confirm the diagnosis of varices and to exclude bleeding from other sites (e.g. gastric ulceration). Portal hypertensive (or congestive) gastropathy is the term used for chronic gastric congestion, punctate erythema and gastric erosions and is a source of bleeding. Varices may or may not be present. Propranolol is the best treatment for this.

A7.2

D

Acute fatty liver of pregnancy (AFLP) presents in the last trimester with symptoms of fulminant hepatitis – jaundice, vomiting, abdominal pain, occasionally haematemesis and coma.

Investigations show hepatocellular damage, hyperuricaemia, thrombocytopenia, and rarely DIC (disseminated intravascular coagulation). CT scanning shows a low density of the liver owing to the high fat content. It can sometimes be difficult to differentiate from the HELLP syndrome (a combination of haemolysis, elevated liver enzymes and a low platelet count) and as LCHAD (long-chain 3-hydroxylacyl-Co-A-dihydroxyl) deficiency has also been shown in HELLP there is a view that there is a spectrum of HELLP to AFLP. Liver biopsy shows fine droplets of fat (microvesicles) in the liver cells with little necrosis, but is not necessary for diagnosis.

A7.3

E

Acute variceal sclerotherapy and banding are the treatment of choice; they arrest bleeding in 80% of cases and reduce early rebleeding. Between 15% and 20% of bleeding comes from gastric varices and here results of endoscopic therapy are poor. The main use of vasoconstrictor agents such as terlipression or somtatoastatin is for emergency control of bleeding while waiting for endoscopy and in combination with endoscopic techniques. Terlipressin should not be given to patients with ischaemic heart disease. Balloon tamponade is used mainly to control bleeding if endoscopic therapy or vasoconstrictor therapy has failed or is contraindicated or if there is exsanguinating haemorrhage. This technique is successful in up to 90% of patients and is very useful in the first few hours of bleeding. However, it can have serious complications such as aspiration pneumonia, oesophageal rupture and mucosal ulceration, which lead to a 5% mortality. The procedure is very unpleasant for the patient.

A7.4

B

Spontaneous bacterial peritonitis (SBP) represents one of the more serious complications of ascites and occurs in approximately 8% of cirrhotics with ascites. The infecting organisms are believed to gain access to the peritoneum by haematogenous spread. The most frequently incriminated bacteria are *Escherichia coli*, *Klebsiella* and enterococci. The condition should be suspected in any patient with ascites with evidence of clinical deterioration. Features such as

Liver, biliary tract and pancreatic disease

pain and pyrexia are frequently absent. Diagnostic aspiration should always be performed in patients with ascites. A raised neutrophil count (>250 cell/mm^3) in ascites is alone sufficient evidence to start treatment immediately. A third-generation cephalosporin, such as cefotaxime or ceftazidime, is used and may be modified on the basis of culture results. The prognosis is grave and depends on the severity of the liver disease. It has a 25% mortality and recurs in 70% of patients within a year. It is an indication for liver transplantation. If the patient survives, an oral quinolone should be prescribed daily to prevent recurrence, and this prolongs survival. Although Gram-positive organisms are subsequently found to be a cause of SBP they are sensitive to third-generation cephalosporins.

A7.5

C

The hepatorenal syndrome occurs typically in a patient with advanced cirrhosis with jaundice and ascites. The urine output is low with a low urinary sodium concentration, a maintained capacity to concentrate urine (i.e. tubular function is intact) and an almost normal renal histology. The renal failure here is described as 'functional'. It is sometimes precipitated by overvigorous diuretic therapy, diarrhoea or paracentesis, but often no precipitating factor is found.

A7.6

B

Ultrasound of the abdomen is a non-invasive, safe and relatively cheap technique and is the investigation of choice in a jaundiced patient.

A7.7

C

Haemobilia (bleeding into the biliary tree) is a well-recognized complication of biopsy of the liver. It produces biliary colic, jaundice and melaena within 3 days of the biopsy.

A7.8

B

Xanthomas (cholesterol deposits) are seen in the palmar creases or above the eyes in primary biliary cirrhosis.

A7.9

D

All patients with Child's grade C (Child's grade C: albumin <30 g/L, bilirubin >50 μmol/L, and ascites) cirrhosis should be considered for liver transplantation. Patients with primary biliary cirrhosis should be transplanted when their serum bilirubin rises above 100 μmol/L.

A7.10

B

Poor prognostic variables in fulminant hepatic failure indicating a need for liver transplantation: a) arterial pH <7.3 (after resuscitation, 7.25 on N-acetylcysteine) or b) serum creatinine >300 μmol/L, PT >100 s, Grade III–V encephalopathy.

A7.11

1) G   2) D   3) A   4) F   5) C
6) B   7) E

Useful blood tests for certain liver diseases

Test	Disease
Antimitochondrial antibody	Primary biliary cirrhosis
Antinuclear, smooth muscle (actin), liver/kidney microsomal antibody	Autoimmune hepatitis
Raised serum immunoglobulins:	
IgG	Autoimmune hepatitis
IgM	Primary biliary cirrhosis
Viral markers	Hepatitis A, B, C, D and others
α-Fetoprotein	Hepatocellular carcinoma
Serum iron, transferrin saturation, serum ferritin	Hereditary haemochromatosis
Serum and urinary copper, serum caeruloplasmin	Wilson's disease
α1-Antitrypsin	Cirrhosis (± emphysema)
Antinuclear cytoplasmic antibodies	Sclerosing cholangitis

A7.12

1) E   2) D   3) C   4) B   5) A

Methyldopa can cause intravascular haemolysis and in haemolytic jaundice the level of unconjugated bilirubin is raised but the serum alkaline phosphatase, transferases and albumin are normal. Serum haptoglobulins are low. Gilbert's syndrome is the most common familial hyperbilirubinaemia and affects 2–7% of the population. It is asymptomatic and is usually detected as an incidental finding of a slightly raised bilirubin (17–102 μmol/L or 1–6 mg/dL) on a routine check. All the other liver biochemistry is normal and no signs of liver disease are seen. There is a family history of jaundice in 5–15% of patients. Crigler–Najjar syndrome is very rare. Only patients with type II (autosomal dominant) with a decrease rather than absence (type I – autosomal recessive) of UDP-glucuronosyl transferase can survive into adult life. Mutation of the gene for UDP-glucuronosyl transferase has been demonstrated in the coding region. Liver histology is normal. Recurrent familial intrahepatic cholestasis or benign recurrent intrahepatic cholestasis is characterized by recurrent attacks of acute cholestasis which occur without progression to chronic liver disease. Jaundice, severe pruritus, steatorrhoea and weight loss develop. Serum γ-GT is normal. The gene has been mapped to the FICI locus, but the precise relation to cholestasis is unclear. Dubin–Johnson syndrome (autosomal recessive) is due to defects in bilirubin handling in the liver. The prognosis is good. The liver is black owing to melanin deposition.

A7.13

1) E   2) B   3) D   4) C   5) A

Infectious mononucleosis is due to the Epstein–Barr (EB) virus. Mild jaundice associated with minor abnormalities of liver biochemistry is extremely common, but 'clinical' hepatitis is rare. Hepatic histological changes occur within 5 days of onset; the sinusoids and portal tracts are infiltrated with large mononuclear cells but the liver architecture is preserved. A Paul–Bunnell or Monospot test is usually positive, and atypical lymphocytes are present in the peripheral blood. Treatment is of the symptoms. Cytomegalovirus (CMV) can cause acute hepatitis, particularly in a patient with an impaired immune response. The virus may be isolated from the urine. The liver biopsy shows intranuclear inclusions and giant cells. Yellow fever viral infection is carried by the mosquito *Aedes aegypti* and can cause acute hepatic necrosis. There is no specific treatment. Very occasionally the herpes simplex virus causes a generalized acute infection, particularly in the immunosuppressed patient, and occasionally in pregnancy. Aminotransferases are usually massively elevated. Liver biopsy shows extensive necrosis. Aciclovir is used for treatment.

A7.14

1) B   2) C   3) A   4) D   5) D

Hepatitis B patients with decompensated liver disease often have severe side-effects with interferons. They should not be routinely treated with this drug but could be treated with lamivudine. Current therapy of hepatitis C is combination therapy with recombinant alpha-interferon (3M units three times a week) and ribavirin (10.6 mg/kg daily) in divided doses for 12 months if genotype 1; and 6 months for non-genotype 1. Treatment of chronic hepatitis D infection is with alpha-interferon, usually at the high dose of 10M units three times weekly for 12 months, but response is poor. There are scanty data about the use of lamivudine. In chronic autoimmune hepatitis prednisolone 30 mg is given daily for 2 weeks, followed by a slow reduction and then a maintenance dose of 10–15 mg daily; azathioprine should be added, 1–2 mg/kg daily, as a steroid-sparing agent and in some patients as sole long-term maintenance therapy.

A7.15

1) E   2) B   3) C   4) A   5) D

Some drugs causing types of liver damage			
Types of liver damage	Drugs	Types of liver damage	Drugs
Zone 3 necrosis	Carbon tetrachloride *Amanita* mushrooms Paracetamol Salicylates Piroxicam Cocaine	Heparlobatum	Combination chemotherapy for metastatic breast cancer
Zone 1 necrosis	Ferrous sulphate	Vascular Sinusoidal dilatation	Contraceptive drugs Anabolic steroids Azathioprine
Microvesicular fat	Sodium valproate Tetracyclines	Pelioses hepatis	Oral contraceptives Anabolic steroids, e.g. danazol Azathioprine
'Alcoholic' hepatitis (phospholipidosis)	Amiodarone Synthetic oestrogens Nifedipine	Veno-occlusive	Pyrrolizidine alkaloids (*Senecio* in bush tea) Cytotoxics – cyclophosphamide, azathioprine
Fibrosis	Methotrexate Other cytotoxic agents Arsenic Vitamin A Retinoids		

Some drugs causing types of liver damage

Types of liver damage	Drugs	Types of liver damage	Drugs
Acute hepatitis	Isoniazid		Allopurinol
	Rifampicin		Antithyroid e.g.
	Methyldopa		propylthiouracil
	Atenolol		carbimazole
	Enalapril		Quinine e.g.
	Verapamil		quinidine
	Ketoconazole		Diltiazem
	Cytotoxic drugs		Anticonvulsants e.g.
	Clonazepam		phenytoin
	Disulfiram	Canalicular cholestasis	Sex hormones
	Niacin		Ciclosporin A
	Volatile liquid anaesthetics,	Hepatocanalicular	Chlorpromazine
	e.g. halothane	cholestasis	Haloperidol
			Erythromycin
Chronic hepatitis	Methyldopa		Cimetidine/ranitidine
	Nitrofurantoin		Nitrofurantoin
	Fenofibrate		Imipramine
	Isoniazid		Azathioprine
			Oral hypoglycaemics
General	Sulphonamides e.g.		Dextropropoxyphene
hypersensitivity	sulfasalazine		
	co-trimoxazole	Ductular cholestasis	Benoxyprofen
	fansidar		
	Penicillins e.g.	Biliary sludge	Ceftriaxone
	flucloxacillin	Sclerosing cholangitis	Hepatic arterial infusion
	ampicillin		of 5-fluorouracil
	amoxicillin		
	co-amoxiclav	Hepatic tumours	Pills with high hormone
	NSAIDs e.g.		content (adenomas)
	salicylates	Hepatocellular	Contraceptive pill
	diclofenac	carcinoma	Danazo

NSAID, non-steroidal anti-inflammatory drug

A7.16

1) D **2)** C **3)** E **4)** A **5)** B

Patients with non-cirrhotic portal hypertension present with portal hypertension and variceal bleeding but without cirrhosis. Histologically, the liver shows mild portal tract fibrosis. The aetiology is unknown, but arsenic, vinyl chloride and other toxic agents have been implicated. A similar disease is found frequently in India. The liver lesion does not progress and the prognosis is therefore good. Schistosomiasis with extensive pipe-stem fibrosis is a common cause of portal hypertension world-wide, but is confined to endemic areas such as Egypt and Brazil. In the chronic form of Budd–Chiari syndrome there is enlargement of the liver (particularly the caudate lobe), mild jaundice, ascites, a negative hepatojugular reflex, and splenomegaly with portal hypertension. In alcoholic hepatitis, in addition to fatty change there is infiltration by polymorphonuclear leucocytes and hepatocyte necrosis mainly

Liver, biliary tract and pancreatic disease

in zone 3. Dense cytoplasmic inclusions called Mallory bodies are sometimes seen in hepatocytes and giant mitochondria are also a feature. Mallory bodies are suggestive of, but not specific for, alcoholic damage as they can be found in other liver disease, such as Wilson's disease and primary biliary cirrhosis (PBC). If alcohol consumption continues, alcoholic hepatitis may progress to cirrhosis. Alcoholic cirrhosis is classically of the micronodular type, but a mixed pattern may also be seen accompanying fatty change, and evidence of pre-existing alcoholic hepatitis may be present. In congenital intrahepatic biliary dilatation (Caroli's disease) there are saccular dilatations of the intrahepatic or extrahepatic ducts. It can present at any age (although usually in childhood) with fever, abdominal pain and recurrent attacks of cholangitis with Gram-negative septicaemia. Jaundice and portal hypertension are absent. Diagnosis is by ultrasound, PTC, ERCP or MRCP.

A7.17

A) F B) F C) T D) T E) F
F) F G) T

Serum antimitochondrial antibodies (AMA) are found in almost all patients with primary biliary cirrhosis (PBC), and of the mitochondrial proteins involved, the antigen M2 is specific to PBC. The presence of AMA in high titre is unrelated to the clinical or histological picture and its role in pathogenesis is unclear. Asymptomatic patients are discovered on routine examination or screening to have hepatomegaly, a raised serum alkaline phosphatase or autoantibodies. Pruritus is often the earliest symptom, preceding jaundice by a few years. Fatigue may accompany pruritus particularly in progressive cases. When jaundice appears,

hepatomegaly is usually found. In the later stages, patients are jaundiced with severe pruritus. Pigmented xanthelasma on eyelids or other deposits of cholesterol in the creases of the hands may be seen. Keratoconjunctivitis sicca (dry eyes and mouth) is seen in 70% of cases. Ursodeoxycholic acid (10–15 mg/kg) improves bilirubin and aminotransferase values. It is not clear if prognosis is altered. Symptoms are not improved. Asymptomatic patients and those presenting with pruritus will survive for more than 20 years. Symptomatic patients with jaundice have a more rapidly progressive course and die of liver failure or bleeding varices in approximately 5 years.

A7.18

A) T B) F C) F D) T E) T
F) T G) T H) F

Hereditary haemochromatosis (HH) is an inherited disease. Between 83% and 90% of patients with overt HH are homozygous for the Cys 282 Tyr mutation. The classic triad of bronze skin pigmentation (due to melanin deposition), hepatomegaly and diabetes mellitus is only present in cases of gross iron overload. Serum iron is elevated (>30 μmol/L), with a reduction in the total iron-binding capacity (TIBC) and complete or almost complete transferrin saturation (>60%). Serum ferritin is elevated (usually >500 μg/L or 240 nmol/L). Venesection prolongs life and may reverse tissue damage; the risk of malignancy still remains if cirrhosis is present. All patients should have excess iron removed as rapidly as possible. Manifestations of the disease usually improve or disappear, except for diabetes, testicular atrophy and chondrocalcinosis. In all cases of HH, all first-degree family members must be screened to detect early and asymptomatic disease. Serum ferritin is an excellent test with only occasional false-positives in hepatocellular necrosis and rare false-negatives in some family studies. Liver biochemistry is often normal, even with established cirrhosis.

A7.19

A) F   B) F   C) F   D) F   E) T
F) T   G) F

Wilson's disease is a very rare inborn error of copper metabolism that results in copper deposition in various organs, including the liver, the basal ganglia of the brain and the cornea. It is an autosomal recessive disorder with a molecular defect within a copper-transporting ATPase encoded by a gene (designated *ATP7B*) located on chromosome 13. The basic problem is a failure of biliary excretion of copper. There is a low serum caeruloplasmin in over 80% of patients owing to poor synthesis, but the precise mechanism for the failure of copper excretion is not known. The liver histology is not diagnostic and varies from that of chronic hepatitis to macronodular cirrhosis. Lifetime treatment with penicillamine, 1–1.5 g daily, is effective in chelating copper. If treatment is started early, clinical and biochemical improvement can occur. Fulminant hepatic failure or decompensated cirrhosis should be treated by liver transplantation.

oxidative deamination to produce ammonia, which is then converted to urea and excreted by the kidneys. This is a major pathway for the elimination of nitrogenous waste. Failure of this process occurs in severe liver disease. The liver also synthesizes all factors involved in coagulation (apart from factor VIII) – that is, fibrinogen, prothrombin, factors V, VII, IX, X and XIII, protein C and S and antithrombin as well as components of the complement system. Glucose homeostasis and the maintenance of the blood sugar is a major function of the liver.

A7.21

A) F   B) F   C) T   D) T   E) T

Triglycerides are mainly of dietary origin but are also formed in the liver from circulating free fatty acids (FFAs) and glycerol and incorporated into very-low-density lipoproteins (VLDLs). Cholesterol may be of dietary origin but most is synthesized from acetyl-CoA mainly in the liver, intestine, adrenal cortex and skin. The liver synthesizes VLDLs and high-density lipoproteins (HDLs). HDLs are the substrate for lecithin–cholesterol acyltransferase (LCAT), which catalyses the conversion of free cholesterol to cholesterol ester. Hepatic lipase removes triglyceride from intermediate-density lipoproteins (IDLs) to produce low-density lipoproteins (LDLs).

A7.20

A) T   B) T   C) T   D) F   E) T

Albumin and fibrinogen are synthesized in the liver. Reduced synthesis of albumin over prolonged periods produces hypoalbuminaemia and is seen in chronic liver disease and malnutrition. Amino acids are degraded by transamination and

A7.22

A) F   B) F   C) T   D) T   E) T

The canalicular multispecific organic anion transporter (cMOAT) also known as multidrug-resistance protein 2 (MRP2) mediates transport of a broad range of compounds including bilirubin diglucuronide, glucuronidated and

Liver, biliary tract and pancreatic disease

sulphated bile acids and other organic anions. Na^+ and water follow the passage of bile salts into the biliary canaliculus by diffusion across the tight junction between hepatocytes (a bile salt-dependent process).

A7.23

A) T   B) T   C) T   D) T   E) T

Bile acids are synthesized in hepatocytes from cholesterol. The rate-limiting step in their production is that catalysed by cholesterol-7α-hydroxylase. The two primary bile acids – cholic acid and chenodeoxycholic acid – are conjugated with glycine or taurine (in a ratio of 3:1 in humans) and this process increases their solubility. Intestinal bacteria convert these acids into secondary bile acids, deoxycholic and lithocholic acid. Bile acids act as detergents; their main function is lipid solubilization.

A7.24

A) F   B) F   C) T   D) T   E) F
F) T   G) T

Bilirubin is produced mainly from the breakdown of mature red cells in the Kupffer cells of the liver and in the reticuloendothelial system; 15% of bilirubin comes from the catabolism of other haem-containing proteins, such as myoglobin, cytochromes and catalase. Normally, 250–300 mg of bilirubin are produced daily. Bilirubin dissociates from albumin and is taken up by the hepatic cell membrane and transported to the endoplasmic reticulum by cytoplasmic proteins, where it is conjugated with glucuronic acid and excreted into bile. The microsomal enzyme, uridine diphosphoglucurosyl transferase, catalyses the formation of bilirubin monoglucuronide and then diglucuronide.

This conjugated bilirubin is water-soluble. It is not absorbed from the small intestine because of its large molecular size. In the terminal ileum, bacterial enzymes hydrolyse the molecule, releasing free bilirubin, which is then reduced to urobilinogen. Some of this is excreted in the stools as stercobilinogen. The remainder is absorbed by the terminal ileum, passes to the liver via the enterohepatic circulation, and is re-excreted into the bile. Urobilinogen bound to albumin enters the circulation and is excreted in the urine via the kidneys. When hepatic excretion of conjugated bilirubin is impaired, a small amount of conjugated bilirubin is found strongly bound to serum albumin. It is not excreted by the kidneys and accounts for the continuing hyperbilirubinaemia for a short time after cholestasis has resolved.

A7.25

A) F   B) F   C) F   D) T   E) F

Serum albumin is a marker of synthetic function and is a valuable guide to the severity of chronic liver disease. A falling serum albumin in liver disease is a bad prognostic sign. In acute liver disease initial albumin levels may be normal. Prothrombin time (PT) is also a marker of synthetic function. Because of its short half-life, it is a sensitive indicator of both acute and chronic liver disease. Vitamin K deficiency should be excluded as the cause of a prolonged PT by giving an intravenous bolus (10 mg) of vitamin K. Aspartate aminotransferase (AST) is primarily a mitochondrial enzyme (80% in mitochondria; 20% in cytoplasm) and is present in heart, muscle, kidney and brain. High levels are seen in hepatic necrosis, myocardial infarction, muscle injury and congestive cardiac failure. Alanine aminotransferase (ALT) is a cytosolic enzyme more specific to the liver so that a rise only occurs with liver disease. Serum alkaline phosphate (ALP) is raised in cholestasis from any cause, whether intrahepatic or extrahepatic disease. The globulin fraction consists of many proteins that can be separated on electrophoresis. A raised globulin fraction, seen in liver disease, is usually due to increased circulating immunoglobulins and is polyclonal.

A7.26

A) F B) T C) T D) T E) T

Liver palms usually indicate chronic disease but they can occur in severe acute disease. Palmar erythema, a non-specific change indicative of a hyperdynamic circulation, is also seen in pregnancy, thyrotoxicosis and rheumatoid arthritis.

A7.27

A) F B) F C) T D) T E) F

This patient's clinical features are typical of viral hepatitis A. Hepatitis A is an RNA virus and belongs to the picorna family. The incubation period is relatively short (2–3 weeks). Spread of infection is mainly by the faeco-oral route. There is no carrier state. Recovery is usually complete and HAV hepatitis never progresses to chronic liver disease.

A7.28

A) T B) T C) T D) T E) T

This patient's clinical features are typical of viral hepatitis A. Extrahepatic complications are rare but include arthritis, vasculitis, myocarditis, renal failure and osteomyelitis.

A7.29

A) F B) F C) T D) T E) T

This patient has hepatitis due to hepatitis B virus (HBV). Mutations occur in the various reading frames of the HBV genome and these mutants can emerge in chronic HBV carriers. Different mutants have also been seen following interferon or lamivudine therapy and in patients with fulminant and fatal hepatitis. Their existence means that serological markers such as the HbeAg are less useful in detecting infectivity and HBV DNA must be always measured. It does not spread by the faecal route. A carrier state has been described and long-term sequelae include liver cancer and chronic liver disease. Active immunization of this condition is with a recombinant yeast vaccine produced by the insertion of a plasmid containing the gene of HbsAg into a yeast.

A7.30

A) F B) T C) T D) T E) T

Hepatitis C virus (HCV) is a single-stranded RNA virus of the Flaviviridae family. The current assay, ELISA-3, incorporates antigens NS3, NS4 and NS5 regions. The virus is transmitted by blood and blood products and it is postulated that 80% of people with haemophilia in the UK may have been infected. The incidence in intravenous drug abusers is high, up to 90%. The low rate of HCV infection in high-risk groups, such as homosexuals, prostitutes and attendees at STD clinics, suggests a limited role for sexual transmission. Most patients will not be diagnosed until they present, years later, with evidence of abnormal transferase values at health checks or with chronic liver disease. There is a higher incidence of diabetes. Interferon has been used in acute

Liver, biliary tract and pancreatic disease

cases with good success, so that needle-stick injuries must be followed and treated early if there is evidence of HCV viraemia. Cirrhosis develops in about 20–30% within 10–30 years and of these patients between 7% and 15% will develop hepatocellular carcinoma.

A7.31

A) F   B) T   C) F   D) F   E) T

The transfer criteria for patients with fulminant hepatic failure to specialized units for patients with acute liver injury include: a) INR >3.0; b) presence of hepatic encephalopathy; c) hypotension after resuscitation with fluid; d) metabolic acidosis; e) prothrombin time (seconds) > interval (hours) from overdose (paracetamol cases).

A7.32

A) T   B) T   C) T   D) F   E) F

An abdominal ultrasound scan is the single most useful investigation for the diagnosis of gallstone-related disease. Cholecystectomy is the treatment of choice for virtually all patients with symptomatic gall bladder stones. Cholecystectomy should not be performed in the absence of typical symptoms just because stones are found on investigation. Pure or near pure cholesterol stones can be solubilized by increasing the bile salt content of bile. Chenodeoxycholic acid and more recently ursodeoxycholic acid are used. For dissolution to occur there must be a functioning gall bladder and optimally the stones should be almost pure cholesterol with a diameter of less than 10 mm. Further benefit may be attained by the addition of an HMG-CoA reductase inhibitor (e.g. simvastatin) to a regimen of ursodeoxycholic acid. This will then combine reduced cholesterol content of bile as well as enhanced bile salt concentration but uses are still limited. A shock wave can be directed either radiologically or by ultrasound on to gall bladder stones (extracorporeal shock wave lithotripsy). This technique has been highly successful but in only a restricted patient population. Fragmentation was limited to a small number of stones only and these had to be greater than 10 mm in diameter.

A7.33

A) T   B) T   C) T   D) F   E) F   F) F

The classical features of common bile duct (CBD) stones are biliary colic, fever and jaundice (acute cholangitis). This triad is only present in the minority of patients. Fever is only present in a minority of cases but indicates biliary sepsis and sometimes an associated septicaemia. The presence of such biliary sepsis is a significant adverse prognostic factor. The raised serum bilirubin tends to be mild and often transient. Very high concentrations of bilirubin (>200 µmol/L) almost always reflect complete bile duct obstruction. The serum amylase levels are often mildly elevated in the presence of bile duct obstruction but are markedly so if stone-related pancreatitis has occurred. Abdominal ultrasound is the initial imaging technique of choice and in most cases the only imaging technique required. Bile duct obstruction is characterized by dilatation of intrahepatic biliary radicals, which are usually easily detected by the ultrasound scan. It may, however, not be possible to identify the cause of obstruction. Stones situated in the distal common bile duct are poorly visualized by transabdominal ultrasound and up to 50%

are missed. The detection of stones within the gall bladder is poorly predictive as to the cause of bile duct obstruction. CT, usually with i.v. contrast, is useful in patients (particularly obese) where the CBD pathology cannot be identified on ultrasound. In experienced hands this will be successful in 98% of cases, providing good documentation of bile duct stones. However, microcalculi can still be missed. Endoscopic retrograde cholangiography (ERC) gives the therapeutic opportunity for sphincterotomy and stone extraction.

A7.34

A) T B) T C) T D) F E) T

Primary sclerosing cholangitis (PSC) is a chronic cholestatic liver disease characterized by fibrosing inflammatory destruction of both the intra- and extrahepatic bile ducts. In 75% of patients PSC is associated with inflammatory bowel disease (usually ulcerative colitis) but it is not unusual for the PSC to predate the onset of the inflammatory bowel disease. The cholangiogram characteristically shows both intra- and extrahepatic bile duct strictures, although either may be involved alone. Liver histology shows inflammation of the intrahepatic biliary radicals with considerable associated scar tissue classically described as being onion skin in appearance. PSC is a slowly progressive disease (symptoms and biochemical tests may fluctuate) ultimately leading to liver cirrhosis and associated decompensation. Cholangiocarcinoma is a well-recognized complication occurring in up to 20% of patients. The only proven treatment is liver transplantation.

A7.35

A) F B) T C) T D) F E) F

Acute pancreatitis is a differential diagnosis in any patient with upper abdominal pain. In such circumstances a serum amylase level is the standard laboratory test carried out to confirm the diagnosis. If this is measured within 24 hours of the onset of pain an elevation of three times the upper limit of normal is an extremely sensitive test. An erect chest X-ray is mandatory to exclude gastroduodenal perforation as a cause of upper abdominal pain, which may also result in an elevated amylase. Endoscopic retrograde cholangiopancreatography (ERCP) is seldom used as a diagnostic tool. Analgesia requirements may be high and in many patients are most appropriately administered by a patient controlled system. Pethidine and tramadol are the drugs of choice. The morphine derivatives should be avoided because of their propensity to cause sphincter of Oddi contraction. Poor prognostic factors include age >55 years, WBC >15×10^9/L, blood glucose <10 mmol/L, serum urea >16 mmol/L, serum albumin <30 g/L, serum calcium <2 mmol/L, serum LDH >600 U/L and P_aO_2 <8.0 kPa (60 mmHg).

A7.36

A) F B) T C) T D) F E) T

Pain is the most common presentation of chronic pancreatitis and is usually epigastric and often radiating through into the back. In established chronic pancreatitis, serum amylase and lipase levels are rarely significantly elevated and have little diagnostic value. MRI with magnetic resonance pancreatography (MRCP) is increasingly utilized to define

Liver, biliary tract and pancreatic disease

more subtle abnormalities of the pancreatic duct which may be seen in non-dilated chronic pancreatitis. Endoscopic retrograde cholangiopancreatography (ERCP) has a diminishing role as a diagnostic tool for chronic pancreatitis. The quality of imaging including ductular definition with MRCP has largely replaced diagnostic ERCP. A faecal elastase level will be abnormal in the majority of patients with moderate to severe pancreatic disease. Tricyclic antidepressants (e.g. amitriptyline) have been widely applied for chronic pain management and appear to be successful in chronic pancreatitis and in particular reduce the need for opiates. The most common structural complication of chronic pancreatitis is a pancreatic pseudocyst, which is where a fluid collection is surrounded by granulation tissue.

A7.37

A) T B) F C) T D) F E) F F) T

Pancreatic adenocarcinoma may be viewed clinically as two diseases – the lesions of the head and lesions of the body and tail. Transabdominal ultrasound is the initial investigation in the majority of patients. CT scanning is also an essential part of tumour assessment prior to possible surgical resection. Several tumour markers have been evaluated for the diagnosis and monitoring of pancreatic cancer. The CA19.9 has a high sensitivity (80%) but a high false-positive rate. The CA242 has a lower sensitivity (70%) but fewer false-positives (less than 10%). The 5-year survival rate for carcinoma of the pancreas is approximately 2% with surgical intervention representing the only chance of long-term survival. In the majority of cases the management is palliative.

A7.38

A) F B) F C) F D) F E) F

Clinically chronic hepatitis is defined as any hepatitis lasting for 6 months or longer. Chronic hepatitis is best classified according to the aetiology: a) due to viral disease; b) due to autoimmune disease; c) drug-induced; d) unknown cause. Chronic viral hepatitis is the principal cause of chronic liver disease, cirrhosis and hepatocellular carcinoma in the world. Chronic inflammatory cell infiltrates comprising lymphocytes, plasma cells and sometimes lymphoid follicles are usually present in the portal tracts. The amount of inflammation varies from mild to severe. In addition, there may be: a) loss of definition of the portal/periportal limiting plate – interface hepatitis (the term 'interface hepatitis' is preferred to 'piecemeal necrosis' because the damage is due to apoptosis rather than necrosis); b) lobular change, focal lytic necrosis, apoptosis and focal inflammation; c) confluent necrosis; d) fibrosis which may be mild, bridging (across portal tracts) or severe; e) cirrhosis. The overall severity of the hepatitis is judged by the degree of the hepatitis and inflammation (grading) and the severity of the fibrosis or cirrhosis (staging) using various scoring systems.

A7.39

A) F B) F C) F D) F E) F

Approximately 90% of patients with cirrhosis will develop gastro-oesophageal varices over 10 years, but only one-third of these will bleed from them. Bleeding is likely to occur with large varices, red signs on varices (diagnosed at endoscopy) and in severe liver disease. Despite all the therapeutic techniques available, the prognosis depends on the severity of the underlying liver disease, with an overall mortality from variceal haemorrhage of 25% – reaching 50% in Child's grade C. Urgent endoscopy should be performed to confirm the diagnosis of varices and to exclude bleeding from other sites.

A7.40

A) F   B) F   C) T   D) T   E) F

Fifty per cent of patients rebled within 10 days. Transjugular intrahepatic portocaval shunt (TIPS) is used in cases where the bleeding cannot be stopped after two sessions of endoscopic therapy within 5 days. It is useful in the short term, but recurrent portal hypertension owing to stent stenosis or thrombosis occurs. Oesophageal transection and ligation of the feeding vessels to the bleeding varices is the most common surgical technique. Acute portosystemic shunt surgery is infrequently performed; encephalopathy is common with these procedures, in contrast to oesophageal transection.

A7.41

A) T   B) T   C) T   D) F   E) T

Hepatocellular carcinoma (HCC) is one of the ten most common cancers world-wide, although it is uncommon in the West. The risk of HCC in HCV is as high or higher than in HBV despite no viral integration. Serum α-fetoprotein may be raised, but is normal in at least a third of patients. Ultrasound scans show filling defects in 90% of cases. Chemotherapy and radiotherapy are unhelpful. Survival, except in very selected groups, is seldom more than 6 months.

A7.42

A) F   B) T   C) T   D) F   E) T

The pathogenesis of the development of ascites in liver disease is controversial, but is probably secondary to renal sodium and water retention. Several factors are involved. a) Sodium and water retention occur as a result of peripheral arterial vasodilatation and consequent reduction in the effective blood volume. Nitric oxide has been postulated as the putative vasodilator, although other substances (e.g. atrial natriuretic peptide and prostaglandins) may be involved. The reduction in effective blood volume activates various neurohumoral pressor systems such as the sympathetic nervous system and the renin–angiotensin system, thus promoting salt and water retention. b) Portal hypertension exerts a local hydrostatic pressure and leads to increased hepatic and splanchnic production of lymph and transudation of fluid into the peritoneal cavity. c) Low serum albumin (a consequence of poor synthetic liver function) may further contribute by a reduction in plasma oncotic pressure.

A7.43

A) F   B) F   C) F   D) F   E) F

The ascitic protein level enables a division into transudative and exudative ascites. For this division the serum albumin must be used as a reference point. An ascitic protein of 11 g/L or more below the serum albumin level suggests a transudate. The maximum rate at which ascites can be mobilized is 500–700 mL in 24 hours. The management is as follows: a) check serum electrolytes and creatinine at the start and every other day; weigh and measure urinary output daily. b) Bed rest alone will lead to a diuresis in a small proportion of

Liver, biliary tract and pancreatic disease

people by improving renal perfusion, but in practice is not helpful. c) By dietary sodium restriction it is possible to reduce sodium intake to 40 mmol in 24 hours and still maintain an adequate protein and calorie intake with a palatable diet. d) Fluid restriction is probably not necessary unless the serum sodium is under 128 mmol/L. e) The diuretic of first choice is the aldosterone antagonist spironolactone, starting at 100 mg daily. However, it is contraindicated when the serum creatinine is greater than 200 μmol/L.

7.44

A) T   B) T   C) F   D) F   E) T

The term 'portosystemic encephalopathy' (PSE) refers to a chronic neuropsychiatric syndrome secondary to chronic liver disease. PSE is seen in patients with portal hypertension that is due to spontaneous 'shunting', or in patients following a portosystemic shunt procedure, e.g. transjugular intrahepatic portocaval shunt (TIPS). Ammonia-induced alteration of brain neurotransmitter balance – especially at the astrocyte–neurone interface – is the leading concept of the causation. Ammonia is produced by the breakdown of protein by intestinal bacteria, and a high blood ammonia is seen in most patients. Electroencephalogram (EEG) shows a decrease in the frequency of the normal α-waves (8–13 Hz) to δ-waves of 1.5–3 Hz. These changes occur before coma supervenes. Management consists of evacuation of the bowels and sterilizing the bowel. Restriction of protein intake is reserved for resistant cases.

7.45

A) T   B) F   C) F   D) F   E) T

The hepatorenal syndrome occurs typically in a patient with advanced cirrhosis with jaundice and ascites. The urine output is low with a low urinary sodium concentration, a maintained capacity to concentrate urine (i.e. tubular function is intact) and an almost normal renal histology. The renal failure here is described as 'functional'. It is sometimes precipitated by overvigorous diuretic therapy, diarrhoea or paracentesis, but often no precipitating factor is found. A number of other mediators have been incriminated in the pathogenesis of the hepatorenal syndrome, in particular the eicosanoids. This has been supported by the precipitation of the syndrome by inhibitors of prostaglandin synthetase such as non-steroidal anti-inflammatory agents. Diuretic therapy should be stopped and intravascular hypovolaemia corrected. Terlipressin has been used as a short-term measure with improvement, but the overall prognosis is poor. Liver transplantation is the best option.

7.46

A) T   B) T   C) T   D) T   E) T

Risk factors for cholesterol gallstones	
Increasing age	Drugs (e.g. contraceptive pill)
Sex (F > M)	Ileal disease or resection
Multiparity	Diabetes mellitus
Obesity	Acromegaly treated with
Rapid weight loss	octreotide
Diet (e.g. high in animal fat)	Liver cirrhosis

A7.47

A) F   B) F   C) T   D) T   E) T

A deficiency of α_1-antitrypsin (α_1AT) is sometimes associated with liver disease and pulmonary emphysema (particularly in smokers). α_1AT is a glycoprotein, part of a family of serine protease inhibitors, or serpin, superfamily. α_1AT is inherited as an autosomal dominant and 1 in 10 northern Europeans carry a deficiency gene. The protein is a 394-amino acid 52 kDa acute phase protein that is synthesized in the liver and constitutes 90% of the serum α_1-globulin seen on electrophoresis. Its main role is to inhibit the proteolytic enzyme, neutrophil elastase. Serum α_1-antritrypsin is low, at 10% of the normal level in the PiZZ phenotypes(60% of normal in the S variant. Patients should be advised to stop smoking.

A7.48

A) T   B) T   C) F   D) T   E) F
F) T   G) F   H) F

Patients with HBsAg, HBeAg and HBV DNA in the serum with abnormal serum aminotransferases and chronic hepatitis on liver biopsy should be treated. Patients with normal aminotransferases and those with decompensated liver disease should not be treated. The main aim of treatment is to eliminate the HBeAg and HBV DNA from the serum with consequent reduction in inflammatory necrosis of the hepatocyte. In patients in whom HBeAg disappears, remission is usually sustained. Both interferon and lamivudine have been shown to be effective. Drug treatment, which often causes transient elevation in aminotransferases, is sometimes accompanied by systemic symptoms, but treatment should be continued, unless these are severe. Pegylated interferon given once weekly is replacing alpha-interferon. Overall, the response rate with disappearance of HBeAg is 25–40%. Those with chronic hepatitis with no HBeAg (i.e. a mutant HBV) generally do not respond to interferon.

8 Haematological disease

Q 8.1

A 42-year-old patient is actively bleeding and is in circulatory shock. He requires blood immediately. Select the best option

A. Fully crossmatched blood
B. Blood of the same ABO group as the patient
C. Blood of the same RhD group as the patient
D. O RhD negative blood
E. Fresh frozen plasma

Q 8.2

A 22-year-old woman with sickle cell disease requires multiple blood transfusions. She is planning to have a baby in the near future. Which one of the following is the best option for transfusion?

A. Same ABO and RhD group as the patient
B. Same ABO and RhD group as the patient which is c-negative and Kell-negative
C. RhD negative blood
D. Same ABO and RhD group as the patient which is Duffy negative
E. Same ABO and RhD group as the patient without IgA antibodies

Q 8.3

A 22-year-old patient is being investigated for a bleeding tendency. His full blood count is: Hb 12 g/dL, white cell count 5.7×10^9/L with a normal differential

count and platelet count is 60×10^9/L. Which of the following is most likely?

A. Prothrombin time 20 s (normal 16–18 s)
B. Bleeding time 13 min (normal 10–12 min)
C. Activated partial thromboplastin time 60 s (normal 30–50 s)
D. Thrombin time 18 s (normal ~12 s)
E. Euglobin clot lysis time 380 min (normal 60–270 min)

Q 8.4

A 35-year-old patient on treatment for thyrotoxicosis is on propylthiouracil. She complains of cough and upper respiratory tract infection. Which one of the following is most likely?

A. Neutrophil leucocytosis
B. Neutropenia
C. Eosinophilia
D. Monocytosis
E. Lymphocytosis

Q 8.5

A 32-year-old woman is being investigated for easy bruising, purpura and epistaxis. Physical examination is normal. She has a history of thyroid disease. Her complete blood count is: Hb 13 g/dL, white cell count 6.7×10^9/L with a normal differential count and platelet count is 55×10^9/L. Select the most likely treatment

A. Factor VIII concentrates
B. Recombinant factor IX
C. Vasopressin
D. Cryoprecipitate
E. Prednisolone

Q8.6

HbA$_{1c}$ is an indicator of blood glucose levels for

A. 7 days
B. 30 days
C. 60 days
D. 90 days
E. 6 weeks

Q8.7

In the normal adult haemopoiesis

A. Is present in the marrow of every bone
B. Partially occurs in the liver
C. Occurs in the spleen
D. Is confined to the central skeleton and the proximal ends of the long bones
E. Occurs in the lymph nodes, central skeleton and proximal ends of long the bones, spleen and liver

Q8.8

Vitamin B$_6$ deficiency causes anaemia because it is required as a co-enzyme for which one of the following?

A. Formation of erythropoeitin
B. Conversion of glycine and succinic acid to δ-aminolaevulinic acid
C. Condensation of two molecules of δ-aminolaevulinic acid to form porphobilinogen
D. Insertion of iron to form haem
E. Formation of protoporphyrins from porphobilinogen

Q8.9

1. The binding of one oxygen molecule to deoxyhaemoglobin to increase oxygen affinity of the remaining binding sites
2. Acidosis resulting in a reduction in oxygen-binding affinity of haemoglobin
3. Oxygenation of haemoglobin reduces its affinity for carbon dioxide
4. Production of red cell 2,3-diphosphoglycerate

Select the best match for each of the above

A. Haldane effect
B. Bohr effect
C. Cooperativity
D. Red cell gluconeogenesis
E. Red cell glycolysis

Q8.10

1. A 52-year-old farmer in India presents with generalized weakness. Haematocrit is 0.20 and mean corpuscular volume (MCV) is 72. On examination he has koilonychia
2. A 28-year-old Greek waiter complains of fatigue. Haematocrit is 0.32. On examination he has bone deformities
3. A 28-year-old Sudanese medical registrar complains of fatigue. Hematocrit is 0.28. On examination he has leg ulcers
4. A 22-year-old presents with shortness of breath. Haematocit is 0.27. Serum bilirubin is elevated

Select the best match for each of the above

A. Sickle cell disease
B. Thalassaemia major
C. Iron deficiency anaemia
D. Sideroblastic anaemia
E. Polycythaemia vera
F. Haemolytic anaemia
G. Spurious polycythaemia

Haematological disease

Q8.11

1. A 45-year-old man with clinical features of lead poisoning
2. A 22-year-old Greek nurse who has a defect in the synthesis of globin genes
3. A 68-year-old woman with long-standing rheumatoid arthritis
4. A 26-year-old woman who has a long history of menorrhagia

Select the best match for each of the above

A. Mean corpuscular volume (MCV) 72 fl, reduced serum iron, raised serum total iron binding capacity (TIBC), reduced serum ferritin, increased serum soluble transfer receptor, iron absent from both bone marrow and erythroblasts
B. MCV 70 fl, reduced serum iron, reduced serum total iron binding capacity (TIBC), normal serum ferritin, normal serum soluble transfer receptor, iron present in bone marrow but absent from erythroblasts
C. MCV 71 fl, normal serum iron, normal serum total iron binding capacity (TIBC), normal serum ferritin, normal serum soluble transfer receptor, iron present in both bone marrow and erythroblasts
D. MCV 96 fl, raised serum iron, normal serum total iron binding capacity (TIBC), raised serum ferritin, normal serum soluble transfer receptor, iron present in bone marrow, iron in ring form in erythroblasts

Q8.12

1. A 28-year-old man is symptom free. Haemoglobin is 11 g/dL, mean corpuscular volume (MCV) is 72, and mean corpuscular haemoglobin (MCH) 25. Serum ferritin levels are normal. Hb A_2 and Hb F are raised

2. A 21-year-old patient complains of fatigue and recurrent leg ulcers. On examination he has splenomegaly and bone deformities. Haemoglobin is 10 g/dL and the patient has not needed a transfusion. Hb A_2 and Hb F are raised
3. A 12-month-old child presents with failure to thrive. Haemoglobin is 6 g/dL. Hb A_2 and Hb F are raised. Skull X-ray shows 'hair on end' appearance
4. A 12-year-old boy presents with fatigue. On examination he has splenomegaly. Haemoglobin is 10 g/dL. Hb A_2 is reduced. Hb A, Hb Barts and haemoglobin with four beta chains are all present. The patient has not required blood transfusion
5. A 22-year-old is asymptomatic. Haemoglobin is 12 g/dL, MCV is 72. On staining the blood film with brilliant cresyl blue, Hb H bodies are seen

Select the best match for each of the above

A. α-Thalassaemia minor
B. Cooley's anaemia
C. Thalassaemia intermedia
D. Hb H disease
E. β-Thalassaemia trait

Q8.13

1. Glucose is metabolized to pyruvate and lactic acid with production of ATP
2. NADPH production
3. 90% of glucose is metabolized by this pathway
4. Maintains glutathione in a reduced form
5. Enables more oxygen to be delivered to the tissues
6. Formation of 2, 3-diphosphoglycerate

Select the best match for each of the above

A. Hexose monophosphate pathway
B. Embden–Meyerhof pathway

C. Shift of oxygen dissociation curve to the right
D. Shift of oxygen dissociation curve to the left
E. Glycogenolysis
F. Gluconeogenesis
G. Rapoport–Luebering shunt

Q8.14

1. A 38-year-old woman has a history of episodes of anaemia and jaundice which often remit and relapse. The spleen is palpable. Investigations confirm haemolytic anaemia. Spherocytes are present in the peripheral blood picture. Direct Coombs' test is positive

2. A 28-year-old woman is diagnosed with mycoplasma pneumonia. Investigations reveal haemolysis. Direct Coombs' test is positive

3. Following surgery, a patient complains that urine voided at night and in the morning on waking is dark in colour. There is a past history of cerebral venous thrombosis

4. A newborn infant has severe jaundice

5. A 7-year-old child develops chickenpox and is noted to have intermittently dark-coloured urine. The antibodies have specificity for P red cell antigen

Select the best match for each of the above

A. Flow cytometric analysis of red cells with anti-CD55 and anti-CD59
B. At birth, cord blood shows anaemia with a high reticulocyte count, and a positive direct antiglobulin test
C. Direct antiglobulin test is positive, with either IgG alone (67%), IgG and complement (20%), or complement alone (13%) being found on the surface of the red cells
D. IgM antibody

E. At birth, cord blood shows anaemia with a low reticulocyte count, and a negative direct antiglobulin test
F. Donath–Landsteiner test

Q8.15

1. Nephrotic syndrome with fluid overload, resistant to diuretic therapy
2. von Willebrand's disease
3. Disseminated intravascular coagulation where plasma fibrinogen levels are low
4. Increased INR due to warfarin requiring urgent surgery
5. Bleeding in a patient whose platelet count is 10×10^9
6. Patient who has a history of severe recurrent urticarial reaction with blood transfusion who requires packed red cells for anaemia
7. Patient with Hb of 6 g/dL who is scheduled for surgery the next day

Select the best option for each of the above

A. Virtually all plasma is removed from blood and replaced by about 100 mL of an additive solution containing sodium chloride, adenine, glucose and mannitol
B. Preparations of red cells suspended in saline, produced by cell separators to remove all but traces of plasma proteins
C. Whole blood from single donors prepared by plateletpheresis (has been stored at 22°C for 2 days)
D. Whole blood from single donors centrifuged to produce platelet concentrates (has been stored at 22°C for 7 days)
E. Plasma prepared from whole blood is subjected to temperature of −30°C within 2 hours of donation
F. Frozen plasma from a single donation thawed at 4–8°C and supernatant removed

Haematological disease

G. Freeze-dried preparations of factor XIII and IX prepared from a large pool of plasma

H. Human albumin solution 20%

Q8.16

A patient would like information about the transmission of infection from blood transfusions. The following statements are correct

A. *Treponema pallidum* spirochaetes are able to proliferate in blood products stored at 4°C for a week

B. *Yersinia enterocolitica* does not survive in red cell concentrates stored at 4°C

C. The risk of transmission of variant Creutzfeldt–Jakob disease can be reduced by a simple screening test

D. The use of leucocyte-depleted blood increases the risk of transmission of variant Creutzfeldt–Jakob disease

E. The risk of transmission of HIV by blood transfusion is extremely low in the UK because of routine testing for anti-HLTV-1

Q8.17

1. Antithrombin

2. Activated protein C

3. Protein S

4. Plasmin

5. High-molecular-weight multimeric forms of von Willebrand factor

Select the best match for each of the above

A. A serine protease which breaks down fibrinogen and fibrin into fragments X, Y, D and E

B. Promotes platelet function

C. Inactivates serine proteases by forming stable complexes and its action is greatly potentiated by heparin

D. Destroys factor V and factor VIII

E. Cofactor for protein C

Q8.18

1. Lack of the platelet membrane glycoprotein IIb/IIIa complex resulting in defective fibrinogen binding and failure of platelet aggregation

2. Lack of the platelet membrane glycoprotein Ib, the binding site for factor vWF. There is failure of platelet adhesion and moderate thrombocytopenia

3. Typically occurs in children. Purpuric rash on legs and buttocks accompanied by haematuria and glomerulonephritis

4. Florid purpura, fever, fluctuating cerebral dysfunction, haemolytic anaemia with red cell fragmentation accompanied by renal failure

5. Arterial or venous thrombosis with risk of abnormal bleeding

Select the best match for each of the above

A. Henoch–Schönlein syndrome

B. Thrombotic thrombocytopenic purpura

C. Essential thrombocythaemia

D. Glanzmann's thrombasthenia

E. Bernard–Soulier syndrome

Q8.19

1. A 29-year-old man has a history of recurrent bleeding with spontaneous trauma. The bleeding is usually in the joints and the joints are deformed. There is a history of muscle bleeds

2. A 45-year-old woman has a history of bleeding following minor trauma. She also has epistaxis and menorrhagia. Despite severe bleeding, there is no history of bleeding in the joints or muscle bleeds

3. A 46-year-old cirrhotic who is severely malnourished and treated with antibiotics has gastrointestinal and cerebral bleeding

4. A 22-year-old woman presents with fever and is toxic. Investigations reveal marked leucocytosis and Gram-negative organisms in blood cultures. She is bleeding from the nose and venepuncture sites

Select the best match for each of the above

A. Bleeding time is normal, prothrombin time is prolonged, APTT is prolonged, factor VIII:C is normal, von Willebrand factor is normal
B. Bleeding time is normal, prothrombin time is normal, APTT is elevated, factor VIII:C is deficient, vonWillebrand factor is deficient, and there is defective platelet aggregation with ristocetin
C. Bleeding time is normal, prothrombin time is normal, APTT is elevated, factor VIII:C is markedly deficient, von Willebrand factor level is normal and platelet aggregation with ristocetin is not defective
D. The prothrombin time, APTT and thrombin time are markedly prolonged. Fibrinogen levels are markedly reduced. There is severe thrombocytopenia and levels of FDPs/D-dimer are elevated. The blood film shows fragmented red blood cells

Q8.20

1. Inhibits the enzyme cyclo-oxygenase, resulting in reduced platelet production of TXA_2
2. Inhibits platelet phosphodiesterase, causing an increase in cyclic AMP with potentiation of the action of PGI_2
3. Blocks ADP-mediated platelet aggregation and transformation of the platelet fibrinogen receptor into a high-affinity form. It is a potential substitute for aspirin but its use has been associated with granulocytopenia and

also, paradoxically, with thrombotic thrombocytopenic purpura (TTP)
4. Affects the ADP-dependent activation of the glycoprotein IIb/IIIa complex
5. Blocks a receptor on the platelet for fibrinogen and von Willebrand factor

Select the best match for each of the above

A. Clopidogrel
B. Glycoprotein IIb/IIIa receptor antagonists
C. Ticlopidine
D. Dipyridamole
E. Aspirin

Q8.21

1. Patients <40 years undergoing major surgery (>30 minutes) with no other risk factors
2. Major general, urological, gynaecological, cardiothoracic, vascular or neurological surgery in patients >40 years or with one or more other risk factor(s)
3. Fracture or major orthopaedic surgery of pelvis, hip or leg
4. Patients undergoing minor surgery (<30 minutes) with no other risk factors
5. Major acute medical illness such as myocardial infarction, heart failure, chest infection, cancer or inflammatory bowel disease
6. Major pelvic or abdominal surgery for cancer
7. Major trauma
8. Major surgery, trauma or illness in patients with previous deep vein thrombosis, pulmonary embolism or thrombophilia
9. Patients with minor trauma or illness with no thrombophilia but with a history of deep vein thrombosis or previous pulmonary embolism

Haematological disease

10. Leg paralysis

11. Minor surgery, trauma or illness in patients with previous deep vein thrombosis, pulmonary embolism or thrombophilia

12. Plastercast immobilization of the leg in patients with minor injury

Select the risk of deep vein thrombosis and pulmonary embolism for each of the above hospitalized patients

A. Low risk (proximal vein thrombosis 0.4%; fatal pulmonary embolism <0.2%)

B. Medium risk (proximal vein thrombosis 2–4%; fatal pulmonary embolism 0.2–0.5%)

C. High risk (proximal vein thrombosis 10–20%; fatal pulmonary embolism 1–5%)

Q8.22

A 33-year-old woman's blood picture is as follows: Hb 9 g/dL reticulocyte count 5%. The following can explain this blood picture

A. Polycythaemia
B. Haemorrhage
C. Haemolysis
D. Treatment with iron
E. Pseudopolycythaemia

Q8.23

A 72-year-old woman's ESR is 32 mm/h. Explanations for this finding include

A. Advanced age
B. Female gender
C. Polycythaemia vera
D. Severe anaemia
E. Infection

Q8.24

A 72-year-old woman's plasma viscosity is markedly elevated. Explanations for this finding include

A. Advanced age
B. Female gender
C. Polycythaemia vera
D. Severe anaemia
E. Infection

Q8.25

C-reactive protein

A. Is exclusively synthesized in the kidney
B. Rises within 6 hours of an acute event
C. Follows the clinical state of the patient much more rapidly than the ESR
D. Is affected by the level of Hb
E. Predicts future cardiovascular disease

Q8.26

The following statements about anticoagulants are correct

A. Heparin is not a single substance but a mixture of unfractionated polysaccharides
B. Low-molecular-weight heparins can be monitored by the use of APTT
C. Heparin-induced thrombocytopenia is associated with severe thrombosis
D. Hirudins can be monitored by the use of APTT
E. Warfarin can be used safely in pregnancy

Q8.27

A 25-year-old woman with pulmonary embolism requires anticoagulant therapy. The following conditions are relative contraindications to initiating warfarin therapy

A. Pregnancy
B. Severe uncontrolled hypertension
C. Peptic ulceration
D. Severe liver disease
E. Non-compliance

C. Haem iron is the major dietary source of iron
D. Non-haem iron is better absorbed than haem iron
E. Absorption of iron is decreased in pregnancy

Q8.28

A 32-year-old woman on oral contraceptives presents with a swollen left leg. She has a past history of venous thrombosis. The following are appropriate tests for determining the cause of thrombophilia

A. Assay for activated protein C resistance
B. Molecular testing for factor V Leiden
C. Lupus anticoagulant
D. Anticardiolipin antibodies
E. Assay for protein S
F. Assay for protein C

Q8.29

A 39-year-old woman complains of fatigue and shortness of breath. Haemoglobin is 9g/dL and MCV is 70. MCHC is 25 pg. The following conditions cause this blood picture

A. Folic acid deficiency
B. Vitamin B_{12} deficiency
C. Long-standing rheumatoid arthritis
D. Haemoglobinopathy with defect in globin synthesis
E. Sideroblastic anaemia

Q8.30

A 25-year-old architect believes in eating health foods. She would like to know which of the following statements regarding iron intake are correct

A. The average daily diet in the UK contains about 100 mg of iron
B. Most of the dietary iron intake is absorbed

Q8.31

The following statements about iron absorption are correct

A. Iron absorption takes place in the terminal ileum
B. Haem iron is absorbed by a protein called divalent metal transporter 1 (DMT1)
C. A transporter protein requiring an accessory multicopper protein, hephaestin, is required for absorption of iron from the basolateral surface of mucosal cells
D. Ferric iron is better absorbed than ferrous iron
E. Gastric acidity retards iron absorption

Q8.32

Correct statements about the regulation of iron absorption include

A. After an intake of dietary iron, mucosal cells are resistant to taking up more iron
B. The stores of iron in the body can influence the levels of divalent metal transporter 1 (DMT1) in the duodenum
C. Anaemia due to hereditary spherocytosis stimulates greater iron absorption than thalassaemia
D. Iron absorption is generally increased in all iron overload states
E. The body tightly regulates the absorption because it is unable to excrete iron once it is absorbed

Haematological disease

Q8.33

Correct statements about iron transport and stores include

A. Iron is transported in plasma bound to serum ferritin
B. About two-thirds of the total body iron is in the liver
C. About two-thirds of the iron in the liver is stored as haemosiderin
D. In an average adult 20 mg of iron/daily is derived chiefly from red cell breakdown in the reticuloendothelial system
E. Ferritin is an insoluble iron–protein complex found in the macrophages in the bone marrow, liver and spleen

Q8.34

A 65-year-old woman with a history of thyroid disease presents with symptoms of anaemia. She also has paraesthesia in the fingers and toes, early loss of vibration sense and proprioception, progressive weakness and ataxia. The following statements are correct

A. Parietal cell antibodies are likely to present in the serum in 90% of patients with this condition
B. Serum bilirubin levels may be raised
C. The Schilling test is likely to show that absorption of vitamin B_{12} is impaired
D. Bone marrow will show megaloblastic erythropoiesis
E. The deficient vitamin is mainly present in leafy vegetables and plants
F. The vitamin is mainly stored in the kidney
G. Treatment with the deficient vitamin should be given for about 4 months to replace body stores

Q8.35

A 29-year-old pregnant woman presents with anaemia. Bone marrow shows macrocytic anaemia. Investigation excludes vitamin B_{12} deficiency. The following statements are correct

A. Green vegetables such as broccoli and spinach contain the deficient vitamin
B. The deficient vitamin is responsible for the conversion of homocysteine to methionine
C. Deficiency of this vitamin in pregnancy increases the incidence of neural tube defects in the fetus
D. Treatment should be given for the rest of the patient's life
E. The amount of the vitamin in the serum, rather than the red cells, is a better measure of tissue level

Q8.36

A 45-year-old man presents with fatigue. Haematocrit is 26 and MCV is 102. Bone marrow shows a normoblastic picture. Likely causes are

A. Iron deficiency anaemia
B. Liver disease
C. Reticulocytosis
D. Hyperthyroidism
E. Alcohol excess

Q8.37

A 25-year-old man presents with anaemia and sore throat. His blood picture shows Hb 7 g/dL, neutrophil count 1×10^9, platelet count 30×10^9/L, reticulocyte count 40×10^9/L. Bone marrow shows hypocellularity. Recognized causes for his blood picture are

A. Hypersplenism
B. Carbimazole
C. Hepatitis A
D. Paroxysmal nocturnal haemoglobinuria
E. Chloramphenicol

Q8.38

A 25-year-old man presents with anaemia and a sore throat. His blood picture shows Hb 7 g/dL, neutrophil count 0.3×10^9, platelet count 15×10^9/L, reticulocyte count 30×10^9/L. Bone marrow shows hypocellularity. The following statements are correct

A. Bone marrow transplantation is the treatment of choice for patients over 50 years of age
B. Immunosuppressive therapy is the treatment of choice for patients under 50 years of age
C. Oxymethalone is sometimes useful in this condition
D. Steroids are very useful for increasing the cellularity of bone marrow
E. This patient has Diamond–Blackfan syndrome

Q8.39

A 22-year-old man presents with fatigue. On examination he has anaemia, jaundice, splenomegaly and leg ulcers. Blood film shows reticulocytes and spherocytes. The following statements are correct

A. Parvovirus infections in these patients result in aplastic anaemia
B. Pigment gallstones are a contraindication to splenectomy
C. When red cells are placed in solutions of increasing hypotonicity, they take in water, swell and eventually lyse
D. Direct antiglobulin (Coombs') test is positive
E. There is an excess of the structural protein spectrin in the red cell membrane

Q8.40

A 29-year-old African man presents with anaemia, jaundice and haemoglobinuria. He is diagnosed to have glucose-6-phosphate dehydrogenase (G6PD) deficiency. The following statements are correct

A. Plasma haptoglobin is typically elevated
B. Heinz bodies may be seen on blood film during an acute attack
C. An acute attack can be precipitated by eating fava beans
D. Splenectomy is recommended in severe cases
E. Chloroquine can precipitate an acute attack

Q8.41

A 22-year-old woman has a white cell count of 7×10^9/L, neutrophils 3.5×10^9/L, lymphocytes 2.5×10^9/L, eosinophil count 1×10^9/L. This picture is associated with the following

A. Hodgkin's disease
B. Urticaria
C. Asthma
D. Churg–Strauss syndrome
E. Hookworm infestation

Q8.42

A 67-year-old man complains of tiredness, depression, angina and intermittent claudication. He develops severe itching after a hot bath. On examination he is plethoric and has a deep dusky cyanosis, hypertension, splenomegaly and hepatomegaly. The following statements are correct

A. Bone marrow shows erythroid hyperplasia
B. Leucocyte alkaline phosphatase is reduced

C. An elevated serum erythropoietin level is diagnostic
D. Venesection will relieve many of the symptoms
E. About two-thirds of patients develop myelofibrosis

8.43

A 35-year-old man complains of lethargy, weakness and weight loss. On examination features include anaemia and massive splenomegaly. Trephine marrow biopsy shows markedly increased fibrosis and increased megakaryocytes. The Philadelphia chromosome is absent. The following statements are correct

A. Chronic myeloid leukaemia is the most likely diagnosis
B. Blood smear shows poikilocytes
C. Median survival is 10 years
D. Splenectomy is contraindicated
E. The leucocyte alkaline phosphatase score is reduced

8.44

A 22-year-old man has blunt trauma of the abdomen which requires splenectomy. The following statements are correct

A. *Haemophilus influenzae* type B vaccine should be avoided in this patient
B. Howell–Jolly bodies may be seen in the peripheral smear
C. Meningococcal immunization is routinely recommended
D. Pappenheimer bodies (containing sideroblastic granules) are seen in the peripheral smear
E. Pitted cells are typically absent

8.45

A 29-year-old Afro-Caribbean man presents with low-grade fever and pleuritic chest pain and bone pains. He has a past history of splenic infarcts and priapism. Haemoglobin is 8 g/dL The following statements are correct

A. Reticulocyte count is typically low
B. When the patient's Hb is mixed with sodium dithionite it gives a turbid appearance
C. The patient is susceptible to *Salmonella* osteomyelitis
D. Aseptic necrosis of femoral heads is a recognized complication
E. Hydroxycarbamide (hydroxyurea) is contraindicated because it can precipitate aplastic crisis

8.46

A 65-year-old man has a haemoglobin of 7 g/dL 2 months after surgery. In order to improve his haematocrit packed red cells are administered. Soon after the transfusion is begun the patient develops severe rigors, lumbar pain and dyspnoea. Urine examination reveals haemoglobinuria. The following statements are correct

A. Reassure the patient that many patients experience such symptoms; administer an antihistamine and continue the blood transfusion
B. Stop the transfusion and return the donor units to the blood transfusion laboratory
C. The presence of elevated D-dimers is a good prognostic sign
D. The most likely cause of his symptoms is urinary tract infection
E. The most likely cause of his symptoms is malaria

A8.1

D

When there is insufficient time for full pre-transfusion testing the options include:

1. Blood required immediately – use of 2 units of O RhD negative blood ('emergency stock'), to allow additional time for the laboratory to group the patient.

2. Blood required in 10–15 minutes – use of blood of the same ABO and RhD groups as the patient.

3. Blood required in 45 minutes – most laboratories will be able to provide fully crossmatched blood within this time.

A8.2

B

For patients who are likely to be multitransfused and at high risk of developing antibodies, e.g. sickle cell disease, many centres routinely provide c-negative and Kell-negative blood for women of child-bearing age to minimize the risk of alloimmunization and subsequent haemolytic disease of the newborn (HDN).

A8.3

B

Prolonged bleeding times are found in patients with platelet function defects and there is a progressive prolongation with platelet counts less than 80×10^9/L. The bleeding time should not be performed at low platelet counts.

A8.4

B

Cough and upper respiratory tract infection in a patient on propylthiouracil suggests bacterial infection due to agranulocytosis. Neutropenia is defined as a circulatory neutrophil count below 1.5×10^9/L. A virtual absence of neutrophils is called agranulocytosis. It should be noted that black patients may have somewhat lower neutrophil counts. Neutropenia caused by viruses is probably the most common type. Chemotherapy and radiotherapy predictably produce neutropenia; many other drugs including propylthiouracil have been known to produce an idiosyncratic cytopenia and a drug cause should always be considered.

A8.5

E

Chronic autoimmune thrombocytopenic purpura (AITP) is characteristically seen in adult women. It is usually idiopathic but may occur in association with other autoimmune disorders such as systemic lupus erythematosus (SLE), thyroid disease and autoimmune haemolytic anaemia (Evans' syndrome), in patients with chronic lymphocytic leukaemia and solid tumours, and after infections with viruses such as HIV. Platelet autoantibodies are detected in about 60–70% of patients, and are presumed to be present, although not detectable, in the remaining patients; the antibodies often have specificity for platelet membrane glycoproteins IIb/IIIa and/or Ib. Spontaneous remissions are rare. The main aims of treatment are to reduce the production of platelet autoantibodies and the removal of antibody-coated platelets. Initial treatment is with prednisolone, 40–60 mg daily in adults, with cautious reduction of the dose after remission has occurred.

Haematological disease

A8.6

D

Red cells survive 120 days, and therefore HbA_{1C} reflects blood sugar for a period of 120 days.

A8.7

D

At birth, haemopoiesis is present in the marrow of nearly every bone. As the child grows the active red marrow is gradually replaced by fat (yellow marrow) so that haemopoiesis in the adult becomes confined to the central skeleton and the proximal ends of the long bones. Only if the demand for blood cells increases and persists do the areas of red marrow extend once again. Pathological processes interfering with normal haemopoiesis may result in resumption of haemopoietic activity in the liver and spleen, which is referred to as extramedullary haemopoiesis.

A8.8

B

Haemoglobin synthesis occurs in the mitochondria of the developing red cell. The major rate-limiting step is the conversion of glycine and succinic acid to δ-aminolaevulinic acid (ALA) by ALA synthetase. Vitamin B_6 is a coenzyme for this reaction, which is inhibited by haem and stimulated by erythropoietin.

A8.9

1) C   2) B   3) A   4) E

The binding of one oxygen molecule to deoxyhaemoglobin increases the oxygen affinity of the remaining binding sites – this property is known as cooperativity and is the reason for the sigmoid shape of the oxygen dissociation curve. Hydrogen ions and carbon dioxide added to blood cause a reduction in the oxygen-binding affinity of haemoglobin (the Bohr effect). Oxygenation of haemoglobin reduces its affinity for carbon dioxide (the Haldane effect). These effects help the exchange of carbon dioxide and oxygen in the tissues. Red cell metabolism produces 2,3-DPG from glycolysis, which accumulates because it is sequestered by binding to deoxyhaemoglobin. The binding of 2,3-DPG stabilizes the T conformation and reduces its affinity for oxygen. The P_{50} increases with 2,3-DPG concentrations, which increase when oxygen availability is reduced in conditions such as hypoxia or anaemia.

A8.10

1) C   2) B   3) A   4) F

Examples of specific signs of different types of anaemia include:

- koilonychia – spoon-shaped nails seen in iron deficiency anaemia
- jaundice – found in haemolytic anaemia
- bone deformities – found in thalassaemia major
- leg ulcers – occur in association with sickle cell disease.

It must be emphasized that anaemia is not a diagnosis, and a cause must be found.

A8.11

1) D   2) C   3) B   4) A

Microcytic anaemia: the differential diagnosis				
	Iron deficiency	Anaemia of chronic disease	Thalassaemia trait (α or β)	Sideroblastic anaemia
MCV	Reduced	Low normal or normal	Very low for degree of anaemia	Low in inherited type but often raised in acquired type
Serum iron	Reduced	Reduced	Normal	Raised
Serum TIBC	Raised	Reduced	Normal	Normal
Serum ferritin	Reduced	Normal or raised	Normal	Raised
Serum soluble transfer receptor	Increased	Normal	Normal or raised	Normal or raised
Iron in marrow	Absent	Present	Present	Present
Iron in erythroblasts	Absent	Absent or reduced	Present	Ring forms

TIBC, total iron binding capacity

A8.12

1) E   2) C   3) B   4) D   5) A

Clinically, β-thalassaemia can be divided into the following: a) thalassaemia minor (or trait), the symptomless heterozygous carrier state; b) thalassaemia intermedia, with moderate anaemia, rarely requiring transfusions; c) thalassaemia major, with severe anaemia requiring regular transfusions. Thalassaemia minor (trait) patients are asymptomatic. Anaemia is mild or absent. The red cells are hypochromic and microcytic with a low MCV and MCH, and it may be confused with iron deficiency. However, the two are easily distinguished as in thalassaemia trait the serum ferritin and the iron stores are normal. Hb electrophoresis usually shows a raised Hb A_2 and often a raised Hb F. Iron should not be given to these patients unless they develop coincidental iron deficiency. Thalassaemia intermedia includes patients who are symptomatic with moderate anaemia (Hb 7–10 g/dL) and who do not require regular transfusions. That is, it is more severe than

in β-thalassaemia trait but milder than in transfusion-dependent thalassaemia major. Patients may have splenomegaly and bone deformities. Recurrent leg ulcers, gallstones and infections are also seen. Thalassaemia major (Cooley's anaemia) affects children during the first year of life with: a) failure to thrive and recurrent bacterial infections; b) severe anaemia from 3–6 months when the switch from γ- to β-chain production should normally occur; c) extramedullary haemopoiesis that soon leads to hepatosplenomegaly and bone expansion, giving rise to the classical thalassaemic facies. Skull X-rays in these children show the characteristic 'hair on end' appearance of bony trabeculation as a result of expansion of the bone marrow into cortical bone.

In contrast to β-thalassaemia, α-thalassaemia is often caused by gene deletions, although mutations also occur. The gene for α chains is duplicated on both chromosomes 16; i.e. there are four genes. Deletion of one α-chain gene ($α^+$) or both α-chain genes ($α^0$) on each chromosome 16 may occur. The former is

Haematological disease

the most common of these abnormalities. If three genes are deleted, there is moderate anaemia (Hb 7–10 g/dL) and splenomegaly (Hb H disease). The patients are not usually transfusion-dependent. Hb A, Hb Barts and Hb H (β_4) are present. Hb A_2 is normal or reduced. If two genes are deleted (α-thalassaemia trait) there is microcytosis with or without mild anaemia. Hb H bodies may be seen on staining a blood film with brilliant cresyl blue. With one gene deletion the blood picture is usually normal.

A8.13

1) B   2) A   3) B   4) A   5) D
6) G

The enzyme systems responsible for producing energy and reducing power are: a) the glycolytic (Embden–Meyerhof) pathway, in which glucose is metabolized to pyruvate and lactic acid with production of ATP; b) the hexose monophosphate (pentosephosphate) pathway, which provides reducing power for the red cell in the form of NADPH. About 90% of glucose is metabolized by the former and 10% by the latter. The importance of the hexose monophosphate shunt is that it maintains glutathione (GSH) in a reduced state. 2,3-DPG (diphosphoglycerate) is formed from a side-arm of the glycolytic pathway. It binds to the central part of the Hb tetramer, fixing it in the low-affinity state. A decreased affinity with a shift in the oxygen dissociation curve to the right enables more oxygen to be delivered to the tissues.

A8.14

1) C   2) D   3) A   4) B   5) F

Warm autoimmune haemolytic anaemias may occur at all ages and in both sexes, although they are most frequent in middle-aged women. They can present as a short episode of anaemia and jaundice but they often remit and relapse and may progress to an intermittent chronic pattern. The spleen is often palpable. Infections or folate deficiency may provoke a profound fall in the haemoglobin level. In more than 30% of cases, the cause remains unknown. These anaemias may be associated with lymphoid malignancies or diseases such as rheumatoid arthritis and SLE or drugs. Spherocytosis is present as a result of red cell damage. Direct antiglobulin test is positive, with either IgG alone (67%), IgG and complement (20%), or complement alone (13%) being found on the surface of the red cells. Autoantibodies may have specificity for the Rh blood group system (e.g. for the e antigen). Autoimmune thrombocytopenia and/or neutropenia may also be present (Evans' syndrome). Normally, low titres of IgM cold agglutinins reacting at 4°C are present in plasma and are harmless. At low temperatures these antibodies can attach to red cells and cause their agglutination in the cold peripheries of the body. In addition, activation of complement may cause intravascular haemolysis when the cells return to the higher temperatures in the core of the body. After certain infections (such as *Mycoplasma*, cytomegalovirus, Epstein–Barr virus (EBV)) there is increased synthesis of polyclonal cold agglutinins producing a mild to moderate transient haemolysis. Paroxysmal cold haemoglobinuria (PCH) is a rare condition associated with common childhood infections, such as measles, mumps and chickenpox. Intravascular haemolysis is associated with polyclonal IgG complement-fixing antibodies. These antibodies are biphasic, reacting with red cells in the cold in the peripheral circulation, with lysis occurring due to complement activation when the cells return to the central circulation. The antibodies have specificity for the P red cell antigen. The lytic reaction is demonstrated in vitro by incubating the patient's red cells and serum at 4°C and then warming the mixture to 37°C (Donath–Landsteiner test). Haemolysis is self-limiting but supportive transfusions of warmed blood may be necessary. Haemolytic disease of the newborn is due to fetomaternal incompatibility for red cell antigens. Maternal alloantibodies against fetal red cell antigens pass from the maternal circulation via the placenta into the fetus, where they destroy the fetal red cells. Only IgG antibodies are capable of transplacental passage from mother to fetus. Clinical features vary from a mild haemolytic anaemia of the newborn to intrauterine death from 18 weeks' gestation with the characteristic appearance of hydrops fetalis (hepatosplenomegaly, oedema and cardiac failure). Kernicterus occurs owing to severe jaundice in the neonatal period, where the unconjugated (lipid-soluble) bilirubin exceeds 250 mmol/L and bile pigment deposition occurs in the basal ganglia. This can result in permanent brain damage, choreoathetosis, and spasticity. In mild cases it may be mainly manifest as deafness. At birth of an affected child the cord blood shows anaemia with a high reticulocyte count, and a positive direct antiglobin test. Paroxysmal nocturnal haemoglobinuria (PNH) is a rare acquired red cell defect in which a clone of red cells is particularly sensitive to destruction by activated complement. These cells are continually haemolysed intravascularly. Platelets and granulocytes are also affected and there may be thrombocytopenia and neutropenia. The underlying defect is an

inability of PNH cells to make glycosylphosphatidylinositol (GPI), which anchors surface proteins such as delay accelerating factor (DAF; CD55) and membrane inhibitor of reactive lysis (MIRL; CD59) to cell membranes. Patients present with haemolysis which may be precipitated by infection, iron therapy or surgery. Characteristically only the urine voided at night and in the morning on waking is dark in colour, although the reason for this phenomenon is not clear. In severe cases all urine samples are dark. Urinary iron loss may be sufficient to cause iron deficiency. Some patients present insidiously with signs of anaemia and recurrent abdominal pains. Venous thrombotic episodes are very common, and unusual and severe thromboses may occur, for example in hepatic (Budd–Chiari syndrome), mesenteric or cerebral veins. The cause of the increased predisposition to thrombosis is not known, but may be due to complement-mediated activation of platelets deficient in CD55 and CD59. Flow cytometric analysis of red cells with anti-CD55 and anti-CD59 has replaced the Ham's test.

A8.15

1) H   2) G   3) F   4) E   5) C
6) B   7) A

The preparation of red cell concentrates involves removal of all the plasma and replacement by about 100 mL of an optimal additive solution, such as SAG-M, which contains sodium chloride, adenine, glucose and mannitol. Washed red cell concentrates are preparations of red cells suspended in saline, produced by cell separators to remove all but traces of plasma proteins. They are used in patients who have had severe recurrent urticarial or anaphylactic reactions. Platelet concentrates are prepared either from whole blood by centrifugation or by plateletpheresis of single donors using cell separators. They may be stored for up to 5 days at 22°C. They are used to treat bleeding in patients with severe thrombocytopenia, and prophylactically to prevent bleeding in patients with bone marrow failure. Fresh frozen plasma (FFP) is prepared by freezing the plasma from 1 unit of blood at −30°C within 6 hours of donation. The volume is approximately 200 mL. FFP contains all the coagulation factors present in fresh plasma and is used mostly for replacement of coagulation factors in acquired coagulation factor deficiencies. The cryoprecipitate is obtained by allowing the frozen plasma from a single donation to thaw at 4–8°C and removing the supernatant. The volume is about 20 mL and it is stored at −30°C. It contains factor VIII:C, von Willebrand factor (vWF) and fibrinogen. It is no longer used for the treatment of haemophilia A and von Willebrand's disease because of the greater risk of virus transmission compared with virus-inactivated coagulation factor concentrates. It may be useful in disseminated intravascular coagulation (DIC) and other conditions where the fibrinogen level is very low. Factor VIII and IX concentrates are freeze-dried preparations of specific coagulation factors prepared from large pools of plasma. They are used for treating patients with haemophilia and von Willebrand's disease, where recombinant coagulation factor concentrates are unavailable. Recombinant coagulation factor concentrates, where they are available, are the treatment of choice for patients with inherited coagulation factor deficiencies. There are two preparations of albumin. a) Human albumin solution 4.5%, previously called plasma protein fraction (PPF),

contains 45g/L albumin and 160 mmol/L sodium. It is available in 50, 100, 250 and 500 mL bottles. b) Human albumin solution 20%, previously called 'salt-poor' albumin, contains approximately 200 g/L albumin and 130 mmol/L sodium and is available in 50 and 100 mL bottles. Human albumin solutions are indicated for treatment of acute severe hypoalbuminaemia and as the replacement fluid for plasma exchange. The 20% albumin solution is particularly useful for patients with nephrotic syndrome or liver disease who are fluid overloaded and resistant to diuretics. Albumin solutions should not be used to treat patients with malnutrition or chronic renal or liver disease.

A8.16

A) F   B) F   C) F   D) F   E) F

In terms of measures to reduce the risk of transmission of variant Creutzfeldt–Jakob disease (vCJD) by blood transfusion, there are no known criteria for exclusion of blood donors, and, as yet, no screening test. The general introduction of leucocyte-depleted blood in the UK aims to minimize the risk of transmission of vCJD by blood transfusion. In the UK the incidence of transmission of HIV by blood transfusion is extremely low – probably under 1 in 3 million units transfused. Prevention is based on self-exclusion of donors in 'high-risk' groups and testing each donation for anti-HIV. Testing for anti-HTLV-1 is not carried out in the UK as it is in other countries, notably Japan and the United States. Only about 1 in 20 000 donors is seropositive, and there is a low risk of developing disease after infection because of the long incubation period. Transfusion-transmitted syphilis is now very rare in the UK. Spirochaetes do not survive for more than 72 hours in blood stored at 4°C, and each donation is tested using the *Treponema pallidum* haemagglutination assay. Bacterial contamination of blood components is potentially a very serious event, and although rare it is one of the most frequent causes of death associated with transfusion, after haemolytic transfusion reactions. Some organisms such as *Yersinia enterocolitica* can proliferate in red cell concentrates stored at 4°C, but platelet concentrates stored at 22°C are a more frequent cause of this problem.

A8.17

1) C   2) D   3) E   4) A   5) B

Von Willebrand factor (vWF) is a glycoprotein with a molecular weight of about 200 000 which readily forms multimers in the circulation with molecular weights of up to 20×10^6. The high-molecular-weight multimeric forms of vWF are the most effective in promoting platelet function. Antithrombin (AT), a member of the serine protease inhibitor (serpin) superfamily, is a potent inhibitor of coagulation. It inactivates the serine proteases by forming stable complexes with them, and its action is greatly potentiated by heparin. Activated protein C is generated from its vitamin K-dependent precursor by the action of thrombin; thrombin activation of protein C is enhanced when thrombin is bound to thrombomodulin, which is an endothelial cell receptor. Activated protein C destroys factor V and factor VIII, reducing further thrombin generation. Protein S is a cofactor for protein C which acts by enhancing binding of activated protein C to the phospholipid surface. It circulates bound to C4b binding protein but some 30–40% remains unbound and active (free protein S). Plasmin is a serine protease which breaks down fibrinogen and fibrin into fragments X, Y, D and E, collectively known as fibrin (and fibrinogen) degradation products (FDPs). Degradation of cross-linked fibrin yields D-dimer and D-dimer-E fragments. Plasmin is also capable of breaking down coagulation factors such as factors V and VIII.

A8.18

1) D   2) E   3) A   4) B   5) C

Henoch–Schönlein purpura is a type III hypersensitivity reaction that is often preceded by an acute upper respiratory tract infection. It occurs mainly in children. Purpura is mainly seen on the legs and buttocks. Abdominal pain, arthritis, haematuria and glomerulonephritis also occur. Recovery is usually spontaneous, but some patients develop renal failure. Thrombotic thrombocytopenic purpura (TTP) is a rare, but very serious condition, in which platelet destruction leads to profound thrombocytopenia. There is a characteristic symptom complex of florid purpura, fever, fluctuating cerebral dysfunction and haemolytic anaemia with red cell fragmentation, often accompanied by renal failure. Glanzmann's thrombasthenia is lack of the platelet membrane glycoprotein IIb/IIIa complex resulting in defective fibrinogen binding and failure of platelet aggregation. Bernard–Soulier syndrome is lack of platelet membrane glycoprotein Ib, the binding site for factor vWF. This causes a failure of platelet adhesion and moderate thrombocytopenia. Essential thrombocythaemia is a myeloproliferative disorder which is associated with a high platelet count. A persistently elevated platelet count can lead to arterial or venous thrombosis. It is usual to treat the underlying cause of the thrombocytosis but a small dose of aspirin (75 mg) is also sometimes given. In myeloproliferative disease there is also a paradoxical risk of abnormal bleeding and specific action to reduce the platelet count, usually with hydroxycarbamide (hydroxyurea), is often taken.

A8.19

1) C   2) B   3) A   4) D

Blood changes in haemophilia A, von Willebrand's disease and vitamin K deficiency			
	Haemophilia A	von Willebrand's disease	Vitamin K deficiency
Bleeding time	Normal	↑	Normal
PT	Normal	Normal	↑
APTT	↑+	↑±	↑
VIII:C	↓++	↓	Normal
vWF	Normal	↓	Normal

PT, prothrombin time; APTT, activated partial prothrombin time; vWF, von Willebrand factor

In DIC with severe bleeding, the PT, APTT and TT (thrombin time) are usually very prolonged and the fibrinogen level markedly reduced, high levels of fibrin degradation products (FDPs)/D-dimer are found owing to the intense fibrinolytic activity stimulated by the presence of fibrin in the circulation, there is severe thrombocytopenia and the blood film may show fragmented red blood cells.

A8.20

1) E   2) D   3) C   4) A   5) B

Aspirin inhibits the enzyme cyclo-oxygenase, resulting in reduced platelet production of TXA_2. Dipyridamole – which inhibits platelet phosphodiesterase, causing an increase in cyclic AMP with potentiation of the action of PGI_2 – has been used widely as an antithrombotic agent. Ticlopidine blocks ADP-mediated platelet aggregation and transformation of the platelet fibrinogen receptor into a high-affinity form. It is a potential substitute for aspirin but its use has been associated with granulocytopenia and also, paradoxically, with thrombotic thrombocytopenic purpura (TTP). Clopidogrel affects the ADP-dependent activation of the glycoprotein IIb/IIIa complex. It is similar to ticlopidine but has fewer side-effects. Glycoprotein IIb/IIIa receptor antagonists block a receptor on the platelet for fibrinogen and von Willebrand factor. Three classes have been described: a) murine–human chimeric antibodies (e.g. abciximab), b) synthetic peptides (e.g. eptifibatide), c) synthetic non-peptides (e.g. tirofiban).

A8.21

1) A   2) B   3) C   4) A   5) B
6) C   7) B   8) C   9) A   10) C
11) B   12) B

Classification of the risk of deep vein thrombosis and pulmonary embolism for hospital patients is as follows:

I) Low risk (proximal vein thrombosis 0.4%; fatal pulmonary embolism <0.2%):
a) patients <40 years undergoing major surgery (>30 minutes) with no other risk factors; b) patients undergoing minor surgery (<30 minutes) with no other risk factors; c) patients with minor trauma or illness with no thrombophilia but with a history of deep vein thrombosis or previous pulmonary embolism

II) Medium risk (proximal vein thrombosis 2–4%; fatal pulmonary embolism 0.2–0.5%):
a) major general, urological, gynaecological, cardiothoracic, vascular, or neurological surgery in patients >40 years or with one or more other risk factor(s); b) major acute medical illness such as myocardial infarction, heart failure, chest infection, cancer or inflammatory bowel disease; c) major trauma; d) minor surgery, trauma or illness in patients with previous deep vein thrombosis, pulmonary embolism, or thrombophilia; e) plastercast immobilization of the leg in patients with minor injury

III) High risk (proximal vein thrombosis 10–20%; fatal pulmonary embolism 1–5%):
a) fracture or major orthopaedic surgery of pelvis, hip or leg; b) major pelvic or abdominal surgery for cancer; c) major surgery, trauma or illness in patients with previous deep vein thrombosis, pulmonary embolism, or thrombophilia; d) leg paralysis; e) critical leg ischaemia or major leg amputation.

A8.22

A) F   B) T   C) T   D) T   E) F

Normally, less than 2% of the red cells are reticulocytes. The reticulocyte count gives a guide to the erythroid activity in the bone marrow. An increased count is seen with haemorrhage or haemolysis, and during the response to treatment with a specific haematinic. A low count in the presence of anaemia indicates an inappropriate response by the bone marrow and may be seen in bone marrow failure (from whatever cause) or where there is a deficiency of a haematinic.

A8.23

A) T   B) T   C) F   D) T   E) T

The erythrocyte sedimentation rate (ESR) is the rate of fall of red cells in a column of blood and is a measure of the acute phase response. The pathological process may be immunological, infective, ischaemic, malignant or traumatic. The ESR increases with age, and is higher in females than in males. It is low in polycythaemia vera, owing to the high red cell concentration, and increased in patients with severe anaemia.

A8.24

A) F   B) F   C) F   D) F   E) T

Plasma viscosity measurement is used instead of the ESR in many laboratories. There is no difference between levels found in males and females, and viscosity increases only slightly in the elderly. It is not affected by the level of Hb.

Haematological disease

A8.25

A) F   B) T   C) T   D) F   E) T

C-reactive protein is a pentraxin, one of the proteins produced in the acute phase response. It is synthesized exclusively in the liver and rises within 6 hours of an acute event. It rises with temperature (possibly triggered by IL-1 and other cytokines) and in inflammatory conditions and after trauma. It follows the clinical state of the patient much more rapidly than does the ESR and is unaffected by the level of Hb, but it is less helpful than the ESR or plasma viscosity in monitoring chronic inflammatory diseases. High-sensitivity assays have recently shown that increased levels predict future cardiovascular disease

A8.26

A) T   B) F   C) T   D) T   E) F

Heparin is not a single substance but a mixture of polysaccharides. Low-molecular-weight (LMW) heparins produce little effect on tests of overall coagulation, such as the APTT at doses recommended for prophylaxis. Heparin-induced thrombocytopenia (HIT) is paradoxically associated with severe thrombosis and when diagnosed all forms of heparin must be discontinued, including heparin flush. Hirudins act directly on thrombin and can be monitored by the use of the APTT. They are excreted by the kidney and must be used with caution in renal failure. Oral anticoagulants should be avoided in pregnancy because they are teratogenic in the first trimester and may be associated with fetal haemorrhage later in pregnancy. When anticoagulation is considered essential in pregnancy, specialist advice should be sought. Self-administered subcutaneous heparin should be used as an alternative, although this may not be as effective for women with prosthetic cardiac valves.

A8.27

A) T   B) T   C) T   D) T   E) T

Contraindications to the use of oral anticoagulants are seldom absolute and include: a) severe uncontrolled hypertension; b) non-thromboembolic strokes; c) peptic ulceration (unless cured by *Helicobacter pylori* eradication); d) severe liver and renal disease; e) pre-existing haemostatic defects; f) non-compliance. Oral anticoagulants should be avoided in pregnancy because they are teratogenic in the first trimester and may be associated with fetal haemorrhage later in pregnancy.

A8.28

A) T   B) T   C) T'   D) T   E) T   F) T

Testing for specific causes of thrombophilia include: a) assays for naturally occurring anticoagulants such as AT, protein C and protein S; b) assay for activated protein C resistance and molecular testing for factor V Leiden and the prothrombin variant; c) screening for a coagulation factor inhibitor including a lupus anticoagulant and anticardiolipin antibodies.

A8.29

A) F   B) F   C) T   D) T   E) T

Causes of a microcytic hypochromic anaemia are iron deficiency, anaemia of chronic disease, sideroblastic anaemia, and thalassaemia.

A8.30

A) F   B) F   C) F   D) F   E) F

The average daily diet in the UK contains 15–20 mg of iron, although normally only 10% of this is absorbed. Absorption may be increased to 20–30% in iron deficiency and pregnancy. Non-haem iron is mainly derived from cereals, which are commonly fortified with iron; it forms the main part of dietary iron. Haem iron is derived from haemoglobin and myoglobin in red or organ meats. Haem iron is better absorbed than non-haem iron, whose availability is more affected by other dietary constituents.

A8.31

A) F   B) F   C) T   D) F   E) F

Iron absorption occurs primarily in the duodenum. Non-haem iron is dissolved in the low pH of the stomach and reduced from the ferric to ferrous form by a brush border ferrireductase. Cells in duodenal crypts are able to sense the body's iron requirements and retain this information as they mature into cells capable of absorbing iron at the tips of the villi. A protein, divalent metal transporter 1 (DMT1), transports iron across the apical (luminal) surface of the mucosal cells in the small intestine. Haem iron is absorbed in a separate less-well-characterized process. The mechanism of transport of iron across the basolateral surface of mucosal cells is uncertain, but probably involves a transporter protein, Ireg1. This transporter protein requires an accessory, multicopper protein, hephaestin.

A8.32

A) T   B) T   C) F   D) F   E) T

The body is unable to excrete iron once it has been absorbed so the regulation of

iron absorption is critical. Iron absorption is regulated in several ways: a) the amount of iron in the diet has an effect. For several days after an intake of a bolus of iron in the diet, mucosal cells are resistant to taking up more iron, probably because the mucosal cells sense their requirements for iron have been met ('dietary regulator'). b) The stores of body iron seem able to influence the levels of DMT1 in duodenal crypt cells ('stores regulator'). c) The requirements for erythropoiesis also influence iron absorption through an unknown mechanism ('erythropoietic regulator'), which may involve a soluble mediator carried in the plasma from the bone marrow to the intestine. Anaemias with increased rates of erythropoiesis do not cause equal increases in iron absorption; for example, conditions with 'ineffective erythropoiesis' such as thalassaemia stimulate greater iron absorption than haemolytic anaemias such as hereditary spherocytosis and autoimmune haemolytic anaemia where red cell destruction occurs in the periphery.

A8.33

A) F   B) F   C) F   D) T   E) F

Most of the iron bound to transferrin comes from macrophages in the reticuloendothelial system and not from iron absorbed by the intestine. About two-thirds of the total body iron is in the circulation as haemoglobin (2.5–3 g in a normal adult man). Iron is stored in reticuloendothelial cells, hepatocytes and skeletal muscle cells (500–1500 mg). About two-thirds of this is stored as ferritin and one-third as haemosiderin in normal individuals. Small amounts of iron are also found in plasma (about 4 mg bound to transferrin), with some in myoglobin and enzymes. Ferritin is a water-soluble complex of iron and protein. It is more easily mobilized than haemosiderin for Hb formation. It is present in small amounts in plasma. Haemosiderin is an insoluble iron–protein complex found in macrophages in the bone marrow, liver and spleen.

A8.34

A) T B) T C) T D) T E) F
F) F G) F

This patient has vitamin B_{12} deficiency due to pernicous anaemia and has the clinical features of subacute combined degeneration. Deoxyuridine suppression is a useful method for rapidly determining the nature and severity of the vitamin B_{12} or folate deficiency in severe or complex cases of megaloblastic anaemia. Tritiated thymidine is added to the patient's bone marrow in vitro. In a normoblastic marrow, the thymidine requirement is supplied by the methylation of deoxyuridine and this 'suppresses' the requirement for preformed tritiated thymidine to less than 5%. In a megaloblastic marrow, however, much more tritiated thymidine is used (5–50%). If the addition of B_{12} corrects the abnormality, it suggests that B_{12} is the cause of the deficiency. Bone marrow shows the typical features of megaloblastic erythropoiesis. Serum bilirubin may be raised as a result of ineffective erythropoiesis. The absorption of B_{12} can be measured using the Schilling test. In pernicious anaemia there is marked gastric atrophy with achlorhydria. Vitamin B_{12} is found in meat, fish, eggs and milk, but not in plants. The average adult stores some 2–3 mg, mainly in the liver, and it may take 2 years or more after absorptive failure before B_{12} deficiency develops, as the daily losses are small (1–2 μg).

Hydroxocobalamin 1000 μg can be given intramuscularly to a total of 5–6 mg over the course of 3 weeks; 1000 μg is then necessary every 3 months for the rest of the patient's life.

A8.35

A) T B) T C) T D) F E) F

This patient has folic acid deficiency. The methylation of homocysteine to methionine requires both methylcobalamin and methyl tetrahydrofolate as coenzymes. Folate is found in green vegetables such as spinach and broccoli, and offal, such as liver and kidney. Cooking causes a loss of 60–90% of the folate. Although there is no simple relationship between maternal folate status and fetal abnormalities, folic acid supplements at the time of conception and in the first 12 weeks of pregnancy reduce the incidence of neural tube defects. The amount of folate in the red cells is a better measure of tissue folate. Folate deficiency can be corrected by giving 5 mg of folic acid daily; the same haematological response occurs as seen after treatment of vitamin B_{12} deficiency. Treatment should be given for about 4 months to replace body stores.

A8.36

A) F B) T C) T D) F E) T

A raised MCV with macrocytosis on the peripheral blood film can occur with a normoblastic rather than a megaloblastic bone marrow. A common physiological cause of macrocytosis is pregnancy, and a newborn may also suffer. Common pathological causes are: a) alcohol excess; b) liver disease; c) reticulocytosis; d) hypothyroidism; e) some haematological disorders (e.g. aplastic anaemia, sideroblastic anaemia, pure red cell aplasia); f) drugs (e.g. cytotoxics – azathioprine); g) spurious (agglutinated red cells measured on red cell counters); h) cold agglutinins due to autoagglutination of red cells (the MCV decreases to normal with warming of the sample to 37°C).

A8.37

A) F B) T C) T D) T E) T

Causes of aplastic anaemia

Primary
Congenital, e.g. Fanconi's anaemia
Idiopathic acquired (67% of cases)

Secondary
Chemicals, e.g. benzene
Drugs
    chemotherapeutic
    idiosyncratic reactions
Insecticides
Ionizing radiation
Infections:
    viral, e.g. hepatitis, EBV, HIV, parvovirus
    other, e.g. tuberculosis
Paroxysmal nocturnal haemoglobinuria

A8.38

A) F B) F C) T D) F E) F

In severe aplastic anaemia, there is a very poor outcome without treatment. Bone marrow transplantation is the treatment of choice for patients under 50 years of age who have an HLA-identical sibling donor, which gives a 75–90% chance of long-term survival and restoring the blood count to normal. Patients over the age of 50 are not eligible for bone marrow transplantation whether an HLA-identical donor is available or not, because of the high risk of graft-versus-host disease as a complication of bone marrow transplantation. Immunosuppressive

therapy is used for patients without HLA-matched siblings and those over the age of 50 years. Androgens (e.g. oxymethalone) are sometimes useful in patients not responding to immunosuppression and in patients with moderately severe aplastic anaemia. Steroids have little activity in severe aplastic anaemia but are used for serum sickness due to antilymphocyte globulin (ALG). They are also used to treat children with congenital pure red cell aplasia (Diamond–Blackfan syndrome).

A8.39

A) T B) F C) T D) F E) F

Hereditary spherocytosis (HS) is inherited in an autosomal dominant manner, but in 25% of patients neither parent is affected and it is presumed that HS has occurred by spontaneous mutation. Several defects in the cell membrane have been identified in HS, the best characterized being a deficiency in the structural protein spectrin. The onset of jaundice can sometimes be delayed for many years and some patients may go through life with no symptoms and are detected only during family studies. The patient may eventually develop anaemia, splenomegaly and ulcers on the leg. Aplastic anaemia usually occurs after infections, particularly with parvovirus. When red cells are placed in solutions of increasing hypotonicity, they take in water, swell, and eventually lyse. Direct antiglobulin (Coombs') test is negative in spherocytosis. The spleen, which is the site of cell destruction, should be removed in all but the mildest cases. The decision about splenectomy in asymptomatic patients is difficult, but a raised bilirubin and especially the presence of gallstones should encourage splenectomy.

Haematological disease

A) F   B) T   C) T   D) T   E) T

Drugs causing haemolysis in glucose-6-phosphate deficiency	
Analgesics, such as: Aspirin Phenacetin (withdrawn in the UK) Acetanilide **Antimalarials,** such as Primaquine Pyrimethamine Quinine Chloroquine Pamaquine	**Antibacterials,** such as: Most sulphonamides Dapsone Nitrofurantoin Nitrofurazone Furazolidone Chloramphenicol Ciprofloxacin **Miscellaneous drugs,** such as: Vitamin K Probenecid Nalidixic acid Quinidine Dimercaprol Phenylhydrazine

An acute attack of intravascular haemolysis can be precipitated by: a) drugs, including chloroquine (see table for complete list); b) ingestion of fava beans (favism); c) infections and acute illnesses. Intravascular haemolysis results in a reduction in plasma haptoglobin levels. During an attack the blood film may show irregularly contracted cells, bite cells (cells with an indentation of the membrane), blister cells (cells in which the Hb appears to have become partially detached from the cell membrane; Heinz bodies (best seen on films stained with methyl violet) and reticulocytosis.

A) T   B) T   C) T   D) T   E) T

Causes of eosinophilia	
Parasitic infestations, such as: Ascaris Hookworm Strongyloides **Allergic disorders,** such as: Hayfever (allergic rhinitis) Other hypersensitivity reactions, including drug reactions **Skin disorders,** such as: Urticaria Pemphigus Eczema	**Pulmonary disorders,** such as: Bronchial asthma Tropical pulmonary eosinophilia Allergic bronchopulmonary aspergillosis Churg–Strauss syndrome **Malignant disorders,** such as: Hodgkin's disease Carcinoma Eosinophilic leukaemia **Miscellaneous,** such as: Hypereosinophilic syndrome Sarcoidosis Hypoadrenalism Eosinophilic gastroenteritis

A) T   B) F   C) F   D) T   E) F

The onset of polycythaemia vera (PV) is insidious. It usually presents in patients aged over 60 years with tiredness, depression, vertigo, tinnitus and visual disturbance. It should be noted that these symptoms are also common in the normal population over the age of 60 and consequently PV is easily missed. These features, together with hypertension, angina, intermittent claudication and a tendency to bleed, are suggestive of PV. Severe itching after a hot bath or when the patient is warm is common. The patient is usually plethoric and has a deep dusky cyanosis. Injection of the conjunctivae is commonly seen. The spleen is palpable in 70% of patients and is useful in distinguishing PV from secondary causes. The liver is enlarged in 50% of patients. Bone marrow shows erythroid hyperplasia and increased numbers of megakaryocytes. Leucocyte alkaline phosphatase (LAP) score is usually high. The serum erythropoietin level is not diagnostic but may be helpful in distinguishing PV from secondary polycythaemia.Venesection will successfully relieve many of the symptoms of PV. PV develops into myelofibrosis in 30% of cases and into acute myeloblastic leukaemia in 5% as part of the natural history of the disease.

A8.43

A) F   B) T   C) F   D) F   E) F

Myelofibrosis presents insidiously with lethargy, weakness and weight loss. Patients often complain of a 'fullness' in the upper abdomen due to splenomegaly. Other physical signs include anaemia, fever and massive splenomegaly. A bone marrow trephine is necessary to show the markedly increased fibrosis. The Philadelphia chromosome is absent; this helps to distinguish myelofibrosis from most cases of chronic myeloid leukaemia (CML). The leucocyte alkaline phosphatase (LAP) score is normal or high. If the spleen becomes very large and painful, and transfusion requirements are high, it may be advisable to perform splenectomy. Splenectomy may also result in relief of severe thrombocytopenia. Median survival is 3 years.

A8.44

A) F   B) T   C) F   D) T   E) F

Following splenectomy, *Haemophilus influenzae* type B vaccine should be given to those who have not previously been immunized. Meningococcal immunization is not routinely recommended, except for travellers to areas where there is an increased risk of group A infection. Abnormalities in red cell morphology are the most prominent changes and include Howell–Jolly bodies, Pappenheimer bodies (contain sideroblastic granules), target cells and irregular contracted red cells. Pitted red cells can be counted.

A8.45

A) F   B) T   C) T   D) T   E) F

Sickle cell anaemia varies from a mild asymptomatic disorder to a severe haemolytic anaemia and recurrent severe painful crises. Reticulocyte count is high (10–20%). The sickle solubility test is positive: a mixture of Hb S in a reducing solution such as sodium dithionite gives a turbid appearance because of precipitation of Hb S, whereas normal Hb gives a clear solution. Long-term problems include: a) susceptibility to infections, particularly to *Streptococcus pneumoniae*, which can cause a fatal meningitis or pneumonia; osteomyelitis can occur in necrotic bone, often due to *Salmonella*; b) chronic leg ulcers, due to ischaemia; c) gallstones: pigment stones from persistent haemolysis; d) aseptic necrosis of bone, particularly of the femoral heads; e) blindness, due to retinal detachment and/or proliferative retinopathy; and f) chronic renal disease. Hydroxycarbamide (hydroxyurea) has been shown in trials to reduce the episodes of pain, the acute chest syndrome, and the need for blood transfusions.

8.46

A) F   B) T   C) F   D) F   E) F

Immediate reaction is the most serious complication of blood transfusion and is usually due to ABO incompatibility. There is complement activation by the antigen–antibody reaction, usually caused by IgM antibodies, leading to rigors, lumbar pain, dyspnoea, hypotension, haemoglobinuria and renal failure. The initial symptoms may occur a few minutes after starting the transfusion. Activation of coagulation may also occur and bleeding due to disseminated intravascular coagulation (DIC) is a bad prognostic sign. At the first suspicion of any serious transfusion reaction, the transfusion should always be stopped and the donor units returned to the blood transfusion laboratory with a new blood sample from the patient to exclude a haemolytic transfusion reaction.

Medical oncology including haematological malignancy

9

Q9.1

A 45-year-old woman has pain in the left iliac region. MRI of the pelvis confirms a mass localized to the ovary and serum CA125 is elevated. Histology reveals that the tumour is a well-differentiated epithelial ovarian cancer. Which one of the following is curative in 80–90% of such cases?

A. Carboplatin
B. Paclitaxel
C. Surgery
D. Doxorubicin
E. Tamoxifen

Q9.2

A 55-year-old woman has a lung mass and biopsy shows small-cell lung cancer. Which one of the following is the best treatment for this condition?

A. Radiotherapy
B. Etoposide and cisplatin
C. Doxorubicin
D. Radiotherapy with doxorubicin
E. Surgery

Q9.3

A 65-year-old woman has metastatic breast cancer. Which one of the following is used to treat this condition?

A. Oophorectomy
B. Radiation-induced ovarian ablation
C. GnRH analogue
D. Tamoxifen
E. Hysterectomy

Q9.4

A 53-year-old woman has metastatic breast cancer and is found to be positive for HER-2 receptors. This indicates that the patient is most likely to respond to

A. Formestane
B. Anastrozole
C. Trastuzumab (Herceptin)
D. Tamoxifen
E. Progesterone

Q9.5

A 48-year-old man with non-Hodgkin's lymphoma presents with difficulty in breathing, stridor, a swollen, oedematous face with venous congestion. The best treatment is

A. Intravenous pamidronate
B. Intravenous steroids with chemotherapy
C. Mediastinal radiotherapy
D. Rib resection
E. Thoracotomy

Medical oncology including haematological malignancy

Q9.6

An 80-year-old man complains of bone pain. Investigation reveals an elevated PSA and prostatectomy confirms prostate cancer. He has multiple bone metastases. Which one of the following is most effective in the palliation of bone pain?

A. Chemotherapy
B. Progesterone
C. Intravenous strontium-labelled bisphosphonate
D. Orchidectomy
E. Tamoxifen

Q9.7

An 88-year-old man complains of severe pain in the epigastrium. He is diagnosed to have gastric cancer. Which one of the following is the drug of choice to relieve his pain?

A. Aspirin
B. Paracetamol
C. Morphine
D. Naproxen
E. Codeine

Q9.8

1. A 67-year-old man who initially smoked cigarettes for decades but has since smoked cigars and now smokes a pipe
2. A 58-year-old farmer in Australia who has spent a lot of time out of doors on his tractor
3. A 65-year-old patient who is a chronic alcoholic
4. A 53-year-old patient on long-term cyclophosphamide therapy for systemic lupus erythematosus
5. A 53-year-old shipyard worker exposed to asbestos

Select the cancer to which each of the above is most susceptible

A. Bladder, bone marrow
B. Lungs, mesothelium
C. Mouth, pharynx, larynx, oesophagus, colorectal
D. Skin, lip
E. Mouth, pharynx, oesophagus, larynx, lung, bladder, lip

Q9.9

1. A 54-year-old woman with pancreatic cancer
2. A 34-year-old woman with breast cancer
3. A 39-year-old patient with chronic myeloid leukaemia
4. A 12-year-old boy with Ewing's sarcoma
5. A 43-year-old man with neuroblastoma

Select the best match for each of the above

A. *BCR-ABL* translocation
B. *EWS* translocation
C. DNA amplification of *HER2*
D. DNA amplification of *myc*
E. Point mutation of *ras*

Q9.10

1. Methotrexate
2. 5-Fluorouracil
3. Vincristine
4. Doxorubicin
5. Cyclophosphamide

Select the mechanism of action of each of the above

A. Blocks thymidylate synthetase
B. Binds preferentially to dihydrofolate reductase
C. Cross-links DNA strands

D. Binds to tubulin and inhibits microtubule formation

E. Intercalates adjoining nucleotide pairs on the same strand of DNA and inhibits DNA repair

Q9.11

1. A 45-year-old woman with breast cancer develops congestive heart failure

2. A 23-year-old patient develops shortness of breath. Chest X-ray and pulmonary function tests suggest pulmonary fibrosis

3. A 38-year-old man with systemic lupus erythematosus on chemotherapy develops sterility

4. A 43-year-old man being treated for stomach cancer develops skin plantar–palmar dermatitis

5. A patient on chemotherapy develops neurotoxicity

Select the most likely cause of each of the above

A. 5-Fluorouracil
B. Bleomycin
C. Doxorubicin
D. Cyclophosphamide
E. Vincristine

Q9.12

1. A 45-year-old woman with metastatic breast cancer

2. A 35-year-old man with chronic myeloid leukaemia and with Philadelphia chromosome-positive cells

3. A 56-year-old patient with bladder cancer

4. A 43-year-old patient with chronic myeloid leukaemia and BCR-ABL

5. A 39-year-old patient with B-cell non-Hodgkin's lymphoma

Select the best match for each of the above

A. Alpha-interferon
B. Bacille Calmette–Guérin (BCG)
C. Tyrosine kinase inhibitor ST1571
D. Monoclonal antibodies (Herceptin (trastuzumab)) against Her2/Neu or C-erbB2 antigen
E. Anti-CD20 surface antigen

Q9.13

1. Acute myeloid leukaemia

2. Acute lymphoblastic leukaemia derived from B cells

3. Acute promyelocytic leukaemia

4. Chronic myeloid leukaemia

5. Chronic lymphocytic leukaemia

Select the best match for each of the above

A. Expression of BCR-ABL oncogene
B. An uncontrolled proliferation and accumulation of mature B lymphocytes
C. Presence of granules and 'Auer rods' in the cytoplasm
D. Disseminated intravascular coagulation
E. CD10 antigen

Q9.14

1. Acute myelogenous leukaemia

2. Acute lymphoblastic leukaemia

3. Acute promyelocytic leukaemia

4. Chronic myeloid leukaemia

5. Chronic lymphocytic leukaemia

Select the best match for each of the above

A. Remission induction with doxorubicin and cytosine arabinoside
B. All-trans-retinoic acid as standard therapy in all patients
C. Cyclical combination therapy comprising vincristine, prednisolone, L-Asparaginase and doxorubicin

Medical oncology including haematological malignancy

D. Alpha-interferons

E. Chlorambucil

D. Melphalan

E. Radiotherapy

Q9.15

1. A 20-year-old man presents with fever and drenching night sweats of several weeks' duration. He has lost weight and on examination cervical lymph nodes are palpable. Lymph node biopsy shows small lymphocytes and histiocytes together with scattered mononuclear cells and binucleate cells

2. A 43-year-old woman complains of fatigue. Her GP finds lymph nodes in the neck and CT shows mediastinal involvement. Biopsy confirms Hodgkin's disease

3. A 45-year-old man presents with weight loss. On examination his right axillary and supratrochlear lymph nodes are palpable. Lymph node biopsy shows follicular lymphoma

4. A 23-year-old man presents with fatigue and anorexia. On examination his left axillary, cervical and supratrochlear lymph nodes are palpable. Lymph node biopsy shows high-grade B cell lymphoma

5. A 53-year-old woman complains of fatigue. On examination cervical lymph nodes are palpable. The spleen is also palpable. Lymph node biopsy shows small lymphocytes and histiocytes together with scattered mononuclear cells and Reed–Sternberg cells

Select the best treatment for each of the above

A. Chlorambucil

B. Alkylating agent with doxorubicin

C. Doxorubicin with cyclophosphamide, vincristine (Oncovin), and prednisolone (CHOP)

Q9.16

A patient undergoes high doses of chemotherapy to ablate the bone marrow followed by transplantation of donor haemopoietic cells to reconstitute the bone marrow and immune system. This therapy has successfully been used in

A. Graft-versus-host disease

B. Acute leukaemias

C. Chronic leukaemias

D. Multiple myeloma

E. Sarcoidosis

Q9.17

The following statements about hormonal management of cancers are correct

A. In patients with advanced metastatic breast cancer, oestrogen deprivation causes tumour regression in 30% of unselected women and in more than 60% of those with oestrogen-receptor-positive tumours for a median duration of 20 months

B. In the adjuvant setting, ovarian ablation and tamoxifen result in a 25% reduction in relative risk of dying from metastatic disease, which is maintained for in excess of 20 years after only 5 years of postoperative treatment

C. Aromatase inhibitors are ineffective in the treatment of metastatic breast cancer in postmenopausal women

D. Endometrial cancers will regress for a median 20 months with tamoxifen

E. In advanced prostate cancer, androgen deprivation induces regression in 70% of cases for a median duration of 24 months

Q9.18

Radiotherapy treatment is used for

A. Adjuvant therapy to primary surgery for teratoma testis
B. Cure of prostatic tumours
C. Reduction in headache and vomiting of raised intracranial pressure from CNS metastases
D. Relief of bronchial obstruction in bronchogenic carcinoma
E. Reversal of neurological impairment from spinal cord compression by metastases

Q9.19

A 64-year-old man has back pain and fatigue. Investigations reveal vertebral collapse and anaemia and bone marrow aspirate shows plasma cells. The following treatments result in a cure

A. Melphalan
B. Cyclophosphamide
C. Doxorubicin
D. Thalidomide
E. High-dose melphalan with autologous bone marrow transplantation

Q9.20

A 48-year-old woman has metastatic breast cancer. Her oncologist wishes to use chemotherapy to provide good quality palliation and prolongation of life. The following regimens are commonly used to achieve this

A. Combination of cyclophosphamide, methotrexate, 5-fluorouracil (CMF)
B. Mitoxantrone (mitozantrone) and methotrexate (MM)
C. Doxorubicin and cyclophosphamide
D. Paclitaxel used as a single agent
E. Vinorelbine

Medical oncology including haematological malignancy

A9.1

C

Surgery has a major role in the treatment of ovarian cancer of all stages. For patients in whom the disease is confined to the ovary, the surgery can be curative in 80–90% of the cases if the histology is well to moderately differentiated.

A9.2

B

Small-cell lung cancers are very chemosensitive and radiosensitive and approximately three-quarters of patients will respond to combination chemotherapy with etoposide and cisplatin with good relief of symptoms and modest prolongation of life. A small proportion of small-cell lung cancer patients with limited disease will be cured. Radiotherapy is used for palliative relief and used to treat the brain prophylactically in patients potentially cured of systemic disease.

A9.3

D

Endocrine therapy of metastatic breast cancer
For premenopausal patients
(a) Suppression of ovarian function by means of oophorectomy, radiation-induced ovarian ablation, or a GnRH analogue, e.g. goserelin
(b) Anti-oestrogen, tamoxifen
(c) Progesterone
For postmenopausal patients
(a) Tamoxifen
(b) Progesterone
(c) Aromatase inhibitors (e.g. anastrozole)

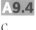
A9.4

C

Herceptin (trastuzumab) is an anti-HER2 antibody which when added to doxorubicin has been shown to provide modest survival advantage in metastatic breast cancer.

A9.5

B

Superior vena caval obstruction can arise from any upper mediastinal mass but is most commonly associated with lung cancer. The patient presents with difficulty breathing and/or swallowing, with stridor, a swollen, oedematous facies and venous congestion. Treatment is with immediate steroids, anticoagulation and mediastinal radiotherapy or chemotherapy. Some tumours, e.g. lymphomas and germ cell tumours, are so sensitive to chemotherapy that this is preferred to radiotherapy as the masses are likely to be both large and associated with more disseminated disease elsewhere.

A9.6

C

Radiotherapy provides a very effective palliation of painful skeletal metastases and can be delivered systematically by intravenous bone-seeking strontium-labelled bisphosphonate for patients with multiple affected sites.

A9.7

C

Morphine is the drug of choice to provide symptomatic relief in pain due to cancer.

A9.8

1) E   2) D   3) C   4) A   5) B

Some causative factors associated with the development of cancer at various sites	
Smoking	Mouth, pharynx, oesophagus, larynx, lung, bladder, lip
Ultraviolet light	Skin, lip
Alcohol	Mouth, pharynx, larynx, oesophagus, colorectal
Drugs (alkylating agents)	Bladder, bone marrow
Asbestos	Lung, mesothelium

A9.9

1) E   2) C   3) A   4) B   5) D

Acquired/somatic mutations and proto-oncogenes	
Point mutation	
ras	Pancreatic cancer
DNA amplification	
myc	Neuroblastoma
HER2	Breast cancer
Chromosome translocation	
BCR-ABL	CML, AML, ALL
EWS	Ewing's sarcoma

CML, chronic myeloid leukaemia; AML, acute myeloid leukaemia; ALL, acute lymphoblastic leukaemia

A9.10

1) B   2) A   3) D   4) E   5) C

The alkylating agents such as cyclophosphamide act by covalently binding alkyl groups, and their major effect is to cross-link DNA strands, interfering with DNA synthesis and causing strand breaks. Methotrexate is structurally very similar to folic acid and binds preferentially to dihydrofolate reductase, the enzyme responsible for the conversion of folic acid to folinic acid. 5-Fluorouracil acts by blocking the enzyme thymidylate synthetase which is essential for pyrimidine synthesis. Vincristine acts by binding to tubulin and inhibiting microtubule formation. Doxorubicin acts by intercalating adjoining nucleotide pairs on the same strand of DNA and by inhibiting DNA repair.

A9.11

1) C   2) B   3) D   4) A   5) E

Drug-specific side-effects of chemotherapy
Cardiotoxicity, e.g. anthracyclines
Pulmonary toxicity, e.g. bleomycin
Neurotoxicity, e.g. platinum, vinca alkaloids, taxanes
Skin plantar–palmar dermatitis, e.g. 5-fluorouracil
Sterility, e.g. alkylating agents

A9.12

1) D   2) A   3) B   4) C   5) E

In chronic myeloid leukaemia, alpha-interferon results in a reduction in the number of Philadelphia (Ph) chromosome-positive cells in at least 50% of patients, with total elimination in 10%. Cytogenetic response has been shown to result in prolongation of survival, but interferon is not curative. Monoclonal antibodies are used in vivo, as treatment for B cell non-Hodgkin's lymphoma (e.g. anti-CD20 surface antigen). Tumour cell lysis occurs by both complement and antibody-dependent cellular cytotoxicity. Monoclonal antibodies (Herceptin (trastuzumab)) against the Her2/Neu or C-erbB2 antigen, a member of the epidermal growth factor receptor family, have both direct anti-breast cancer activity in clinical trials and increase the apoptotic response to cytotoxics. Activation of the immune system using bacille Calmette–Guérin

Medical oncology including haematological malignancy

(BCG) for bladder cancer or interleukin-2 for renal cancer are successful in 60% and 10% of patients respectively. Tyrosine kinase inhibitor STI571 (which specifically inhibits the fusion oncoprotein *BCR-ABL*), is an extremely effective treatment for chronic myeloid leukaemia, a disease characterized by the presence of the *BCR-ABL* fusion protein.

A9.13

1) C   2) E   3) D   4) A   5) B

Acute myeloid leukaemia (AML) is distinguished by the presence of granules and 'Auer rods' in the cytoplasm, the presence of enzymes such as myeloperoxidase, expression of myeloid antigens (CD13, CD33) and the presence of typical cytogenetic abnormalities. Most cases of acute lymphoblastic leukaemia (ALL) are derived from B cells, and will express the CD10 antigen. Acute promyelocytic leukaemia (APML) is associated with disseminated intravascular coagulation (DIC). Expression of the *BCR-ABL* oncogene can be detected by reverse transcriptase polymerase chain reaction (RT-PCR) in all patients with chronic myeloid leukaemia (CML); if it is absent, the diagnosis is called into doubt. Chronic lymphoblastic leukaemia (CLL) is characterized by an uncontrolled proliferation and accumulation of mature B lymphocytes (although T-cell CLL does occur).

A9.14

1) A   2) C   3) B   4) D   5) E

In acute myelogenous leukaemia remission induction therapy usually includes an anthracycline drug such as daunorubicin or doxorubicin (or a newer analogue such as idarubicin), given in conjunction with cytosine arabinoside (cytarabine) with or without another drug such as etoposide. The administration of all-*trans*-retinoic acid (ATRA) is standard in all patients with acute promyelocytic leukemia (APML). ATRA differentiates the leukaemic cells of APML into mature granulocytes, which ameliorates both the disseminated intravascular coagulation (DIC) and the marrow failure associated with the disease. In acute lymphoblastic leukaemia, cyclical combination chemotherapy comprising vincristine, prednisolone, L-asparaginase and an anthracycline such as doxorubicin forms the basis of most treatment regimens. Alpha-interferons have been shown to induce haematological remission in the majority of patients with chronic myeloid leukaemia and cytogenetic remission in about 10%. Chronic lymphocytic leukaemia may remain stable for several years. There is no advantage in starting treatment before there is a clinical indication, such as anaemia, recurrent infections, bleeding, 'bulky' lymphadenopathy or increasing splenomegaly. Chlorambucil is most often used, with or without prednisolone. Treatment is given intermittently, as and when necessary. Chlorambucil may be effective repeatedly.

A9.15

1) B   2) E   3) A   4) C   5) B

The majority of patients with Stage IA and IIA Hodgkin's lymphoma are treated with radiotherapy. Stage IIB, IIIA or B, IVA/B Hodgkin's lymphoma is treated with chemotherapy comprising alkylating agents and doxorubicin. Follicular lymphomas are low grade lymphomas where repeated remissions can be achieved with chlorambucil. High grade lymphomas are usually treated with an anthracycline (e.g. doxorubicin) and cyclophosphamide, vincristine (Oncovin) and prednisolone (CHOP).

androgen deprivation induces regression in 70% of cases for a median duration of 24 months.

A9.16

A) F   B) T   C) T   D) T   E) F

Allogeneic haemopoietic transplantation has been successfully used in acute and chronic leukaemias, and myeloma.

A9.17

A) T   B) T   C) F   D) F   E) T

In patients with advanced metastatic breast cancer, oestrogen deprivation causes tumour regression in 30% of unselected women and in more than 60% of those with oestrogen-receptor-positive tumours for a median duration of 20 months. In the adjuvant setting, ovarian ablation and tamoxifen result in a 25% reduction in relative risk of dying from metastatic disease, which is maintained for in excess of 20 years after only 5 years of postoperative treatment. Aromatase inhibitors, for example anastrozole and exemestane, reduce circulating oestrogen levels and oestrogen synthesis in tumour cells and have recently shown even greater efficacy than tamoxifen in the treatment of metastatic breast cancer in the postmenopausal woman. Endometrial cancers have receptors for both oestrogens and progestogens. Approximately 20% of receptor-positive metastases will regress for a median 20 months with synthetic progestogens such as medroxyprogesterone acetate but paradoxically tamoxifen has little effect. Trials to date with adjuvant progestogens have not been successful in increasing survival. In advanced prostate cancer,

A9.18

A) F   B) T   C) T   D) T   E) T

Curative radiotherapy treatment

Primary modality
Retina
CNS
Skin
Oropharynx and larynx
Oesophagus
Cervix and vagina
Prostate
Lymphoma

Adjuvant to primary surgery
Lung
Breast
Uterus
Bladder
Rectum
Testis seminoma
Sarcoma

Palliative benefits of radiotherapy include: a) reduction of headache and vomiting of raised intracranial pressure from CNS metastases; b) relief of obstruction of bronchus, oesophagus, ureter, and lymphatics; c) reversal of neurological impairment from spinal cord or optic nerve compression by metastases.

A9.19

1) F   2) F   3) F   4) F   5) F

Multiple myeloma is incurable – no known therapy, including allogeneic bone marrow transplantation, is associated with indefinite remission. Although chemotherapy rarely eradicates the disease it may induce periods of freedom from disease progression known as the plateau phase. Relapse from plateau phase is inevitable after a number of months to years and although further therapy is possible, it becomes less effective.

A9.20

A) T B) T C) T D) T E) T

All these regimens are used commonly and there is very little difference in efficacy between the different regimens for metastatic disease, with response rates varying from 40–60% for a median duration of 8 months. The addition of Taxotere (docetaxel) or Herceptin (trastuzumab) to doxorubicin is the only example of improved survival for metastatic breast cancer in recent years. The regimens do differ in toxicity, however, with MM being one of the least toxic.

10

Q10.1

A 5-year-old boy develops high, swinging, early-evening fever, arthralgia and an evanescent pink maculopapular rash. On examination there is hepatosplenomegaly. Laboratory tests show a high ESR, and C-reactive protein, neutrophilia and thrombocytosis. Autoantibodies are negative. The most likely diagnosis is

A. Henoch–Schönlein purpura
B. Perthes' disease
C. Still's disease
D. Rheumatic fever
E. Enthesitis-related arthritis

Q10.2

A 69-year-old man has back pain. X-ray of the spine reveals osteosclerotic areas with bone destruction. He has hypercalcaemia and raised acid phosphatase. Which one of the following is most likely to be associated with this condition?

A. Raised carcinoembryonic antigen (CEA)
B. Elevated levels of blood urea nitrogen (BUN) and creatinine
C. Raised prostate specific antigen (PSA)
D. Raised serum angiotensin-converting enzyme (ACE) level
E. Raised adrenocorticotrophic hormone (ACTH)

Q10.3

A 45-year-old woman develops arthralgia, and dryness of the skin, vagina and mouth. The salivary and parotid glands are enlarged. In patients with this condition the antibody most likely to cross the placenta and cause congenital heart block is

A. Rheumatoid factor
B. Antinuclear antibodies
C. Antimitochondrial antibodies
D. Anti-Ro (SSA) antibodies
E. Anti-dsDNA antibodies

Q10.4

A 69-year-old woman develops fever, systemic malaise, tenderness of the scalp while combing her hair and claudication of the jaw. ESR is 100 mm/1st hour. The best treatment is

A. Observe the patient and start prednisolone at the first sign of visual loss
B. Initiate high dose prednisolone therapy immediately
C. Beta-blocker therapy
D. Intravenous glycoprotein IIB/IIIA inhibitors
E. High dose salicylate

Rheumatology and bone disease

Q10.5

A middle-aged man who is positive for hepatitis B antigen develops fever, malaise, weight loss and myalgia. He has mononeuritis multiplex and an elevated ESR. A renal angiogram is most likely to show

A. Unilateral renal artery stenosis
B. Bilateral renal artery stenosis
C. Aneurysms
D. Dissection of the renal artery
E. Agenesis of the kidney

Q10.6

A 27-year-old woman has had three abortions. She also has thrombocytopenia, a positive Coombs' test and livedo reticularis. Which one of the following tests is most likely to be positive in this condition?

A. Elevated ESR
B. Elevated C-reactive protein
C. Anticardiolipin antibodies detected by ELISA
D. Anti-Ro antibodies
E. Anti-La antibodies

Q10.7

A 65-year-old woman notices that the skin over her fingers feels tight. She first noticed Raynaud's phenomenon at the age of 40 years. She now has a beak-like nose and microstomia. Over two-thirds of such patients have

A. Anti-topoisomerase-1 antibodies
B. Rheumatoid factor
C. VDRL (Venereal Disease Research Laboratory) positive
D. Anti-RNA polymerase antibodies
E. Anticentromere antibodies

Q10.8

A 43-year-old woman develops difficulty climbing stairs, getting up from a squatting position or raising her hand above her head. On examination she has purplish discoloration of the eyelids and periorbital oedema. Which one of the following tests is the best predictor of the patient developing pulmonary fibrosis subsequently?

A. Anti-topoisomerase-1 antibodies
B. Rheumatoid factor
C. Myositis-specific antibodies
D. Antinuclear antibodies
E. Antibodies to Jo-1

Q10.9

A 43-year-old coal-miner complains of pain and stiffness of the small joints of the hands, wrists, elbows, shoulders, knees and ankles that is typically worse in the morning and improves with gentle activity. The patient complains that he has generally been feeling tired for over 3 months. The rheumatologist diagnoses Caplan's syndrome. This condition is characterized by

A. Mononeuritis multiplex
B. Amyloidosis
C. Dry mouth and dry eyes
D. Splenomegaly and neutropenia
E. Large cavitating lung nodules

Q10.10

A 49-year-old woman has a 16-week history of pain and stiffness of the small joints of the hands, wrists, elbows, shoulders, knees and ankles that is typically worse in the morning and improves with gentle activity. The rheumatologist also diagnoses sicca syndrome. This condition is characterized by

A. Mononeuritis multiplex
B. Amyloidosis
C. Dry mouth and dry eyes
D. Splenomegaly and neutropenia
E. Large cavitating lung nodules

Q10.11

A 29-year-old man has since his late teens had low back pain and stiffness that is typically worse in the morning and relieved by exercise. Now the lordosis of his lumbar spine persists in flexion. He has recently been diagnosed to have anterior uveitis. Which one of the following features is most likely to confirm the diagnosis?

A. HLA-B27 on HLA testing
B. Beak-like osteophytes on X-ray of spine
C. Response to NSAIDs
D. Response to sulfasalazine
E. Vertically oriented syndesmophytes, with preserved spinal disc

Q10.12

A 42-year-old man develops urethritis, arthritis and conjunctivitis following an episode of dysentery. This condition is known as

A. Pott's disease
B. Jaccoud's arthropathy
C. Reiter's disease
D. Poncet's disease
E. CREST syndrome

Q10.13

A 49-year-old patient with heart failure develops acute tenderness and redness in the right metacarpophalangeal joint after initiation of diuretic therapy. The best option for treatment is

A. Naproxen
B. Diclofenac
C. Indometacin
D. Colchicine
E. Phenylbutazone

Q10.14

A 45-year-old white male has generalized pigmentation of the skin, diabetes and hepatomegaly. He develops fever, joint pains and a raised white cell count. Liver biopsy reveals elevated ferritin levels. Aspiration of joint fluid reveals rhomboidal, weakly positively birefringent crystals. The most likely aetiology for his joint symptoms is

A. Gout
B. Calcium pyrophosphate arthropathy
C. Septic arthritis
D. Palindromic rheumatoid arthritis
E. Gonococcal arthritis

Q10.15

A 49-year-old patient has recurrent attacks of gout. His primary care physician starts him on allopurinol to reduce these recurrent attacks. The mechanism of action of allopurinol is

A. Inhibtion of pyramidine synthesis
B. Uricosuric drug
C. Inhibits xanthine oxidase
D. Cyclo-oxygenase inhibitor
E. Inhibits DNA gyrase B

Q10.16

A 33-year-old man trekking through the woods in Connecticut in the month of May develops a fever and headache, and an expanding, erythematous rash. The test which is most likely to confirm the diagnosis is

A. Presence of uric acids crystals in the joint fluid
B. The detection of IgM antibodies against the spirochaete *Borrelia burgdorferi*
C. Serum VDRL (Venereal Disease Research Laboratory) is positive
D. Presence of calcium pyrophosphate crystals in the joint fluid
E. HLA B27 on HLA testing

Q10.17

A 19-year-old soldier engaged in the first Gulf War hurts his left leg. The leg initially recovers but subsequently is painful and he has hyperaesthesia. A few months later he complains of leg stiffness, and on examination the skin over the leg is cold and shows trophic changes. Finally, his condition is extremely disabling and he develops muscle atrophy and contractures requiring an orthopaedic shoe. A three-phase bone scan of the left leg in this patient is most likely to show

A. Loss of joint space in the knee joint
B. Loss of joint space in the ankle joint
C. Diffuse or patchy uptake in all three phases
D. Periarticular osteoporosis
E. Lytic lesions in the tibia and fibula

Q10.18

A 45-year-old woman complains of joint stiffness in the early morning. On examination she has active arthritis of the interphalangeal joints and nodules on the elbow. Which one of the following tests indicates a poor prognosis in this condition

A. Low complement levels
B. High titres of IgM antibody detected by agglutination test using IgG-coated latex particles
C. Elevated anti-DNA/histone (homogeneous) antibodies
D. Elevated anticentromere antibodies
E. Elevated antibodies to the enzyme histidyl tRNA synthetase

Q10.19

A 45-year-old woman has pain and swelling of her left knee joint. Examination of her synovial fluid under polarized light reveals weakly positively birefringent crystals. The most likely diagnosis is

A. Palindromic rheumatoid arthritis
B. Gout
C. Pyrophosphate arthropathy
D. Osteoarthritis
E. Fibromyalgia

Q10.20

A 29-year-old secretary complains of pain in her right shoulder. On examination she is unable to actively abduct the right arm, but if she uses her left arm to elevate the right arm she is able to hold it in place without help from the left arm. The most likely diagnosis is

A. Supraspinatus tendonitis
B. Acute cervical disc prolapse
C. Whiplash injury to the neck
D. Torn rotator cuff
E. Frozen shoulder

Q10.21

A 39-year-old white woman with history of smoking and premature menopause wishes to prevent osteoporosis. She also has a family history of oestrogen-receptor-positive breast cancer. Select the best option for her treatment

A. Alendronate
B. Risedronate
C. Hormone replacement therapy
D. Raloxifene
E. Androgens

Q10.22

1. Point where a tendon or ligament joins to a bone
2. The type of collagen which comprises the majority of the collagen in the body
3. Cross-linkages with desmosine and isodesmosine are specific to this substance
4. The major non-collagenous glycoprotein in the extracellular matrix
5. Proteins which contain glycosaminoglycan

Select the best match for each of the above

A. Cartilage
B. Enthesis
C. Type III collagen
D. Type I collagen
E. Fibronectin
F. Proteoglycans
G. Elastin

Q10.23

1. Oral contraceptives
2. Diuretics
3. Steroids
4. Hydralazine

Select the best match for each of the above

A. May precipitate gout
B. May cause lupus-like syndrome
C. May precipitate systemic lupus erythematosus
D. May cause avascular necrosis of the hip

Q10.24

1. High titres indicate a poor prognosis and are specific to systemic lupus erythematosus (SLE)
2. These antibodies are non-specific for SLE
3. Low levels indicate consumption and suggest an active disease process in SLE
4. Used as a screening test for SLE but low titres occur in rheumatoid arthritis, in chronic infections and in elderly individuals
5. Present in SLE with Sjögren's syndrome
6. Occurs in a range of diseases including SLE and overlap syndrome

Select the best match for each of the above

A. Anti-Ro (SS-A)
B. Anti-single-stranded DNA antibodies
C. Anti-U1-RNP antibodies
D. Antinuclear antibodies
E. Anti-double-stranded DNA antibodies
F. Complement levels
G. Rheumatoid factor

Q10.25

1. A 69-year-old woman has difficulty in abducting her left shoulder. On examination the muscles that flex her left elbow are weak, the left biceps jerk is absent and there is loss of sensation on the lateral aspect of the left upper arm

2. An 88-year-old man on examination has weakness of the abductors and adductors of small muscles of his right hand and loss of sensation on the medial side of the upper arm

3. A 73-year-old woman complains of pain on the right side of the neck and upper arm. On examination she has weakness of extension of her right elbow, loss of sensation over the middle finger and the triceps jerk is absent

4. A 78-year-old man complains of pain on the right side of the neck. On examination there is weakness of the flexors of the right elbow and wrist. The biceps jerk is absent on that side and there is loss of sensation on the lateral side of the right forearm, thumb and index finger

5. An 82-year-old man known to have cervical spondylosis has weakness of the flexors of the fingers and sensory loss over the little and ring fingers

For each of the above select the best match for cervical nerve root entrapment

A. C8 nerve root
B. T1 nerve root
C. C7 nerve root
D. C6 nerve root
E. C5 nerve root

Q10.26

A 45-year-old woman complains of acute onset of pain in the right knee joint. Differential diagnosis includes

A. Gout
B. Pseudogout
C. Palindromic rheumatoid arthritis
D. Septic arthritis
E. Osteoarthroses

Q10.27

An 85-year-old woman complains of pain and stiffness of both her knees, making it difficult to walk. On examination both joints are tender, there is crepitus on movement, limitation in the range of movement and wasting of the muscles. Rheumatoid factor and antinuclear factor antibodies are negative. Factors known to influence the pathogenesis of this condition include

A. Action of matrix metalloproteinases on the matrix of joint cartilage
B. Action of tissue inhibitors of matrix metalloproteinases on the matrix of joint cartilage
C. Mutations in the gene for type II collagen
D. High intake of vitamin B
E. Body mass index more than 35

Q10.28

A 43-year-old woman complains of pain and stiffness of the small joints of the hands, wrists, elbows, shoulders, knees and ankles that is typically worse in the morning and improves with gentle activity. The patient complains that she feels tired. Complications of this condition include

A. Transthyretin variant of amyloidosis
B. Separation of the odontoid peg from the anterior arch of the atlas vertebra
C. Septic arthritis
D. Rupture of Baker's cysts
E. A sudden onset of finger drop of little and ring fingers

Q10.29

A 49-year-old woman has a 16-week history of pain and stiffness of the small joints of the hands, wrists, elbows, shoulders, knees and ankles that is typically worse in the morning and improves with gentle activity. On examination she has inflamed joints, a large spleen and neutropenia. This condition is characterized by

A. Mononeuritis multiplex
B. Sepsis
C. Leg ulcers
D. Increased incidence of HLA-DRW4 compared to rheumatoid arthritis alone
E. Decreased incidence of HLA-DRW4 compared to rheumatoid arthritis alone

Q10.30

A 45-year-old woman develops joint pains, fever and weight loss. Her rheumatologist is certain that the has systemic lupus erythematosus despite being negative for anti-dsDNA. The following agents could have caused this clinical picture

A. Hydralazine
B. Methyldopa
C. Isoniazid
D. D-Penicillamine
E. Minocycline

Q10.31

A 45-year-old woman develops joint pains, fever and weight loss. She has a 'butterfly rash' on her face, livedo reticularis on her shins, and also has Raynaud's phenomenon. The following statements regarding this condition are correct

A. C-reactive protein is often raised particularly during active disease
B. Serum complement levels are elevated during active disease

C. Double-stranded DNA is positive in almost all cases
D. Antinuclear antigen is positive in less than 25% of patients
E. Rheumatoid factor is positive in almost all cases
F. Anticardiolipin antibodies are present in 35–45% of cases
G. A third of patients test false-positive for syphilis

Q10.32

A 45-year-old woman develops arthralgia together with dryness of the skin, vagina and mouth. The salivary and parotid glands are enlarged. Associated systemic features of this condition include

A. Increased incidence of Hodgkin's T cell lymphoma
B. Renal tubular acidosis
C. Myasthenia gravis
D. Primary biliary cirrhosis
E. Autoimmune hepatitis

Q10.33

ANCA-negative small-vessel vasculitis includes

A. Wegener's granulomatosis
B. Churg–Strauss granulomatosis
C. Microscopic polyangiitis
D. Henoch–Schönlein purpura
E. Cutaneous leucocytoclastic angiitis

Q10.34

Parathyroid hormone increases renal phosphate excretion and raises plasma calcium by increasing

A. The levels of colecalciferol in the skin
B. Osteoclastic resorption of bone
C. Intestinal absorption of calcium
D. Synthesis of $1,25\text{-}(OH)_2D_3$
E. Renal tubular reabsorption of calcium

Rheumatology and bone disease

Q10.35

A 92-year-old man has asymptomatic elevation of alkaline phosphatase. Skull X-ray reveals osteoporosis circumscripta. On examination he has bowed tibia and skull changes. Complications of this condition include

A. Deafness due to compression of the VIIIth cranial nerve
B. High-output cardiac failure
C. Pathological fractures
D. 30-fold increased risk of osteogenic sarcoma
E. VIIth cranial nerve palsy

Q10.36

A 33-year-old Asian woman who traditionally wears a veil now has a waddling gait and weakness of the proximal muscles. She has clinical features of tetany. The following are likely to be seen in this condition

A. Decreased serum alkaline phosphatase
B. Raised serum acid phosphatase
C. Low serum 25-hydroxyvitamin D_3
D. Linear areas of low density surrounded by sclerotic borders on skeletal X-ray
E. Raised plasma calcium

A10.1

C

Still's disease accounts for 10% of cases of juvenile idiopathic arthritis (JIA). It affects boys and girls equally up to 5 years of age; then girls are more commonly affected. Adult-onset Still's disease is extremely rare. Clinical features include a high, swinging, early-evening pyrexia, an evanescent pink maculopapular rash with arthralgia and arthritis, myalgia and generalized lymphadenopathy. Hepatosplenomegaly, pericarditis and pleurisy occur. The differential diagnoses include malignancy, in particular leukaemia and neuroblastoma, and infection. Laboratory tests show a high ESR and CRP, neutrophilia and thrombocytosis. Autoantibodies are negative.

A10.2

C

Osteosclerotic metastases are characteristic of prostatic carcinoma. Prostate specific antigen (PSA) and serum acid phosphate are raised in the presence of prostatic metastases.

A10.3

D

Laboratory abnormalities in Sjögren's syndrome include raised immunoglobulin levels, circulating immune complexes and many autoantibodies. Rheumatoid factor is usually positive. Antinuclear antibodies are found in 60–70% of cases and antimitochondrial antibodies in 10%. Anti-Ro (SSA) antibodies are found in 70%, compared with 10% of cases of rheumatoid arthritis (RA) and secondary Sjögren's syndrome. This antibody is of

particular interest because it can cross the placenta and cause congenital heart block.

A10.4

B

In giant cell arteritis, corticosteroids are obligatory because they significantly reduce the risk of irreversible visual loss and other focal ischaemic lesions, but much higher doses are needed. The disease settles after between 12 and 36 months of treatment in about 75% of patients, but the remaining 25% continue to require low doses of corticosteroids for years. The starting dose of prednisolone is 60–100 mg prednisolone, usually in divided doses.

A10.5

C

In polyarteritis nodosa angiography shows aneurysms in hepatic, intestinal or renal vessels.

A10.6

C

The antiphospholipid syndrome is associated with autoantibodies which have specificity for negatively charged phospholipids. The terms lupus anticoagulant and anticardiolipin are used to describe these antibodies. A small proportion of these patients have systemic lupus erythematosus (SLE). Recurrent arterial and venous thromboses and miscarriages are the hallmark of the syndrome. The paradoxical association between a prothrombotic state and the presence of autoantibodies with in-vitro anticoagulant effects is not fully understood. However, B_2-glycoprotein

(B$_2$GP1), also known as apolipoprotein H, has been identified as the target for both anticardiolipin antibodies and lupus anticoagulant. Anticardiolipin antibodies (detected by ELISA) are diagnostic. Lupus anticoagulant antibodies are found in coagulation assays and these antibodies, directed against B$_2$GP1, can be detected by ELISA. The ESR is usually normal and antinuclear antibodies are usually negative.

A10.7

E

Limited cutaneous scleroderma (LcSSc) usually starts with Raynaud's phenomenon many years (up to 15) before any skin changes. The skin involvement is limited to the hands, face, feet and forearms. The skin is tight over the fingers and often produces flexion deformities of the fingers. Involvement of the skin of the face produces a characteristic 'beak'-like nose and a small mouth (microstomia). Painful digital ulcers and telangiectasia with dilated nail-fold capillary loops are seen. Digital ischaemia may lead to gangrene. Gastrointestinal tract involvement is common in this group. Pulmonary hypertension develops in 10–15% of this group and pulmonary interstitial disease may occur. Speckled, nucleolar or anticentromere antibodies (ACAs) occur in 70–80% of cases.

A10.8

E

Antinuclear antibody testing is commonly positive in patients with dermatomyositis. Rheumatoid factor is present in up to 50% and many myositis-specific antibodies (MSAs) have been recognized and correlate with certain subsets. Antibodies to Jo-1 (antibodies to histidyl tRNA synthetase) are predictive of pulmonary fibrosis but are rarely seen in patients with dermatomyositis.

A10.9

E

In rheumatoid arthritis peripheral, intrapulmonary nodules are usually asymptomatic but may cavitate. When pneumoconiosis is present (Caplan's syndrome), large cavitating lung nodules develop.

A10.10

C

Sicca syndrome (Sjogren syndrome, or keratoconjunctivitis sicca) causes dry mouth and eyes. It is seen in menopausal women and often associated with rheumatoid arthritis.

A10.11

E

Human lymphocyte antigen (HLA) testing is rarely of value in ankylosing spondylitis because of the high frequency of HLA-B27 in the population, but may give supporting evidence in a difficult case. Persistent inflammatory enthesitis causes bony spurs (syndesmophytes). Syndesmophytes are more vertically oriented than the beak-like osteophytes of spondylosis and the disc is preserved, unlike in spondylosis.

A10.12

C

The triad of Reiter's disease comprises urethritis, arthritis and conjunctivitis. Poncet's disease is a reactive arthritis seen in tuberculosis. Jaccoud's arthropathy is the rheumatoid arthritis-like picture seen in systemic lupus erythematosus (SLE). Pott's disease is tuberculosis of the spine, and CREST syndrome represents calcinosis, Raynaud's phenomenon, oesophageal involvement, sclerodactyly and telangiectasia. Reactive arthritis is a sterile synovitis, which occurs following an infection. Reiter's disease comprises the triad of urethritis, arthritis and conjunctivitis.

A10.13

D

This patient has acute gout. Diuretics can precipitate gout. In the setting of heart failure NSAIDs are best avoided and colchicine is the best option for treatment of acute gout.

A10.14

B

Calcium pyrophosphate deposits in hyaline and fibrocartilage produce the radiological appearance of chondrocalcinosis. Shedding of crystals into a joint precipitates acute synovitis which resembles gout, except that it is more common in elderly women and usually affects the knee or wrist. The attacks are often very painful. The attacks may be associated with fever and a raised white blood cell count. In young people it may be associated with haemochromatosis, hyperparathyroidism, Wilson's disease or alkaptonuria. The diagnosis is made by detecting rhomboidal, weakly positively birefringent crystals in joint fluid, or deduced from the presence of chondrocalcinosis on X-ray. The joint fluid looks purulent. Septic arthritis must be excluded and joint fluid should be sent for culture.

A10.15

C

Allopurinol (300–600 mg) blocks the enzyme xanthine oxidase, which converts xanthine into urate. It reduces serum urate levels rapidly and is relatively non-toxic.

A10.16

B

Diagnosis of Lyme disease is by the detection of IgM antibodies against the spirochaete *Borrelia burgdorferi*.

A10.17

C

Reflex sympathetic dystrophy (RSD), Sudek's atrophy or chronic regional pain syndrome type I leads to structural changes of superficial and deep tissues (trophic changes). Not all components need be present. The sensory, motor and sympathetic nerve changes are not restricted to the distribution of a single nerve and may be remote from the site of injury. Diagnosis is initially clinical – a high index of suspicion and recognizing the unusual distribution of the pain. A three-phase bone scan shows diffuse or patchy increase in uptake in the affected limb in all three phases: early (a few seconds – arterial); middle (a few minutes – soft tissue); and late (several hours – mineral). The bone phase abnormalities appear early and well before demineralization is seen on X-ray. There is never loss of joint space, which distinguishes the appearances from the periarticular osteoporosis of inflammatory joint disease.

A10.18

B

IgM rheumatoid factors (RFs) are detected by agglutination tests using IgG-coated latex particles (the Rose–Waaler test) or sensitized sheep red cells (sheep cell agglutination test or SCAT). They are antibodies (usually IgM, but occasionally IgG or IgA) against the Fc portion of IgG and are detected in 70% of patients with rheumatoid arthritis (RA), but are not diagnostic. A high titre in early RA indicates a poor prognosis. Positive titres occasionally predate the onset of RA. Titres may fluctuate. Rheumatoid factor is detected in many autoimmune rheumatic disorders (e.g. systemic lupus erythematosus), in chronic infections, and in asymptomatic older people.

A10.19

C

In pyrophosphate arthropathy shedding of crystals into a joint precipitates acute synovitis which resembles gout, except that it is more common in elderly women and usually affects the knee or wrist. The attacks are often very painful. In young people it may be associated with haemochromatosis, hyperparathyroidism, Wilson's disease or alkaptonuria. The diagnosis is made by detecting rhomboidal, weakly positively birefringent crystals in joint fluid, or deduced from the presence of chondrocalcinosis on X-ray. The joint fluid looks purulent. Septic arthritis must be excluded and joint fluid should be sent for culture. The attacks may be associated with fever and a raised white blood cell count.

A10.20

D

Torn rotator cuff is caused by trauma in the young but also occurs spontaneously in the elderly and in rheumatoid arthritis (RA). It prevents active abduction of the arm, but patients learn to initiate elevation using the unaffected arm. Once elevated, the arm can be held in place by the deltoid muscle.

A10.21

D

Raloxifene is a selective oestrogen-receptor modulator (SERM) for osteoporosis. It has no stimulatory effect on endometrium but activates oestrogen receptors in bone (i.e. physiologically similar to hormone replacement therapy). It prevents bone mineral density loss at spine and hip in postmenopausal women, though fracture rates were only reduced in the spine. It also reduced the incidence of oestrogen-receptor-positive breast carcinoma by 90% over 3 years. Leg cramps and flushing occur more commonly than with hormone replacement therapy, the risk of thromboembolic complications being comparable.

A10.22

1) B   2) D   3) G   4) E   5) F

The point where a tendon or ligament joins a bone is called an enthesis and may be the site of inflammation. Fibronectin is the major non-collagenous glycoprotein in the extracellular matrix. Proteoglycans are proteins which contain glycosaminoglycan side-chains and are of variable form and size. Elastin is an insoluble protein polymer and is the main component of elastic fibres. Tropoelastin, its precursor, is synthesized by vascular smooth muscle cells and skin fibroblasts. Cross-linkages with desmosine and isodesmosine are specific to elastin fibres. Most collagen in the body is type I – the major component of bone, tendon, ligament, skin, sclera, cornea, blood vessels and the hollow organs.

A10.23

1) C   2) A   3) D   4) B

Diuretics may precipitate gout in men and older women. Hormone replacement therapy or the oral contraceptive pill may precipitate systemic lupus erythematosus (SLE). Steroids can cause avascular necrosis. Some drugs (e.g. hydralazine and procainamide) can cause a lupus-like syndrome.

Low complement levels indicate consumption and suggest an active disease process in systemic lupus erythematosus (SLE). Anti-single-stranded DNA antibodies are non-specific whereas anti-double-stranded DNA antibodies are diagnostic of active SLE but may be negative in mild or inactive disease. High titres of IgG anti-dsDNA indicate a poor prognosis and are specific to SLE. Anti-extractable nuclear antigen (ENA) antibodies produce a speckled ANA fluorescent pattern and can be distinguished by ELISA:

- anti-Ro (SS-A) – SLE + Sjögren's
- anti-La (SS-B) – Sjögren's
- anti-Sm – SLE
- anti-U1-RNP – a range of diseases, including SLE, overlap syndrome.

A10.24

1) E   2) B   3) F   4) D   5) A   6) C

A10.25

1) E   2) B   3) C   4) D   5) A

Cervical nerve root entrapment – symptoms and signs			
Nerve root	Sensory changes	Reflex loss	Weakness
C5	Lateral arm	Biceps	Shoulder abduction Elbow flexion
C6	Lateral forearm Thumb and index finger	Biceps Supinator	Elbow flexion Wrist extension
C7	Middle finger	Triceps	Elbow extension
C8	Medial forearm Little and ring fingers	None	Finger flexion
T1	Medial upper arm	None	Finger ab- and adduction

Rheumatology and bone disease

A10.26

A) T   B) T   C) T   D) T   E) T

Pattern of joint involvement in inflammatory arthritis

Diseases presenting as an inflammatory monarthritis
Crystal arthritis, e.g. gout, pseudogout
Septic arthritis
Palindromic rheumatism
Traumatic + haemarthrosis
Arthritis due to juxta-articular bone tumour
Occasionally, psoriatic, reactive, rheumatoid may present as monarthritis

Diseases presenting as an inflammatory polyarthritis
Rheumatoid arthritis
Reactive arthritis
Seronegative arthritis associated with psoriasis or ankylosing spondylitis
Postviral arthritis
Lyme arthritis
Enteropathic arthritis
Athritis associated with erythema nodosum

A10.27

A) T   B) T   C) T   D) F   E) T

Several mechanisms have been suggested for the pathogenesis of osteoarthritis (OA) including:

a) Matrix loss is caused by the action of matrix metalloproteinases such as collagenase (MMP-1), gelatinase (MMP-2) and stromelysin (MMP-3). These are secreted by chrondrocytes in an inactive form. Extracellular activation then leads to the degradation of collagen and proteoglycans

b) Mutations in the gene for type II collagen (COL2A1) have been associated with early polyarticular OA

c) Obesity (BMI>30) is a risk factor for developing OA in later life.

A10.28

A) F   B) T   C) T   D) T   E) T

Complications of rheumatoid arthritis include: a) ruptured tendons; b) ruptured joints (Baker's cysts); c) joint infection; d) spinal cord compression (atlanto-axial or upper cervical spine); and e) AA (reactive or secondary) amyloidosis.

A10.29

A) F   B) T   C) T   D) T   E) F

Felty's syndrome is splenomegaly and neutropenia in a patient with rheumatoid arthritis (RA). Leg ulcers or sepsis are complications. HLA-DRW4 is found in 95% of patients, compared with 70% of patients with RA alone.

A10.30

A) T   B) T   C) T   D) T   E) T

Drugs such as hydralazine, methyldopa, isoniazid, D-penicillamine and minocycline can induce lupus not associated with anti-dsDNA. Flare-ups can be induced by the contraceptive pill and hormone replacement therapy.

A10.31

A) F   B) F   C) F   D) F   E) F
F) T   G) T

In systemic lupus erythematosus (SLE) the erythrocyte sedimentation rate is raised in proportion to the disease activity. In contrast, the C-reactive protein is normal. Serum antinuclear antibodies (ANA) are positive in almost all cases. Double-stranded DNA (dsDNA) binding is specific for SLE, although it is only present in 50% of cases, particularly those with severe systemic involvement (e.g. renal disease).

Antinucleosome antibodies predate anti-dsDNA antibodies. Antibodies to RNA (ss and ds) anti-Ro and anti-La can also be detected. Rheumatoid factor is positive in 25% of the patients. Serum complement levels are reduced during active disease. Anticardiolipin antibodies are present in 35–45% of the patients. A third of patients have a false-positive test for syphilis owing to the anticardiolipin antibody.

A10.32

A) F B) T C) T D) T E) T

Associated systemic features of Sjögren's syndrome include: a) arthralgia and occasional non-progressive polyarthritis, like that seen in systemic lupus erythematosus (but much less common); b) Raynaud's phenomenon; c) dysphagia and abnormal oesophageal motility as seen in systemic sclerosis (but less common); d) other organ-specific autoimmune disease, including thyroid disease, myasthenia gravis, primary biliary cirrhosis and autoimmune hepatitis; e) renal tubular defects (uncommon) causing nephrogenic diabetes insipidus and renal tubular acidosis; f) pulmonary diffusion defects and fibrosis; g) polyneuropathy, fits and depression; h) vasculitis; i) increased incidence of non-Hodgkin's B cell lymphoma.

A10.33

A) F B) F C) F D) T E) T

ANCA-positive vasculitis

- Wegener's granulomatosis.
- Churg–Strauss granulomatosis.
- Microscopic polyangiitis.

ANCA-negative small-vessel vasculitis
This includes Henoch–Schönlein purpura and cutaneous leucocytoclastic angiitis.

A10.34

A) F B) T C) T D) T E) T

Parathyroid hormone (PTH) increases renal phosphate excretion, and increases plasma calcium by increasing: a) osteoclastic resorption of bone (occurring rapidly); b) intestinal absorption of calcium (a slow response); c) synthesis of $1,25\text{-}(OH)_2D_3$; d) renal tubular reabsorption of calcium.

A10.35

A) T B) T C) T D) T E) T

Complications from Paget's disease include:

a) Nerve compression (deafness from VIIIth cranial nerve; also cranial nerves II, V, VII; spinal stenosis, hydrocephalus)

b) Increased bone blood flow (myocardial hypertrophy and high-output cardiac failure)

c) Pathological fractures

d) Osteogenic sarcoma in pagetic bone (fewer than 1% of cases, but a 30-fold increased risk compared with non-pagetic patients).

A10.36

A) F B) F C) T D) T E) F

In adult osteomalacia the following may be seen. a) Increased serum alkaline phosphatase, indicating increased osteoblast activity, is the most common abnormality (note: alkaline phosphatase is elevated during skeletal growth). b) Plasma calcium is low or normal, in association with secondary hyperparathyroidism and a raised parathyroid hormone (PTH). c) Serum phosphate may be low, owing to increased

Rheumatology and bone disease

PTH-dependent phosphaturia, though this is variable. d) Serum 25-hydroxyvitamin D$_3$ is usually low (exceptions being vitamin-D-resistant rickets). e) X-rays are often normal in adults, but may show defective mineralization, especially in the pelvis, long bones and ribs, with 'Looser's zones' – linear areas of low density surrounded by sclerotic borders.

Q11.1

A 47-year-old woman is being considered for heart transplant. The protocol requires that her glomerular filteration rate is adequate. One of the following tests is used routinely in hospitals to determine this function?

A. Inulin clearance
B. Serum creatinine divided BUN
C. Creatinine clearance
D. Urea clearance
E. BUN corrected for 24-hour urine output

Q11.2

A 25-year-old doctor complains of a painful swelling in the testis. Investigations reveal localized seminoma of the testis. The best therapeutic option is

A. Orchidectomy
B. Chemotherapy
C. Radiotherapy
D. Buserelin
E. Goserelin

Q11.3

A 34-year-old diabetic, 2 months after her renal transplant from an identical twin, develops acute rejection. The primary treatment for acute rejection in this patient is

A. Do nothing since the donor is an identical twin and, therefore it should resolve spontaneously

B. Ciclosporin
C. Mycophenolate mofetil
D. Tacrolimus
E. Corticosteroids
F. Azathioprine

Q11.4

A 23-year-old man complains of colicky pain in the left flank. The pain radiates from the flank to the iliac fossa and the testis. Plain X-ray of the abdomen shows renal stones. Serum calcium levels are elevated. Which one of the following conditions is the most common cause of this clinical picture?

A. Hypoparathyroidism
B. Hypohypoparathyroidism
C. Primary hyperparathyroidism
D. Vitamin D ingestion
E. Sarcoidosis

Q11.5

A 53-year-old diabetic on haemodialysis develops nausea, vomiting, restlessness, headache, hypertension, myoclonic jerking, seizures and coma. The most likely diagnosis is

A. Diabetic ketoacidosis
B. Hyperosmolar coma
C. Hypertensive encephalopathy
D. Dialysis disequlibrium
E. Grand mal epilepsy

Renal disease

Q11.6

A 42-year-old patient has been admitted for cardiogenic shock and requires haemofiltration. The buffer used in this process is

A. Calcium carbonate
B. Sodium carbonate
C. Sodium bicarbonate
D. Lactate
E. Aluminium bicarbonate

Q11.7

A 65-year-old patient on long-term haemodialysis develops disabling stiffness in the hips, hand and knees. The best test to confirm the extent of the disorder is

A. Urine microalbuminuria
B. Arthroscopy
C. A trial of NSAIDs
D. A trial of prednisolone
E. Radiolabelled serum amyloid P component

Q11.8

A 40-year-old man presents with haematuria, loin pain and a mass in the flank. There is a left-sided varicocele and ultrasound reveals a solid lesion in the left kidney. Biopsy reveals carcinoma arising from proximal tubular epithelium. There is a deletion of the short arm of chromosome 3. This condition is associated with

A. Tuberous sclerosis
B. Von Hippel–Lindau disease
C. Von Recklinghausen's disease
D. Van Harrison's disease
E. Sturge–Weber syndrome

Q11.9

A 48-year-old patient on chronic haemodialysis requires right hip replacement. Serum Na 142, K 6 mmol/L, chloride 100 and glucose 6 mmol/L. The best option is

A. Perform surgery with measurement of central venous pressure
B. Perform surgey with careful monitoring of urea, electrolyte and creatinine concentrations
C. Administer mannitol before surgery and perform surgery with careful monitoring of urea, electrolyte and creatinine concentrations and central venous pressure
D. Perform surgery with careful monitoring of urea, electrolyte and creatinine concentrations and central venous pressure
E. Delay surgery

Q11.10

A 55-year-old executive with hypertension undergoes routine urine examination and the Stix test for blood is positive. Examination of fresh urine under the microscope does not show any red cells. Which of the following is the most likely cause of these findings?

A. A high urine specific gravity
B. Decreased urine osmolality
C. Haemoglobinuria
D. Proteinuria
E. Microalbuminuria

Q11.11

A 73-year-old man complains of loin pain which worsens on drinking alcohol. He has intermittent polyuria and anuria. On examination there is loin tenderness and an enlarged left kidney is palpable. Which one of the following is a reliable means of ruling out upper urinary tract dilatation as an initial investigation in such a patient?

A. Biochemical investigation showing azotemia
B. Hyperkalaemia
C. Blood in the urine
D. Ultrasound of the abdomen
E. Radionuclide studies

Q11.12

On routine examination of the urine of a diabetic patient the Stix test does not detect any urinary albumin. However, further testing reveals that urine albumin concentration is around 75 mg/L. Which one of the following statements is correct?

A. This suggests that the patient has associated distal tubular disease
B. Normal individuals excrete less than 175 mg of albumin in 24 h and therefore this can be ignored
C. This is an early indicator of diabetic glomerular disease
D. The patient should be treated with a beta-blocker
E. This finding suggests that the patient has a urinary tract infection

Q11.13

A 22-year-old man presents with sore throat, fever, puffiness of face, haematuria, oliguria, hypertension and worsening azotemia. Renal biopsy shows that the glomeruli are swollen, packed with cells, and bulge into the opening of the proximal tubule. There is proliferation of the endothelial and mesangial cells, and polymorphonuclear leucocytes are present. Immunofluorescence shows granular deposits of immunoglobulin and C3. Electron microscopy reveals electron-dense deposits. Select the best option for this clinical picture

A. Membranous glomerulonephritis
B. Minimal change nephropathy
C. IgA nephropathy
D. Diffuse proliferative glomerulonephritis
E. Focal glomerulosclerosis

Q11.14

1. A 24-year-old man presents with puffiness of face, haematuria and is found have 6 g of protein in a 24-hour urine sample. Renal biopsy shows mesangial cell proliferation with electron-dense, linear intramembranous deposits that stain for C3 only

2. A 33-year-old woman presents with puffiness of face and has 7 g of protein in a 24-h urine sample. Renal biopsy shows mesangial cell proliferation with subendothelial immune complex deposition and the capillary basement membrane shows a 'tram-line' effect

3. A 49-year-old man presents with puffiness of face and has features of nephrotic syndrome. Renal biopsy shows thickening of the capillary basement membrane because of immune complex deposition

4. A 26-year-old boy presents with puffiness of face and his 24 h urine protein is 8 g. Renal biopsy shows that glomeruli appear normal on light microscopy and on electron microscopy there is fusion of the foot processes of epithelial cells

5. A 17-year-old boy notices discoloration of his urine following an upper

respiratory tract infection. Urine microscopy shows haematuria. The blood pressure is normal, and proteinuria is absent. Renal biopsy shows focal proliferative glomerulonephritis

6. A 17-year-old girl presents with skin rash, abdominal colic, joint pain and glomerulonephritis following a respiratory tract infection. Serum concentrations of IgA are elevated. Kidney biopsy reveals a focal segmental glomerulonephritis and IgA deposits are seen in the glomerular mesangium

7. A 29-year-old cigarette smoker presents with a history of recurrent haemoptysis and a severe progressive glomerulonephritis

Select the best for each of the above

A. Henoch–Schönlein syndrome
B. Mediated by antiglomerular basement membrane antibody
C. Mediated by antiglomerular basement membrane antigen
D. IgA nephropathy
E. Minimal change glomerular lesion
F. *Plasmodium malariae* infection
G. Partial lipodystrophy
H. Shunt nephritis

Q11.15

1. A 33-year-old man has glomerulonephritis together with necrotizing lesions affecting the nasopharynx, lungs and kidneys. The necrotizing glomerular lesions do not appear be due to immune complex deposition

2. A 45-year-old diabetic has frequency of micturition, dysuria and fever. Urine culture reveals that *Proteus mirabilis* is the organism causing urinary tract infection and this has been successfully treated

3. A 22-year-old pregnant woman is asymptomatic. Routine urine studies reveal $>10^5$ organisms/mL of urine on two occasions

4. An 18-year-old woman is asymptomatic. Routine urine studies reveal 10^5 organisms/mL of urine on two occasions

Select the best match for each of the above

A. Proteinase-3 antineutrophil cytoplasmic antibodies (PR3-ANCA) positivity
B. Myeloperoxidase MPO-ANCA positivity
C. This patient is more predisposed to renal stones
D. No treatment required despite bacteriuria
E. Antibiotic treatment required for bacteriuria

Q11.16

1. A 22-year-old patient with polycystic kidney disease is treated for urinary tract infection. Five days after completion of antibiotic treatment urine examination reveals bacteriuria with the same organism as before

2. A 23-year-old woman presents with urinary tract infection and is successfully treated. Repeat urine culture 10 days after completion of antibacterial treatment shows no organisms. Five days after this she develops symptoms and urine culture reveals that the infection is due to the same organism as before

3. A 43-year-old diabetic woman presents with fever, loin pain and tenderness. Urine examination reveals significant bacteriuria. CT shows a wedge-shaped area of renal inflammation in the renal cortex

4. A 22-year-old patient has a history of vesicoureteric reflux and urinary tract

infection acquired in early childhood. Excretion urography shows irregular renal outlines, clubbed calyces and a reduction in renal size

5. A 43-year-old man, following treatment with NSAIDs, presents with fever, arthralgia, skin rashes and acute renal failure with urine output less than 10 mL/hour. In addition laboratory tests show an elevated eosinophil count and eosinophiluria

6. A 63-year-old immigrant from the Indian subcontinent presents with haematuria. Urine microscopy shows red blood cells, white blood cells but no organisms

Select the best match for each of the above

A. Typically there is papillary damage, interstitial nephritis and cortical scarring in areas adjacent to 'clubbed calyces'
B. Typically in such patients there are small renal cortical abscesses and streaks of pus in the renal medulla. Histologically there is focal infiltration by polymorphonuclear leucocytes and many polymorphs in the tubular lumina
C. Relapse of urinary tract infection
D. Reinfection
E. Renal biopsy shows an intense interstitial cellular infiltrate including eosinophils and variable tubular necrosis
F. Excretion urography shows cavitating lesions in the renal papillary areas with calcification

Q11.17

1. A 58-year-old woman, following renal transplantation, develops fracture of the femoral neck due to avascular necrosis, diabetes, skin fragility and ecchymoses

2. A 19-year-old woman develops rash, tremor, hairiness and nephrotoxicity 2 years after renal transplantation

3. A 33-year-old man develops pancytopenia and hepatoxicity 6 months after renal transplantation. Investigations reveal bone marrow depression

4. A 43-year-old patient after renal transplantation is allergic to ciclosporin and has been weaned off steroids several years ago. He is 10 years post-transplant and develops neurotoxicity, nephrotoxicity and diabetes.

Select the best match for each of the above

A. Azathioprine
B. Corticosteroids
C. Ciclosporin
D. Tacrolimus
E. Antithymocyte globulin

Q11.18

A 78-year-old woman presents with chest pain. She requires cardiac catheterization. Serum urea is 2.5 mmol/L and serum creatinine is 79 μmol/L. Urinary sodium is normal. This biochemical picture can be explained by

A. Corticosteroid therapy
B. Low-protein diet
C. Old age
D. Liver failure
E. Gastrointestinal bleeding

Q11.19

The following statements about serum creatinine are correct

A. A normal level suggests that the glomerular filtration rate is normal
B. Spironolactone reduces tubular secretion of creatinine
C. The serum creatinine does not rise above the normal until there is a reduction of 50–60% in the glomerular filtration rate
D. It is a very sensitive measure of proximal tubular function
E. Serum levels are low when distal tubular function is impaired

Q11.20

The following reflect impaired distal tubular function

A. Hypokalaemia
B. Hypophosphataemia
C. Generalized aminoaciduria
D. Impaired urinary concentrating capacity in response to water deprivation
E. Low pH of urine

Q11.21

A healthy man notices that his urine is discoloured after standing for some time. The most likely causes include

A. L-Dopa
B. Beta-blockers
C. Porphyria
D. Alkaptonuria
E. Endapril

Q11.22

The patient reports to the nurse that his urine is discolored. Examination of the urine excludes haematuria. The following can explain these findings

A. Angiotensin-converting enzyme inhibitors
B. Rifampicin
C. Ingestion of beetroot
D. Cholestatic jaundice
E. Spironolactone

Q11.23

Correct statements about urine microscopy include

A. The presence of even one white blood cell per cubic millimetre in a fresh unspun mid-stream urine sample indicates an inflammatory reaction within the urinary tract
B. The presence of even one red blood cell per cubic millimetre in a fresh unspun mid-stream urine sample indicates an inflammatory reaction within the urinary tract
C. Even one red cell cast indicates renal disease
D. Stix testing for blood or protein is of considerable value in the diagnosis of urinary tract infection
E. The demonstration of bacteria on Gram staining of the centrifuged deposit of a clean-catch mid-stream urine sample is highly suggestive of urinary tract infection

Q11.24

A fresh unspun mid-stream urine sample of a 32-year-old man shows 15 white blood cells per cubic millimetre. Gram staining does not reveal any bacteria and quantitative bacterial culture excludes bacterial infection. Likely causes for this finding include

A. Renal stones
B. Tubulointersititial nephritis
C. Papillary necrosis
D. Tuberculosis
E. Interstitial cystitis

Q11.25

A 35-year-old man presents with puffiness of the face, haematuria, oliguria, elevated blood pressure and worsening renal function. Renal biopsy reveals that only some of the glomeruli are affected and changes are present only in one or two parts of the affected glomeruli. The affected portions of these glomeruli show proliferation of the endothelial and mesangial cells. This condition can be seen in

A. Systemic lupus erythematosus
B. Subacute infective bacterial endocarditis
C. Shunt nephritis
D. Henoch–Schönlein nephropathy
E. Diffuse proliferative glomerulonephritis

Q11.26

A 12-year-old boy has haematuria, marked hypertension, puffiness of face, swelling of the feet, oliguria and uraemia following a streptococcal pharyngitis. The following statements about this child's condition are correct

A. The infecting organism is a Lancefield A β-haemolytic streptococcus

B. Although the diagnosis of post-streptococcal glomerulonephritis is clear-cut, renal imaging and renal biopsy are necessary
C. In the majority of patients, either corticosteroid or immunosuppressive therapy is of benefit
D. Spontaneous remission usually occurs in these patients
E. Hospital admission is advisable for this patient

Q11.27

A 29-year-old patient with systemic lupus erythematosus develops glomerulonephritis. The urine sediment contains red cells and red cell casts, and she has an elevated creatinine. The following statements about this condition are correct

A. Corticosteroid therapy substantially improves renal prognosis
B. Pregnancy decreases the risk to the lupus patient
C. Cyclophosphamide improves renal function
D. Evidence is lacking that corticosteroid therapy improves extrarenal manifestations
E. Histological diagnosis should be obtained before commencing treatment with azathioprine

Q11.28

A 22-year-old pregnant woman has dysuria. Routine urine studies reveal $>10^5$ organisms/mL of urine on two occasions. The following antibiotics can be safely used to treat her urinary tract infection

A. Tetracycline
B. Trimethoprim
C. Sulphonamides
D. 4-Quinolones

Renal disease

E. Amoxicillin

F. Ampicillin

G. Nitrofurantoin

H. Oral cephalosporins

Q11.29

A 45-year-old patient presents with proteinuria. Renal biopsy shows eosinophilic deposits in the mesangium, capillary loops and arteriolar walls. Staining with Congo red renders these deposits pink and they show green birefrigence under polarized light. Serum electrophoresis reveals immunoglobulin light chains. This condition is found in

A. Haemochromatosis

B. Sarcoidosis

C. Myeloma

D. Waldenstrom's macroglobulinaemia

E. Non-Hodgkin's lymphoma

Q11.30

A 65-year-old patient presents with puffiness of face and swelling of the feet. Twenty-four-hour urine examination reveals heavy proteinuria. Renal biopsy shows eosinophilic deposits in the mesangium, capillary loops and arteriolar walls. Staining with Congo red renders these deposits pink and they show green birefrigence under polarized light. The protein found is amyloid protein A. This condition is found following

A. Nephrotic syndrome

B. Renal infarcts

C. Long-standing lung abscess

D. Rheumatoid arthritis

E. Familial Mediterranean fever

Q11.31

A 58-year-old diabetic with multiple myeloma is undergoing cardiac catheterization. The following statements about contrast nephropathy are correct

A. The risk and severity of contrast nephropathy are amplified by the presence of hypovolaemia and renal impairment due to diabetic nephropathy

B. Diabetes *per se* is a risk factor for contrast nephropathy

C. Hyperviscosity in myeloma may decrease the risk of contrast-induced nephropathy

D. Acetylcysteine worsens renal impairment following intravenous contrast

E. Prevention of hypovolaemia before administration of contrast medium has been proven to reduce risk of contrast-induced nephropathy

F. The use of low-osmolality contrast medium reduces the risk of contrast-induced nephropathy

Q11.32

A 68-year-old man has malaise, bone pain, lethargy and weight loss. Skeletal survey reveals osteolytic lesions and serum protein electrophoresis reveals monoclonal M band. Bone marrow shows 40% plasma cells. Causes of renal impairment in this condition include

A. Blockage of tubules by casts

B. Renal amyloid deposition

C. Hypercalcaemia

D. Renal sepsis

E. Urinary tract obstruction

Q11.33

A 29-year-old nurse has a butterfly rash on the face and her face is puffy. Urine microscopy reveals proteinuria. Antinuclear and antinative DNA antibodies is also present. She undergoes a renal biopsy. The following histological types can be expected in this condition

A. Normal on light microscopy
B. Mesangial change not seen on light microscopy but detectable only by immunological staining
C. Mesangial change seen on light microscopy
D. Focal proliferative glomerulonephritis
E. Diffuse proliferative glomerulonephritis
F. Membranous nephritis

Q11.34

A 45-year-old woman presents with puffiness of the face. Laboratory studies reveal that serum albumin concentration is 25 g/L. The following would explain these findings

A. Inadequate protein intake
B. Chronic liver disease
C. Protein-losing enteropathy
D. Urinary protein of 6 g per day
E. Extensive burns
F. Pregnancy

Q11.35

A patient presents with puffiness of face. Urine examinations reveals that 24-hour urinary protein excretion is 6 g daily. Renal biopsy is indicated in the following

A. In male children who have a highly selective protein leak, no hypertension, and no red cells or red-cell casts in the urine

B. In long-standing insulin-dependent diabetes with associated retinopathy or neuropathy
C. The patient is on long-term pencillamine therapy
D. In all patients with this clinical picture
E. When the question is whether a steroid-sensitive minimal-change lesion is present or not.

Q11.36

A 48-year-old woman complains of puffiness of face. Urine examination reveals that her 24-hour urinary protein is 6.5 g daily. The following statements regarding her condition are correct

A. Prolonged bed rest should be encouraged
B. Pneumococcal vaccine should be avoided
C. When her urine output is less than 15 mL/hour then albumin infusion combined with mannitol may initiate diuresis
D. HMG-CoA reductase inhibitors should be avoided when these patients have hypercholesterolaemia
E. Renal vein thrombosis is both a cause and a complication of this condition

Q11.37

A 13-year-old boy presents with puffiness of face. On examination he has periorbital oedema, swelling of feet and arms. The jugular venous pressure is not elevated and there is no pulmonary oedema. His 24-hour urinary protein is 6 g per day, serum albumin is 29 g/L, low-density lipoprotein is elevated, high-density lipoprotein is normal, and serum triglycerides are elevated. Renal biopsy shows minimal-change glomerular lesion.

Renal disease

The following statements about the management of this condition are correct

A. Initial treatment should be with dietary sodium restriction and a thiazide diuretic
B. High protein diet (80–90 g/day) is recommended since it confers benefit
C. Steroid therapy in this patient should be withheld because his age and laboratory findings suggest that he has a more benign variant of the disease
D. Children, even if in remission for 4 years after steroid therapy, tend in general to have further relapse
E. At least six courses of cyclophosphamide when it is indicated in male children
F. Ciclosporin therapy, when used instead of cyclophosphamide, is effective but must be continued long term to prevent relapse on stopping treatment

Q11.38

The following clinical scenarios meet the criteria for bacteriuria

A. A 23-year-old woman with dysuria and $\geq 10^2$ coliform organisms/mL plus pyuria (>10 WCC/mm^3)
B. A 45-year-old woman with dysuria and $\geq 10^5$ of any pathogenic organism/mL urine
C. Any growth of pathogenic organisms in urine by suprapubic aspiration in a 55-year-old woman with dysuria
D. A 55-year-old man with $\geq 10^3$ pathogenic organisms/mL urine
E. An asymptomatic adult with $\geq 10^5$ pathogenic organisms/mL of urine on two occasions

Q11.39

After reviewing the renal biopsy of a 38-year-old black African patient with benign essential hypertension the pathologist concludes that she has nephrosclerosis. The following are consistent with these observations

A. Cavitary lesions in the renal cortex
B. In small vessels and arterioles, intimal thickening with reduplication of the internal elastic lamina occurs and the vessel wall becomes hyalinized
C. In large vessels, concentric reduplication of the internal elastic lamina and endothelial proliferation produce an 'onion skin' appearance
D. Reduction in size of both kidneys may occur; this may be asymmetrical if one major renal artery is more affected than the other
E. The proportion of sclerotic glomeruli is increased compared with age-matched controls

Q11.40

A 23-year-old man complains of colicky pain in the left flank. The pain radiates from the flank to the iliac fossa and the testis. Plain X-ray of the abdomen shows renal stones. The following stones are clearly radiopaque on a plain X-ray of the abdomen

A. Pure uric acid stones
B. Mixed infective stones in which organic matrix predominates
C. Calcium-containing stones
D. Cystine stones
E. Staghorn calculi

Q11.41

A 33-year-old woman complains of colicky pain in the left flank. The pain radiates from the flank to the left iliac fossa and the labia. Urinary examination reveals mild hyperoxaluria. The causes are

A. Excessive ingestion of spinach
B. Excessive ingestion of tea
C. Excessive dietary calcium
D. Crohn's disease with resection of intestine
E. Excessive ingestion of rhubarb

Q11.42

A 43-year-old patient with chronic renal impairment becomes severely uraemic after initiation of new medications. The following medications cause this by their catabolic effect

A. Doxycycline
B. Oxytetracycline
C. Amoxicillin
D. Corticosteroids
E. Propranolol

Q11.43

A 21-year-old man develops oliguria following prolonged hypotension. Factors postulated in the development of this condition include

A. Entry of calcium into cells with an increase in cytosolic cell calcium concentration
B. Induction by hypoxia of nitric oxide synthases with increased production of nitric oxide
C. Increased production of intracellular proteases such as calpain
D. Activation of phospholipase A_2 with increased production of free fatty acids and consequent damage to cell membranes

E. Cell injury resulting from reperfusion with blood after initial ischaemia
F. Vasoconstriction
G. Liberation of toxic endothelial factors
H. Damage from the vasodilator effects of endotoxins
I. Reduced prostaglandin production
J. Tubular obstruction by desquamated cells and casts

Q11.44

A 47-year-old patient develops acute tubular necrosis. The nephrologist decides that the patient is a candidate for haemodialysis. The following indications would lead her to make this decision

A. Uraemic pericarditis
B. Pulmonary oedema
C. Rising creatinine in an anuric patient
D. Severe respiratory acidosis
E. To remove gentamicin

Q11.45

A 48-year-old diabetic patient with uraemia has marked pruritus. The causes of pruritus include

A. Hypercalcaemia
B. Hyperphosphataemia
C. Retention of nitrogenous waste products of protein metabolism
D. Elevated calcium × phosphate product
E. Hyperparathyroidism even when calcium and phosphate levels are normal
F. Iron deficiency

Q11.46

A 66-year-old patient has chronic renal failure and anaemia. Factors which have been implicated in the pathogenesis of anaemia in renal failure include

Renal disease

A. Bone marrow fibrosis secondary to hyperparathyroidism
B. Deficiency of haematinics such as iron, folate and vitamin B_{12}
C. Increased destruction of red cells
D. Abnormal red cell membranes
E. Erythropoietin deficiency
F. ACE inhibitors

Q11.47

A 47-year-old patient has long-standing hypertension and now complains of itching and generalized lethargy. She is anaemic and has a creatinine of 700 mmol/L. This patient is at increased risk of the following gastrointestinal conditions

A. Reflux oesophagitis
B. Peptic ulcer
C. Acute pancreatitis
D. Constipation
E. Elevations of serum amylase

Q11.48

Cardiovascular disease reduces life expectancy of patients with chronic renal failure compared to the normal population because of an increased incidence of

A. Myocardial infarction
B. Cardiac failure
C. Sudden cardiac death
D. Stroke
E. Coronary artery calcification

Q11.49

A 45-year-old patient with chronic renal failure develops anaemia and is treated with erythropoietin 300 U/kg per week. There is an initial satisfactory response of haemoglobin to treatment but subsequently there is a fall in haemoglobin. This can be due to

A. Iron deficiency
B. Bleeding
C. Infection
D. Malignancy

Q11.50

A 55-year-old patient in chronic renal failure and on haemodialysis is treated with erythropoietin for his anaemia. Partial correction of anaemia with erythropoietin results in

A. Hypotension
B. Improvement in exercise tolerance
C. Improvement in sexual function
D. Improvement in cognitive function
E. Regression of left ventricular hypertrophy

Q11.51

A 25-year-old patient on long-term haemodialysis requires emergency bowel surgery. The following can be used without adjusting the dosage

A. Morphine
B. Atropine
C. Diazepam
D. Halothane
E. Nitrous oxide

Q11.52

A 45-year-old woman develops recurrence of the disease which caused renal failure 2 years after her renal transplant. The following can lead to recurring disease in the graft

A. Primary oxalosis
B. Mesangiocapillary glomerulonephritis
C. Focal segmental glomerulosclerosis
D. Goodpasture's syndrome
E. Polycystic kidney disease

Q 11.53

A 25-year-old patient presents with acute loin pain, haematuria and hypertension. Physical examination reveals large and irregular kidneys. The gene responsible for this condition is located on chromosome 16. Complications and associations of this condition include

A. Subarachnoid haemorrhage
B. Hepatic cysts
C. Hypertension
D. Renal calculi
E. Mitral valve prolapse

Q 11.54

A 40-year-old man presents with haematuria, severe flank pain, and a mass in the flank. There is a left-sided varicocele and ultrasound reveals a solid lesion in the left kidney. Biopsy reveals carcinoma arising from proximal tubular epithelium. Liver biopsy shows metastases. Treatment modalities which have value include

A. Radiotherapy
B. Nephrectomy
C. Medroxyprogesterone acetate
D. Interleukin-2
E. α-Interferon

Q 11.55

A 55-year-old patient presents with painless haematuria. Cytological examination of the urine reveals malignant cells. Cystoscopy shows a bladder mass. Predisposing factors to this condition include

A. Alcohol dependence
B. Cyclophosphamide
C. Cigarette smoking
D. β-Naphthylamine
E. Schistosomiasis

Q 11.56

A 67-year-old patient presents with nocturia, difficulty in initiating urination and post-void dribbling. There is no haematuria. The following investigations are essential

A. Cystourethroscopy
B. Excretion urography
C. Renal ultrasonography
D. Prostate-specific antigen
E. Plain X-ray of the abdomen

Q 11.57

A 75-year-old patient on routine examination has a serum prostate-specific antigen level of 20 μg/L. Prostate biopsy reveals adenocarcinoma. Bone scan shows osteosclerotic lesions. The following are treatment options

A. Orchidectomy
B. Buserelin
C. Goserelin
D. Local radiotherapy with androgens
E. Radical prostatectomy alone

Renal disease

A11.1

C

The most widely used measurement of glomerular filtration rate (GFR) is the creatinine clearance. Creatinine clearance is a reasonably accurate measure of GFR in those situations in which it is most required. With progressive renal failure, creatinine clearance may overestimate GFR but, in clinical practice, this is seldom important. Inulin clearance – the gold standard of physiologists – is not practical or necessary in clinical practice. Two tests of distal tubular function are commonly applied in clinical practice: measurement of urinary concentrating capacity in response to water deprivation, and measurement of urinary acidification. Hypokalaemia, hypophosphataemia and generalized aminoaciduria suggest impaired proximal tubular function.

A11.2

C

Seminomas are radiosensitive, so tumours confined to the testis or with metastases below the diaphragm only are treated by radiotherapy. More widespread tumours require chemotherapy. Teratomas are treated by orchidectomy if the growth is confined to the testis. Chemotherapy is required for more widespread disease.

A11.3

E

Corticosteroids have a non-specific immunosuppressive action. High-dose methylprednisolone is used as the primary treatment for acute rejection.

A11.4

C

The common causes of hypercalcaemia leading to stone formation are: a) primary hyperparathyroidism; b) vitamin D ingestion; c) sarcoidosis. Of these, primary hyperparathyroidism is the most common cause of stones.

A11.5

D

Haemodialysis is the most efficient way of achieving rapid biochemical improvement, for instance in the treatment of acute renal failure or severe hyperkalaemia. This advantage is offset by disadvantages such as haemodynamic instability, especially in acutely ill patients with multiorgan disease, and over-rapid correction of uraemia can lead to 'dialysis disequilibrium'. This is characterized by nausea and vomiting, restlessness, headache, hypertension, myoclonic jerking, and in severe instances seizures and coma owing to rapid changes in plasma osmolality leading to cerebral oedema.

A11.6

D

Haemofiltration involves removal of plasma water and its dissolved constituents (e.g. K^+, Na^+, urea, phosphate) by convective flow across a high-flux semipermeable membrane, and replacing it with a solution of the desired biochemical composition. Lactate is used as buffer in the replacement solution because rapid infusion of acetate causes vasodilatation and bicarbonate may cause precipitation of calcium carbonate.

A11.7

E

Dialysis amyloidosis is the accumulation of amyloid protein as a result of failure of clearance of β_2-microglobulin. This protein is the light chain of the class I HLA antigens and is normally freely filtered at the glomerulus but is not removed by cellulose-based haemodialysis membranes. Complement activation resulting from the use of cellulose-based membranes may increase the generation rate of the protein. The protein polymerizes to form amyloid deposits, which may cause median nerve compression in the carpal tunnel or a dialysis arthropathy – a clinical syndrome of pain and disabling stiffness in the shoulders, hips, hands, wrists and knees. The extent of amyloid deposition is best assessed by nuclear imaging, either using [^{99m}Tc]DMSA, or, more specifically, by the use of radiolabelled serum amyloid P component.

A11.8

B

Polymorphic probes from the short arm of chromosome 3, the region implicated in renal cell carcinoma, have demonstrated genetic linkage between them and von Hippel–Lindau disease.

A11.9

E

To reduce the risk of worsening renal failure and the risk of morbidity and mortality, the following measures are undertaken. a) Ensure that blood volume is normal, employing measurement of central venous pressure if necessary. b) Ensure an adequate diuresis in the perioperative period, using intravenous fluid infusion as necessary. c) Avoid hypotension, using inotropes if necessary. d) Delay surgery if hyperkalaemia (serum potassium >5.5 mmol/L) or fluid overload is present preoperatively until these have been corrected. e) Monitor urea, electrolyte and creatinine concentrations carefully. Serum potassium should be checked immediately postoperatively (or intraoperatively if surgery is prolonged) and 4–6 hours later, and urea, electrolyte and creatinine concentrations should be checked daily thereafter. If possible weigh the patient daily to monitor fluid balance. f) Prior mannitol infusion may reduce the risk of acute renal tubular necrosis in patients with extrahepatic cholestatic jaundice.

A11.10

C

Currently used Stix tests for blood are very sensitive, being positive if two or more red cells are visible under the high-power field of a light microscope. Indeed, the test is too sensitive, sometimes giving positive results in normal individuals. A further disadvantage is that Stix testing cannot distinguish between blood and free haemoglobin. A positive Stix test must always be followed by microscopy of fresh urine to confirm the presence of red cells and so exclude the relatively rare conditions of haemoglobinuria or myoglobinuria. In females with a positive Stix test result for blood, it is essential to enquire whether the patient is menstruating.

A11.11

D

Routine blood and biochemical investigations may be abnormal; for example, there may be a raised serum urea

Renal disease

or creatinine, hyperkalaemia, anaemia of chronic disease or blood in the urine. Nevertheless, the diagnosis of obstruction cannot be made on these tests alone and further investigations must be performed. Ultrasonography is a reliable means of ruling out upper urinary tract dilatation. Ultrasound cannot distinguish a baggy, low-pressure unobstructed system from a tense, high-pressure obstructed one, so that false-positive scans are seen. However, in the hands of an experienced observer, a normal scan does rule out urinary tract obstruction, except in very rare circumstances such as, for example, encasement of the kidney by fibrous or malignant tissue.

A11.12

C

The term microalbuminuria is an unfortunate one since the albumin referred to is of normal molecular size and weight. Normal individuals excrete less than 30 µg of albumin per minute (43 mg in 24 hours). Dipsticks, however, detect albumin only in a concentration around 100 mg/L (150 mg per 24 hours if urine volume is normal). An increase in albumin excretion between these two levels – so-called microalbuminuria – is now known to be an early indicator of diabetic glomerular disease. It is widely used as a predictor of the development of nephropathy in diabetics and may be extended to other conditions.

A11.13

D

The clinical picture and biopsy are typical of diffuse proliferative glomerulonephritis.

A11.14

1) G   2) H   3) F   4) E   5) D
6) A   7) B

In type 1 mesangiocapillary (membranoproliferative) glomerulonephritis (MCGN) there is mesangial cell proliferation, with mainly subendothelial immune complex deposition and apparent splitting of the capillary basement membrane, giving a 'tram-line' effect. It may be idiopathic or may occur with shunt nephritis. In type 2 MCGN there is mesangial cell proliferation with electron-dense, linear intramembranous deposits that usually stain for C3 only. This type may be idiopathic or may occur after measles. Partial lipodystrophy (loss of subcutaneous fat in various parts of the body) may be seen. Thickening of the capillary basement membrane because of immune complex deposition is the main feature of membranous glomerulonephritis. *Plasmodium malariae* is a common cause in the tropics. In minimal-change glomerular lesion the glomeruli appear normal on light microscopy. The only abnormality seen on electron microscopy is fusion of the foot processes of epithelial cells (podocytes). IgA nephropathy consists of focal proliferative glomerulonephritis with mesangial deposits of IgA. IgA nephropathy tends to occur in children and young males. They present with asymptomatic microscopic haematuria or recurrent macroscopic haematuria sometimes following an upper respiratory or gastrointestinal viral infection. Proteinuria occurs and 5% can be nephrotic. Henoch–Schönlein comprises a characteristic skin rash, abdominal colic, joint pain and glomerulonephritis. Goodpasture's syndrome is mediated by anti-GBM antibody. It presents with recurrent haemoptysis and a severe progressive proliferative, often crescentic, glomerulonephritis.

A11.15

1) A   2) C   3) E   4) D

PR3-ANCA (c-ANCA) positivity is the rule in Wegener's granulomatosis. The urine of pregnant women must always be cultured as 2–6% have asymptomatic bacteriuria. While asymptomatic bacteriuria in the non-pregnant female seldom leads on to acute pyelonephritis and often does not require treatment, acute pyelonephritis frequently occurs in pregnancy under these circumstances. Failure to treat may thus result in severe symptomatic pyelonephritis later in pregnancy, with the possibility of premature labour. Asymptomatic bacteriuria, in the presence of previous renal disease, may predispose to pre-eclamptic toxaemia, anaemia of pregnancy, and small or premature babies. Therefore bacteriuria must always be treated and be shown to be eradicated. Reinfection may require prophylactic therapy.

A11.16

1) C   2) D   3) B   4) A   5) E   6) F

Relapse is diagnosed by recurrence of bacteriuria with the same organism within 7 days of completion of antibacterial treatment and implies failure to eradicate infection. It usually occurs in conditions in which it is difficult to eradicate the bacteria, such as stones, scarred kidneys, polycystic disease or bacterial prostatitis. Reinfection is when bacteriuria is absent after treatment for at least 14 days, usually longer, followed by recurrence of infection with the same or different organisms. This is not due to failure to eradicate infection, but is the result of reinvasion of a susceptible tract with new organisms. Approximately 80% of recurrent infections are due to reinfection. The combination of fever, loin pain and tenderness and significant bacteriuria is usually regarded as indicating bacterial infection of the kidney (acute pyelonephritis). Small renal cortical abscesses and streaks of pus in the renal medulla are often present. Histologically there is focal infiltration by polymorphonuclear leucocytes and many polymorphs in tubular lumina. Reflux nephropathy was called chronic pyelonephritis or atrophic pyelonephritis and it results from a combination of vesicoureteric reflux, and infection acquired in infancy or early childhood. Typically there is papillary damage, interstitial nephritis and cortical scarring in areas adjacent to 'clubbed calyces'. Diagnosis is based on excretion urography, which shows irregular renal outlines, clubbed calyces and a variable reduction in renal size. Acute tubulointerstitial nephritis is most often due to a hypersensitivity reaction to drugs, most commonly drugs of the penicillin family and non-steroidal anti-inflammatory drugs (NSAIDs). Patients present with fever, arthralgia, skin rashes and acute oliguric or non-oliguric renal failure. Many have eosinophilia and eosinophiluria. Renal biopsy shows an intense interstitial cellular infiltrate, often including eosinophils, with variable tubular necrosis. Tuberculosis of the urinary tract should be kept in mind in patients presenting with frequency, dysuria or haematuria, particularly in the Asian immigrant population of the UK. Diagnosis depends on constant awareness, especially in patients with sterile pyuria. Excretion urography may show cavitating lesions in the renal papillary areas, commonly with calcification.

Renal disease

A11.17

1) B   2) C   3) A   4) D

Corticosteroid therapy can lead to weight gain, 'mooning' of the face, skin striae, increased skin fragility with ecchymoses, diabetes, osteoporosis and fractures, particularly of the femoral neck owing to avascular necrosis of bone. Ciclosporin therapy can produce nephrotoxicity, rash, tremor, increased hairiness and diabetes. Tacrolimus therapy can lead to neurotoxicity and nephrotoxicity that appear to be greater than with ciclosporin. The incidence of drug-induced diabetes is much higher than with ciclosporin. Azathioprine therapy can lead to bone marrow depression and hepatotoxicity.

A11.18

A) F   B) T   C) T   D) T   E) F

Factors influencing serum urea levels	
Production	Elimination
Increased by	**Increased by**
High-protein diet	Elevated GFR, e.g. pregnancy
Increased catabolism	
Surgery	**Decreased by**
Infection	Glomerular disease
Trauma	Reduced renal blood flow
Corticosteroid therapy	Hypotension
Tetracyclines	Dehydration
Gastrointestinal bleeding	Urinary obstruction
Cancer	Tubulointerstitial nephritis
Decreased by	
Low-protein diet	
Reduced catabolism, e.g. old age	
Liver failure	

GFR, glomerular filtration rate

A11.19

A) F   B) T   C) T   D) F   E) F

Serum creatinine does not rise above the normal range until there is a reduction of 50–60% in the glomerular filtration rate. Certain drugs – for example cimetidine, trimethoprim, spironolactone and amiloride – reduce tubular secretion of creatinine, leading to a rise in serum creatinine and a fall in measured clearance.

A11.20

A) F   B) F   C) F   D) T   E) T

Two tests of distal tubular function are commonly applied in clinical practice: measurement of urinary concentrating capacity in response to water deprivation, and measurement of urinary acidification. Five tests of proximal tubular function are employed in clinical practice:

- Hypokalaemia in the face of a normal or increased urinary potassium excretion (>40 mmol in 24 hours) is indicative of proximal tubular failure of potassium reabsorption. Other explanations such as treatment with thiazide diuretics or hyperaldosteronism must be ruled out.

- Hypophosphataemia is attributed to a proximal tubular abnormality provided alternative explanations, such as the use of gut phosphorus binders and primary hyperparathyroidism, can be ruled out.

- Glycosuria in the absence of hyperglycaemia.

- Generalized aminoaciduria.

- Proteins derived from tubular cells, such as β_2-microglobulin, are reabsorbed in the proximal nephron. If proteinuria is present, and urine electrophoresis shows the characteristic 'tubular' as distinct from 'glomerular' pattern (i.e. albumin), a proximal tubular defect is demonstrated.

A11.21

A) T   B) F   C) T   D) T   E) F

Discoloration of urine after standing for some time occurs in porphyria, alkaptonuria and in patients ingesting the drug L-dopa.

A11.22

A) F   B) T   C) T   D) T   E) F

Very concentrated urine may also appear dark or smoky. Other causes of discoloration of urine include cholestatic jaundice, haemoglobinuria, drugs such as rifampicin, use of fluorescein or methylthioninium chloride (methylene blue), and ingestion of beetroot.

A11.23

A) F   B) T   C) T   D) F   E) T

The presence of 10 or more white blood cells (WBCs) per cubic millimetre in fresh unspun mid-stream urine samples is abnormal and indicates an inflammatory reaction within the urinary tract. Most commonly it is due to urinary tract infection (UTI), but it may also be found in sterile urine in patients during antibiotic treatment of urinary infection or within 14 days of treatment. The presence of one or more red cells per cubic millimetre in unspun urine samples results in a positive Stix test for blood and is abnormal. Red-cell casts – even one – always indicate renal disease. If red cells degenerate, a rusty coloured 'haemoglobin' granular cast is seen. White cell casts may be seen in acute pyelonephritis. They may be confused with the tubular cell casts that occur in patients with acute tubular necrosis. The demonstration of bacteria on Gram staining of the centrifuged deposit of a clean-catch mid-stream urine sample is highly suggestive of urinary infection and can be of value in the immediate differential diagnosis of UTI. Stix testing for blood or protein is of no value in the diagnosis of UTI, as both are absent from the urine of many patients with bacteriuria.

A11.24

A) T   B) T   C) T   D) T   E) T

Sterile pyuria occurs during antibiotic treatment of urinary infection or within 14 days of treatment, and in patients with stones, tubulointerstitial nephritis, papillary necrosis, tuberculosis, and interstitial cystitis.

Renal disease

A11.25

A) T   B) T   C) T   D) T   E) F

Focal segmental glomerulonephritis occurs as a primary renal disease, and also in systemic lupus erythematosus (SLE), subacute infective endocarditis, with infected atrioventricular shunts (shunt nephritis), and in disorders with IgA deposits (e.g. Henoch–Schönlein purpura and IgA nephropathy). A severe focal necrotizing form is seen in microscopic polyarteritis and Wegener's granulomatosis.

A11.26

A) T   B) F   C) F   D) T   E) T

The infecting organism is a Lancefield group A β-haemolytic streptococcus of a nephritogenic type. If the clinical diagnosis of a nephritic illness is clear-cut (e.g. in post-streptococcal glomerulonephritis), renal imaging and renal biopsy are usually unnecessary. In the majority of patients with glomerulonephritis, neither corticosteroid nor immunosuppressive therapy is of benefit. Spontaneous remissions usually occur in acute glomerulonephritis. Hospital admission is advisable for all children with oliguria and marked hypertension; levels of blood pressure that are of no risk to adults may be associated with hypertensive fits in the young.

A11.27

A) F   B) F   C) T   D) F   E) T

Pregnancy is associated with significant risk to the lupus patient, not only owing to hypertension and premature delivery, but also to more rapid progression of the glomerular lesion following delivery. While corticosteroid therapy improves the extrarenal manifestations of SLE, evidence is lacking that this treatment alters the renal prognosis. Both azathioprine and cyclophosphamide improve renal function, but long-term studies suggest that cyclophosphamide is better. A histological diagnosis should be obtained before commencing such potentially hazardous treatment.

A11.28

A) F   B) F   C) F   D) F   E) T
F) T   G) T   H) T

Tetracycline, trimethoprim, sulphonamides and 4-quinolones must be avoided in pregnancy. Amoxicillin and ampicillin, nitrofurantoin and oral cephalosporins may safely be used in pregnancy.

A11.29

A) F   B) F   C) T   D) T   E) T

AL amyloid (consisting of immunoglobulin light chains) is found in disorders associated with lymphoproliferative diseases such as myeloma, Waldenström's macroglobulinaemia or non-Hodgkin's lymphoma. It is also present in cases of so-called primary amyloidosis where an abnormal clone of cells is presumed to be responsible, although at present not identifiable.

A11.30

A) F   B) F   C) T   D) T   E) T

AA amyloid is found following long-standing inflammatory conditions such as suppurative infections, rheumatoid arthritis and familial Mediterranean fever.

A11.31

A) T   B) F   C) F   D) F   E) T   F) T

The risk and severity of contrast nephropathy is amplified by the presence of hypovolaemia and renal impairment due to diabetic nephropathy. Diabetes *per se* is not a risk factor. Hyperviscosity in patients with myeloma may also be associated with an increased risk of contrast-induced nephropathy. Prevention involves minimization as far as possible of the dose of contrast employed and use of low-osmolality contrast medium. The only proven preventative measure is prevention of hypovolaemia before administration of contrast. Recent evidence that oral acetylcysteine may be of benefit in preventing worsening of pre-existing renal impairment following intravenous contrast requires confirmation.

A11.32

A) T   B) T   C) T   D) T   E) T

In myeloma, free κ and λ light chains are excreted. Blockage of tubules by casts composed in part at least of light chains, and their toxic effects upon tubular cells, account for the proteinuria and chronic renal impairment associated with 'myeloma kidney'. Renal amyloid deposition often complicates myeloma, accounting both for proteinuria – sometimes of nephrotic proportions – and chronic renal failure. Hypercalcaemia, renal sepsis and (rarely) urinary tract obstruction due to bulky myeloma deposits are further causes of renal impairment in myelomatosis.

A11.33

A) T   B) T   C) T   D) T   E) T   F) T

All varieties of histological abnormality are seen in systemic lupus erythematosus, ranging from a minimal-change lesion to crescentic glomerulonephritis. The World Health Organization classification of histological types is:

- Type I – Normal on light microscopy
- Type II – Mesangial change, whether seen on light microscopy or detectable only by immunological staining and/or electron microscopy
- Type III – Focal proliferative
- Type IV – Diffuse proliferative
- Type V – Membranous

Serial renal biopsies show that in approximately 25% of patients, histological appearances alter from one histological classification to another during the interbiopsy interval. The prognosis is better in patients with Types I and V.

A11.34

A) T   B) T   C) T   D) T   E) T   F) T

Causes of hypoalbuminaemia
Inadequate protein intake: protein–energy malnutrition
Failure of protein production: liver disease
Excessive protein loss: nephrotic syndrome, protein-losing enteropathy, extensive burns
Pregnancy

A11.35

A) F   B) F   C) F   D) F   E) T

Transcutaneous renal biopsy is performed to make a histological diagnosis when management will be affected, particularly when the major question is whether a steroid-sensitive minimal-change lesion is present or not. It is not indicated in three groups of patients: a) in young children (particularly males) who have a highly selective protein leak, no hypertension and no red cells or red-cell casts in the urine (the diagnosis is almost certain to be a minimal-change lesion, so a trial of steroids should be instituted first); b) in long-standing, insulin-dependent diabetes with associated retinopathy or neuropathy, since the diagnosis is in little doubt; c) in patients on drugs such as penicillamine, which should be stopped first.

A11.36

A) F   B) F   C) T   D) F   E) T

In nephrotic syndrome hypovolaemia and a hypercoagulable state predispose to venous thrombosis. Prolonged bed rest should therefore be avoided. Sepsis is an important cause of death in nephrotic patients. Pneumococcal infections are particularly common and pneumococcal vaccine should be given. A low blood volume and hypotension may lead to underperfused kidneys. Albumin infusion combined with mannitol or another diuretic may initiate a diuresis in oliguric renal failure. Treatment of hypercholesterolaemia is best achieved with an HMG-CoA reductase inhibitor. Renal vein thrombosis can cause nephrotic syndrome and is also a complication of this condition!

A11.37

A) T   B) F   C) F   D) F   E) F   F) T

In the nephrotic syndrome, initial treatment should be with dietary sodium restriction and a thiazide diuretic (e.g. bendroflumethazide (bendrofluazide)). A

high-protein diet (approximately 80–90 g protein daily) confers no benefit and normal protein intake is advisable. High-dose corticosteroid therapy with prednisolone 60 mg daily (dose corrected to a normal body surface area of 1.73 m^2) for 8 weeks corrects the urinary protein leak in more than 95% of children. Spontaneous remission also occurs and steroid therapy should, in general, be withheld if urinary protein loss is insufficient to cause hypoalbuminaemia or oedema. In both children and adults, if remission lasts for 4 years after steroid therapy, further relapse is very rare. In children, approximately one-third do not subsequently relapse, but in the remainder further courses of corticosteroids are indicated. No more than two courses of cyclophosphamide should be prescribed in children because of the risk of side-effects, which include azoospermia. An alternative to cyclophosphamide is ciclosporin, which is effective but must be continued long term to prevent relapse on stopping treatment.

A11.38

A) T   B) T   C) T   D) T   E) T

Criteria for diagnosis of bacteriuria

Symptomatic young women
$\geq 10^2$ coliform organisms/mL urine plus pyuria
(> 10 WCC/m^3)
OR
$\geq 10^5$ any pathogenic organism/mL urine
OR
any growth of pathogenic organism in urine by suprapubic aspiration

Symptomatic men
$\geq 10^3$ pathogenic organisms/mL urine

Asymptomatic patients
$\geq 10^5$ pathogenic organisms/mL of urine on two occasions

A11.39

A) F   B) T   C) T   D) T   E) T

In benign essential hypertension, arteriosclerosis of major renal arteries and changes in the intrarenal vasculature (nephrosclerosis) occur as follows. a) In small vessels and arterioles, intimal thickening with reduplication of the internal elastic lamina occurs and the vessel wall becomes hyalinized. b) In large vessels, concentric reduplication of the internal elastic lamina and endothelial proliferation produce an 'onion skin' appearance. c) Reduction in size of both kidneys may occur; this may be asymmetrical if one major renal artery is more affected than the other. d) The proportion of sclerotic glomeruli is increased compared with age-matched controls.

A11.40

A) F   B) F   C) T   D) T   E) T

Pure uric acid stones are radiolucent. Mixed infective stones in which organic matrix predominates are barely radiopaque. Calcium-containing and cystine stones are radiopaque. Calculi overlying bone are easily missed. Staghorn calculi may be missed if the plain abdominal X-ray carried out before contrast injection during urography is not inspected. Uric acid stones may present as a filling defect after injection of contrast medium. Such stones are readily seen on CT scanning.

A11.41

A) T   B) T   C) F   D) T   E) T

Common causes of mild hyperoxaluria are: a) excess ingestion of foodstuffs high in oxalate, such as spinach, rhubarb and tea; b) dietary calcium restriction, with compensatory increased absorption of oxalate; c) gastrointestinal disease (e.g. Crohn's), usually with an intestinal resection, associated with increased absorption of oxalate from the colon.

A11.42

A) F   B) T   C) F   D) T   E) F

Tetracyclines, with the exception of doxycycline, have a catabolic effect and as a result the concentration of nitrogenous waste products is increased. They may also cause impairment of glomerular filtration rate by a direct effect. Corticosteroids have a catabolic effect and so also increase the production of nitrogenous wastes. A patient with moderate impairment of renal function may therefore become severely uraemic if given tetracyclines or corticosteroid therapy.

A11.43

A) T   B) T   C) T   D) T   E) T
F) T   G) T   H) T   I) T   J) T

Factors postulated to be involved in the development of acute tubular necrosis include: a) entry of calcium into cells with an increase in cytosolic cell calcium concentration; b) induction by hypoxia of nitric oxide synthases with increased production of nitric oxide; c) increased production of intracellular proteases such as calpain (fairly strong evidence exists that this mechanism operates in ciclosporin-induced nephrotoxicity); d) activation of phospholipase A_2 with increased production of free fatty acids and consequent damage to cell membranes; e) cell injury resulting from reperfusion with blood after initial ischaemia; f) vasoconstriction; g) liberation of toxic endothelial factors; h) damage from the vasodilator effects of endotoxins; i) reduced prostaglandin production; (j) tubular obstruction by desquamated cells and casts.

A11.44

A) T   B) T   C) T   D) F   E) T

The main indications for blood purification and/or excess fluid removal are: a) symptoms of uraemia; b) complications of uraemia, such as pericarditis; c) severe biochemical derangement in the absence of symptoms (especially if a rising trend is observed in an oliguric patient and in hypercatabolic patients); d) hyperkalaemia not controlled by conservative measures; e) pulmonary oedema; f) severe metabolic acidosis; h) and for removal of drugs causing the acute renal failure, e.g. gentamicin, lithium, severe aspirin overdose.

A11.45

A) T   B) T   C) T   D) T   E) T   F) T

Pruritus (itching) is common in severe renal failure and is usually attributed in the main to retention of nitrogenous waste products of protein catabolism. Certainly, marked improvement often follows the institution of dialysis. Other causes of pruritus include: hypercalcaemia, hyperphosphataemia, elevated calcium × phosphate product, hyperparathyroidism (even if calcium and phosphate levels are normal) and iron deficiency. In dialysis patients, inadequate dialysis is a cause of pruritus. Nevertheless, a significant number of dialysis patients who are well dialysed and in whom other causes of pruritus can be excluded suffer persistent itching. The cause is unknown and no effective treatment exists.

A11.46

A) T   B) T   C) T   D) T   E) T   F) T

Anaemia is present in the great majority of patients with chronic renal failure. Several factors have been implicated: erythropoietin deficiency (the most important), bone marrow toxins retained in renal failure, bone marrow fibrosis secondary to hyperparathyroidism, haematinic deficiency – iron, vitamin B_{12}, folate, increased red cell destruction, abnormal red cell membranes causing increased osmotic fragility, increased blood loss – occult gastrointestinal bleeding, blood sampling, blood loss during haemodialysis or because of platelet dysfunction and ACE inhibitors (may cause anaemia in chronic renal failure, probably by interfering with the control of endogenous erythropoietin release).

A11.47

A) T   B) T   C) T   D) T   E) T

Gastrointestinal complications of chronic renal failure include decreased gastric emptying and increased risk of reflux oesophagitis, increased risk of peptic ulceration, increased risk of acute pancreatitis and constipation – particularly in patients on continuous ambulatory peritoneal dialysis (CAPD). However, elevations of serum amylase of up to three times normal may be found in chronic renal failure without any evidence of pancreatic disease, owing to retention of high-molecular-weight forms of amylase normally excreted in the urine.

A11.48

A) T   B) T   C) T   D) T   E) T

Life expectancy remains severely reduced compared with the normal population owing to a greatly increased (16-fold) incidence of cardiovascular disease, particularly myocardial infarction, cardiac failure, sudden cardiac death and stroke. Coronary artery calcification is more common in patients with end-stage renal failure than in normal individuals and it is highly likely that this contributes significantly to cardiovascular mortality.

A11.49

A) T   B) T   C) T   D) T

Failure to respond to 300 U/kg weekly, or a fall in haemoglobin after a satisfactory response, may be due to iron deficiency, bleeding, malignancy or infection. The demand for iron by the bone marrow is enormous when erythropoietin is commenced. Recently available intravenous (rather than oral) iron supplements optimize response to treatment.

A11.50

A) F   B) T   C) T   D) T   E) T

Partial correction of anaemia with erythropoietin improves quality of life, exercise tolerance, sexual function and cognitive function in dialysis patients, and leads to regression of left ventricular hypertrophy. The disadvantages of erythropoietin therapy are that it is expensive and causes a rise in blood pressure in up to 30% of patients, particularly in the first 6 months. Peripheral resistance rises in all patients, owing to loss of hypoxic vasodilatation and to increased blood viscosity. A rare complication is encephalopathy with fits, transient cortical blindness and hypertension.

A11.51

A) F   B) T   C) T   D) T   E) T

The action of some anaesthetic agents such as muscle relaxants and opiates are prolonged in renal impairment. Appropriate precautions should be taken. Anaesthetic agents that are safe in renal failure and can be used without alteration in dosage include fentanyl, atropine, diazepam, halothane and nitrous oxide.

A11.52

A) T   B) T   C) T   D) T   E) F

Recurrence of the disease which caused renal failure, although uncommon, may occur in specific diseases. Examples are primary oxalosis, mesangiocapillary glomerulonephritis, focal segmental glomerulosclerosis, and Goodpasture's syndrome.

A11.53

A) T   B) T   C) T   D) T   E) T

Hypertension is an early and very common feature of autosomal-dominant polycystic kidney disease (ADPKD). Approximately 30% of patients have hepatic cysts and in a minority of patients massive enlargement of the polycystic liver is seen. About 8% of ADPKD patients have an asymptomatic intracranial aneurysm and the prevalence is twice as high in the subgroup of patients with a family history of such aneurysms or of subarachnoid haemorrhage. Such haemorrhage is preceded in from 20–40% of cases by premonitory headaches from a few hours

Renal disease

up to 2 weeks before the onset of subarachnoid bleeding. Mitral valve prolapse is found in 20% of individuals with ADPKD, whereas it is present in only 2–3% of the general population. Renal calculi are diagnosed in about 10–20% of patients with ADPKD.

A11.54

A) F   B) T   C) T   D) T   E) T

If metastases are present, nephrectomy may still be warranted since regression of metastases has been reported after removal of the main tumour mass. Severe flank pain may also demand nephrectomy despite the presence of metastases. Radiotherapy has no proven value. Medroxyprogesterone acetate is of some value in controlling metastatic disease. Treatment with interleukin-2 and α-interferon produces a remission in about 20% of cases.

A11.55

A) F   B) T   C) T   D) T   E) T

Predisposing factors to urothelial tumours include: a) cigarette smoking; b) exposure to industrial carcinogens such as β-naphthylamine and benzidene (workers in the chemical, cable and rubber industries are at particular risk); c) exposure to drugs (e.g. phenacetin, cyclophosphamide); d) chronic inflammation (e.g. schistosomiasis, usually associated with squamous carcinoma).

A11.56

A) F   B) F   C) T   D) T   E) T

Investigations in suspected benign enlargement of the prostate gland include urine culture, assessment of renal function by measuring serum urea and creatinine concentrations, measurement of prostate-specific antigen (markedly raised in prostatic cancer), a plain abdominal X-ray, and renal ultrasonography to define whether upper tract dilatation is present. Excretion urography is not usually necessary. Cystourethroscopy is only essential in patients with haematuria.

A11.57

A) T   B) T   C) T   D) F   E) F

Microscopic, impalpable tumour can sometimes be managed expectantly. Treatment for disease confined to the gland is radical prostatectomy (provided the patient is fit for the procedure) or radiotherapy. Evidence is accumulating that radical prostatectomy is the treatment of choice in younger patients with poorly differentiated tumours. There have, however, been no controlled trials of this therapy and survival may be good without therapy. Locally extensive disease is managed with radiotherapy with or without androgen ablation therapy. Metastatic disease can be treated with orchidectomy, but many men refuse. Luteinizing hormone-releasing hormone (LHRH) analogues such as buserelin or goserelin are equally effective and preferred by many. Non-hormonal chemotherapy is unhelpful.

Water, electrolytes and acid–base balance

12

Q 12.1

In a 70 kg man plasma fluid constitutes

A. Almost all the extracellular volume
B. About two-thirds of the extracellular volume
C. About half the extracellular volume
D. About a third of the extracellular volume
E. A minimal amount of the extracellular volume

Q 12.2

A 45-year-old patient with cirrhosis has ascites. Which of the following mechanisms is the most likely explanation for persistent aldosterone-mediated sodium retention, absence of escape phenomenon and resistance to natriuretic peptides in such patients

A. Increased sodium delivery to the proximal tubule
B. Decreased sodium delivery to the proximal tubule
C. Decreased sodium delivery to the collecting duct
D. Increased sodium delivery to the collecting duct
E. Decreased sodium delivery to the loop of Henle

Q 12.3

Before she starts exercising, an athlete's plasma osmolality is 275 mOsm/kg. She starts sweating profusely on exertion. Which one of the following is most likely to occur as she continues to exercise in the heat

A. Plasma osmolality is going to decrease to 260 mOsm/kg
B. Plasma osmolality is going to remain the same
C. Plasma osmolality is going to decrease to 250 mOsm/kg
D. Plasma osmolality is going to increase to 280 mOsm/kg
E. Plasma osmolality is going to initially decrease and then increase

Q 12.4

The plasma osmolality of a 22-year-old healthy waiter is 275 mOsm/kg. He now eats salted crisps and peanuts without drinking water. Which of the following is most likely to occur?

A. Plasma osmolality is going to decrease to 260 mOsm/kg
B. Plasma osmolality is going to remain the same
C. Plasma osmolality is going to decrease to 250 mOsm/kg
D. Plasma osmolality is going to increase to 280 mOsm/kg
E. Plasma osmolality is going to initially decrease and then increase

Water, electrolytes and acid–base balance

Q12.5

Normal saline is administered to a healthy adult. Which of the following is most likely to occur?

A. Plasma osmolality is going to decrease to 260 mOsm/kg
B. Plasma osmolality is going to remain the same
C. Plasma osmolality is going to decrease to 250 mOsm/kg
D. Plasma osmolality is going to increase to 280 mOsm/kg
E. Plasma osmolality is going to initially decrease and then increase

Q12.6

A 43-year-old woman with idiopathic dilated cardiomyopathy presents with shortness of breath and pink frothy sputum. The emergency department doctor administers intravenous furosemide (frusemide) and she feels better within minutes. The most likely mechanism of action by which her symptoms improved is

A. Arterial dilatation
B. Reduction of Na^+ reabsorption (in exchange for K^+) in collecting duct
C. Venous dilatation
D. Reduction of Na^+ HCO_3^- reabsorption in the proximal tubule
E. Reduction of Na^+ Cl^- cotransport in the early distal tubule

Q12.7

Renal reabsorption of magnesium mainly occurs in

A. Proximal tubule
B. Thick ascending loop of Henle
C. Glomerulus
D. Collecting duct
E. Descending loop of Henle

Q12.8

A 55-year-old patient on a loop diuretic for congestive heart failure presents with confusion, irritability and tremor. On examination he has carpopedal spasms and hyperreflexia. ECG shows prolonged QT interval and broad flattened T waves. The most likely cause for this clinical picture is

A. Hypermanganesaemia
B. Hyperkalaemia
C. Hypernatraemia
D. Hyponatraemia
E. Hypomagnesaemia

Q12.9

An alcoholic patient presents with confusion and hallucinations. He is intubated because of respiratory distress. Attempts to wean him off the respirator are unsuccessful. A pulmonologist confirms that he has diaphragmatic weakness. In addition he has rhabdomyolysis and mild haemolysis. The most likely cause for this clinical picture is

A. Hyperphosphataemia
B. Left phrenic nerve palsy
C. Right phrenic nerve palsy
D. Hypophosphataemia
E. Hypernatraemia

Q12.10

A 29-year-old man following a cardiac arrest has a bicarbonate of 15 mmol/L. In this patient the most important buffer system is

A. Potassium
B. Sodium
C. Ammonia
D. Phosphoric acid
E. Alpha-ketoglutaric acid

Q12.11

1. Administration of 1 L of 5% dextrose
2. Administration of 1 L of normal saline
3. Administration of 1 L of a colloid solution

Select the best match for each of the above

A. Remains in the extracellular compartment
B. Stays in the intravascular compartment
C. Distributed equally in the intravascular, extracellular and cellular compartment

Q12.12

1. Proximal tubule
2. Loop of Henle
3. Distal tubule
4. Collecting tubule

Select the best option for major mechanism of luminal sodium entry

A. Na–Cl cotransport
B. Na–K–2Cl cotransport
C. Na channels
D. Na–H exchange and cotransport of Na with glucose, phosphate and other organic solutes

Q12.13

1. Furosemide (frusemide)
2. Metolazone
3. Spironolactone
4. Acetazolamide
5. Mannitol
6. Amiloride

Select the best match for each of the above

A. Decreases Na^+ Cl^- cotransport in the early distal tubule
B. Acts on loop of Henle to promote osmotic diuresis

C. Decreases Na^+ Cl–K^+ cotransport in the thick ascending limb of Henle
D. Decreases Na^+ reabsorption (in exchange for K^+) in collecting duct
E. Decreases Na^+ HCO_3^- reabsorption in the proximal tubule
F. Blocks sodium epithelial channels and reduces lumen negative transepithelial voltage in the collecting duct

Q12.14

1. 43-year-old man who presents with serum calcium level of 3.2 mmol/L (12 mg/dL)
2. A 45-year-old man with oliguria, ascites and decompensated congestive heart failure with serum creatinine of 200 μmol/L (2.3 mg/dL)
3. A 52-year-old woman with hypercalciuria
4. A 79-year-old woman with mild hypertension
5. A 23-year-old nurse who wishes to avoid mountain sickness while climbing in the Himalayas
6. A 49-year-old alcoholic who presents with ascites due to cirrhosis
7. A 33-year-old who develops cerebral oedema following a motor cycle accident
8. A 58-year-old with glaucoma

Select the best option for each of the above

A. Spironolactone
B. Acetazolamide
C. Bendroflumethiazide (bendrofluazide)
D. Furosemide (frusemide)
E. Mannitol
F. Amiloride

Water, electrolytes and acid–base balance

Q 12.15

1. A 32-year-old woman with severe diarrhoea has a heart rate of 112, blood pressure of 100/70 mmHg on lying down and there is a 20 mmHg fall in systolic blood pressure when she is upright

2. A 65-year-old woman is recovering from a stroke and is unable to eat. On examination her blood pressure is 120/80 mmHg, and her heart rate is 70 beats/minute. She has no signs of dehydration or fluid overload. Her sodium is 146 mmol/L, K 4 mmol/L and chloride 100 mmol/L. Urea and serum creatinine are normal. The neurologist wishes to maintain fluid balance

3. A 97-year-old woman is confused. Her sodium is 150 mmol/L, K 3.5 mEq/L, chloride 100 mmol/L. Urea and serum creatinine are normal

4. A 52-year-old woman has ingested an overdose of aspirin. Blood gases reveal pH 7.4, P_aO_2 11 kPa, P_{CO_2} 5 kPa, chloride 100 mmol/L and bicarbonate is normal

Select the best option for each of the above

A. Sodium bicarbonate 1.26%
B. Glucose 5% + potassium chloride 0.3%
C. Sodium chloride 0.18% + glucose 4%
D. Sodium chloride 0.9%

Q 12.16

1. A 23-year-old man has normal blood pressure. Serum sodium is 140 mmol/L, potassium is 2.8 mmol/L, bicarbonate is 40 mmol/L, pH is 7.45 and he has hypercalciuria. Plasma renin and aldosterone are elevated

2. A 16-year-old boy complains of fatigue. Blood pressure is normal, serum sodium is 140 mmol/L, potassium is 2.8 mmol/L, bicarbonate is 40 mmol/L, there is hypomagnesaemia, pH is 7.45, and he has hypocalciuria. Plasma renin and aldosterone are elevated

3. An 18-year-old boy has hypertension. Serum sodium is 140 mmol/L, potassium is 2.8 mmol/L, bicarbonate is 40 mmol/L, there is hypomagnesaemia, pH is 7.45. Plasma renin and aldosterone are low

4. A 23-year-old Chinese woman presents with weakness precipitated whenever she has sugary drinks

5. A 28-year-old patient presents with hypertension. On examination there is peripheral oedema. Serum sodium is 140 mmol/L, potassium is 6.8 mmol/L, bicarbonate is 20 mmol/L, pH is 7.30. Plasma renin and aldosterone are low

Select the best match for each of the above

A. Liddle's syndrome
B. Gordon's syndrome
C. Bartter's syndrome
D. Gitelman's syndrome
E. Hyperkalaemic periodic paralysis
F. Hypokalaemic periodic paralysis

Q 12.17

A 75-year-old man with congestive heart failure and osteoarthrosis presents with fatigue. He is currently on furosemide (frusemide), digoxin, lisinopril, NSAIDs, and spironolactone. Serum Na 140 mmol/L, K$^+$ 7.1 mmol/L, chloride 100, bicarbonate 25 mmol/L. Serum digoxin level is normal. The following medications could have contributed to this clinical picture

A. Digoxin
B. Furosemide (frusemide)
C. NSAIDs
D. Lisinopril
E. Spironolactone

Q12.18

A 75-year-old man with congestive heart failure and osteoarthrosis presents with fatigue. He is currently on furosemide (frusemide), digoxin, lisinopril, NSAIDs, and spironolactone. Serum Na 140 mmol/L, K^+ 7.1 mmol/L, chloride 100, bicarbonate 15 mmol/L. Serum digoxin level is normal. ECG shows tented T waves. Treatment includes

A. Intravenous metoprolol
B. Intravenous calcium gluconate
C. Insulin–dextrose infusions
D. Polystyrene sulphonate resin
E. Intravenous sodium bicarbonate

Q12.19

A 45-year-old patient with chronic renal failure has elevated phosphate levels. This can result in

A. Itching
B. Hyperthyroidism
C. Hyperparathyroidism
D. Periarticular calcification
E. Vascular calcification

Q12.20

The proximal renal tubule

A. Reabsorbs bicarbonate, which is catalysed by the sodium–potassium ATPase pump
B. Contributes significantly to the elimination of hydrogen ions from the body

C. Has the principal cell with an aldosterone-sensitive sodium absorption site
D. Has the alpha-intercalated cell that possesses the proton pump for the active secretion of hydrogen ions in exchange for reabsorption of potassium ions
E. Has a greater quantity of luminal carbonic anhydrase than the distal nephron

Q12.21

A 28-year-old woman has pH 7.2, P_aco_2 is decreased and HCO_3 is 15 mmol/L. Sodium is 138 mEq/L, K is 4 mEq/L, chloride is 110 mmol/L. Conditions which can cause this clinical picture include

A. Diarrhoea
B. Acetazolamide
C. Respiratory acidosis
D. Distal renal tubular acidosis
E. Ammonium chloride ingestion

Q12.22

A 25-year-old man presents with weakness and lassitude. pH is 7.2, plasma bicarbonate 18 mmol/L, Na 144, K 3.5, chloride 100. Conditions which can result in this clinical picture include

A. Diabetes
B. Sepsis
C. Metformin accumulation
D. Uraemia
E. Salicylate overdose

Q12.23

A 43-year-old woman has pH 7.5, chloride 90 mmol/L, and bicarbonate is 38 mmol/L. Likely causes include

Water, electrolytes and acid–base balance

A. Bulimia
B. Metolazone
C. Villous adenoma
D. Cystic fibrosis
E. Metformin overdose

Q12.24

A 43-year-old woman has pH 7.5, chloride 110 mmol/L, potassium 3.2 mmol/L and bicarbonate is 38 mmol/L. Likely causes include

A. Liquorice
B. Laxative abuse
C. Bartter's syndrome
D. Conn's syndrome
E. Ethylene glycol poisoning

Q12.25

In a patient with cirrhosis, sodium and water retention occurs despite increased extracellular volume. Arterial underfilling seen in this condition promotes sodium and water retention by

A. Increased secretion of corticosteroids
B. Activation of sympathetic nervous system
C. Activation of the renin–angiotensin–aldosterone system
D. Nonosmotic release of antidiuretic hormone
E. Increased secretion of follicle-stimulating hormone/luteinizing hormone

Q12.26

A 55-year-old woman develops confusion following initiation of an antipsychotic medication. Her physician correctly diagnoses SIADH (syndrome of inappropriate secretion of antidiuretic hormone). The following are true about SIADH

A. Impaired water excretion
B. Hypernatraemia
C. Release of aldosterone is impaired
D. Release of ANP is impaired
E. Sodium handling is intact

Q12.27

A 68-year-old woman presents with confusion, drowsiness and clonic jerks. On examination she has no signs of increased extracellular volume. Her sodium is 120 mmol/L, K 4.5 mol/L and chloride and bicarbonate are normal. The following can explain her clinical picture

A. Addison's disease
B. Hypothyroidism
C. Hyperosmolar diabetic coma
D. Diabetes insipidus
E. Administration of hypertonic sodium solutions

A 12.1

D

In a 70 kg man, plasma fluid constitutes one-third of extracellular volume (4.6 L), of which 85% (3.9 L) lies in the venous side and only 15% (0.7 L) resides in the arterial circulation.

A 12.2

C

In patients with oedematous conditions such as cardiac failure, hepatic cirrhosis and hypoalbuminaemia escape from the sodium-retaining actions of aldosterone does not occur and therefore they continue to retain sodium in response to aldosterone. Accordingly they have substantial natriuresis when given spironolactone, which blocks mineralocorticoid receptors. Alpha-adrenergic stimulation and elevated angiotensin II increase sodium transport in the proximal tubule, and reduced renal hypoperfusion and glomerular filtration rate further increase sodium absorption from the proximal tubules by presenting less sodium and water in the tubular fluid. Sodium delivery to the distal portion of the nephron, and thus the collecting duct, is reduced. Similarly, increased cardiac atrial natriuretic peptide release in these conditions requires optimum sodium concentration at the site of its action in the collecting duct for its desired natriuretic effects. Decreased sodium delivery to the collecting duct is therefore the most likely explanation for the persistent aldosterone-mediated sodium retention, absence of escape phenomenon and resistance to natriuretic peptides in these patients.

A 12.3

D

Water loss resulting from sweating is followed by, in sequence, a rise in both plasma osmolality and antidiuretic hormone (ADH) secretion, enhanced water reabsorption, and the appropriate excretion of a small volume of concentrated urine.

A 12.4

D

If a person with normal renal function eats salted snacks without drinking any water, the excess Na^+ will increase the plasma osmolality, leading to osmotic water movement out of the cells and increased extracellular volume. The rise in osmolality will stimulate both antidiuretic hormone (ADH) release and thirst (the main reason why many restaurants and bars supply free salted foods), whereas the hypervolaemia will enhance the secretion of atrial natriuretic peptide and suppress that of aldosterone. The net effect is increased excretion of Na^+ without water.

A 12.5

B

The administration of isotonic saline causes an increase in volume but no change in plasma osmolality. In this setting, atrial natriuretic peptide (ANP) secretion is increased, aldosterone secretion is reduced, and antidiuretic hormone (ADH) secretion does not change. The net effect is the appropriate excretion of the excess Na^+ in a relatively iso-osmotic urine.

Water, electrolytes and acid–base balance

A12.6

C

In acute pulmonary oedema due to congestive heart failure intravenous furosemide (frusemide) initially acts by increasing venous capacitance and thereby decreasing preload. It also acts by reducing Na^+ Cl^- K^+ cotransport in the thick ascending limb of Henle.

A12.7

B

Magnesium transport differs from that of most other ions in that the proximal tubule is not the major site of reabsorption. Only 15–25% of the filtered magnesium is reabsorbed passively in the proximal tubule and 5–10% in the distal tubule. The major site of magnesium transport is the thick ascending limb of the loop of Henle, where 60–70% of the filtered load is reabsorbed.

A12.8

E

Symptoms and signs of hypomagnesaemia include irritability, tremor, ataxia, carpopedal spasm, hyperreflexia, confusional and hallucinatory states and epileptiform convulsions. An ECG may show a prolonged QT interval, broad flattened T waves, and occasional shortening of the ST segment.

A12.9

D

Significant hypophosphataemia (<0.4 mmol/L) may occur in a number of clinical situations, owing to redistribution into cells, to renal losses, or to decreased intake (alcoholics). It may cause: a) muscle weakness – diaphragmatic weakness, decreased cardiac contractility, skeletal muscle rhabdomyolysis; b) a left-shift in the oxyhaemoglobin dissociation curve (reduced 2,3-diphosphoglycerate (2,3-DPG)) and rarely haemolysis; c) confusion, hallucinations and convulsions.

A12.10

C

In the setting of metabolic acidosis, titratable acids cannot increase significantly because availability of the titratable acid is fixed by the plasma concentration of the buffer and by the glomerular filtration rate. The ammonia buffer system, in contrast, can increase several hundred-fold when necessary. Consequently, impaired renal excretion of hydrogen ions is always associated with a defect in ammonium excretion.

A12.11

1) C 2) A 3) B

1 L of water given intravenously as 5% dextrose is distributed equally into all compartments, whereas the same amount of 0.9% saline remains in the extracellular compartment. The latter is thus the correct treatment for extracellular water depletion – sodium keeping the water in this compartment. The addition of 1 L of colloid with its high oncotic pressure stays in the vascular compartment and is the treatment for hypovolaemia.

A 12.12

1) D   2) B   3) A   4) C

Mechanisms of sodium transport in the various nephron segments	
Tubule segment	Major mechanism of luminal Na$^+$ entry
Proximal tubule	Na$^+$–H$^+$ exchange and cotransport of Na+ with glucose, phosphate and other organic solutes
Loop of Henle	Na$^+$–K$^+$–2Cl$^-$ cotransport
Distal tubule	Na$^+$–Cl$^-$ cotransport
Collecting tubules	Na+ channels

A 12.13

1) C   2) A   3) D   4) E   5) B   6) F

Types of diuretics	
Major action	Examples
↓ Na$^+$ Cl$^-$ K$^+$ cotransport in thick ascending limb	Furosemide (frusemide) Bumetanide Torasemide
↓ Na$^+$ Cl$^-$ cotransport in early distal tubule	Bendroflumethiazide (bendrofluazide) Chlorthalidone Metolazone Indapamide
↓ Na$^+$ reabsorption (in exchange for K$^+$) in collecting duct	Aldosterone antagonist, e.g. oral spironolactone or i.v. potassium canrenoate Others: Amiloride Triamterene
↓ Na$^+$ HCO$_3^-$ reabsorption in proximal tubule ↓ Aqueous humour formation	Acetazolamide

A12.14

1) D   2) D   3) C   4) C   5) B
6) A   7) E   8) B

Clinical uses of diuretics

Examples	Clinical uses
Furosemide (frusemide) Bumetanide Torasemide	Volume overload (CCF, nephrotic syndrome, CRF) Sodium-dependent hypertension Hypercalcaemia ?Acute renal failure SIADH
Bendroflumethiazide (bendrofluazide) Chlorthalidone Metolazone Indapamide	Hypertension Volume overload (CCF) Hypercalciuria

Aldosterone antagonist e.g. oral
spironolactone or i.v. potassium canrenoate
Others:
  Amiloride
  Triamterene
	Hyperaldosteronism (primary and secondary)
	Bartter's syndrome
	Prevention of K^+ deficiency in combination with loop
	or thiazide
	Heart failure
	Cirrhosis with fluid overload

Acetazolamide	Metabolic alkalosis Glaucoma

CCF, congestive cardiac failure; CRF, chronic renal failure; SIADH, syndrome of inappropriate antidiuretic hormone secretion

A12.15

1) D   2) C   3) B   4) A

Intravenous fluids in general use for fluid and electrolyte disturbances

	Indication (see footnote)
Normal plasma values	
Sodium chloride 0.9%	1
Sodium chloride 0.18% + glucose 4%	2
Glucose 5% + potassium chloride 0.3%	3
Sodium bicarbonate 1.26%	4

1. Volume expansion in hypovolaemic patients. Rarely to maintain fluid balance when there are large losses of sodium. The sodium (150 mmol/L) is greater than plasma and hypernatraemia can result. It is often necessary to add KCl 20–40 mmol/L.
2. Maintenance of fluid balance in normovolaemic, normonatraemic patients.
3. To replace water. Can be given with or without potassium chloride. May be alternated with normal saline as an alternative to (2).
4. For volume expansion in hypovolaemic, acidotic patients alternating with (1). Occasionally for maintenance of fluid balance combined with (2) in salt-wasting, acidotic patients. To induce forced alkaline diuresis, e.g. in severe salicylate poisoning.

A12.16

1) C 2) D 3) A 4) F 5) B

Bartter's syndrome consists of metabolic hypokalaemia, alkalosis, hypercalciuria, normal blood pressure, and elevated plasma renin and aldosterone. The primary defect in this disorder appears to be an impairment in sodium and chloride reabsorption in the thick ascending limb. Gitelman's syndrome is a phenotype variant of Bartter's syndrome characterized by hypokalaemia, metabolic alkalosis, hypocalciuria, hypomagnesaemia, normal blood pressure, and elevated plasma renin and aldosterone. There are striking similarities between the Gitelman syndrome and the biochemical abnormalities induced by chronic thiazide diuretic administration. Liddle's syndrome is characterized by potassium wasting, hypokalaemia, and alkalosis, but is associated with low renin and aldosterone production, and high blood pressure. Hypokalaemic periodic paralysis may be precipitated by carbohydrate intake, suggesting that insulin-mediated potassium influx into cells may be responsible. This syndrome also occurs in association with hyperthyroidism in Chinese patients. Gordon's syndrome appears to be a mirror image of Bartter's syndrome, in which primary renal retention of sodium causes hypertension, volume expansion, low renin/aldosterone, hyperkalaemia and metabolic acidosis.

A12.17

A) F B) F C) T D) T E) T

Digoxin results in hyperkalaemia only at toxic doses. Furosemide (frusemide) causes hypokalaemia. NSAIDs, ACE inhibitors and spironolactone all cause hyperkalaemia and should be temporarily discontinued.

A12.18

A) F B) T C) T D) T E) T

Correction of hyperkalaemia

IMMEDIATE
Protect myocardium
10 mL of 10% calcium gluconate given in the presence of ECG change
Effect is temporary but dose can be repeated

Drive K^+ into cells
Insulin 10 units + 50 mL of 50% glucose followed by regular checks of blood glucose and plasma K^+
Repeat as necessary

and/or correction of severe acidosis (pH < 6.9) – $NaHCO_3$ (1.26%)

and/or salbumatol 0.5 mg in 100 mL of 5% glucose over 15 min (rarely used)

LATER
Deplete body K^+ (to decrease plasma K^+ over next 24 h)
Polystryrene sulphonate resins:
　15 g orally up to three times daily with laxatives
　30 g rectally followed 3–6 hours later by an enema
Haemodialysis or peritoneal dialysis

A12.19

A) T B) F C) T D) T E) T

Hyperphosphataemia is usually asymptomatic but may result in precipitation of calcium phosphate, particularly in the presence of a normal or raised calcium or of alkalosis. Uraemic itching may be caused by a raised calcium × phosphate product. Prolonged hyperphosphataemia causes hyperparathyroidism, and periarticular and vascular calcification.

Water, electrolytes and acid–base balance

A12.20

A) T   B) F   C) F   D) F   E) T

The proximal convoluted tubule reclaims 85–90% of filtered bicarbonate; in contrast, the distal nephron reclaims very little. This difference is caused by the greater quantity of luminal carbonic anhydrase in the proximal tubule than in the distal nephron. Proximal tubular bicarbonate reabsorption is catalysed by the Na^+–K^+-ATPase pump located in the basolateral cell membrane. More acid is secreted into the proximal tubule (up to 4500 nmol of hydrogen ions each day) than into any other nephron segment.

However, the hydrogen ions secreted into the proximal tubule are almost completely reabsorbed with bicarbonate; consequently, proximal tubular hydrogen ion secretion does not contribute significantly to hydrogen ion elimination from the body. The collecting tubule has two types of cells: a) the principal cell with an aldosterone-sensitive Na absorption site. These cells reabsorb Na^+ and H_2O and secrete K^+ under the influence of aldosterone. b) The α-intercalated cell, which possesses the proton pump for the active secretion of hydrogen ions in exchange for reabsorption of K^+ ions. Aldosterone increases H^+ ion secretion.

A12.21

A) T   B) T   C) F   D) T   E) T

Causes of metabolic acidosis with a normal anion gap	
Increased gastrointestinal bicarbonate loss	**Decreased renal hydrogen ion excretion**
Diarrhoea	Distal (type 1) renal tubular acidosis
Ileostomy	Type 4 renal tubular acidosis (aldosterone deficiency)
Ureterosigmoidostomy	
Increased renal bicarbonate loss	**Increased HCl production**
Acetazolamide	Ammonium chloride ingestion
Proximal (type 2) renal tubular acidosis	Increased catabolism of lysine, arginine
Hyperparathyroidism	
Tubular damage, e.g. drugs, heavy metals, paraproteins	

A12.22

A) T B) T C) T D) T E) T

Causes of metabolic acidosis with an increased anion gap

Renal failure (sulphate, phosphate)

Accumulation of organic acids

Lactic acidosis
L-lactic
Type A – anaerobic metabolism in tissues
Hypotension/cardiac arrest
Sepsis
Poisoning – e.g. ethylene glycol, methanol
Type B – decreased hepatic lactate metabolism
Insulin deficiency (decreased pyruvate dehydrogenase activity)
Metformin accumulation (chronic renal failure)
Haematological malignancies
Rare inherited enzyme defects
D-lactic (fermentation of glucose in bowel by abnormal bowel flora, complicating abnormal small bowel anatomy, e.g. blind loops)

Ketoacidosis
Insulin deficiency
Alcohol excess
Starvation

Exogenous acids
Salicylate

A12.23

A) T B) T C) T D) T E) F

Causes of metabolic alkalosis

Chloride depletion
Gastric losses: vomiting, mechanical drainage, bulimia
Chloruretic diuretics: e.g. bumetanide, furosemide (frusemide), chlorothiazide, metolazone
Diarrhoeal states: villous adenoma, congenital chloridorrhoea
Cystic fibrosis (high sweat chloride)

A12.24

A) T B) T C) T D) T E) F

Causes of metabolic alkalosis

Potassium depletion/mineralocorticoid excess
Primary aldosteronism
Secondary aldosteronism
Apparent mineralocorticoid excess
Primary deoxycorticosterone excess: 11α- and 17α-hydroxylase deficiencies
Drugs: liquorice (glycyrrhizic acid) as a confection or flavouring, carbenoxolone
Liddle's syndrome
Bartter's and Gitelman's syndromes and their variants
Laxative abuse, clay ingestion

A12.25

A) F B) T C) T D) T E) F

Arterial underfilling in cirrhosis leads to reduction of pressure or stretch (i.e. 'unloading' of arterial volume receptors) which results in the activation of the sympathetic nervous system, activation of the renin–angiotensin–aldosterone system and nonosmotic release of antidiuretic hormone (ADH). These neurohumoral mediators promote salt and water retention in the face of increased extracellular volume.

Water, electrolytes and acid–base balance

A 12.26

A) T B) F C) F D) F E) T

Patients with the syndrome of inappropriate ADH secretion (SIADH) have impaired water excretion and hyponatraemia caused by the persistent presence of antidiuretic hormone (ADH); but the release of atrial natriuretic peptide (ANP) and aldosterone is not impaired; thus, Na^+ handling remains intact. These findings have implications for the correction of the hyponatraemia in this setting and require restriction of water intake.

A 12.27

A) T B) T C) F D) F E) F

The cause of hyponatraemia with apparently normal extracellular volume is usually not obvious. Causes include Addison's disease, hypothyroidism, the syndrome of inappropriate ADH secretion (SIADH) and drug-induced water retention. Diabetes insipidus, administration of hypertonic sodium solutions and hyperosmolar diabetic coma are causes of hypernatraemia.

Cardiovascular disease 13

13

Q 13.1

A 63-year-old hospital doctor develops central crushing chest pain. He is seen by a cardiologist within 15 minutes. ECG shows ST elevation in leads II, III and avF. He is given oxygen, aspirin and a beta-blocker. The cardiologist then does an emergency coronary angiography and finds a clot in the proximal right coronary artery and 80% stenosis of the artery. All other vessels have insignificant disease. The next step is

A. Percutaneous transluminal coronary angioplasty of proximal right coronary artery lesion without stent
B. Percutaneous transluminal coronary angioplasty of proximal right coronary artery lesion with stent
C. Spinal cord stimulation
D. Single vessel coronary artery bypass grafting
E. Transmyocardial laser revascularization

Q 13.2

A 71-year-old diabetic presents to the emergency department with prolonged chest pain at rest for 30 minutes. His blood pressure is 100/60 mmHg (usually it is 160/90 mmHg). His ECG is normal. He is administered aspirin and intravenous unfractionated heparin. The most appropriate next step is

A. Observe the patient overnight and discharge him with an appointment for outpatient exercise test

B. Coronary angiography
C. Initiate subcutaneous low-molecular-weight heparin and discharge him the next day with a 3-month prescription
D. Intravenous glycoprotein IIb/IIIa antagonist for 1 week
E. Thrombolytic therapy

Q 13.3

A 14-year-old boy has been told from a young age that he has a murmur. He is asymptomatic. On auscultation he has normal first and second heart sounds and a harsh pansystolic murmur along the left lower sternal border. Chest X-ray and ECG are normal. He most likely has

A. Atrial septal defect
B. Papillary muscle dysfunction
C. Mitral valve prolapse
D. Small ventricular septal defect
E. Pulmonary stenosis

Q 13.4

A 68-year-old smoker complains of pain in the right upper quadrant. The pain subsides spontaneously. His gastroenterologist requests a plain X-ray of the abdomen and an abdominal ultrasound. The abdominal ultrasound reveals gallstones and an aneurysm of the abdominal aorta measuring 6 cm in diameter. He is referred to a cardiologist for an opinion regarding the management of the aneurysm. Which one of the following is most likely

Cardiovascular disease

A. Since it is asymptomatic he should be reassured and monitored every year
B. Steroids should be administered if the C-reactive protein is elevated
C. He should be treated surgically even though he is asymptomatic
D. He should be administered coumarin to prevent thromboemboli
E. Since it is asymptomatic he should be reassured and monitored in 6 months

Q13.5

A 45-year-old woman develops idiopathic dilated cardiomyopathy and congestive heart failure. The strongest independent predictor of mortality is

A. Kerley B lines on chest X-ray
B. An ejection fraction of 0.25
C. Peak oxygen consumption less than 50% predicted
D. Elevated serum brain natriuretic peptide levels
E. Non-sustained ventricular arrhythmia

Q13.6

A 56-year-old patient complains of central chest pain radiating to the back. The chest pain also radiates down the arms and into the neck. The patient is hypertensive and all peripheral pulses are felt. Which one of the following investigations is the gold standard for diagnosis of this condition

A. Chest X-ray showing widened mediastinum
B. CT scanning of the chest
C. Emergency surgery
D. Transthoracic echocardiogram
E. MRI of the aorta

Q13.7

A 20-year-old psychology student on routine examination has normal blood pressure. He wants to know how frequently he should record his blood pressure. Which one of the following recommendations is currently accepted

A. He should use a home blood pressure machine and record his blood pressure at least once a day
B. He should have his blood pressure recorded every 10 years
C. He should have his blood pressure measured at least every 5 years
D. His should have his blood pressure measured every month
E. He should have his blood pressure measured at least three times a year

Q13.8

A 46-year-old barman has angina pectoris. He has hypertension, reduced levels of high-density lipoprotein cholesterol, hypertriglyceridaemia hyperinsulinaemia and central obesity. This patient has which one of the following?

A. Conn's syndrome
B. Phaeochromocytoma
C. Nelson's syndrome
D. Metabolic syndrome X
E. Addison's disease

Q13.9

A 45-year-old hospital employee presents with headaches. His blood pressure is 180/100 mmHg and he has normal peripheral pulses. Fundoscopy reveals arteriovenous nipping, flame-shaped haemorrhages and soft (cotton wool) exudates. There is no papilloedema. His electrolytes are normal. Abdominal ultrasound reveals normal kidneys and liver. The ECG is normal and chest X-ray does not show any evidence of rib notching. He most likely has which one of the following?

A. Conn's syndrome
B. Malignant hypertension

C. Polycystic kidney disease

D. Grade 2 Keith–Wagener's hypertensive fundus

E. Grade 4 Keith–Wagener's hypertensive fundus

Q13.10

A 38-year-old patient is seen by her GP who finds her blood pressure is 220/120 mmHg. The patient is not compliant with her medications or diet. As a consquence of her blood pressure she is most likely to suffer from which one of the following?

A. Congestive heart failure

B. Coronary heart disease

C. Stroke

D. Azotemia

E. Peripheral vascular disease

Q13.11

A 32-year-old woman with asthma who has been non-compliant with her medications and has continued to smoke now presents to the chest physician with shortness of breath. On examination there is a prominent 'a' wave in the jugular venous pulse. She has a barrel-shaped chest with a right ventricular heave and a loud pulmonary second sound. She has bilateral leg oedema. Echocardiography shows right ventricular dilatation with normal left ventricular ejection fraction. Select one of the following

A. The diagnosis is primary pulmonary hypertension

B. Long-term oxygen therapy improves prognosis

C. Angiotensin-converting enzyme inhibitors substantially reduce mortality

D. Diuretic therapy should be avoided

E. This patient has left ventricular systolic failure

Q13.12

A 49-year-old patient is admitted with angina. His ECG shows that there is no ST elevation. His cardiac enzymes show elevated troponins. In the coronary care unit he develops a rapid heart rate of 220 b.p.m. with wide (>0.14 s) and abnormal QRS complexes. His blood pressure begins to fall and he is haemodynamically unstable. The management of choice is which one of the following?

A. Intravenous esmolol

B. Intravenous verapamil

C. Emergency DC cardioversion

D. Intravenous lidocaine (lignocaine)

E. Intravenous amiodarone

Q13.13

A 38-year-old patient with Marfan's syndrome presents with syncope and central chest pain radiating to the back. Her blood pressure is stable. The investigation of first choice is which one of the following?

A. 24-hour ambulatory taped electrocardiography

B. Tilt testing

C. Transthoracic echocardiogram

D. Transoesophageal echocardiogram

E. Carotid sinus massage

Q13.14

A 21-year-old patient tells you that she has been told that she has a short PR interval with a delta wave in the QRS complex. Which one of the following statements about the PR interval is correct?

A. It is the length of time from the end of the P wave to the start of the QRS complex

B. It is the time taken for the activation to pass from the sinus node through the atrium, AV node and the His–Purkinje system to the ventricle

C. It is due to atrial repolarization
D. It represents ventricular repolarization
E. It represents ventricular depolarization

Q13.15

When a young healthy adult exercises there are increases in pulmonary capillary wedge pressure. The increase in pulmonary wedge pressure results in an increase in cardiac output. This is known as which one of the following?

A. Somogyi phenomenon
B. Treppe phenomenon
C. Frank–Starling relationship
D. Bowditch phenomenon
E. Law of Laplace

Q13.16

The increase in heart rate on vigorous exercise in a healthy adult is initiated at which one of the following?

A. Atrioventricular node
B. The His bundle
C. The right bundle
D. The main left bundle
E. Sinoatrial node

Q13.17

A 68-year-old man with hypertension is found to have left ventricular hypertrophy on an echocardiogram. The mitogen-activated protein (MAP) kinases which are most likely to promote growth of the cardiac myocytes are which one of the following?

A. The c-Jun N-terminal kinase/stress-activated protein kinases (JNK/SAPK)
B. Extracellular signal-regulated kinases (ERK-1 and ERK-2)
C. The p38 kinase pathway
D. cAMP kinase
E. Troponin kinase

Q13.18

A 58-year-old woman has crushing central chest pain. Her ECG shows ST elevation in ECG leads II, III and aVF. The vessel which is most likely to be obstructed on coronary angiography is which one of the following?

A. Left main coronary artery
B. Left circumflex artery
C. Coronary sinus
D. Left anterior descending artery
E. Right coronary artery

Q13.19

A 52-year-old patient has been admitted to the local hospital with crushing central chest pain. Investigations confirm that he has had an uncomplicated acute myocardial infarction. He has been walking around and the cardiologist plans to discharge him soon. A day before scheduled discharge he develops central chest pain. Investigations rule out a second myocardial infarction. The next step in the management is

A. Reassure the patient that he may have angina occasionally and recommend sublingual nitrate
B. Treadmill exercise test
C. Thallium-201 cardiac scintigraphy
D. Coronary angiography
E. Stress echocardiography

Q13.20

For a 55-year-old patient with ischaemic cardiomyopathy, a history of ventricular arrhythmia and left ventricular ejection fraction less than 35%, the intervention of first choice for secondary prevention of sudden death is which one of the following?

A. Amiodarone
B. Carvedilol
C. Sotalol

D. Implantable defibrillator

E. Cardiac pacemaker

Q13.21

A 35-year-old woman with peripartum cardiomyopathy is being evaluated for cardiac transplantation. Which one of the following is a contraindication for cardiac transplantation?

A. High systemic vascular resistance

B. High pulmonary vascular resistance

C. Creatinine clearance of 90 ml/h

D. History of breast cancer 8 years ago, now in full remission

E. History of alcohol abuse while she was a teenager

Q13.22

A 57-year-old patient with two-vessel coronary artery disease is seen in clinic. He has a 6-month history of developing central retrosternal chest pain on heavy exertion, relieved within minutes by rest. The pain radiates to the jaw. The most likely cause for his symptoms is which one of the following?

A. Unstable angina

B. Cardiac syndrome X

C. Variant angina

D. Prinzmetal's angina

E. Stable angina pectoris

Q13.23

A 75-year-old diabetic presents with profuse sweating and palpitations but denies pain. His ECG shows ST elevation in leads II, III and AVF and ST depression in leads in V_2–V_3. Serum cardiac troponins are elevated. Which one of the following is the most appropriate conclusion made by the emergency room house officer

A. The ECG changes are normal in leads II, III and AVF and the patient can be reassured and discharged

B. The ECG changes are typical of Wolff–Parkinson–White syndrome

C. The patient has developed an inferior wall myocardial infarction

D. The ECG changes rule out right ventricular infarction

E. The patient has developed an anterior wall myocardial infarction

Q13.24

A 67-year-old man develops crushing central chest pain and he presents to the emergency department of a major teaching hospital within 1 hour. Heart rate is 60 beats per minute and blood pressure is 210/110 mmHg. ECG shows >1 mm ST elevation in chest leads V_2–V_5. There is a past history of proliferative diabetic retinopathy but this was successfully treated with laser therapy. He developed a small haemorrhagic stroke 6 weeks ago and has minimal residual hemiparesis. He has been able to walk unaided for the past 3 weeks. An urgent echocardiogram shows clot in the left ventricle. The best option for reperfusion is which one of the following?

A. Thrombolysis with streptokinase

B. Thrombolysis with front-loaded tissue-type plasminogen activatior (t-PA)

C. Primary percutaneous transluminal coronary angiography

D. Intravenous nitrates

E. Intravenous morphine

Q13.25

A 28-year-old Indian woman who has recently arrived in the UK has a history of rheumatic fever. Eight years ago she developed shortness of breath at the end of

Cardiovascular disease

the second trimester of her pregnancy. On auscultation she has a mid-diastolic murmur at the apex. She had an echocardiogram in India and was told that she has severe mitral stenosis. An echocardiogram done in the UK reveals a mitral valve area of 0.8 cm^2. Which one of the following is the most likely?

A. She has a normal mitral valve orifice area
B. She has minimally reduced mitral valve orifice area
C. She has severe mitral stenosis
D. She has a flow murmur
E. Her mitral valve orifice is moderately stenosed

Q13.26

1. A 77-year-old woman known to have dilated cardiomyopathy is progressively short of breath. She is breathless during activities of daily living (e.g. walking from her bed to the bathroom)

2. A 67-year-old woman wakes up from sleep fighting for breath. She gets up and opens a window to gasp for fresh air before she calls the ambulance. She had a similar episode 3 days ago

3. An 89-year-old woman without heart failure, living in a nursing home, is found by her nurse to have alternate hyperventilation and apnoea

4. A 43-year-old tennis player complains of central chest pain. The pain is sharp and severe and is aggravated by coughing and deep breaths. The pain is relieved by sitting forwards

5. A 35-year-old pregnant woman with Marfan's syndrome develops central chest pain that is radiating to the back

6. A 42-year-old doctor develops palpitations in the middle of the night. These last for an hour before he requests his GP to make a house call. He feels his own pulse and finds that his heart is racing. He also passes copious quantities of urine following the episode

7. A 78-year-old man falls to the ground without warning during a church service. A paramedic in the congregation rushes to his side and finds that his pulse is 38 beats/minute. After a few seconds the pulse quickens and the man flushes and recovers consciousness

8. A 78-year-old smoker, diabetic and hypertensive complains of a 10-day history of central chest pain radiating to the neck and jaw which is typically provoked by exercise and relieved by rest. The pain has been worse during the last 24 hours, is increasing in frequency, and has been coming on at rest

Select the best match for each of the above

A. New York Heart Association grade III congestive heart failure
B. New York Heart Association grade II congestive heart failure
C. New York Heart Association grade IV congestive heart failure
D. Paroxysmal nocturnal dyspnoea
E. Cheyne–Stokes respiration
F. Sleep apnoea syndrome
G. Acute pericarditis
H. Aortic dissection
I. Acute myocardial infarction
J. Chronic stable angina
K. Unstable angina
L. Pulmonary embolism
M. Da Costa's syndrome
N. Stokes–Adams attack
O. Supraventricular tachycardia
P. Ventricular tachycardia

Q13.27

1. A 78-year-old patient complains of syncope. On ausculatation he has an ejection systolic murmur in the right second intercostal space radiating to the carotids

2. A 67-year-old woman with hypertension is complaining of shortness of breath. Her blood pressure is 140/40 mmHg and she has an early diastolic murmur along the left third intercostal space. The murmur is best heard on sitting forwards and deep expiration

3. A 58-year-old ice-skater has pericardial tamponade

4. A 25-year-old woman has grossly dilated cardiomyopathy with New York Heart Association class IV symptoms and ejection fraction of less than 10%

5. A 72-year-old patient complains of palpitations. His echocardiogram reveals a grossly enlarged left atrium. He has a tachyarrhythmia which reverses with ibutilide

6. A 28-year-old patient with rheumatic heart disease complains of shortness of breath. On auscultation he has an ejection systolic murmur in the right second intercostal space conducted to the carotids and an early diastolic murmur in the left third intercostal space which is better heard on expiration

Select the best match for each of the above

A. Corrigan's pulse
B. Pulsus bigeminus
C. Pulsus bisferiens
D. Pulsus alternans
E. Irregularly irregular pulse
F. Pulsus paradoxus
G. Anacrotic pulse

Q13.28

1. A 53-year-old patient complains of dizziness. On examination he has an irregular pulse with a rate of 36 beats per minute

2. An 18-year-old patient is diagnosed to have Ebstein's anomaly. On auscultation he has a pansystolic murmur along the left lower sternal border which is better heard on inspiration

3. A 68-year-old man complains of palpitations. He has an irregularly irregular pulse

4. A 59-year-old woman is diagnosed to have constrictive pericarditis

5. A 32-year-old woman has primary pulmonary hypertension

Match each of the above with the following changes in the jugular venous pulse

A. Steep y descent
B. Large v waves
C. Large a waves
D. Cannon waves
E. Absent a waves
F. Prominent c wave

Q13.29

1. A 55-year-old woman had rheumatic heart disease as a child. On auscultation she has a mid-diastolic rumbling murmur at the apex

2. An 89-year-old woman complains of recurrent syncope. On auscultation she has an ejection systolic murmur conducted to the carotids

3. A 28-year-old woman has a body mass index of 40

4. A 35-year-old man has a family history of sudden death. His echocardiogram shows a cardiomyopathy with asymmetrical hypertrophy of the interventricular septum

5. A 32-year-old woman complains of chest pain on exertion. On auscultation a loud pulmonary second heart sound may be felt

Select the best match for each of the above

A. Sustained parasternal heave
B. Double apical impulse

C. Impalpable apex beat

D. Heaving apex beat

E. Tapping apex beat

Q13.30

1. A 28-year-old patient with primary pulmonary hypertension

2. A 58-year-old Afro-Caribbean patient with a blood pressure of 170/120 mmHg

3. A 73-year-old patient with an ejection systolic murmur in the right second intercostal space conducted to the carotids. Her blood pressure is 100/90 mmHg

4. A 22-year-old doctor who has been told that he has a defect in the septum between his left and right atrium

5. An extra heart sound heard at the apex in a 58-year-old patient who presents with heart failure. His heart failure is due to mitral regurgitation

6. An 89-year-old patient who is said to have a stiff heart

7. A 28-year-old patient with rheumatic heart disease has a mid-diastolic murmur at the apex

8. A 26-year-old medical student who has been told that she has a bicuspid aortic valve

Select the best match for each of the above

A. Opening snap

B. An ejection click that occurs immediately after the first heart sound

C. Fourth heart sound

D. Third heart sound

E. Fixed splitting of second heart sound

F. Reversed splitting of second heart sound

G. Loud pulmonary second heart sound

H. Loud aortic second sound

Q13.31

1. A 20-year-old patient has a short early systolic murmur heard well at the lower left sternal edge

2. A patient with severe aortic regurgitation has a mid-diastolic murmur at the apex

3. A 23-year-old woman with an early diastolic murmur louder on inspiration

4. A 17-year-old boy complains of severe, sharp pain of 1 day's duration. He has a scratching or crunching noise, best heard with the diaphragm and most obvious in systole

Select the best match for each of the above

A. Austin Flint murmur

B. Graham Steell murmur

C. Venous hum

D. Pericardial rub

E. Ventricular septal defect

Q13.32

A student doctor is called to a cardiac arrest. The following statements about the management of cardiac arrest are correct

A. Adrenaline (epinephrine) should be avoided if the arrest is due to ventricular fibrillation

B. A bolus dose of intravenous amiodarone may be beneficial in refractory ventricular tachycardia

C. Transcutaneous pacing may useful in asystole

D. Toxic levels of beta-blockers may cause electromechanical dissociation

E. Initially in ventricular fibrillation an electric shock of 50 J is used for defibrillation

Q13.33

1. A fisherman is brought to the emergency room having fallen in ice-cold water

while sailing in the sea. His heart rate is 40 beats per minute and ECG shows sinus rhythm

2. A 45-year-old patient with congestive heart failure is found to have atrial tachycardia. Digoxin level is 3.5

3. A 45-year-old woman is diagnosed with Graves' disease. Her heart rate is 120 beats per minute and ECG shows sinus rhythm

4. A 41-year-old patient has a history of regular paroxysmal supraventricular tachycardia

5. A patient with long QT syndrome develops ventricular arrhythmia on initiation of drug therapy

6. A patient is found to have progressive PR prolongation until a P wave fails to conduct

7. A patient develops myocardial infarction. He is found to have a heart rate of 50 beats per minute. The ECG shows dropped QRS complex that is not preceded by progressive PR interval prolongation

Match the above clinical scenarios with the following mechanisms of arrhythmia production

A. Accelerated automaticity
B. Abnormal conduction within the atrioventricular node
C. Abnormally slow automaticity
D. Triggered activity
E. Re-entry or circus movements
F. Abnormal conduction within the His bundle

Q13.34

1. Following myocardial infarction, the patient develops complete heart block which lies in the atrioventricular node

2. An 87-year-old faints in church. Her heart rate is 36 beats per minute and

she is suspected to have fibrosis of the distal conduction system. The escape rhythm originates below the His bundle

3. A 24-year-old doctor is known to have a congenital heart defect. He has a wide fixed split second heart sound. The ECG shows deep S waves in leads I and V_6 and a tall late R wave in lead V_1

4. A 73-year-old hypertensive has a deep S wave in lead V_1 and a tall late R wave in leads I and V_6

5. Following a myocardial infarction, a patient is suspected to have a block in the posteroinferior division of the left bundle of His

6. A patient with coronary artery disease has a block in the anterior division of the left bundle of His

7. A patient has a family history of sudden death. He has a mutation in the gene that encodes for sudden death

Select the best match of each of the above

A. Right bundle branch block
B. Narrow complex escape rhythm
C. Broad complex escape rhythm
D. Right axis deviation
E. Right bundle branch block with ST elevation in right precordial leads
F. Left ventricular hypertrophy
G. Left axis deviation

Q13.35

1. A 45-year-old smoker with coronary artery disease has a history of paroxysmal palpitations precipitated by drinking coffee. During an acute episode the ECG shows QRS complexes at a rate of 200 beats/minute. Inverted P waves are visible just before the QRS complexes

2. A 22-year-old patient with Wolff–Parkinson–White syndrome complains of paroxysmal palpitations. ECG shows

Cardiovascular disease

a narrow complex QRS tachcardia and the P wave is clearly seen between the QRS complex and T wave

3. A 75-year-old patient has recent-onset palpitations. RR intervals are irregular and there is absence of organized atrial activity

4. A 28-year-old patient with hypertrophic cardiomyopathy presents with sawtooth waves at a rate of 300 per minute. Ventricular rate is 150 beats per minute

5. A 45-year-old patient with cardiomyopathy complains of a sudden history of dizziness, and palpitations which last for a minute. Her Holter monitor shows rapid irregular sharp QRS complexes that continously change from an upright to an inverted position. Before the onset of tachycardia the QT interval is prolonged

6. A 69-year-old patient with chronic lung disease complains of palpitations. The heart rate is 120 beats per minute. The ECG shows multiple P wave morphologies and the RR intervals are irregular

Select the best match for each of the above

A. Atrioventricular nodal re-entry tachycardia (AVNRT)
B. Atrioventricular reciprocating tachycardia (AVRT)
C. Atrial fibrillation
D. Atrial flutter with 2:1 varying block
E. Atrial flutter with with 1:2 varying block
F. Multifocal atrial tachycardia
G. Torsades de pointes
H. Ventricular fibrillation
I. Ventricular tachycardia

Q13.36

1. Lengthen action potential
2. Shorten action potential
3. No effect on duration of action potential
4. Widen duration of action potential

5. Predominant action on the atrioventricular node

Match the predominant mechanism of action with the following anti-arrhythmic drugs

A. Quinidine
B. Lidocaine (lignocaine)
C. Flecainide
D. Sotalol
E. Verapamil

Q13.37

The following tachyarrhythmias can be readily ablated by radiofrequency

A. Atrioventricular node re-entry tachycardia (AVNRT)
B. Accessory-pathway-mediated tachycardias
C. Atrioventricular reciprocating tachycardia (AVRT)
D. Wolff–Parkinson–White syndrome
E. Atrial flutter
F. Atrial tachycardia

Q13.38

A 35-year-old Afro-Caribbean patient develops congestive heart failure. Pathophysiological changes that occur in this condition include

A. Decreased collagen synthesis
B. Decreased secretion of atrial natriuretic peptide
C. Sympathetic stimulation
D. Peripheral vasoconstriction
E. Salt and water retention

Q13.39

Causes of left ventricular failure include

A. Tricuspid regurgitation
B. Atrial septal defect with left-to-right shunt

C. Mitral stenosis with pulmonary hypertension

D. Ischaemic heart disease

E. Systemic hypertension

Q13.40

A 69-year-old woman develops acute pulmonary oedema. She is diuresed and an echocardiogram shows an ejection fraction of 65%. The cardiologist proceeds to look for an underlying cause. Possible causes include

A. Coronary artery disease

B. Hypertension

C. Hypertrophic cardiomyopathy

D. Amyloidosis

E. Sarcoidosis

Q13.41

A 42-year-old patient develops dilated cardiomyopathy, is short of breath while climbing stairs and walking 400 metres. He is not short of breath with activities of daily living. Drugs which have been shown to reduce mortality include

A. Digoxin

B. Beta-blockers

C. Spironolactone

D. Loop diuretics

E. Hydralazine plus nitrate

Q13.42

1. A 33-year-old patient with dilated cardiomyopathy develops acute pulmonary oedema. He receives intravenous furosemide (frusemide)

2. A 45-year-old patient with ischaemic cardiomyopathy is initiated on diuretics and enalapril. The patient develops a dry cough

3. An 18-year-old with mild heart failure occasionally develops swelling in his feet. His doctor initiates bendroflumethiazide (bendrofluazide)

4. A 45-year-old is diagnosed with New York Heart Association (NYHA) class II congestive heart failure. His cardiologist initiates therapy with carvedilol

5. A 52-year-old patient with congestive heart failure develops shortness of breath at rest. He is admitted to the coronary care unit and intravenous dobutamine is started

6. A 52-year-old patient with congestive heart failure develops shortness of breath at rest. He is admitted to the coronary care unit and intravenous milrinone therapy is initiated

7. A 45-year-old patient with ischaemic cardiomyopathy is initiated on digoxin

Select the best association for each of the above

A. Non-selective vasodilator beta-blocker

B. Beta$_1$-adrenoceptor agonist

C. Inhibition of phosphodiesterase

D. Competitive inhibition of sodium–potassium-ATPase

E. Arteriolar vasodilatation by reducing afterload

F. Inhibition of bradykinin metabolism

G. Stimulation of bradykinin metabolism

H. Reduces sodium reabsorption in distal convoluted tubule

Q13.43

A 28-year-old man who has undergone cardiac transplantation wishes to know about the possible complications. He has obtained some information off the internet and wishes to know whether it is accurate. The following items on the patient's list are complications of cardiac transplantation

Cardiovascular disease

A. Hypertension
B. Hypercholesterolaemia
C. Malignancy
D. Opportunistic infection
E. Coronary artery disease

Q13.44

A 67-year-old asthmatic develops flash pulmonary oedema due to acute left ventricular failure. The following treatments are potentially beneficial in this patient

A. Administration of aminophylline (5 mg/kg i.v.) over 60 seconds
B. Intravenous morphine with metoclopramide
C. Intravenous glyceryl trinitrate
D. Intra-arterial hydralazine
E. 60% oxygen via a variable performance mask

Q13.45

A 78-year-old patient with coronary artery disease is found by his family in the early hours of the morning barely rousable. He is seen in the emergency department where his blood pressure is found to be 90/60 mmHg. His extremities are cold and he is not alert. A pulmonary artery catheter is floated into the right side of the heart and pulmonary capillary wedge pressure is 27 mmHg. The likely causes for this clinical picture include

A. Acute myocardial infarction
B. Severe sepsis
C. Pericardial tamponade
D. Acute mitral regurgitation
E. Upper gastrointestinal haemorrhage

Q13.46

A 14-year-old schoolboy's father died of acute myocardial infarction at the age of 42 about 5 years ago. The boy has

researched the process of atherosclerosis and approaches his general practitioner regarding the accuracy of his research. The following statements are correct

A. 'Fatty streak' is the layman's term for complicated plaque
B. A 50% reduction in luminal diameter causes a haemodynamically significant stenosis
C. Superficial endothelial injury of the plaque results in clot formation on the surface of the plaque
D. Fissures in the plaque result in thrombus formation within the plaque
E. Smooth muscle proliferation is a feature of plaque formation

Q13.47

A 39-year-old pilot is having his annual check. He has a family history of coronary artery disease. He has read about this condition and would like to know whether any of the following are *independent* risk factors for coronary artery disease

A. Deletion polymorphism in the angiotensin-converting enzyme gene
B. Homocysteinaemia
C. Central obesity
D. High plasma Lp(a) concentrations
E. High serum fibrinogen

Q13.48

1. A 66-year-old patient develops acute myocardial infarction. On the second day in the coronary care unit she has ventricular extrasystoles which are frequent and multiform, and many exhibit the R-on-T phenomenon

2. A 38-year-old patient presents with acute myocardial infarction; within hours he develops ventricular fibrillation

3. A 67-year-old patient with acute myocardial infarction develops sustained wide complex tachycardia 18 hours after admission and blood pressure begins to fall

4. A 72-year-old patient with acute myocardial infarction develops an irregularly irregular rhythm. The P waves are not seen and his ventricular rate is 130 beats/minute

5. A 44-year-old patient develops an acute myocardial infarction with ST elevation in leads II, III and AVF. Three hours after admission he develops an uneasy sensation and his heart rate is 40 beats per minute and he is in sinus rhythm

6. A 55-year-old woman develops acute myocardial infarction. She is very anxious and her heart rate is 104 beats per minute and in sinus rhythm

7. A 49-year-old patient with acute anterior wall myocardial infarction has a heart rate of 36 beats/per minute with atrioventricular dissociation and wide QRS complexes which are irregular

8. A 69-year-old man is admitted with chest pain and ST segment elevation in leads II, III, AVF and V_4R. Blood pressure is 80/60 mmHg and jugular venous pressure is elevated

9. A 64-year-old patient develops an acute anterior wall myocardial infarction. An echocardiogram shows a large mural thrombus in the left ventricle and ejection fraction of 0.35

10. A 42-year-old man is admitted with central chest pain and ECG shows acute anterior wall myocardial infarction. He is successfuly treated. Three days after admission he complains of sharp chest pain aggravated by deep inspiration and typically worse on lying down. ECG shows generalized ST segment elevation (concave upward) with upright peaked T waves

Select the best option for each of the above

A. No specific treatment
B. Anti-inflammatory drugs
C. Thrombolysis
D. Aspirin only
E. Warfarin therapy
F. Synchronized cardioversion with 100 J
G. Unsynchronized cardioversion with 200 J
H. Intravenous digoxin
I. Intravenous amiodarone
J. Intravenous atropine
K. Temporary pacemaker
L. Intravenous fluids
M. Intravenous dobutamine
N. Beta-blockers

Q13.49

1. A 42-year-old patient with Marfan's syndrome and a holosystolic murmur at the apex conducted to the axilla

2. A 36-year-old patient with rumbling mid-diastolic murmur at the apex

3. A 45-year-old patient with a history of bicuspid aortic valve has an ejection systolic murmur at the base of the heart conducted to the carotids

4. A 45-year-old patient with ankylosing spondylitis has an early diastolic mumur best heard at the left sternal edge in the fourth intercostal space with the patient leaning forward and the breath held in expiration

5. A 42-year-old patient with rheumatic fever has a mid-diastolic murmur along the left lower sternal border and the murmur is louder on inspiration

Select the most likely cardiac catheterization finding for each of the above

A. Diastolic pressure in the left atrium exceeds left-ventricular end-diastolic pressure

B. Prominent left atrial systolic pressure wave
C. The peak systolic pressure changes from 250 mmHg in the left ventricle to 130 mmHg in the aorta
D. This demonstrates a diastolic pressure gradient between the right atrium and the right ventricle. Contrast injection will demonstrate a large right atrium
E. Injection of contrast material in the aorta results in the appearance of the contrast in the left ventricle

Q13.50

1. A 56-year-old patient with ischaemic cardiomyopathy and a holosystolic murmur at the apex conducted to the axilla
2. A 36-year-old woman with shortness of breath. On auscultation she has a loud first heart sound and a rumbling mid-diastolic murmur at the apex
3. A 35-year-old patient with a history of bicuspid aortic valve has an ejection systolic murmur at the base of the heart conducted to the carotids. There is no shortness of breath
4. A 40-year-old patient with a past history of syphilis has an early diastolic murmur best heard at the left sternal edge in the fourth intercostal space with the patient leaning forward and the breath held in expiration. The patient is short of breath on exertion
5. A 32-year-old patient with rheumatic fever has a mid-diastolic murmur along the left lower sternal border and the murmur is louder on inspiration

Select the most likely chest X-ray finding for each of the above

A. A small heart with an enlarged left atrium. Pulmonary venous hypertension is present

B. Left atrial and left ventricular enlargement. There is an increase in the cardiothoracic ratio, and the mitral valve is calcified
C. A relatively small heart with a prominent, dilated, ascending aorta. The aortic valve is calcified
D. Large dilated heart with left ventricular enlargement and dilatation of the ascending aorta
E. Prominent right atrial bulge

Q13.51

1. A 56-year-old patient with ischaemic cardiomyopathy and a holosystolic murmur at the apex conducted to the axilla
2. A 36-year-old woman with shortness of breath. On auscultation she has a loud first heart sound and a rumbling mid-diastolic murmur at the apex
3. A 35-year-old patient with a history of bicuspid aortic valve has an ejection systolic murmur at the base of the heart conducted to the carotids
4. A 40-year-old patient with a past history of syphilis has an early diastolic murmur best heard at the left sternal edge in the fourth intercostal space with the patient leaning forward and the breath held in expiration. The patient is short of breath on exertion
5. A 32-year-old patient with rheumatic fever has a mid-diastolic murmur along the left lower sternal border and the murmur is louder on inspiration

Select the most likely ECG finding for each of the above

A. Peaked, tall P waves (>3 mm) in lead II
B. Tall R waves and deeply inverted T waves in the left-sided chest leads, and deep S waves in the right-sided leads
C. Depressed ST segments and T wave inversion in leads I, AVL, V_5 and V_6

D. Bifid P waves and tall R waves in leads I and V_6 and deep S waves in leads V_1 and V_2

E. Bifid P wave owing to delayed left atrial activation. As the disease progresses right axis deviation and tall R waves in lead V_1 may develop

Q13.52

1. A 56-year-old patient with infective endocarditis and a holosystolic murmur at the apex conducted to the axilla and rapidly progressive congestive heart failure

2. A 36-year-old woman with shortness of breath. On auscultation she has a loud first heart sound and a rumbling mid-diastolic murmur at the apex

3. A 46-year-old woman with shortness of breath. On auscultation she has a normal first heart sound and a rumbling mid-diastolic murmur at the apex best heard with the bell of the stethoscope

4. A 35-year-old patient with a history of bicuspid aortic valve has an ejection systolic murmur at the base of the heart conducted to the carotids. She has a history of syncope

5. A 40-year-old asymptomatic patient has an early diastolic murmur best heard at the left sternal edge in the fourth intercostal space with the patient leaning forward and the breath held in expiration. Echocardiography shows normal ejection fraction and left ventricular end-diastolic diameter of 50 mm

Select the best treatment for each of the above conditions when indicated

A. Trans-septal balloon valvotomy
B. Open mitral valvotomy
C. Mitral valve replacement
D. Aortic valve replacement
E. Medical treatment and observation

Q13.53

1. A 35-year-old intravenous drug abuser who presents with progressive shortness of breath

2. A 22-year-old patient who dissolves heroin in lemon juice before injecting it into her veins

3. A 65-year old patient who has a history of rheumatic mitral regurgitation and has now developed bowel malignancy

4. A 47-year-old with a history of rheumatic mitral regurgitation undergoes a dental procedure without adequate antibiotic prophylaxis

5. A 45-year-old patient with a prosthetic heart valve and fever

6. A 65-year-old patient with endocarditis and negative blood cultures

Select the most likely organism in each of the above cases of infective endocarditis

A. Staphylococcus
B. Streptococcus bovis
C. Candida
D. *Coxiella burnetii*
E. *Streptococcus viridans*

Q13.54

1. A 35-year-old intravenous drug abuser who presents with progressive shortness of breath

2. A 22-year-old patient who dissolves heroin in lemon juice before injecting it into her veins

3. A 47-year-old with a history of rheumatic mitral regurgitation undergoes a dental procedure without adequate antibiotic prophylaxis

4. A 45-year-old patient with a prosthetic heart valve and fever

Select the best treatment for each of the above cases of endocarditis

A. Vancomycin and gentamycin
B. Valve surgery
C. Penicillin and gentamycin
D. Valve replacement

Q13.55

1. A 26-year-old doctor has a right ventricular heave, loud P2, fixed split S2, a mid-systolic ejection murmur in the pulmonary area and diastolic murmur along the left lower sternal border

2. A 12-year-old boy has a continuous machinery murmur best heard below the left clavicle in the first interspace or over the rib. A thrill is felt. He has a large volume (bounding) pulse

3. An 18-year-old complains of nosebleeds, headaches and claudication in both his legs. He has hypertension in the upper limbs and weak delayed pulses in the legs. He has a mid-systolic murmur over the upper precordium and vascular bruits over the back

4. An 8-year-old immigrant from Bangladesh complains of frequent episodes of dyspnoea and turns blue on exertion. His symptoms are relieved by squatting. On examination he has finger clubbing and he is short in stature. He has a left parasternal heave and a systolic ejection murmur with a thrill in the second left interspace close to the sternum

Select the most likely diagnosis for each of the above

A. Mitral stenosis
B. Tricuspid stenosis
C. Atrial septal defect
D. Pulmonary stenosis
E. Coarctation of the aorta
F. Patent ductus arteriosus
G. Fallot's tetralogy
H. Eisenmenger's syndrome
I. Ventricular septal defect

Q13.56

1. A 13-year-old boy has a continuous machinery murmur best heard below the left clavicle in the first interspace or over the rib. A thrill is felt. He has a large volume (bounding) pulse

2. A 29-year-old weightlifter complains of nosebleeds, headaches and claudication in both his legs. He has hypertension in the upper limbs and weak delayed pulses in the legs. He has a mid-systolic murmur over the upper precordium and vascular bruits over the back

3. An 18-year-old immigrant from Africa complains of frequent episodes of dyspnoea and and turns blue on exertion. His symptoms are relieved by squatting. On examination he has finger clubbing and he is short in stature. He has a left parasternal heave and a systolic ejection murmur with a thrill in the second left interspace close to the sternum

4. A 36-year-old lawyer has a right ventricular heave, fixed split S2, a mid-systolic ejection murmur in the pulmonary area and diastolic murmur along the left lower sternal border

Select the most likely chest X-ray finding for each of the above

A. A large right ventricle and a small pulmonary artery ('boot-shaped' heart)
B. A dilated aorta (seen in the upper right mediastinum) shaped like a figure '3'. Tortuous and dilated collateral intercostal arteries erode the undersurfaces of the ribs
C. Prominent aorta and pulmonary arterial system
D. Prominent pulmonary artery and pulmonary plethora
E. 'Pruned' pulmonary arteries

Q13.57

1. A 42-year-old patient complains of shortness of breath. Echocardiogram shows a dilated left ventricle. Left ventricular ejection fraction is 30%. He has a family history of cardiomyopathy. Genetic studies have identified the dystrophin gene responsible

2. A 26-year-old patient complains of shortness of breath. Echocardiogram shows a dilated left ventricle. Left ventricular ejection fraction is 20%. He has a family history of cardiomyopathy. Genetic studies have identified the desmin gene responsible

3. A 29-year-old athlete has syncope. His echocardiogram shows marked left ventricular hypertrophy and left ejection fraction is 75% and rapid. There is systolic anterior movement of the anterior mitral valve leaflet

4. A 19-year-old basketball player complains of syncope. His echocardiogram shows mild left ventricular hypertrophy and left ventricular ejection fraction is normal. There is systolic anterior movement of the anterior mitral valve leaflet. Genetic studies have revealed he has a high risk of sudden death

5. A 56-year-old patient is newly diagnosed as having hypertrophic cardiomyopathy

Select the best match for each of the above

A. X-linked
B. Autosomal dominant cardiomyopathy
C. Mutations of the beta-myosin heavy chain
D. Mutations in troponin T
E. Mutations of the myosin-binding protein C

Q13.58

1. A 56-year-old woman with systemic amyloidosis presents with shortness of breath. The jugular venous pressure is elevated with diastolic collapse

2. A 45-year-old African-American with sarcoidosis presents with shortness of breath. There is elevation of the jugular venous pressure with inspiration. MRI shows normal pericardium

3. The patient presents with right ventricular failure. There is a family history of similar disease. Endomyocardial biopsy shows fibrofatty replacement of the right ventricular myocardium. There are associated dermatological abnormalities with mutation in the gene encoding the protein plakoglobin

4. A 45-year-old patient with a past history of tuberculosis has the following clinical features: ascites, dependent oedema, hepatomegaly, jugular venous distension, and minimal shortness of breath. Cardiac catheterization reveals that diastolic pressure is equal in all four chambers

Select the best match for each of the above

A. Kussmaul's sign
B. Friedreich's sign
C. Pulsus paradoxus
D. Naxos disease
E. Constrictive pericarditis
F. Buerger's disease

Q13.59

1. A 28-year-old weightlifter has a blood pressure of 220/110 mmHg. His upper torso is well developed. He complains of claudication in both his lower legs. His primary care physician did not feel his peripheral pulses. His chest X-ray shows rib notching

Cardiovascular disease

2. A 27-year-old patient is found to have elevated blood pressure of 180/120 mmHg. She is not on any medications. Her serum sodium is 142 mEq/L, potassium 3.0 mEq/L, normal urea and creatinine

3. A 45-year-old school head was diagnosed as having hypertension 18 months ago. She complains of attacks of sweating, headache and palpitations. Blood pressure, despite regular treatment, varies from 240/180 mmHg to 140/90 mmHg. She has normal kidney function and normal electrolytes

4. A 65-year-old patient with coronary artery disease and peripheral vascular disease is started on captopril for the treatment of hypertension. Her first dose was administered before she went to bed. Overnight she developed oliguria

5. A 22-year-old patient is diagnosed as having hypertension. She has a family history of kidney disease. Her urine examination reveals red blood cells and the serum creatinine is elevated

Select the most likely aetiology for each of the above

A. Polycystic kidney disease
B. Bilateral renal artery stenosis
C. Coarctation of aorta
D. Conn's syndrome
E. Addison's disease
F. Phaeochromocytoma

Q13.60

1. A 42-year-old asthmatic has a blood pressure of 130/100 mmHg

2. A 38-year-old woman with a blood pressure of 170/120 mmHg is diagnosed as having phaeochromocytoma

3. A 22-year-old woman with a blood pressure of 180/120 mmHg is

diagnosed as having fibromuscular dysplasia of both renal arteries

4. A 38-year-old with a blood pressure of 150/100 mmHg and left ventricular ejection fraction of 30%

5. A 58-year-old patient with a blood pressure of 158/112 mmHg and a history of recurrent gouty arthritis

Select which of the following medications you would avoid in each of the above instances

A. Angiotensin-converting enzyme inhibitors
B. Beta-blockers
C. Nifedipine
D. Amlodipine
E. Thiazide diuretics

Q13.61

1. A 29-year-old woman complains of attacks of pallor of both hands followed by bluish discoloration and finally redness. Numbness and burning of fingers occurs initially followed by severe pain when the hands turn red

2. A 45-year-old patient with chest pain undergoes MRI which shows aortic dissection originating in the ascending aorta and confined to the ascending aorta

3. A 25-year-old woman complains of fever and systemic illness. She has hypertension and absent peripheral pulses

4. A 35-year-old smoker has claudication in both legs of 2 years' duration. Now he has rest pain in his feet and gangrene of the toes. He has thrombophlebitis

5. A 7-year-old child has a 4-day history of fever. The child has central chest pain and elevated cardiac troponin levels. General examination reveals lymphadenopathy and absent peripheral pulses

A. Buerger's disease
B. Kawasaki disease
C. Takayasu's syndrome
E. DeBakey type II aortic dissection
E. DeBakey type I aortic dissection
F. Raynaud's phenomenon

Q13.62

A 37-year-old Asian man has a 3-month history of central chest pain on exertion. He has a family history of coronary artery disease and has been smoking two packs of cigarettes per day since the age of 20. His general practitioner requests a treadmill exercise test. Findings suggesting an adverse prognosis include

A. Up-sloping ST segment depression
B. Total exercise time of 10 minutes
C. A slow recovery of heart rate to basal levels
D. Frequent premature ventricular depolarizations
E. A sustained fall in blood pressure

Q13.63

You are looking at a posteroanterior view of a chest film done on end inspiration. The cardiothoracic ratio is about 60%. This may be seen in

A. Neonates
B. Athletes
C. Patients with scoliosis
D. Pericardial effusion with 100 mL of pericardial fluid
E. Pure mitral stenosis without pulmonary hypertension

Q13.64

A 19-year-old woman presents with haemoptysis and shortness of breath. On examination she has a tapping apex beat, loud first heart sound, an opening snap

and mid-diastolic rumbling murmur. Her physician orders posteroanterior and lateral chest films. Recognized features on chest X-ray in this condition include

A. Kerley B lines
B. Straightening of the upper left heart border
C. A double atrial shadow to the right of the sternum
D. On lateral film a calcified valve above the line joining the carina to the sternophrenic angle
E. Splaying of the carina due to elevation of the left main bronchus

Q13.65

The radiologist reports that the chest film shows a paucity of vascular markings and a reduction in the width of the arteries. These features are seen in

A. Atrial septal defect with left-to-right shunt
B. Ventricular septal defect with left-to-right shunt
C. Pulmonary embolism
D. Severe pulmonary stenosis
E. Fallot's tetralogy

Q13.66

On auscultation a loud first heart sound may be heard in

A. Pericardial effusion
B. Short PR interval
C. Mitral stenosis
D. Calcific mitral stenosis
E. Mitral regurgitation

Q13.67

The increase in catecholamine activity on vigorous exercise

A. Decreases calcium flux in the myocyte
B. Strengthens force of contraction of the cardiac myocyte

Cardiovascular disease

C. Inhibits membrane-bound adenlyate kinases

D. Phosphorylates phospholamban

E. Results in phosphorylation of troponin-I

Q13.68

Your patient with ischaemic cardiomyopathy in the outpatient clinic would like to know which of the following interventions would improve his endothelium-dependent coronary vasodilatation

A. Angiotensin-converting enzyme inhibitors

B. Statins

C. Antioxidants

D. Regular physical exercise

E. α_2-Agonists

Q13.69

A 22-year-old medical student is pregnant. She sees her obstetrician in the outpatient clinic and would like to know whether the following 'facts' about the circulation of the fetus and changes at birth are correct

A. *In utero*, fetal blood that passes through the right ventricle is diverted from the aorta through the ductus arteriosus to the pulmonary artery

B. The systemic venous return of the fetus is a mixture of oxygentated and deoxygenated blood

C. At birth there is a dramatic increase in pulmonary vascular resistance

D. At birth increased levels of prostaglandins trigger the closure of the patent ductus arteriosus

E. In the fetus both the left and right heart propel blood from the systemic arteries to the systemic veins

Q13.70

The student technician in the cardiac catheterization laboratory is trying to understand the cardiac cycle. She would like to know whether the following facts are correct

A. Right ventricular contraction oocurs shortly before left ventricular contraction

B. The tricuspid valve closes just before the mitral valve

C. There is no change in the volume of the ventricles during systole until the aortic and pulmonary valves open

D. The mitral and triscupid valves open after the ventricular pressures exceed the right and left atrial pressures

E. Isovolumetric relaxation of the ventricles occurs just before the closure of the aortic and pulmonary valves

Q13.71

Indications for carotid sinus massage include

A. Ventricular tachycardia

B. Ventricular fibrillation

C. Junctional tachycardia

D. To reveal on the ECG the P wave pattern of an atrial arrhythmia by reducing the frequency of AV nodal conduction during the tachycardia

E. To test for carotid sinus hypersensitivity

Q13.72

A 37-year-old asthmatic complains of palpitations. His ECG was correctly diagnosed by the emergency department physician to be narrow complex tachycardia. The following treatments can be used in this patient

A. Intravenous adenosine

B. Carotid sinus massage

C. Intravenous verapamil

D. Intravenous esmolol

E. Intravenous lidocaine (lignocaine)

D. Mutation in fibrillin gene

E. Retinal detachment

Q13.73

A 45-year-old woman has a corrected QT interval of 0.48 seconds. She develops a polymorphic ventricular tachyarrhythmia. The following can precipitate this arrhythmia

A. Hypokalaemia

B. Erythromycin

C. Cisapride

D. Terfenadine

E. Chlorpromazine

Q13.74

Intra-aortic balloon pulsation is indicated in the following situations

A. Patient with severe mitral regurgitation and an ejection fraction of 10% awaiting mitral valve surgery

B. Patient with severe aortic valve regurgitation with an ejection fraction of 10% awaiting aortic valve surgery

C. Patient with aortic dissection and hypotension awaiting repair of the aorta

D. Patient with unstable angina refractory to medical therapy awaiting coronary artery bypass grafting

E. Patient with haemodynamic instability due to a ventricular septal defect following myocardial infarction awaiting cardiac surgery

Q13.75

A 45-year-old man is seen in clinic. He has a tall, thin body with long arms, legs and fingers. He has scoliosis and pectus carinatum. Recognized features of this condition include

A. Mitral valve prolapse

B. Aortic aneurysm

C. Dislocated lenses

Q13.76

A 33-year-old woman has a tall, thin body with long arms and legs. She has scoliosis and a pectus deformity. She has a family history of aortic dissection. Her aortic root diameter is 3.9 cm. She has hypermobile joints. The following statements regarding her management are correct

A. Beta-blockade therapy is recommended

B. She should avoid pregnancy

C. She should be monitored with echocardiograms every 5 years

D. Elective aortic root replacement is recommended at a diameter of 5 cm even if she is asymptomatic

E. The patient wishes to do cross-country running and she should not be discouraged

Q13.77

A 28-year-old woman complains of pleuritic chest pain which began suddenly 3 days ago. She is now breathless and woke up this morning with haemoptysis. She is seen in the accident and emergency department. The physician may be able to elicit the following clinical signs

A. Tachypnoea

B. Pleural rub

C. Crackles

D. Stony dull note over the affected area

E. Fever

Q13.78

A 28-year-old woman complains of pleuritic chest pain which began suddenly 3 days ago. She is now breathless and woke up this morning with haemoptysis. She is seen in the accident and emergency department.

Cardiovascular disease

The physician can expect the following from the results of the investigations

A. Chest X-ray usually shows wedge-shaped pulmonary infarcts
B. ECG is usually normal
C. If plasma D-dimer is undetectable, it excludes a diagnosis of pulmonary embolism
D. A ventilation/perfusion scan which shows a ventilation defect with normally perfused area is highly suggestive of pulmonary embolus
E. Spiral chest CT with intravenous contrast is useful to exclude emboli in small pulmonary arteries

---

Q13.79

A 48-year-old man, 3 days after abdominal surgery, has acute central chest pain. He is pale and hypotensive and the jugular venous pressure is raised with prominent 'a' wave. He has a right ventricular heave, a gallop rhythm and a widely split second heart sound. Clinical examination of the chest reveals no abnormal signs. The following may occur

A. The ECG shows tall peaked T waves in lead II
B. Plasma D-dimer is undetectable
C. The ECG shows S wave in lead I, a Q wave in lead III and an inverted T wave in lead III
D. ECG shows right axis deviation, incomplete right bundle branch block and T wave inversion in right precordial leads
E. Blood gases show hypocapnia

Q13.80

A 35-year-old rugby player loses consciousness and dies suddenly while playing a game. The following conditions could be the cause of his sudden death

A. Acute myocardial infarction
B. Hypertrophic cardiomyopathy
C. Ischaemic cardiomyopathy
D. Idiopathic cardiomyopathy
E. Aortic stenosis

Q13.81

A 35-year-old woman develops flash pulmonary oedema at the end of the second trimester of her pregnancy. A Doppler echocardiogram confirms pure mitral stenosis. The patient has searched the internet and has a list of complications and would like to check the accuracy of the information. The following are recognized complications of this condition

A. Left ventricular systolic dysfunction
B. Left ventricular diastolic dysfunction
C. Atrial fibrillation
D. Pulmonary hypertension
E. Right ventricular failure

Q13.82

A 67-year-old patient has a history of mitral stenosis. The doctor can expect to detect the following signs

A. A holosystolic murmur at the apex radiating to the axilla
B. Tapping apex beat
C. Opening snap
D. Malar flush
E. Loud second aortic second heart sound

Q13.83

A 45-year-old is found to have severe mitral stenosis. The following signs detected by the cardiologist are indicators of the severity of mitral stenosis

A. Loud mid-diastolic murmur
B. Graham Steell murmur
C. Closeness of the opening snap to the first heart sound

D. Heaving apex beat
E. 'Rumbling' quality of mid-diastolic murmur

Q13.84

A 55-year-old bus driver develops an acute ST elevation myocardial infarction. His ejection fraction is 0.30. The following recommendations, prescribed by the doctor on discharge, are correct

A. Beta-blockers should be prescribed as they reduce the incidence of sudden death
B. The patient should undergo symptom-limited treadmill exercise testing 6 weeks post-infarction
C. Aspirin should be continued indefinitely
D. ACE inhibitors should be continued indefinitely
E. The patient cannot drive his car for 3 months

Q13.85

A 52-year-old patient undergoes exercise testing because he has central chest pain which occurs sometimes at rest and at other times on exertion. He also has a family history of heart disease. The following statements about exercise testing are true

A. ST segment depression of ≥1 mm suggests myocardial ischaemia, particularly if typical chest pain occurs at the same time
B. A positive test (within 6 minutes of starting the Bruce protocol) helps to identify patients who should be considered for coronary angiography
C. A normal test excludes coronary artery disease
D. About half of the patients with positive exercise tests are subsequently found to have no evidence of coronary artery disease (so-called false-positive test) and

the patient should be reassured regarding this
E. Exercise testing is not indicated for this patient and the patient should have undergone emergency coronary angiography

Q13.86

A 68-year-old woman with a past history of breast cancer and severe reactive airways disease has chronic stable angina pectoris. Drugs which can be safely used to control her angina include

A. High dose metoprolol
B. High dose nifedipine
C. Slow release amlodipine
D. Hormone replacement therapy
E. Nicorandil

Q13.87

A 37-year-old patient had an inferior wall myocardial infarction about 4 hours ago. His past history includes myocardial infarction of the anterior wall 2 days ago and myocardial infarction in the circumflex territory about 3 months ago. He dies in the coronary care unit within hours of admission and undergoes autopsy. The pathology house officer writes the preliminary report and is awaiting the final approval. The patient's history correlates with the following findings of the house officer

A. The occlusive thrombus in the coronary artery has a platelet-rich core
B. The inferior myocardium is swollen and pale
C. The anterior myocardium is necrotic tissue which is deep red
D. The myocardium supplied by the circumflex is thin and has a fibrous scar
E. The occclusive thrombus in the coronary artery has a fibrin-rich cortex

Cardiovascular disease

A13.1

B

The BENESTENT study demonstrated that percutaneous transluminal coronary angioplasty (PTCA) plus stent implantation is significantly better than PTCA alone in terms of death, myocardial infarction, occurrence of cerebrovascular accident, the need for coronary artery bypass grafting (CABG) or a repeat percutaneous intervention. There are two principal indications for coronary artery bypass grafting. The first is symptom control in patients who remain symptomatic despite optimal medical therapy and whose disease is not suitable for PTCA. Surgery provides dramatic relief from angina in about 90% of cases. The second is improved survival in patients with severe three-vessel coronary artery disease (significant proximal stenoses in all three main coronary vessels), particularly those with impaired left ventricular function, and in those with left main stem artery disease. These patients obtain prognostic benefit from CABG, irrespective of symptoms. Several studies have compared PTCA with bypass surgery. Both techniques provide excellent symptomatic relief with a similar incidence of major ischaemic complications. The major short-term advantage of PTCA is the avoidance of major open-heart surgery (and a shorter hospital stay). However, up to 50% of patients will require a repeat revascularization procedure within the next 2 years. There is some evidence that diabetic patients have a better 5-year survival after treatment with bypass surgery than with PTCA. Some patients remain symptomatic despite medication and are not suitable for (further) revascularization. Transmyocardial laser revascularization (TMR), whereby a laser is used to form channels in the myocardium to allow direct perfusion of the myocardium from blood within the ventricular cavity, has been used in some centres but in controlled trials it has not been beneficial. Spinal cord stimulation (SCS) is accomplished using a flexible electrode in the epidural space at the mid-thoracic level. Stimulation via a pacemaker-like generator reduces angina and has been shown to reduce indices of ischaemia. Similarly, transcutaneous electrical nerve stimulation has been shown to reduce angina and increase exercise capacity in selected patients.

A13.2

B

In terms of the short-term risk of death or myocardial infarction, it is possible to risk-stratify patients with unstable angina into high risk, intermediate risk and low risk. Those at high risk should proceed promptly to angiography with a view to proceeding to revascularization, when appropriate, during that admission. Those at low risk can be discharged and then assessed electively as outpatients. In between, there is much controversy regarding the optimal management of patients at intermediate risk, and in particular those who settle on initial medical therapy. Thrombolytic therapy has not been shown to be of benefit in patients with unstable angina.

A13.3

D

A small ventricular septal defect (VSD) ('maladie de Roger') presents with a loud and sometimes long systolic murmur in an asymptomatic patient. Such VSDs usually close spontaneously, with 90% no longer patent by 10 years of age. A small VSD produces no abnormal X-ray or ECG findings.

A13.4

C

Large, asymptomatic aneurysms should also be treated surgically (except in patients with severe comorbid disease) because those larger than 5 cm diameter have a high risk of rupture. Follow-up with ultrasound is required with small aneurysms and surgery offered when the aneurysm reaches 5 cm.

A13.5

C

Peak oxygen consumption (Vo_2 max) is a strong independent predictor of hospital admission and death in patients with heart failure but is not widely available. Serum brain natriuretic peptide (BNP) levels are over 70% sensitive and specific for detecting left ventricular systolic dysfunction. An ejection fraction of <0.45 is generally accepted as evidence for systolic dysfunction.

A13.6

E

In aortic dissection the major symptom is severe and central chest pain, often radiating to the back. The pain radiates down the arms and into the neck and can be difficult to distinguish from myocardial infarction. On examination, the patient is usually shocked and there may be neurological signs owing to the involvement of the spinal vessels or carotid arteries. The peripheral pulses may be absent, but this is not invariable. Half of the patients are hypertensive and this

should be controlled immediately. The diagnosis is suggested by the presence of back pain in addition to chest pain. The chest X-ray may show a wide mediastinum, and CT scanning and ultrasonography with transoesophageal echocardiography (if available) are diagnostic. MRI is highly accurate and is the gold standard. Aortography is now rarely necessary to confirm the diagnosis.

A13.7

C

All adults should have blood pressure measured routinely at least every 5 years.

A13.8

D

An association between diabetes and hypertension has long been recognized, but more recently a syndrome has been described of hyperinsulinaemia, glucose intolerance, reduced levels of high-density lipoprotein (HDL) cholesterol, hypertriglyceridaemia and central obesity (all of which are related to insulin resistance) in association with hypertension. This association (also called the 'metabolic syndrome' or 'syndrome X') is a major risk factor for cardiovascular disease.

A13.9

B

Fundoscopy is an essential part of the examination of any hypertensive patient. The abnormalities are graded according to the Keith–Wagener classification:

Grade 1 – tortuosity of the retinal arteries with increased reflectiveness (silver wiring)

Cardiovascular disease

Grade 2 – grade 1 plus the appearance of arteriovenous nipping produced when thickened retinal arteries pass over the retinal veins

Grade 3 – grade 2 plus flame-shaped haemorrhages and soft ('cotton wool') exudates actually due to small infarcts

Grade 4 – grade 3 plus papilloedema (blurring of the margins of the optic disc)

Grades 3 and 4 are diagnostic of malignant hypertension.

A13.10

C

In the Framingham study, hypertensives had a sixfold increase in stroke (both haemorrhagic and atherothrombotic) compared with normotensives. In the same study, there was a threefold increase in cardiac death (due either to coronary events or to cardiac failure). Furthermore, peripheral arterial disease was twice as common in hypertensives.

A13.11

B

This patient has chronic cor pulmonale due to chronic obstructive pulmonary disease (COPD). Diuretic treatment may be used for right ventricular failure, but care should be taken to avoid excessive fluid depletion as this will result in reduced output from the impaired right ventricle. Hypoxia is avoided by the use of oxygen therapy when safe and necessary. In those with COPD and some others, long-term oxygen therapy (LTOT) improves symptoms and prognosis. In contrast to their enormous value in those with left ventricular impairment, angiotensin-converting enzyme inhibitors are seldom useful and may make matters worse.

A13.12

C

Treatment of sustained ventricular tachycardia may be urgent, depending on the haemodynamic situation. If the patient is haemodynamically compromised (e.g. hypotensive or pulmonary oedema) emergency DC cardioversion must be considered. On the other hand, if the blood pressure and cardiac output are well maintained, intravenous therapy with class I drugs or amiodarone is usually advised. First-line drug treatment consists of amiodarone (300 mg over 1 h) followed by 900 mg amiodarone (900 mg over 23 h). DC cardioversion may be necessary if medical therapy is unsuccessful.

A13.13

D

This patient probably has an aortic dissection which is a surgical emergency. Transoesophageal views are particularly suitable for detecting pathology in the ascending and descending aorta. In many hospitals this is the investigation of first choice when aortic dissection is suspected. Magnetic resonance imaging (MRI) or computed tomography (CT) may also be used as an investigation of first choice. 24-hour ambulatory taped electrocardiography is recorded generally when tachy- or bradyarrhythmias are suspected. Although transthoracic echocardiography may detect aortic dissection it is not sensitive for aortic dissection. Carotid sinus massage is only done when carotid sinus hypersensitivity is suspected.

A 13.14

B

The PR interval is the length of time from the start of the P wave to the start of the QRS complex. It is the time taken for activation to pass from the sinus node, through the atrium, AV node and the His–Purkinje system to the ventricle. The P wave is caused by atrial depolarization. The QRS complex reflects ventricular activation or depolarization and is sharper and larger in amplitude than the P wave. The QT interval extends from the start of the QRS complex to the end of the T wave. This interval represents the time taken to depolarize and repolarize the ventricular myocardium. The ST segment is the period between the end of the QRS complex and the start of the T wave. In the normal heart, all cells are depolarized by this phase of the ECG, i.e. the ST segment represents ventricular repolarization.

A 13.15

C

'Starling's law of the heart' or the 'Frank–Starling relationship' is described in the intact heart as an increase of stroke volume (ventricular performance) with an enlargement of the diastolic volume (preload). It has been transcribed into more clinically relevant indices. Thus, stroke work (aortic pressure × stroke volume) is increased as ventricular end-diastolic volume is raised. Alternatively, within certain limits, cardiac output rises as pulmonary capillary wedge pressure increases.

A 13.16

E

The increase in heart rate on exercise in a healthy adult begins at the heart's natural pacemaker – the sinoatrial node. This is a crescent-shaped structure that is located around the medial and anterior aspect of the junction between the superior vena cava and the right atrium. Progressive loss of the diastolic resting membrane potential is followed, when the threshold potential has been reached, by a more rapid depolarization of the sinus node tissue. This depolarization triggers successively depolarization of the atrial myocardium, atrioventricular node, the His bundle, the right and left bundle and the ventricle. Impulse conduction through the atrioventricular node is slow and depends on action potentials largely produced by slow transmembrane calcium flux. In the atria, ventricles and His–Purkinje system conduction is rapid and is due to action potentials generated by rapid transmembrane sodium diffusion.

A 13.17

B

The mitogen-activated protein (MAP) kinases are a family of serine–threonine kinases involved in numerous types of intracellular signalling. Mammalian MAP kinases can be divided into three families according to their structure and function: a) the extracellular signal-regulated kinases (ERK-1 and 2) are related to promotion of cell growth in response to growth factor receptor activation; b) the c-Jun N-terminal kinase/stress-activated protein kinases (JNK/SAPK), whose activation is associated with arrest of cell growth and apoptosis; and c) the p38 kinase, activation of which is associated with apoptosis in a variety of cell systems and may be related to JNK/SAPK activation. cAMP kinase and troponin kinase are not MAP kinases.

A13.18

E

The right coronary artery arises from the right coronary sinus and courses through the right side of the atrioventricular groove, giving off vessels that supply the right atrium and the right ventricle. The vessel usually continues as the posterior descending coronary artery, which runs in the posterior interventricular groove and supplies the posterior part of the interventricular septum and the posterior left ventricular wall. The left main coronary divides into the left anterior descending artery and the circumflex artery. The left anterior descending artery runs in the anterior interventricular groove and supplies the anterior septum and the anterior left ventricular wall. The left circumflex artery travels along the left atrioventricular groove and gives off branches to the left atrium and the left ventricle (marginal branches). ECG changes are usually confined to the ECG leads that 'face' the infarction. Therefore, an inferior wall myocardial infarction (MI) is diagnosed when the ECG findings are seen in leads II, III and AVF. Lateral infarction produces changes in leads I, AVL and $V_{5/6}$. In anterior infarction, leads V_2–V_5 may be affected. Because there are no posterior leads, a true posterior wall infarct is usually diagnosed by the appearance of a mirror image or reciprocal changes in leads V_1 and V_2 (i.e. the development of a tall initial R wave, ST segment depression and tall, upright T waves). These reciprocal changes can also be seen in association with other infarctions. For example, in an inferior wall myocardial infarction, anterior ST segment depression may be seen. In right ventricular infarction the ST segment is raised in lead V_4R.

A13.19

D

The patient has angina following myocardial infarction and the investigation of choice in such instances is coronary angiography.

A13.20

D

The implantable cardiac defibrillator (ICD) is superior to all other treatment options at preventing sudden cardiac death. The use of this device has cut the sudden death rate in patients with a history of serious ventricular arrhythmias to approximately 2% per year. However, the majority of these patients have significant structural heart disease and overall cardiac mortality due to progressive heart failure remains high. Large multicentred prospective trials such as the Antiarrhythmics (amiodarone) Versus Implantable Defibrillator (AVID) trial have proven that implantable defibrillators improve overall survival in patients who have experienced an episode of life-threatening ventricular tachyarrhythmia. As a result ICDs are now first-line therapy in the secondary prevention of sudden death.

A13.21

B

Contraindications for cardiac transplantation
Age > 60 years (some variations between centres)
Alcohol/drug abuse
Uncontrolled psychiatric illness
Uncontrolled infection
Severe renal/liver failure
High pulmonary vascular resistance
Systemic disease with multiorgan involvement
Treated cancer in remission but with < 5 years' follow-up
Recent thromboembolism
Other disease with a poor prognosis

There are specific contraindications to cardiac transplantation (see table); notably, high pulmonary vascular resistance is an absolute contraindication.

A13.22

E

The diagnosis of angina is largely based on the clinical history. The chest pain is generally described as 'heavy', 'tight' or 'gripping'. Typically, the pain is central/retrosternal and may radiate to the jaw and/or arms. Angina can range from a mild ache to a most severe pain that provokes sweating and fear. Classical or exertional angina pectoris is provoked by physical exertion, especially after meals and in cold, windy weather, and is commonly aggravated by anger or excitement. The pain fades quickly (usually within minutes) with rest. Occasionally it disappears with continued exertion ('walking through the pain'). While in some patients the pain occurs predictably at a certain level of exertion, in most patients the threshold for developing pain is variable. Variant (Prinzmetal's) angina refers to an angina that occurs

without provocation, usually at rest, as a result of coronary artery spasm. It occurs more frequently in women. Characteristically, there is ST segment elevation during the pain. Cardiac syndrome X refers to those patients with a good history of angina, a positive exercise test and angiographically normal coronary arteries. Unstable angina refers to angina of recent onset (less than 1 month), worsening angina or angina at rest.

A13.23

C

'Silent' myocardial infarctions (MI) are more common in diabetics and the elderly, and as many as 20% of patients with MI have no pain. Diagnosis requires at least two of the following: a) a history of ischaemic-type chest pain; b) evolving ECG changes; c) a rise in cardiac enzymes or troponins. ECG changes are usually confined to the ECG leads that 'face' the infarction. Therefore, an inferior wall MI is diagnosed when the ECG findings are seen in leads II, III and AVF. Lateral infarction produces changes in leads I, AVL and $V_{5/6}$. In anterior infarction, leads V_2–V_5 may be affected. Reciprocal changes can also be seen. For example, in an inferior wall myocardial infarction, anterior ST segment depression may be seen. In right ventricular infarction the ST segment is raised in lead V_4R.

A13.24

C

If the diagnosis of myocardial infarction is suspected, an ECG should be obtained immediately. If diagnostic ST elevation is present, thrombolysis should be commenced without delay (unless contraindicated). Contraindications

Cardiovascular disease

include stroke or active bleeding in the last 2 months, systolic blood pressure >200 mmHg, proliferative diabetic retinopathy and pregnancy. An increasing number of interventional centres are performing 'primary PTCA' – immediate cardiac catheterization and percutaneous transluminal coronary angioplasty – in patients with evolving myocardial infarction. Primary PTCA is indicated when thrombolysis is contraindicated. Intravenous nitrates and morphine are also given, but for pain not for reperfusion.

A13.25

C

When the normal valve orifice area of 5 cm^2 is reduced to approximately 1 cm^2, severe mitral stenosis is present. Usually there are no symptoms until the valve orifice is moderately stenosed (i.e. has an area of 2 cm^2). In Europe this does not usually occur until several decades after the first attack of rheumatic fever, but children of 10–20 years of age in the Middle or Far East may have severe calcific mitral stenosis.

A13.26

1) A   2) D   3) E   4) G   5) H
6) O   7) N   8) K

The New York Heart Association functional and therapeutic classification applied to dyspnoea

Grade 1 No breathlessness
Grade 2 Breathlessness on severe exertion
Grade 3 Breathlessness on mild exertion
Grade 4 Breathlessness at rest

Dyspnoea is an abnormal awareness of breathlessness, and can be due to cardiac or respiratory causes. It can occur on exertion or may be present at rest. The New York Heart Association has graded this symptom (see table). Paroxysmal nocturnal dyspnoea (PND) occurs when there is an accumulation of fluid in the lungs (pulmonary oedema) at night. The patient is woken from sleep fighting for breath, a dramatic and frightening experience. Sitting on the side of the bed or getting up may relieve the breathlessness. Sometimes the patient will get up and open a window to gasp for fresh air. In very severe heart failure, alternate hyperventilation and apnoea known as Cheyne–Stokes respiration may occur. This may also develop in the elderly without obvious heart failure. Angina pectoris literally means a strangling sensation (angina) in the chest (pectoris). It is a gripping or crushing central chest pain (or discomfort) that may be felt around the whole chest or deep within the chest. The pain may radiate into the neck or jaw and, rarely, into the teeth, back or abdomen. It is associated with heaviness, paraesthesia or pain in one (usually the left) or both arms. It is typically provoked by exercise and is promptly relieved by rest. Angina of increasing frequency, or coming on at rest or unpredictably is called unstable (or crescendo) angina. The pain of pericarditis is felt in the centre of the chest and, like that of pleurisy, is aggravated by movement, posture, respiration and coughing, but may be relieved by sitting forwards. It is sharp and severe. Central chest pain that radiates to the back is characteristic of a dissecting or enlarging aortic aneurysm and can mimic the pain of myocardial infarction. Supraventricular tachycardias, such as atrial fibrillation or junctional tachycardias, may produce polyuria. A Stokes–Adams attack is due to a disturbance of cardiac rhythm (e.g. a profound bradycardia related to complete heart block). Without warning, the patient falls to the ground, pale and deeply unconscious. The pulse is usually very slow or absent. After a few seconds the patient flushes brightly and recovers consciousness as the pulse quickens.

A13.27

1) G 2) A 3) F 4) D 5) E 6) C

Pulsus bisferiens is found in hypertrophic obstructive cardiomyopathy and in mixed aortic valve disease (regurgitation combined with stenosis). Alternating pulse (pulsus alternans) is characterized by regular alternate beats that are weak and strong. It is a feature of severe myocardial failure and is due to the prolonged recovery time of damaged myocardium; it indicates a very poor prognosis. Paradoxical pulse is a misnomer as it is actually an exaggeration of the normal pattern. In normal subjects, the systolic pressure and the pulse pressure (the difference between the systolic and diastolic blood pressures) fall during inspiration. In patients with cardiac tamponade, the fluid in the pericardium increases the intrapericardial pressure, thereby impeding diastolic filling of the heart. The normal inspiratory increase in venous return to the right ventricle is at the expense of the left ventricle, as both ventricles are confined by the accumulated pericardial fluid within the pericardial space. Carotid pulsations are not normally apparent on inspection of the neck but may be visible (Corrigan's sign) in conditions associated with a large-volume pulse, including high output states (such as thyrotoxicosis, anaemia or fever) and in aortic regurgitation. Irregularly irregular pattern of pulse in which no pattern is recognizable occurs in atrial fibrillation.

A13.28

1) D 2) B 3) E 4) A 5) C

The jugular venous pressure wave consists of three peaks and two troughs. The peaks are described as *a*, *c* and *v* waves and the troughs are known as *x* and *y* descents. Large *a* waves are caused by increased resistance to ventricular filling, as seen with right ventricular hypertrophy due to pulmonary hypertension or pulmonary stenosis. A very large *a* wave occurs when the atrium contracts against a closed tricuspid valve; this is known as a 'cannon wave'. Tricuspid regurgitation results in giant *v* waves (systolic waves) because the right ventricular pressure is transmitted directly to the right atrium and the great veins. Steep *y* descent or diastolic collapse of elevated venous pressure can occur in right ventricular failure but is more dramatic in constrictive pericarditis and tricuspid regurgitation. The *a* wave is produced by atrial systole and hence is absent in atrial fibrillation.

A13.29

1) E 2) D 3) C 4) B 5) A

The apex beat is normally just palpable and confined to a point that can be covered by one finger. There are several abnormal forms. a) Tapping is a sudden but brief cardiac impulse felt in mitral stenosis. This suggests that the anterior mitral valve leaflet is pliable. b) Heaving (sustained) is a vigorous and sustained pulsation due to 'pressure overload' as in aortic stenosis and systemic hypertension. There is often confusion about the terms thrusting and heaving. c) An impalpable apex occurs in emphysema, pleural effusion, obesity and pericardial effusion. d) Double pulsation – two apical pulsations with each heartbeat – may be felt in hypertrophic cardiomyopathy. This may be due to a palpable atrial impulse. A double apex can also be due to accentuated outward movement in late systole in a ventricular aneurysm. A sustained parasternal impulse (heave) is elicited by pressing the outstretched hand flat against the sternum or against the costal cartilages just to the left of the sternum. It occurs because of right ventricular hypertrophy due to pulmonary hypertension.

A13.30

1) G   2) H or C   3) F   4) E   5) D
6) C   7) A   8) B

The second heart sound is caused by the closure of the aortic and pulmonary valves. Splitting of the second heart sound on inspiration is known as normal or physiological splitting and is most commonly heard in children or young adults. Reversed splitting of the second heart sound (when the aortic component follows the pulmonary component) is more marked on expiration. It is due to a delay in left heart emptying caused by aortic stenosis, left bundle branch block or left ventricular failure. Thus, when right heart emptying is delayed during inspiration, the two sounds move together, and when the right heart empties more quickly during expiration, the sounds move apart. Wide splitting of the second heart sound is characteristic of conditions associated with delayed emptying of the right ventricle such as right bundle branch block or pulmonary stenosis. The second heart sound is also widely split in the presence of an uncomplicated atrial septal defect due to shunting of blood from the left to the right heart (and the presence of some degree of right bundle branch block in many cases). In such circumstances, the widely split second heart sound is also fixed owing to respiratory variation in

shunting at the atrial level which counterbalances the normal respiratory variation in systemic venous return responsible for physiological splitting. The aortic second sound is louder in systemic hypertension and when a hyperdynamic circulation is present. It is soft in aortic stenosis because the valve is relatively immobile, and it is soft in cardiac failure because of low blood flow. Similarly, the pulmonary component of the second heart sound is loud in pulmonary hypertension and soft in pulmonary stenosis.

Third and fourth heart sounds are additional diastolic heart sounds. The presence of a third or fourth sound produces a triple rhythm that, when associated with sinus tachycardia, sounds like a galloping horse – a gallop rhythm. A third heart sound is heard immediately after the second heart sound during the early, passive filling phase of ventricular diastole. This is due to rapid ventricular filling as soon as the mitral and tricuspid valves open. It is a normal finding in children and young adults when it is heard at the apex, especially in the left lateral position. In those over 40 years it represents heart failure or volume overload, for example due to mitral regurgitation. A fourth heart sound is heard immediately before the first sound and is associated with atrial contraction during the late, active filling phase of ventricular diastole. This is caused by the surge of ventricular filling that accompanies atrial systole. It may be a normal finding in an elderly subject, but in younger patients it usually indicates increased ventricular stiffness associated with hypertension, aortic stenosis or acute myocardial infarction. An ejection click occurs immediately after the first heart sound and is produced by the sudden opening of a deformed but mobile aortic or pulmonary valve. It is most commonly heard in association with a bicuspid aortic valve when it is easily heard throughout the respiratory cycle. A stenotic mitral or tricuspid valve may produce a high-frequency opening snap that occurs just after the second heart sound. It can be distinguished from a split second sound or a third sound by the site at which it is best heard, its higher frequency and its lack of respiratory variation.

A13.31

1) E   2) A   3) B   4) D

Heart murmurs are caused by turbulent blood flow. Systolic murmurs occur synchronously with carotid pulsation. There are three main varieties of pathological systolic murmur. a) Ejection mid-systolic murmurs are heard separately from the first and second heart sounds. Their intensity rises then falls, being greatest in mid-systole e.g. aortic stenosis, pulmonary stenosis. b) Pansystolic murmurs extend from the first to the second heart sound and tend to be of constant intensity throughout the whole of systole, e.g. mitral regurgitation, tricuspid regurgitation, ventricular septal defect. c) Late systolic murmurs are separated from the first sound but extend up to the second sound. Diastolic murmurs are always associated with cardiac disease. They are of two types. a) Mid-diastolic murmurs usually arise from the mitral and tricuspid valves. In aortic regurgitation the flow of blood back into the left ventricle may partially close and obstruct the mitral valve, producing a mitral mid-diastolic murmur (Austin Flint murmur). b) Early diastolic murmurs usually result from aortic regurgitation and rarely from pulmonary regurgitation. These murmurs begin with the second heart sound and are

blowing (high-pitched) in quality. Pulmonary hypertension secondary to mitral stenosis may lead to pulmonary valve regurgitation (Graham Steell murmur). A continuous murmur may occur because of a combination of systolic and diastolic murmurs, owing to connections between the aorta and pulmonary artery (e.g. in patent ductus arteriosus) or owing to arteriovenous anastomoses and collateral circulations (such as those associated with coarctation of the aorta). High venous flow, especially in young children, can produce a continuous venous hum in the neck. This is reduced by occluding the vein or by laying the child flat. Similarly, high mammary blood flow in pregnant or lactating women can produce a continuous murmur known as a 'mammary souffle'. A pericardial friction rub is a scratching or crunching noise produced by the movement of inflamed pericardium. Since it is relatively high frequency, it is best heard with the diaphragm. It is most obvious in systole but may also be heard in early diastole or synchronously with atrial contraction. It should be listened for during both held inspiration and expiration.

A13.32

A) F   B) T   C) T   D) T   E) F

Ventricular fibrillation is readily treated with defibrillation (initially 200 J is used for defibrillation), antiarrhythmic drugs and adrenaline (epinephrine). Antiarrhythmic drugs, which are routinely employed, include intravenous lidocaine (lignocaine) and amiodarone. A bolus dose of intravenous amiodarone may be of benefit in refractory VF/VT. Asystole is more difficult to treat but the heart may respond to atropine or

Cardiovascular disease

adrenaline (epinephrine). If there is any sign of slow electromechanical activity (e.g. bradycardia with a weak pulse), emergency pacing should be used. Transcutaneous pacing may be life-saving for patients in whom a cardiac arrest is precipitated by bradycardia. Toxic levels of cardiodepressant drugs, such as beta-blockers, may cause electromechanical dissociation, nowadays referred to as pulseless electrical activity (PEA).

A13.33

1) C   2) D   3) A   4) E   5) D
6) B   7) F

Acclerated automaticity is thought to produce sinus tachycardia, escape rhythms and accelerated atrioventricular (AV) nodal (junctional) rhythms. The atrial tachycardias produced by digoxin toxicity are due to triggered activity. The initiation of ventricular arrhythmia in the long QT syndrome may be caused by this mechanism. The majority of regular paroxysmal tachycardias are produced by re-entry or circus movements. Sinus bradycardia is a result of abnormally slow automaticity while bradycardia due to AV block is caused by abnormal conduction within the AV node or the distal AV conduction system. Mobitz I block (Wenckebach block phenomenon) is progressive PR interval prolongation until a P wave fails to conduct. The PR interval before the blocked P wave is much longer than the PR interval after the blocked P wave. Mobitz II block occurs when a dropped QRS complex is not preceded by progressive PR interval prolongation. Wenckebach AV block is due to block in the AV node whereas Mobitz II block signifies block at an infranodal level such as the His bundle.

A13.34

1) B   2) C   3) A   4) F   5) D
6) G   7) E

Complete heart block occurs when all atrial activity fails to conduct to the ventricles. In this situation, life is maintained by a spontaneous escape rhythm that has either broad (>0.12 s) or narrow (<0.12 s) QRS complexes. If the patient has a narrow complex escape rhythm, it implies that it originates in the His bundle and therefore that the region of block lies more proximally in the atrioventricular (AV) node. If the patient has a broad complex escape rhythm, it implies that the escape rhythm originates below the His bundle and therefore that the region of block lies more distally in the His–Purkinje system. In the elderly, it is usually caused by degenerative fibrosis of the distal conduction system (Lev's disease). In younger patients, broad-complex AV block may be caused by ischaemic heart disease. Right bundle branch block produces late activation of the right ventricle. This is seen as deep S waves in leads I and V_6 and as a tall late R wave in lead V_1. Left bundle branch block produces the opposite – a deep S wave in lead V_1 and a tall late R wave in leads I and V_6. Right bundle branch block and left bundle branch block both produce a broad QRS complex (>0.12 s). Because left bundle branch conduction is normally responsible for the initial ventricular activation, left bundle branch block also produces abnormal Q waves. Delay or block in the divisions of the left bundle branch produces a swing in the direction of depolarization (electrical axis) of the heart. When the anterior division is blocked (left anterior hemiblock), the left ventricle is activated from inferior to superior. This produces a superior and leftwards movement of the axis (left axis deviation). Delay or block in the posteroinferior division swings the QRS axis inferiorly to the right (right axis deviation).

A13.35

1) A   2) B   3) C   4) D   5) G   6) F

Atrioventricular node re-entry tachycardia (AVNRT) is the commonest cause of supraventricular tachycardia (SVT) in patients with structurally normal hearts. Clinically, the tachycardia often strikes suddenly without obvious provocation, but exertion, coffee, tea and alcohol may aggravate or induce the arrhythmia. The rhythm is rapid (140–280 per minute) and regular. An attack may stop spontaneously or may continue indefinitely until medical intervention. The predominant symptom is palpitations, but chest pain, dyspnoea, presyncope and polyuria may develop. The polyuria occurs because tachycardia leads to an elevated atrial pressure and the release of atrial natriuretic peptide and other hormones. The rhythm is recognized on ECG by normal regular QRS complexes usually at a rate of 140–240 per minute. Sometimes the QRS complexes will show typical bundle branch block (aberration). P waves are either not visible or are seen immediately before or after the QRS complex because of simultaneous atrial and ventricular activation. In atrioventricular reciprocating tachycardia (AVRT) there is a large circuit comprising the AV node, the His bundle, the ventricle and an abnormal connection from the ventricle back to the atrium. This abnormal connection consists of myocardial fibres that span the atrioventricular groove and is called an accessory pathway or bypass tract. In contrast to AVNRT, this tachycardia is due to a macro-reentry circuit and each part of

the circuit is activated sequentially. As a result atrial activation occurs after ventricular activation and the P wave is usually clearly seen between the QRS and T complexes. In atrial fibrillation the ECG shows fine oscillations of the baseline (so-called fibrillation or φ waves) and no clear P waves. The QRS rhythm is rapid and irregular. Untreated, the ventricular rate is usually 120–180 per minute, but it slows with treatment. This is a rhythm disturbance that is usually associated with structural heart disease. The atrial rate is usually around 300 per minute. Symptoms are largely related to the degree of AV block. Most often, every second flutter beat conducts, giving a ventricular rate of 150 per minute. Occasionally, every beat conducts, producing a heart rate of 300 b.p.m. More often, especially when patients are receiving treatment, AV conduction block reduces the heart rate to approximately 75 b.p.m. The ECG shows regular sawtooth-like atrial flutter waves (F waves) between QRST complexes. Torsades de pointes arises when ventricular repolarization (QT interval) is greatly prolonged (long QT syndrome). It is characterized on the ECG by rapid, irregular, sharp complexes that continuously change from an upright to an inverted position. Between spells of tachycardia or immediately preceding the onset of tachycardia the ECG shows a prolonged QT interval; the corrected QT is equal to or greater than 0.44 s.

A13.36

1) A   2) B   3) C   4) D   5) E

Vaughan Williams Singh Class Ia drugs (e.g. disopyramide) lengthen the action potential. Class Ib drugs (e.g. lidocaine (lignocaine)) shorten the action potential. Class Ic (flecainide, propafenone) do not

Cardiovascular disease

affect the duration of the action potential. Class III drugs prolong the action potential and do not affect sodium transport through the membrane. The drugs in this class include amiodarone and sotalol. Sotalol is also a beta-blocker. The non-dihydropyridine calcium antagonists that reduce the plateau phase of the action potential are particularly effective at slowing conduction in nodal tissue. Verapamil and diltiazem are two drugs in this group.

13.37

A) T   B) T   C) T   D) T   E) T   F) T

Radiofrequency catheter ablation is frequently employed in the management of symptomatic tachyarrhythmias. Ablations are performed by placing three or four electrode catheters into the heart chambers in order to record and pace from various sites. The following tachyarrhythmias can be readily ablated: a) AV node re-entry tachycardia (AVNRT); b) accessory-pathway-mediated tachycardias; c) AV reciprocating tachycardia (AVRT); d) Wolff–Parkinson–White syndrome; e) normal heart ventricular tachycardia; f) atrial flutter; g) atrial tachycardia.

13.38

A) F   B) F   C) T   D) T   E) T

Pathophysiological changes in heart failure
Ventricular dilatation
Myocyte hypertrophy
Increased collagen synthesis
Altered myosin gene expression
Altered sarcoplasmic Ca^{2+}-ATPase density
Increased ANP secretion
Salt and water retention
Sympathetic stimulation
Peripheral vasoconstriction

When the heart fails, considerable changes occur to the heart and peripheral vascular system in response to the haemodynamic changes associated with heart failure (see table). These physiological changes are compensatory and maintain cardiac output and peripheral perfusion. However, as heart failure progresses, these mechanisms are overwhelmed and become pathophysiological. The development of pathological peripheral vasoconstriction and sodium retention in heart failure by activation of the renin–angiotensin–aldosterone system, is a loss of beneficial compensatory mechanisms and represents cardiac decompensation. Factors involved are venous return, outflow resistance, contractility of the myocardium, and salt and water retention. The sympathetic nervous system is activated in heart failure via baroreceptors as an early compensatory mechanism, which provides inotropic support and maintains cardiac output. The increase in venous pressure that occurs when the ventricles fail leads to retention of salt and water and their accumulation in the interstitium, producing many of the physical signs of heart failure. Collagen synthesis may also be increased. Levels of circulating atrial natriuretic peptide (ANP) are increased in congestive cardiac failure and correlate with functional class, prognosis and haemodynamic state.

13.39

A) F   B) F   C) F   D) T   E) T

Causes of left heart failure include:

- Ischaemic heart disease (the most common cause)

- Systemic hypertension (chronic or 'malignant')

- Mitral and aortic valve disease

- Cardiomyopathies.

Mitral stenosis causes left atrial hypertension and signs of left heart failure but does not itself cause failure of the left ventricle.

Right heart failure occurs in association with:

- Left heart failure

- Chronic lung disease (cor pulmonale)

- Pulmonary embolism or pulmonary hypertension

- Tricuspid valve disease

- Pulmonary valve disease

- Left-to-right shunts (e.g. atrial or ventricular septal defects)

- Isolated right ventricular cardiomyopathy

- Mitral valve disease with pulmonary hypertension.

A13.40

A) T   B) T   C) T   D) T   E) T

Diastolic ventricular dysfunction results from impaired myocardial relaxation, with increased stiffness in the ventricular wall and decreased left ventricular compliance leading to impairment of diastolic ventricular filling and hence decreased cardiac output. Coronary artery disease, hypertension and hypertrophic cardiomyopathy are common causes although infiltrative disease such as amyloid may lead to pure diastolic dysfunction.

A13.41

A) F   B) T   C) F   D) F   E) T

A recent large prospective trial (Digoxin Investigation Group (DIG) trial) showed that digoxin combined with ACE inhibitors and diuretics reduced death and hospitalization resulting from progressive heart failure in patients in sinus rhythm. A significant increase in deaths presumed to be secondary to myocardial infarction and/or arrhythmia meant that the effect on overall mortality was neutral. Spironolactone is a specific competitive antagonist to aldosterone, producing a weak diuresis but with a potassium-sparing action. A randomized placebo-controlled study, the Randomized Aldactone Evaluation Study (RALES) showed a 30% reduction in all cause mortality when spironolactone (up to 25 mg) was added to conventional treatment in patients with moderate to severe heart failure (New York Heart Association class III and IV). However, this study did not study the benefits of spironolactone in New York Heart Association class I and class II congestive heart failure. The studies MERIT and CIBIS 2 using the beta-blockers metoprolol and bisoprolol respectively have shown improved symptomatic class, exercise tolerance, left ventricular function and mortality in patients with heart failure of any cause. The US Carvedilol Studies using carvedilol, a non-selective vasodilator beta-blocker with additional vasodilator and antioxidant properties, has also demonstrated a significant improvement in mortality. Beta-blocker use should be restricted to those with stable heart failure and their introduction should be cautious because of the potential to cause heart failure decompensation. Combination therapy of nitrate with hydralazine (Veterans Heart Failure Trials, VHeFT) has

Cardiovascular disease

been shown to improve mortality and exercise performance, and may be useful when angiotensin-converting enzyme inhibitors (ACEI) are contraindicated. The benefit of vasodilators is not as great as with ACEI (VHeFT 2). Although heart failure symptoms are improved by loop diuretic treatment, loop diuretics are not proven to have any survival benefit.

A13.42

1) E   2) F   3) H   4) A   5) B
6) C   7) D

The intravenous administration of loop diuretics such as furosemide (frusemide) relieves pulmonary oedema rapidly by means of arteriolar vasodilatation reducing afterload, an action that is independent of its diuretic effect. Thiazide diuretics such as bendroflumethiazide (bendrofluazide) have a mild diuretic effect and act on the distal convoluted tubule, reducing sodium reabsorption. Between 10 and 15% of patients on ACE inhibitors develop a cough, owing to the inhibition of bradykinin metabolism. The US Carvedilol Studies using carvedilol, a non-selective vasodilator beta-blocker with additional vasodilator and antioxidant properties, have also demonstrated a significant improvement in mortality. Dobutamine is a selective agonist of the β_1-adrenoceptor, increasing intracellular cyclic AMP, which in turn increases calcium availability for myocardial contraction. Digoxin acts as a positive inotrope by competitive inhibition of Na^+–K^+-ATPase, producing high levels of intracellular sodium. This is then exchanged for extracellular calcium. High levels of intracellular calcium result in enhanced actin–myosin interaction and

increased contractility. Milrinone acts by inhibiting phosphodiesterase, thus preventing breakdown of cyclic AMP. Accumulation of cAMP produces an increase in contractility and peripheral vasodilatation. The Starling curve is shifted upwards.

A13.43

A) T   B) T   C) T   D) T   E) T

The complications of heart transplantation include those related to immunosuppression (infection, malignancy, hypertension and hyperlipidaemia). Allograft coronary atherosclerosis is the major cause of long-term graft failure and is present in 30–50% of patients at 5 years. It is due to a 'vascular' rejection process in conjunction with hypertension and hyperlipidaemia.

A13.44

A) F   B) T   C) T   D) F   E) T

In pulmonary oedema high-concentration oxygen (60% via a variable performance mask) and morphine (10–20 mg i.v. depending on the size of the patient) together with an antiemetic such as metoclopramide (10 mg i.v.) are given. Venous vasodilators, such as glyceryl trinitrate, may produce prompt relief by reducing the preload. Cardiac output may be increased by using arterial vasodilatation, such as occurs with hydralazine but hydralazine is not administered intra-arterially. Aminophylline (250–500 mg or 5 mg/kg i.v.) is infused slowly over 10 minutes.

A13.45

A) T   B) F   C) T   D) T   E) F

Shock is a severe failure of tissue perfusion, usually characterized by hypotension, a low cardiac output and signs of poor tissue perfusion such as oliguria, cold extremities and poor cerebral function. Its most common cause is myocardial infarction (MI) and it complicates up to 10% of MI. Other causes are acute massive pulmonary embolus, pericardial tamponade and sudden-onset valvular regurgitation. In cardiogenic shock the wedge pressure is normal or elevated whereas the wedge pressure is low when there is loss of fluid.

A13.46

A) F   B) T   C) T   D) T   E) T

The development of atherosclerosis begins following endothelial dysfunction, with increased permeability to and accumulation of oxidized lipoproteins, which are taken up by macrophages at focal sites within the endothelium to produce lipid-laden foam cells. Macroscopically, these lesions are seen as flat yellow dots or lines on the endothelium of the artery and are known as 'fatty streaks'. The 'fatty streak' progresses with the appearance of extracellular lipid within the endothelium ('transitional plaque'). Release of cytokines by monocytes, macrophages or the damaged endothelium promotes further accumulation of macrophages as well as smooth muscle cell migration and proliferation. The proliferation of smooth muscle with the formation of a layer of cells covering the extracellular lipid separates it from the adaptive smooth muscle thickening in the endothelium. Collagen is produced in larger and larger quantities by the smooth muscle and the whole sequence of events cumulates as an 'advanced or raised fibrolipid plaque'. The 'advanced plaque' may grow slowly and encroach on the lumen or become unstable, undergo thrombosis and produce an obstruction ('complicated plaque').

Two different mechanisms are responsible for thrombosis on the plaques. The first process is superficial endothelial injury, which involves denudation of the endothelial covering over the plaque. Subendocardial connective tissue matrix is then exposed and platelet adhesion occurs because of reaction with collagen. The thrombus is adherent to the surface of the plaque. The second process is deep endothelial fissuring, which involves an advanced plaque with a lipid core. The plaque cap tears (ulcerates, fissures or ruptures), allowing blood from the lumen to enter the inside of the plaque itself. The core with lamellar lipid surfaces, tissue factor (which triggers platelet adhesion and activation) produced by macrophages and exposed collagen, is highly thrombogenic. Thrombus forms within the plaque, expanding its volume and distorting its shape. Thrombosis may then extend into the lumen.

A 50% reduction in luminal diameter (producing a reduction in luminal cross-sectional area of approximately 70%) causes a haemodynamically significant stenosis. At this point the smaller distal intramyocardial arteries and arterioles are maximally dilated (coronary flow reserve is near zero), and any increase in myocardial oxygen demand provokes ischaemia.

Cardiovascular disease

A13.47

A) T   B) T   C) F   D) F   E) T

Risk factors for coronary disease

Fixed
Age
Male sex
Positive family history
Deletion polymorphism in the ACE gene (DD)

Potentially changeable with treatment
Hyperlipidaemia
Cigarette smoking
Hypertension
Diabetes mellitus
Lack of exercise
Blood coagulation factors – high fibrinogen, factor VII
C-reactive protein
Homocysteinaemia
Personality
Obesity
Gout
Soft water
Contraceptive pill
Heavy alcohol consumption

ACE, angiotensin-converting enzyme

The aetiology of coronary artery disease (CAD) is multifactorial, and a number of 'risk' factors are known to predispose to the condition (see table). Some of these – such as age, gender, race and family history – cannot be changed, whereas other major risk factors, such as serum cholesterol, smoking habits, diabetes and hypertension, can be modified. However, not all patients with myocardial infarction are identified by these risk factors. High plasma lipoprotein (a) (Lp(a)) concentrations are associated with CAD and, although probably not an independent risk factor, elevated plasma Lp(a) increases the CAD risk associated with more traditional risk factors. Obesity, particularly central obesity, is associated with CAD, but it is not certain whether obesity itself is independently linked to the condition. Serum fibrinogen is strongly, consistently and independently related to CAD risk.

A13.48

1) A   2) G   3) F   4) I or H   5) J
6) N   7) K   8) L   9) E   10) B

Ventricular extrasystoles. These commonly occur after myocardial infarction (MI). Their occurrence may precede the development of ventricular fibrillation, particularly if they are frequent (more than five per minute), multiform (different shapes) or R-on-T (falling on the upstroke or peak of the preceding T wave). Treatment has not been shown to reduce the likelihood of subsequent ventricular tachycardia or fibrillation.

Sustained ventricular tachycardia. This may degenerate into ventricular fibrillation or may itself produce serious haemodynamic consequences. It can be treated with intravenous amiodarone or lidocaine (lignocaine) or, if haemodynamic deterioration occurs, synchronized cardioversion (initially 200 J).

Ventricular fibrillation. This may occur in the first few hours or days following an MI in the absence of severe cardiac failure or cardiogenic shock. It is treated with prompt defibrillation (200–360 J).

Atrial fibrillation. This occurs in about 10% of patients with MI. It is due to atrial irritation caused by heart failure, pericarditis and atrial ischaemia or infarction. It may be managed with intravenous digoxin (to reduce ventricular rate in 1–2 h) or with intravenous amiodarone.

Sinus bradycardia. This is especially associated with acute inferior wall MI. Symptoms emerge only when the bradycardia is severe. When symptomatic, the treatment consists of elevating the foot of the bed and giving intravenous atropine, 600 mg if necessary.

Sinus tachycardia. This is produced by heart failure, fever and anxiety. Reassurance for anxiety should be given, together with beta blockade, if there is no overt heart failure or contraindications.

Acute anterior wall MI may produce damage to the distal conduction system (the His bundle or bundle branches). The development of complete heart block usually implies a large MI and a poor prognosis. The ventricular escape rhythm is slow and unreliable, and a temporary pacemaker is necessary. This form of block is often permanent.

Hypotension and raised right-heart filling pressures are characteristically seen in right ventricular infarction that may accompany inferior infarcts. ST segment elevation is seen in V_4R leads on ECG. Echocardiography should be performed to exclude pericardial effusion. Initial treatment is with volume expansion.

Left ventricular mural thrombus may form on the endocardial surface of the infarcted region. Anticoagulant therapy appears to protect against stroke and should be considered in a patient with documented mural thrombus and in those patients with significant left ventricular dysfunction.

Pericarditis. This is characterized by sharp chest pain, aggravated by movement and respiration. It is characteristically worse on lying down. It is common in the first few days, particularly in anterior wall infarction. ECG shows generalized ST segment elevation (concave upward) with upright, peaked T waves. Anti-inflammatory drugs are usually effective.

A13.49

1) B   2) A   3) C   4) E   5) D

The typical finding in mitral stenosis is a diastolic pressure that is higher in the left atrium than in the left ventricle. This gradient of pressure is usually proportional to the degree of the stenosis. In mitral regurgitation this demonstrates a prominent left atrial systolic pressure wave, and when contrast is injected into the left ventricle it may be seen regurgitating into an enlarged left atrium during systole. Cardiac catheterization can be used to document the systolic pressure difference (gradient) between the aorta and the left ventricle and assess left ventricular function. This is rarely necessary since all of this information can be gained non-invasively with echocardiography. In aortic regurgitation during cardiac catheterization, injection of contrast medium into the aorta (aortography) will outline aortic valvular abnormalities and allow assessment of the degree of regurgitation. Tricuspid stenosis demonstrates a diastolic pressure gradient between the right atrium and the right ventricle. Contrast injection will demonstrate a large right atrium.

A13.50

1) B   2) A   3) C   4) D   5) E

Mitral stenosis: The chest X-ray usually shows a generally small heart with an enlarged left atrium. Pulmonary venous hypertension is usually also present. Late in the course of the disease a calcified mitral valve may be seen on a penetrated or lateral view. The signs of pulmonary oedema or pulmonary hypertension may also be apparent when the disease is severe.

Mitral regurgitation: The chest X-ray may show left atrial and left ventricular enlargement. There is an increase in the cardiothoracic ratio (CTR), and valve calcification is seen.

Aortic stenosis: The chest X-ray usually reveals a relatively small heart with a

Cardiovascular disease

prominent, dilated, ascending aorta. This occurs because turbulent blood flow above the stenosed aortic valve produces so-called 'post-stenotic dilatation'. The aortic valve may be calcified. When heart failure occurs, the CTR increases.

Aortic regurgitation: The chest X-ray features are those of left ventricular enlargement and possibly of dilatation of the ascending aorta. The ascending aortic wall may be calcified in syphilis, and the aortic valve may be calcified if valvular disease is responsible for the regurgitation.

Tricuspid stenosis: On the chest X-ray there may be a prominent right atrial bulge.

A 13.51

1) D   2) E   3) C   4) B   5) A

Tricuspid stenosis: The enlarged right atrium may be manifested on the ECG by peaked, tall P waves (>3 mm) in lead II.

Aortic regurgitation: The ECG appearances are those of left ventricular hypertrophy due to 'volume overload' – tall R waves and deeply inverted T waves in the left-sided chest leads, and deep S waves in the right-sided leads. Normally, sinus rhythm is present.

Aortic stenosis: The ECG shows left ventricular hypertrophy and left atrial delay. A left ventricular 'strain' pattern due to 'pressure overload' (depressed ST segments and T wave inversion in leads orientated towards the left ventricle, i.e. leads I, AVL, V_5 and V_6) is common when the disease is severe. Usually, sinus rhythm is present, but ventricular arrhythmias may be recorded.

Mitral regurgitation: The ECG shows the features of left atrial delay (bifid P waves) and left ventricular hypertrophy as manifested by tall R waves in the left lateral leads (e.g. leads I and V_6) and deep S waves in the right-sided precordial leads

(e.g. leads V_1 and V_2). (Note that SV_1 plus RV_5 or RV_6 >35 mm indicates left ventricular hypertrophy.) Left ventricular hypertrophy occurs in about 50% of patients with mitral regurgitation. Atrial fibrillation may be present.

Mitral stenosis: In sinus rhythm the ECG shows a bifid P wave owing to delayed left atrial activation. However, atrial fibrillation is frequently present. As the disease progresses, the ECG features of right ventricular hypertrophy (right axis deviation and perhaps tall R waves in lead V_1) may develop.

A 13.52

1) C   2) A   3) B   4) D   5) E

Mitral stenosis: There are four operative measures: trans-septal balloon valvotomy, closed valvotomy, open valvotomy and mitral valve replacement. Trans-septal balloon valvotomy cannot be performed when there is heavy calcification or more than mild mitral regurgitation. Closed valvotomy is advised for patients with mobile, non-calcified and non-regurgitant mitral valves.

Mitral regurgitation: Sudden torrential mitral regurgitation, as seen with chordal or papillary muscle rupture or infective endocarditis, may necessitate emergency mitral valve replacement.

Aortic stenosis: In patients with aortic stenosis, symptoms are a good index of severity and all symptomatic patients should have aortic valve replacement.

Aortic regurgitation: The treatment of aortic regurgitation usually requires aortic valve replacement but the timing of surgery is critical. Because symptoms do not develop until the myocardium fails and because the myocardium does not recover fully after surgery, operation is performed before significant symptoms occur.

A13.53

1) A   2) C   3) B   4) E   5) A   6) D

The oral streptococci account for between a third and a half of cases of infective endocarditis, and more in undeveloped countries, where iatrogenic endocarditis is rare. This group of α haemolytic streptococci includes species such as *Streptococcus mutans* and *Strep. sanguis*; they are often collectively but somewhat inaccurately known as 'Strep. viridans'. They are obviously often associated with dental disease or procedures.

Staphylococci cause up to a third of cases of native valve endocarditis, and about a half of prosthetic valve infections. Increasingly cases are seen in intravenous drug abusers (IVDAs) and patients with intravenous catheters, especially if these are long-standing and poorly cared for. Candidal endocarditis is rare: it is seen in i.v. drug users who dissolve heroin in (infected) lemon juice. *Strep. bovis* endocarditis is even rarer, but as there is a well-documented association with bowel malignancy, it should prompt consideration of this diagnosis. Culture-negative endocarditis accounts for 5–10% of cases. The usual cause is prior antibiotic therapy, but some cases are due to a variety of fastidious organisms that fail to grow in normal blood cultures. These include *Coxiella burnetii*, the cause of Q fever, *Chlamydia* spp., *Bartonella* spp. (recently recognized organisms that cause trench fever and cat-scratch-disease) and *Legionella*.

A13.54

1) A   2) B   3) C   4) D

Endocarditis is treated with bactericidal antibiotics chosen on the basis of the results of the blood culture and antibiotic sensitivity, where possible. The treatment should continue for 4–6 weeks, although recent studies of 2-week short-course therapy have shown that it is highly effective in uncomplicated penicillin-sensitive *Strep. viridans* endocarditis. There are several situations in which surgery is necessary: a) extensive damage to a valve; b) prosthetic valve endocarditis – valve replacement is usually required; c) persistent infection despite therapy; d) serious embolization; e) large vegetations; f) myocardial abscesses; g) fungal endocarditis – this is often refractory to antimicrobial therapy; h) progressive cardiac failure.

A13.55

1) C   2) F   3) E   4) G

The physical signs of atrial septal defect reflect the volume overloading of the right ventricle. Therefore, the splitting of the second sound is wide and fixed. The increased flow through the right heart produces a loud ejection systolic pulmonary flow murmur, and sometimes a diastolic tricuspid flow murmur may be heard. A right ventricular heave can usually be felt. In patent ductus arteriosus, the characteristic physical sign is a continuous 'machinery' murmur (due to turbulent aorta-to-pulmonary artery shunting in both systole and diastole), best heard below the left clavicle in the first interspace or over the first rib. A thrill may often be felt. This lessens or disappears as pulmonary hypertension develops leading to shunt reversal. The peripheral pulse is large in volume ('bounding') because of the increased left heart blood flow and the decompression of the aorta into the pulmonary artery. Coarctation of the aorta is often asymptomatic for many years. Headaches and nosebleeds (due to hypertension) and claudication and cold legs (due to poor blood flow in the lower limbs) may be present. Physical examination reveals hypertension in the upper limbs, and weak, delayed (radiofemoral delay) pulses in the legs. A mid-to-late systolic murmur due to turbulent flow through the coarctation may be heard over the upper precordium or the back. Vascular bruits from the collateral circulation may also be heard. Children with Fallot's tetralogy may present with dyspnoea or fatigue, or with hypoxic episodes on exertion (Fallot's spells) – deep cyanosis and possible syncope. These can even result in seizures, cerebrovascular events or sudden death. Squatting is common. Adults tend not to suffer 'spells' but fatigue easily with dyspnoea on exertion. Erythrocytosis (polycythaemia) secondary to chronic hypoxaemia commonly results in thrombotic strokes. Endocarditis is common. Physical signs include a parasternal sustained heave and a systolic ejection murmur, often associated with a thrill in the second left interspace close to the sternum. The second heart sound is usually single because the pulmonary component is too soft to be heard. Central cyanosis is commonly present from birth, and finger clubbing and polycythaemia are obvious after about 12 months. Growth is usually retarded.

A13.56

1) C   2) B   3) A   4) D

In coarctation of the aorta the chest X-ray may reveal a dilated aorta indented at the site of the coarctation. This is manifested by an aorta (seen in the upper right mediastinum) shaped like a figure '3'. In adults, tortuous and dilated collateral intercostal arteries may erode the

undersurfaces of the ribs ('rib notching'). In Fallot's tetralogy the chest X-ray shows a large right ventricle and a small pulmonary artery (classically described as 'boot-shaped'). In patent ductus arteriosus the aorta and pulmonary arterial system are usually prominent on X-ray, although a small ductus shows no abnormality. There is both a left atrial abnormality and left ventricular hypertrophy on the ECG. In atrial septal defect there is a prominent pulmonary artery and pulmonary plethora. There may be noticeable right ventricular enlargement.

A13.57

1) A   2) B   3) C   4) D   5) E

Dilated cardiomyopathy (DCM) is characterized by dilatation and impaired systolic function of the left ventricle and/or right ventricle, in the absence of abnormal loading conditions (e.g. hypertension, valve disease). At least 25% of 'idiopathic' cases are now known to be familial. In the majority of familial cases inheritance is autosomal dominant, but X-linked and recessive cases occur. In a limited number of cases the responsible genes have been identified. Many of these are genes encoding cytoskeletal or associated myocyte proteins (dystrophin in X-linked cardiomyopathy, actin, desmin and lamin a/c in autosomal dominant DCM). Twenty-five percent of patients with hypertrophic cardiomyopathy have dynamic left ventricular outflow tract obstruction due to the combined effects of hypertrophy, systolic anterior motion (SAM) of the anterior mitral valve leaflet and rapid ventricular ejection. The majority of cases of hypertrophic cardiomyopathy are familial, autosomal dominant, and due to mutations in the genes encoding sarcomeric proteins. The salient clinical and morphological features of the disease vary according to the underlying genetic mutation. For example, marked hypertrophy is common with beta-myosin heavy chain mutations whereas mutations in troponin T may be associated with mild hypertrophy but a high risk of sudden death. Hypertrophic cardiomyopathy (HCM) due to myosin-binding protein C may not manifest until the sixth decade of life or later.

A13.58

1) B   2) A   3) D   4) E

Conditions associated with restrictive cardiomyopathy include amyloidosis, sarcoidosis, Loeffler's endocarditis and endomyocardial fibrosis. Physical signs are similar to those of constrictive pericarditis – a high jugular venous pressure with diastolic collapse (Friedreich's sign) and elevation of venous pressure with inspiration (Kussmaul's sign). Arrhythmogenic right ventricular cardiomyopathy (ARVC) is characterized by progressive fibrofatty replacement of the right ventricular myocardium. It is familial in at least 50% of cases, most commonly with an autosomal dominant pattern of inheritance. A rare form of ARVC which is associated with dermatological abnormalities (Naxos disease) is caused by a mutation in a gene encoding a myocyte structural protein (plakoglobin) found in desmosomes and gap junctions. Following certain forms of pericarditis (tuberculous effusion, haemopericardium, bacterial infection or rheumatic heart disease), the pericardium may become thick, fibrous and calcified. The heart is then encased in a solid shell and cannot fill properly. Myocardial contractility is usually preserved but is impaired at late stages owing to fibrosis,

atrophy, and calcification of subepicardial layers of myocardium. Constrictive pericarditis also develops late after open-heart surgery. Typical signs are of systemic venous congestion – ascites, dependent oedema, hepatomegaly and jugular venous distension, without much breathlessness or pulmonary venous distension. There are signs of impaired ventricular filling (Kussmaul's sign), Friedreich's sign and pulsus paradoxus. Fatigue and exercise intolerance are common symptoms. Sinus tachycardia often occurs to compensate for low cardiac output.

A13.59

1) C   2) D   3) F   4) B   5) A

Features in the history such as attacks of sweating, headaches and palpitations may point towards the diagnosis of phaeochromocytoma, while angina or symptoms of peripheral arterial occlusive disease suggest the diagnosis of atheromatous renal artery stenosis. If the urea or creatinine is elevated, more specific renal investigations are indicated – creatinine clearance, renal ultrasound (in case of polycystic kidney disease, or parenchymal renal artery disease) and a renal isotope scan or renal angiography if renovascular disease (either atheromatous or fibromuscular dysplasia) is suspected. A low serum potassium may indicate an endocrine disorder (either primary hyperaldosteronism or glucocorticoid excess), and aldosterone, cortisol and renin measurements must then be made, preferably prior to initiating pharmacological therapy. Rib notching on the X-ray may be a sign of coarctation of the aorta and should be investigated further with an MRI scan.

Cardiovascular disease

A13.60

1) B   2) B   3) A   4) C   5) E

Beta-blockers should be used cautiously in patients with reactive airways disease including asthma. They should be avoided in phaeochromocytoma because beta-blockade will result in unopposed stimualtion of alpha-adrenergic receptors and a possible worsening of hypertension. ACEI are contraindicated in patients with bilateral renal artery stenosis. Calcium-channel blockers also reduce afterload, but first-generation calcium antagonists (diltiazem, nifedipine) may have a detrimental effect on left ventricular function in patients with heart failure. The PRAISE 2 trial showed that the second-generation calcium antagonist amlodipine showed no prognostic benefit in patients with heart failure. The use of thiazide diuretics may be complicated by overdiuresis and electrolyte depletion (potassium and magnesium), which may predispose to the development of lethal ventricular arrhythmias, hyperkalaemia (potassium-sparing diuretics) and other metabolic disturbances (hyperuricaemia and dyslipidaemia).

A13.61

1) F   2) D   3) C   4) A   5) B

Aortic dissections are of three types: a) DeBakey I – originates in the ascending aorta, propagates at least to the aortic arch and often beyond; b) DeBakey II – originates in, and is confined to, the ascending aorta; c) DeBakey III – originates in the distal aorta and extends distally down the aorta. Buerger's disease, involving the small vessels of the lower limbs, occurs in young men who smoke. Clinically it presents with severe claudication and rest pain leading to

gangrene. A thrombophlebitis is sometimes present. Takayasu's syndrome is known as 'pulseless disease' or the aortic arch syndrome. It is of unknown aetiology and occurs in young females. There is a vasculitis involving the aortic arch as well as other major arteries. There is also a systemic illness, with pain and tenderness over the affected arteries. Absent peripheral pulses and hypertension are usually found. Kawaski's disease is an uncommon acute febrile illness of early childhood. There is a generalized vasculitis with involvement of the coronary arteries and lymphadenopathy. Raynaud's phenomenon consists of spasm of the arteries supplying the fingers or toes and is usually precipitated by cold and relieved by heat. When Raynaud's phenomenon occurs without any underlying disorder, it is then known as Raynaud's disease. This is a common disease affecting 5% of the population and occurring predominantly in young women. The disorder is usually bilateral and fingers are affected more commonly than toes. There is an initial pallor of the skin resulting from vasoconstriction and this is followed by cyanosis due to sluggish blood flow. Redness finally occurs owing to hyperaemia. The duration of the attacks can be variable and can sometimes last for hours. Numbness and burning of the fingers usually occurs and pain can be severe, particularly in the rewarming phase.

A13.62

A) F   B) F   C) T   D) T   E) T

Patients who can exercise for less than 6 minutes generally have a poorer prognosis. The form of ST segment depression provoked by ischaemia is characteristic: it is either planar or shows down-sloping depression. Up-sloping depression is a non-specific finding. Exercise normally causes an increase in heart rate and blood pressure. A sustained fall in blood pressure usually indicates severe coronary artery disease. A slow recovery of the heart rate to basal levels has also been reported to be a predictor of mortality. Frequent premature ventricular depolarizations during the test are associated with a long-term increase in the risk of death from cardiovascular causes and further testing is required in these patients.

A) T   B) T   C) T   D) F   E) F

The cardiothoracic ratio (CTR) is usually less than 50%, except in neonates, infants, athletes and patients with skeletal abnormalities such as scoliosis and funnel chest. A transverse cardiac diameter of more than 15.5 cm is abnormal. Pericardial effusion or cardiac dilatation causes an increase in the ratio; however, at least 250 mL of fluid must accumulate before X-ray changes are apparent. Pure mitral stenosis without pulmonary hypertension is associated with left atrial enlargement and the CTR is normal.

A) T   B) T   C) T   D) F   E) T

This patient has mitral stenosis and typical features of accompanying left atrial dilatation. This results in prominence of the left atrial appendage and a straightening or convex bulging of the upper left heart border, a double atrial shadow to the right of the sternum, and splaying of the carina because a large left atrium elevates the left main bronchus. On the lateral film, a calcified aortic valve is seen on or above a line joining the carina

to the sternophrenic angle. Mitral valvular calcification is seen below and behind this line. Pulmonary venous hypertension occurs in left ventricular failure or mitral valve disease. Normal pulmonary venous pressure is 5–14 mmHg at rest. Mild pulmonary venous hypertension (15–20 mmHg) produces isolated dilatation of the upper zone vessels. Interstitial oedema occurs when the pressure is between 21 and 30 mmHg. This manifests as fluid collections in the interlobar fissures, interlobular septa (Kerley B lines) and pleural spaces. This gives rise to indistinctness of the hilar regions and haziness of the lung fields.

A) F   B) F   C) T   D) T   E) T

Pulmonary oligaemia is a paucity of vascular markings and a reduction in the width of the arteries. It occurs in situations where there is reduced pulmonary blood flow, such as pulmonary embolism, severe pulmonary stenosis and Fallot's tetralogy. Pulmonary arterial hypertension may result from pulmonary embolism, chronic lung disease or chronic left heart disease, such as shunts due to a ventricular septal defect or mitral valve stenosis. In addition to X-ray features of these conditions, the pulmonary arteries are prominent close to the hila but are very reduced in size (pruned) in the peripheral lung fields. This pattern is usually symmetrical. Pulmonary plethora results from left-to-right shunts (e.g. atrial or ventricular septal defects). It is seen as a general increase in the vascularity of the lung fields and as an increase in the size of hilar vessels (e.g. in the right lower lobe artery), which normally should not exceed 16 mm diameter.

Cardiovascular disease

A13.66

A) F B) T C) T D) F E) F

The first heart sound is caused by the closure of the mitral and tricuspid valves and is best heard at the cardiac apex. The first heart sound is loud when the patient is thin and when the circulation is hyperdynamic (e.g. due to anaemia or thyrotoxicosis). The sound is also loud if the valve is still open when ventricular systole begins (e.g. in mitral stenosis). A soft first heart sound occurs in patients with obesity, emphysema or pericardial effusion. It is also present when the valve leaflets are immobile (e.g. in severe calcific mitral stenosis), or when the leaflets are partly closed when systole begins, which occurs when the PR interval is long. A soft first heart sound also occurs when the valve does not close properly, as in mitral regurgitation. Heart failure and cardiogenic shock are also associated with a soft first heart sound. The intensity of the first heart sound is variable when the relationship between atrial and ventricular systole is not constant (e.g. during ventricular tachycardia or complete heart block). When the PR interval is short the sound is loud, and when the PR interval is long the sound is soft.

A13.67

A) F B) T C) F D) T E) T

On exercise there is an increase in catecholamine activity and stimulation of the β-adrenergic receptors. β-Adrenergic stimulation enhances Ca^{2+} flux in the myocyte and thereby strengthens the force of contraction. Binding of catecholamines (e.g. noradrenaline (norepinephrine)) to the myocyte $β_1$-adrenergic receptor stimulates membrane-bound adenylate kinases. These enzymes enhance production of cyclic AMP that activates intracellular protein kinases, which in turn phosphorylate cellular proteins, including L-type calcium channels within the cell membrane. β-Adrenergic stimulation of the myocyte also enhances myocyte relaxation. The return of calcium from the cytosol to the sarcoplasmic reticulum (SR) is regulated by phospholamban (PL), a low molecular weight protein in the SR membrane. In its dephosphorylated state, PL inhibits Ca^{2+} uptake by the SR ATPase pump. However, $β_1$-adrenergic activation of protein kinase phosphorylates PL, and blunts its inhibitory effect. The subsequently greater uptake of calcium ions by the SR hastens Ca^{2+} removal from the cytosol and promotes myocyte relaxation. The increased cAMP activity also results in phosphorylation of troponin-I, an action that inhibits actin–myosin interaction, and further enhances myocyte relaxation.

A13.68

A) T B) T C) T D) T E) F

Endothelium-dependent coronary vasodilatation can be improved by a variety of interventions, including the use of agents such as angiotensin-converting enzyme inhibitors, β-hydroxymethyl-glutaryl-coenzyme A reductase inhibitors (statins) and antioxidants. Among the non-pharmacological therapeutic options for patients with coronary artery disease, regular physical exercise improves endothelium-dependent vasodilatation both in epicardial and resistance vessels. $α_2$-agonists are vasoconstrictors.

A13.69

A) F   B) T   C) F   D) F   E) F

In the fetus the left and right heart both propel blood from the systemic veins to the systemic arteries; thus, severe abnormalities of the heart may not compromise fetal blood flow. Blood that passes through the right ventricle is diverted from the pulmonary artery to the aorta through the ductus arteriosus. Thus, the systemic venous return, which is a mixture of oxygenated and deoxygenated blood, is mostly returned to the systemic arterial system. At birth, inspiration dilates the pulmonary arterioles, resulting in a dramatic reduction of pulmonary vascular resistance. Blood therefore flows through the pulmonary circulation. The increased oxygen tension and reduced levels of prostaglandins trigger closure of the ductus arteriosus, and the reduced right atrial pressure and increasing left atrial pressure tend to close the foramen ovale.

A13.70

A) F   B) F   C) T   D) F   E) F

Left ventricular contraction starts and shortly thereafter right ventricular contraction begins. The increased ventricular pressures exceed the atrial pressures, and close first the mitral and then the tricuspid valves. Until the aortic and pulmonary valves open, the ventricles contract with no change of volume (isovolumetric contraction). When ventricular pressures rise above the aortic and pulmonary artery pressures, the pulmonary valve and then the aortic valve open and ventricular ejection occurs. As the ventricles begin to relax, their pressures fall below the aortic and

pulmonary arterial pressures, and aortic valve closure is followed by pulmonary valve closure. Isovolumetric relaxation then occurs. After the ventricular pressures have fallen below the right atrial and left atrial pressures, the tricuspid and mitral valves open.

A13.71

A) F   B) F   C) T   D) T   E) T

Carotid sinus massage may be used in supraventricular tachycardia to stimulate the vagal efferent discharge. In atrial flutter if F waves are not clearly visible, it is worth accentuating them by slowing AV conduction by carotid sinus massage. In atrial tachycardia carotid sinus massage may increase AV block during tachycardia thereby facilitating the diagnosis but does not usually terminate the arrhythmia. Diagnosis of carotid sinus hypersensitivity is made by carotid sinus massage (after excluding carotid stenosis by auscultation). Carotid sinus massage has no role in ventricular tachyarrhythmias.

A13.72

A) F   B) T   C) T   D) F   E) F

In narrow complex tachycardia carotid sinus massage, and the Valsalva manoeuvre may be used to stimulate the vagal efferent discharge. If physical manoeuvres have not been successful, intravenous adenosine (up to 0.25 mg/kg) may be tried. It is contraindicated in patients with a history of asthma. An alternative treatment is verapamil 10 mg i.v. over 5–10 minutes. Verapamil must not be given if beta-blockers have been previously administered or if the

Cardiovascular disease

tachycardia presents with broad (>0.12 s) QRS complexes. Intravenous beta-blockers should be avoided in patients with history of bronchospasm. Lidocaine (lignocaine) is not indicated in supraventricular tachycardia.

A13.73

A) T   B) T   C) T   D) T   E) T

Causes of long QT syndrome and torsades de pointes tachycardia

Congenital syndromes
Jervell–Lange–Nielsen (autosomal recessive)
Romano–Ward (autosomal dominant)

Electrolyte abnormalities
Hypokalaemia
Hypomagnesaemia
Hypocalcaemia

Drugs
Quinidine (and other class Ia antiarrhythmic drugs)
Sotalol (and other class III antiarrhythmic drugs)
Amitriptyline (and other tricyclic antidepressants)
Chlorpromazine (and other phenothiazine drugs)
Terfenadine and astemizole
Erythromycin and the macrolides
Cisapride (withdrawn in the UK)

Poisons
Organophosphate insecticides

Miscellaneous
Bradycardia
Mitral valve prolapse
Acute myocardial infarction
Prolonged fasting and liquid protein diets (long term)
Central nervous system diseases e.g. dystrophia myotonica

A13.74

A) T   B) F   C) F   D) T   E) T

Balloon pumping is used to improve cardiac output when there is a transient or reversible depression of left ventricular function, such as in a patient with severe mitral valve regurgitation who is awaiting surgical replacement of the mitral valve, or in a patient with a ventricular septal defect that is due to septal infarction. Balloon pumping is used to treat unstable angina pectoris by improving coronary flow and decreasing myocardial oxygen consumption by reducing the 'afterload'. This technique may be successful, even when medical therapy has failed. Balloon pumping should not be used in patients with aortic valve regurgitation or dissection of the aorta.

A13.75

A) T   B) T   C) T   D) T   E) T

Marfan's syndrome (MFS) is one of the most common autosomal dominant inherited disorders of connective tissue, affecting the heart (aortic aneurysm and dissection, mitral valve prolapse), eye (dislocated lenses, retinal detachment) and skeleton (tall, thin body build with long arms, legs and fingers; scoliosis and pectus deformity). Diagnosis may be confirmed by studying family linkage to the causative gene, or by demonstrating a mutation in the Marfan's syndrome gene (*MFS1*) for fibrillin (FBN-1) on chromosome 15q21.

A13.76

A) T B) F C) F D) T E) F

In Marfan's syndrome beta-blocker therapy slows the rate of dilatation of the aortic root. Lifestyle alterations, involving sports and career choice, may be indicated, because of ocular, cardiac or skeletal involvement. Sports that necessitate prolonged exertion at maximum cardiac output, such as cross-country running, are to be avoided. Sedentary occupations are usually best, as patients tend to suffer from easy fatigability and hypermobile painful joints. The patient should be monitored with yearly echocardiograms up to aortic root diameter 4.5 cm, 6-monthly from 4.5–5 cm, and then referred directly to a surgeon who is experienced in aortic root replacement in Marfan's syndrome. Pregnancy is generally well tolerated if no serious cardiac problems are present, but is preferably avoided if the aortic root diameter is over 4 cm, with aortic regurgitation. Caesarean section at 39 weeks' gestation is the recommended method of delivery when the aortic root is over 4.5 cm. Beta-blocker therapy may be safely instituted or continued throughout pregnancy, to help prevent aortic dissection. Elective aortic root replacement is recommended at a diameter of 5 cm.

A13.77

A) T B) T C) T D) T E) T

In this situation a small/medium-sized embolus has impacted in a terminal pulmonary vessel. Symptoms are pleuritic chest pain and breathlessness. Haemoptysis occurs in 30%, often 3 or more days after the initial event. On examination, the patient may be tachypnoeic with a localized pleural rub and often coarse crackles over the area involved. A pleural effusion (occasionally blood-stained) can develop. The patient may have a fever and cardiovascular examination is normal.

A13.78

A) F B) T C) T D) F E) F

In small/medium-sized pulmonary emboli, chest X-ray is often normal, but linear atelectasis or blunting of a costophrenic angle (due to a small effusion) is not uncommon. ECG is usually normal, except for sinus tachycardia, but sometimes atrial fibrillation or another tachycardia occurs. If plasma D-dimer is undetectable, it excludes a diagnosis of pulmonary embolism. Radionuclide ventilation/perfusion scan ($\dot{V}/\dot{Q}$ scan) is a good and widely available diagnostic investigation. The pulmonary ^{99m}Tc scintigram demonstrates underperfused areas which, if not accompanied by a ventilation defect on a ventilation scintigram performed after inhalation of radioactive xenon gas, is highly suggestive of a pulmonary embolus. Spiral CT scans with intravenous contrast show good sensitivity and specificity for medium-sized pulmonary emboli. They do not exclude pulmonary emboli in small arteries.

A13.79

A) T B) F C) T D) T E) T

In massive pulmonary embolus ECG shows right atrial dilatation with tall peaked T waves in lead II. Right ventricular strain and dilatation give rise to right axis deviation, some degree of right bundle

Cardiovascular disease

branch block, and T wave inversion in the right precordial leads. The 'classic' ECG pattern with an S wave in lead I, and a Q wave and inverted T waves in lead III (S^1, Q^{iii}, T^{iii}), is rare. Blood gases show hypoxia and hypocapnia.

A13.80

A) T B) T C) T D) T E) T

Causes of sudden cardiac death

Coronary
Acute myocardial infarction
Chronic ischaemic heart disease
Post-coronary-artery bypass surgery
Post-successful resuscitation for cardiac arrest
Congenital anomaly of coronary arteries
Coronary artery embolism
Coronary arteritis

Non-coronary
Hypertrophic cardiomyopathy
Dilated cardiomyopathy (ischaemic or idiopathic)
Arrhythmogenic right ventricular cardiomyopathy
Congenital long QT syndrome
Brugada's syndrome
Valvular heart disease (aortic stenosis, mitral valve prolapse)
Cyanotic heart disease (tetralogy of Fallot, transposition)
Acyanotic heart disease (ventricular septal defect, patent ductus arteriosus)

A13.81

A) F B) F C) T D) T E) T

Complications of mitral stenosis

Atrial fibrillation
Systemic embolization
Pulmonary hypertension
Pulmonary infarction
Chest infections
Infective endocarditis (rare)
Tricuspid regurgitation
Right ventricular failure

Left ventricular function is preserved in pure mitral stenosis. Both left ventricular systolic and diastolic function are typically unaffected unless there is associated mitral regurgitation or aortic valve involvement. Mitral stenosis is frequently associated with complications (see table).

A13.82

A) F B) T C) T D) T E) F

Severe mitral stenosis with pulmonary hypertension is associated with the so-called mitral facies or malar flush. This is a bilateral, cyanotic or dusky pink discoloration over the upper cheeks that is due to arteriovenous anastomoses and vascular stasis. There is a tapping impulse felt parasternally on the left side which is not localized. This is the result of a palpable first heart sound combined with left ventricular backward displacement produced by an enlarging right ventricle. Auscultation reveals a loud first heart sound if the mitral valve is pliable, but it will not occur in calcific mitral stenosis. As the valve suddenly opens with the force of the increased left atrial pressure, an 'opening snap' will be heard. This is followed by a low-pitched 'rumbling' mid-diastolic murmur best heard with the bell of the stethoscope held lightly at the apex with the patient lying on the left side. If the patient is in sinus rhythm, the murmur becomes louder at the end of diastole as a result of atrial contraction (presystolic accentuation). Pulmonary hypertension is recognized by a right ventricular heave, a loud pulmonary component of the second heart sound, with eventually signs of right-sided heart failure, such as oedema and hepatomegaly.

A13.83

A) F   B) T   C) T   D) F   E) F

The severity of mitral stenosis is judged clinically on the basis of several criteria. a) The presence of pulmonary hypertension implies that mitral stenosis is severe. Pulmonary hypertension is recognized by a right ventricular heave, a loud pulmonary component of the second heart sound, with eventually signs of right-sided heart failure, such as oedema and hepatomegaly. Pulmonary hypertension results in pulmonary valvular regurgitation that causes an early diastolic murmur in the pulmonary area, known as a Graham Steell murmur. b) The closeness of the opening snap to the second heart sound is proportional to the severity of mitral stenosis. c) The length of the mid-diastolic murmur is also proportional to the severity. d) As the valve cusps become immobile, the loud first heart sound softens and the opening snap disappears. When pulmonary hypertension occurs, the pulmonary component of the second sound is increased in intensity and the mitral diastolic murmur may become quieter because of the reduction of cardiac output.

A13.84

A) T   B) T   C) T   D) T   E) F

Aspirin 75–150 mg daily is given unless contraindicated. Beta-blockers have been shown to reduce the incidence of sudden death following myocardial infarction by 20–25% (about 10 lives saved per 1000 patients yearly). All patients – except those with ongoing clinical heart failure – should be treated with beta-blockers for at least 1 year unless contraindicated (e.g. COPD). ACE inhibitors should be continued indefinitely in patients with persistent impairment of left ventricular function (i.e. an ejection fraction <0.4). Patients need to be advised that they cannot drive for 1 month, and heavy goods and public service driving licences are withdrawn prior to special assessment. Prior to discharge, patients should undergo submaximal exercise-tolerance testing. An exercise-tolerance test is used to identify the presence of residual ischaemia and has short- and long-term prognostic value. It is useful for the prescription of rehabilitation programmes. It normally entails submaximal treadmill testing (70% of age-predicted maximal heart rate) at 4–6 days post-MI or symptom-limited treadmill testing at 10–14 days post-MI. Patients with test results suggesting ischaemia should be referred for coronary angiography.

A13.85

A) T   B) T   C) F   D) F   E) F

Exercise testing can be very useful both in confirming the diagnosis of angina and in giving some indication as to the severity of the coronary artery disease (CAD). ST segment depression of ≥1 mm suggests myocardial ischaemia, particularly if typical chest pain occurs at the same time. The test has a specificity of 80% and a sensitivity of about 70% for CAD. A strongly positive test (within 6 minutes of starting the Bruce protocol) suggests 'prognostic' disease and helps to identify patients who should be considered for coronary angiography. Exercise testing, however, can be misleading. a) A normal test does not exclude CAD (so-called false-negative test) although these patients, as a group, have a good prognosis. b) Up to 20% of patients with positive exercise tests are subsequently found to have no

Cardiovascular disease

evidence of coronary artery disease
(so-called false-positive test). Coronary
angiography should be performed only
when the benefit in terms of diagnosis and
potential treatment outweighs the small
risk of the procedure (a mortality rate of
less than 1 in 1000 cases).

A13.86

A) F   B) F   C) T   D) F   E) T

Metoprolol is best avoided in asthma and
severe reactive airways disease. High dose
nifedipine is associated with adverse
outcome. Slow release amlodipine is a
calcium-channel blocker which can safely
be used since they have no significant
effect on heart rate and it has no
significant negative inotropic effect.
Hormone replacement therapy should be
avoided in patients with a high risk of
breast cancer. Nicorandil is a potassium-
channel activator which is not used as a
first-line drug but may be used when there
are contraindications to first-line agents.

A13.87

A) T   B) T   C) T   D) T   E) T

Myocardial infarction almost always
occurs in patients with coronary atheroma
as a result of plaque rupture with
superadded thrombus. This occlusive
thrombus consists of a platelet-rich core
('white clot') and a bulkier surrounding
fibrin-rich ('red') clot. About 6 hours after
the onset of infarction, the myocardium is
swollen and pale, and at 24 hours the
necrotic tissue appears deep red owing to
haemorrhage. In the next few weeks, an
inflammatory reaction develops and the
infarcted tissue turns grey and gradually
forms a thin, fibrous scar.

Respiratory disease

Q14.1

A 49-year-old patient with recently diagnosed bronchogenic carcinoma develops mental confusion. Her blood chemistry reveals Na 120 mEq/L, K. 4.5 mEq/L, urea 30 mmol/L, creatinine 90 μmol/L, blood sugar 9 mmol/L, serum calcium 2.60 mmol/L, and TSH 4 U/L. The most likely cause for her symptoms is which one of the following?

A. Thyrotoxicosis
B. Hypercalcaemia
C. Syndrome of inappropriate secretion of antidiuretic hormone (SIADH)
D. Hypoglycaemia
E. Ectopic adrenocorticotrophic hormone (ACTH) syndrome

Q14.2

The majority of all primary lung carcinomas arise in which one of the following regions?

A. Periphery
B. Lateral segment of lower lobe
C. Right middle lobe
D. Lingular lobe
E. Hilar region

Q14.3

A 49-year-old man has bronchogenic carcinoma. Biopsy shows non-small-cell cancer of the lung. His haematocrit is 35, FEV_1 is 1.4 L, carbon monoxide gas transfer is 75% predicted. Select the best option for management

A. Chemotherapy with etoposide
B. Exploratory thoracotomy
C. Pneumonectomy
D. Radiotherapy
E. Palliative care

Q14.4

A 52-year-old man develops sudden onset of right-sided chest pain followed by progressive shortness of breath. On examination the patient is breathless at rest and his heart rate is 120 beats/minute. ECG shows sinus tachycardia and chest X-ray shows the right lung is grossly deflated. The best step in the management of this patient is now to

A. Reassure the patient and administer morphine
B. Administer an intravenous beta-blocker to control the heart rate
C. Aspirate air from the right side
D. Aspirate air from the left side
E. Initiate cardiac massage

303

Respiratory disease

Q14.5

A 58-year-old thoracic surgeon has a routine chest X-ray. He is asymptomatic. The chest X-ray shows a solitary round shadow which on biopsy, is metastatic carcinoma. The most common primary tumour is

A. Carcinoma of the thyroid
B. Renal cell carcinoma
C. Carcinoma of the liver
D. Carcinoma of the bladder
E. Carcinoma of the adrenal glands

Q14.6

A 42-year-old Afro-Caribbean woman has a history of sarcoidosis treated 20 years ago. Currently the only medication she is taking is an oral contraceptive. She now complains of a 4-week history of fever, night sweats and haemoptysis. Her chest X-ray shows numerous minute opacities in all lung fields, about 2 mm in size. The most likely cause for her clinical picture is

A. Recurrent sarcoidosis
B. Pulmonary embolism
C. Miliary tuberculosis
D. Pneumoconiosis
E. Pulmonary microlithiasis

Q14.7

A 29-year-old woman has noticed progressive shortness of breath and dysphagia. She now also complains of hoarseness of voice. CT of the chest shows a mediastinal mass. The most common mediastinal mass is

A. Thymoma
B. Dermoid cyst
C. Lipoma
D. Retrosternal thyroid
E. Hernia through the foramen of Morgagni

Q14.8

A 43-year-old smoker is known to have emphysema. Chest X-ray shows hyperlucency of lungs and increase in lung fields. These findings suggest which one of the following?

A. There is associated chronic bronchitis
B. More than 40% of the lung tissue is destroyed
C. There is associated consolidation
D. Emphysema is the wrong diagnosis
E. This patient has associated bronchial asthma

Q14.9

A 23-year-old woman is known to have brittle asthma. Which one of the following is the best option in the event of a life-threatening attack while at work?

A. Breathe into a closed bag to suppress hyperventilation
B. Ask a colleague to inject 100 mg intravenous aminophylline rapidly
C. Self-inject 0.3mg adrenaline (epinephrine)
D. Take several slow deep breaths while a colleague contacts emergency services
E. Self-inject esmolol rapidly

Q14.10

A 55-year-old smoker staying in a hotel develops malaise, myalgia, headaches and fever. He also develops a dry cough, nausea, vomiting and diarrhoea. He is confused and appears ill. Urine examination reveals haematuria. Blood count reveals lymphopenia with marked leucocytosis. Serum sodium is 125 mEq/L. Chest X-ray shows lobar consolidation with a small pleural effusion. The quickest way of diagnosis is which one of the following?

A. Blood cultures
B. Sputum cultures
C. Immunofluorescent staining of the organism in sputum
D. A fourfold increase in antibody titre
E. Complement fixation tests

Q14.11

A 55-year-old smoker staying in a hotel develops malaise, myalgia, headaches and fever. He also develops a dry cough, nausea, vomiting and diarrhoea. He is confused and appears ill. Urine examination reveals haematuria. Blood count reveals lymphopenia with marked leucocytosis. Serum sodium is 125 mEq/L. Chest X-ray shows lobar consolidation with a small pleural ellusion. The antibiotic choice for this patient is which one of the following?

A. Penicillin
B. Pyrimethamine
C. Tetracycline
D. Clarithromycin
E. Trimpethoprim with sulfamethoxazole

Q14.12

A 42-year-old homosexual man who is HIV-infected develops purple skin lesions. Subsequently he develops progressive shortness of breath and cough. Bronchoscopy shows multiple red lesions. Histological diagnosis is not obtained because of the risk of haemorrhage. Select the best option for treatment from the following

A. Intravenous piperacillin
B. Vincristine and bleomycin every 3 weeks
C. Intravenous amphotericin B
D. Combination of rifampicin, ethambutol and clofazimine
E. Corticosteroids and zidovudine

Q14.13

A previously healthy 32-year-old man develops a temperature of 39°C, pleuritic pain and a dry cough. A day later he develops rusty-coloured sputum and a herpes simplex infection around the mouth. His breathing is rapid and shallow. Chext X-ray shows lobar pneumonia. White blood cell count is 15×10^9/L, with 90% polymorphonuclear leucocytosis. Erythrocyte sedimentation rate is 110 mm/h. The most sensitive test for confirming the diagnosis is which one of the following?

A. Sputum culture for pneumococcus
B. Blood culture for pneumococcus
C. Cold agglutinins in serum
D. Counterimmunoelectrophoresis of sputum for pneumococcal antigen
E. Cultures of bronchoscopy washing for pneumococcus

Q14.14

A previously healthy 32-year-old man develops a temperature of 39°C, pleuritic pain and a dry cough. A day later he develops rusty-coloured sputum and a herpes simplex infection around the mouth. His breathing is rapid and shallow. Chest X-ray shows lobar pneumonia. White blood cell count is 15×10^9/L, with 90% polymorphonuclear leucocytosis. Erythrocyte sedimentation rate is 110 mm/h. The most appropriate treatment is which one of the following?

A. Intravenous metronidazole
B. Parenteral ampicillin with clarithromycin
C. Intravenous flucloxacillin with sodium fusidate
D. Oral erythromcyin
E. Oral erythromcyin with rifampicin

Respiratory disease

Q14.15

The patient in question 14.14 is allergic to penicillin and macrolides. The most appropriate therapy is

A. Intravenous metronidazole
B. Oral tetracycline
C. Levofloxacin
D. Oral erythromcyin
E. Oral erythromcyin with rifampicin

Q14.16

A 69-year-old patient with a history of alcoholism, diabetes and coronary artery disease presents with sudden onset of systemic symptoms including fever and malaise. He has a cough with purulent sputum which is blood-stained. Chest X-ray shows that the right upper lobe is involved. On lateral chest X-ray the lobe is swollen as evidenced by the bulging of the fissures. The most likely organism is

A. Anaerobic bacteria
B. *Nocardia asteroides*
C. *Cryptococcus* sp.
D. *Klebsiella pneumoniae*
E. *Coxiella burnetii*

Q14.17

A 65-year-old patient has worsening signs of pneumonia despite treatment. He begins to produce foul-smelling sputum and develops a swinging fever. He complains of generalized malaise and is losing weight. Chest examination reveals some dullness in the right axilla but is otherwise unremarkable. He is also noted to have clubbing of the fingernails. His haemoglobin falls to 9 g/dL, serum albumin is low and ESR is 75 mm/h. The most likely diagnosis is which one of the following?

A. Bronchopneumonia
B. Cryptogenic organizing pneumonia
C. Bronchiolitis obliterans organizing pneumonia
D. Lung abscess
E. Lymphoid interstitial pneumonia

Q14.18

A 48-year-old doctor from India has X-ray changes compatible with previous tuberculosis. He has known about these changes on X-ray for 10 years and has not required anti-tuberculosis treatment. He now has chronic renal failure and requires haemodialysis. Select the best management option

A. Observation only, no treatment required since he has old TB
B. Isoniazid 200 mg daily
C. Six months' treatment with once-daily rifampicin 450 mg and isoniazid 300 mg. Initial 2 months with daily pyrazinamide 1.5 g/daily
D. BCG vaccine before haemodialysis is initiated
E. Rifampicin 450 mg daily

Q14.19

A 26-year-old man is diagnosed to have tuberculosis. His wife is asymptomatic. The best option for the management of his wife is which one of the following?

A. Initiate chemoprophylaxis with isoniazid
B. Do a chest X-ray and a tuberculin test
C. Do a chest X-ray at first and do a tuberculin test if the X-ray is positive
D. Do a tuberculin test initially and do a chest X-ray if the tuberculin test is positive
E. Reassure the man's wife that until she is symptomatic nothing needs to be done

Q14.20

A 26-year-old man is diagnosed to have tuberculosis. His 9-year-old son is asymptomatic and tuberculin test and chest X-ray are negative. The best option for the management of his son is which one of the following?

A. Reassure the parents that since the tuberculin test is negative he needs no further intervention
B. Administer BCG vaccination
C. Repeat the tuberculin test in 6 weeks
D. Repeat the chest X-ray in 6 weeks
E. Perform bronchoscopy to obtain bronchial washing for acid and alcohol-fast bacilli

Q14.21

A 26-year-old man is diagnosed to have tuberculosis. His 10-month-old son is asymptomatic. The best option for the management of his son is which one of the following?

A. Do a chest X-ray only
B. Do a chest X-ray and a tuberculin test
C. Do a tuberculin test only
D. Prescribe daily isoniazid together with a strain of BCG that is resistant to isoniazid
E. Reassure the parents that since their son is asymptomatic no further intervention is required until he develops symptoms

Q14.22

A 26-year-old man is diagnosed to have tuberculosis. His 12-year-old daughter is asymptomatic. Her chest X-ray is negative but the tuberculin test is positive The best option for the management of his daughter is which one of the following?

A. Administer BCG vaccination
B. Repeat the tuberculin test in 4–6 weeks to confirm that it is positive
C. Repeat the chest X-ray in 4–6 weeks to determine whether the patient has tuberculosis
D. Initiate anti-tuberculosis treatment
E. Prescribe anti-tuberculosis chemoprophylaxis with BCG vaccination

Q14.23

A 26-year-old man is diagnosed to have tuberculosis. His wife is asymptomatic. Her tuberculin test is positive and her chest X-ray is negative. The best option for the management of his wife is which one of the following?

A. Repeat the tuberculin test in 4–6 weeks to confirm that it is positive
B. Repeat the chest X-ray in 4–6 weeks to determine whether the patient has tuberculosis
C. Initiate anti-tuberculosis treatment
D. Prescribe anti-tuberculosis chemoprophylaxis with BCG vaccination
E. Nothing more needs to be done

Q14.24

A 38-year-old West Indian woman presents with fatigue, weight loss, mild fever and cough. Her skin shows erythema nodosum. Her chest X-ray shows bilateral hilar adenopathy. The most likely diagnosis is which one of the following?

A. Lymphoma
B. Pulmonary tuberculosis
C. Carcinoma of the bronchus
D. Sarcoidosis
E. Pneumococcal pneumonia

Respiratory disease

Q14.25

A 47-year-old Afro-Caribbean patient complains of fever and red eye. On examination he has parotid enlargement and bilateral uveitis. He also has a left seventh cranial nerve palsy. Which one of the following is the the most likely cause for these clinical features?

A. Bell's palsy
B. Ramsay Hunt syndrome
C. Sarcoidosis
D. Keratoconjunctivitis sicca
E. Gradenigo's syndrome

Q14.26

A 38-year-old West Indian woman presents with fatigue, weight loss, mild fever and cough. Her chest X-ray shows bilateral hilar adenopathy and pulmonary infiltrates. The most useful investigation in confirming the diagnosis is which one of the following?

A. CT scan of chest
B. Transbronchial biopsy
C. Serum angiotensin-converting enzyme level
D. Lung function test
E. Tuberculin skin test

Q14.27

A 17-year-old boy has progressive shortness of breath and unifocal bone lesions. Chest X-ray shows honeycomb lung, and histology shows typical cells with Birbeck granules on electron-microscopy and CD1$_a$ antigen on the surface of the cells. These features suggest that the most likely diagnosis is which one of the following?

A. Churg–Strauss syndrome
B. Caplan's syndrome
C. Wegener's granulomatosis
D. Langerhans' cell histiocytosis
E. Goodpasture's syndrome

Q14.28

A 45-year-old coal miner has a long history of rheumatoid arthritis. On a routine physical examination his chest X-ray shows several 5 cm rounded nodules in both lung fields. These features suggest that the most likely diagnosis is which one of the following?

A. Churg–Strauss syndrome
B. Caplan's syndrome
C. Wegener's granulomatosis
D. Langerhans' cell histiocytosis
E. Goodpasture's syndrome

Q14.29

A retired coal miner has a history of rheumatoid arthritis. On a routine physical examination his chest X-ray shows several 3 cm rounded nodules in both lung fields. The most constant feature in the serum in this condition is which one of the following?

A. Proteinase-3 (PR3) ANCA
B. Myeloperoxidase (MPO) ANCA
C. Rheumatoid factor
D. Eosinophilia
E. CD1$_a$ antigen

Q14.30

A 29-year-old man complains of rhinorrhoea followed by cough and haemoptysis. Routine urine examination reveals haematuria. Chest X-ray shows pneumonic infiltrates with cavitation. ANCA is positive. Kidney biopsy shows glomerulonephritis. The most likely diagnosis is which one of the following?

A. Churg–Strauss syndrome
B. Caplan's syndrome

C. Wegener's granulomatosis
D. Langerhans' cell histiocytosis
E. Goodpasture's syndrome

Q14.31

A 36-year-old man has a long-standing history of asthma and is on steroid therapy. Withdrawal of steroids results in rhinitis and exacerbation of the asthma. He also notices painful petechial skin lesions. Peripheral smear shows eosinophilia. Chest X-ray shows patchy pneumonia. ANCA is positive. Biopsy of the skin lesion shows vasculitis of small arteries and veins dominated by eosinophilic infiltration. Extravascular granulomas are also seen. The most likely diagnosis is which one of the following?

A. Churg–Strauss syndrome
B. Caplan's syndrome
C. Wegener's granulomatosis
D. Langerhans' cell histiocytosis
E. Goodpasture's syndrome

Q14.32

A 48-year-old man complains of several episodes of wheeze, cough, fever and malaise. The expectoration contains firm sputum plugs containing mycelia. The peripheral blood eosinophil count is raised and total levels of IgE are raised. The most likely diagnosis is which one of the following?

A. Churg–Strauss syndrome
B. Allergic bronchopulmonary aspergillosis
C. Wegener's granulomatosis
D. Langerhans' cell histiocytosis
E. Goodpasture's syndrome

Q14.33

A 21-year-old woman initially had an upper respiratory tract infection. This was followed by cough and intermittent haemoptysis. She now complains of tiredness and the haematocrit is low. She also has oliguria, and urine examination shows red cells and red cell casts. Both urea and creatinine are elevated. Chest X-ray shows transient blotchy shadows. ANCA is positive. Antibodies against the basement membrane of the kidney and lung are elevated. The most likely diagnosis is which one of the following?

A. Churg–Strauss syndrome
B. Allergic bronchopulmonary aspergillosis
C. Wegener's granulomatosis
D. Langerhans' cell histiocytosis
E. Goodpasture's syndrome

Q14.34

A 49-year-old man has bronchogenic carcinoma. Biopsy shows small-cell cancer of the lung. His haematocrit is 35, FEV_1 is 1.4 L, carbon monoxide gas transfer is 75% predicted. The best option for management is which one of the following?

A. Exploratory thoracotomy
B. Pneumonectomy
C. Chemotherapy with etoposide and cisplatin
D. Radiotherapy
E. Palliative care

Q14.35

1. A 16-year-old patient complains of shortness of breath. He has had recurrent attacks of this requiring salbutamol inhalers, with complete reversal of symptoms with therapy

2. A child develops shortness of breath suddenly while eating peanuts

3. A 42-year-old patient with ischaemic cardiomyopathy has ingested a high salt meal a few hours before. He complains of shortness of breath and has pink, frothy sputum at the mouth

4. A 19-year-old patient complains of fever, cough and chest pain on deep inspiration

5. A 75-year-old patient complains of shortness of breath. On examination there is a stony dull note on percussion

Select the best match for each of the above

A. Absent breath sounds
B. Polyphonic wheeze
C. Late inspiratory crackles
D. Monophonic wheeze
E. Localized creaking sound

14.36

1. A 35-year-old woman on oral contraceptives complains of shortness of breath which started suddenly. She also has haemoptysis

2. A 33-year-old patient complains of shortness of breath which is gradually getting worse. On examination she has fine crackles at both bases on end-inspiration

3. A 22-year-old patient with Kartagener's syndrome complains of shortness of breath and cough with purulent expectoration

4. A 67-year-old smoker is found to have a mass in the lungs. The surgeon wants imaging studies for staging

5. A 54-year-old woman with breast cancer complains of shortness of breath. The chest X-ray shows streaky opacities and the oncologist wants to better define this condition

6. A 52-year-old woman complains of shortness of breath. Her lung function tests are normal except for a low gas transfer factor

7. A 42-year-old patient has a mass at the apex of the lung and the surgeon wishes to know whether the tumour is invading the mediastinum

Select the most valuable investigation for each of the above

A. Spiral CT with contrast injection
B. Conventional CT
C. High-resolution CT
D. Bronchography
E. Six-minute walk test
F. MRI

14.37

1. A 28-year-old patient complains of recurrent wheeze which is reversible with inhaled bronchodilators

2. A 69-year-old smoker complains of shortness of breath. On examination he has a barrel-shaped chest and a resonant note on percussion

3. A 55-year-old woman complains of shortness of breath. On examination she has fine, end-inspiratory crackles

Select the best match for each of the above

A. Increased peak expiratory flow rate
B. Increased FEV_1
C. FEV_1 falls proportionately more than the FVC
D. Increased total lung capacity with decreased transfer factor
E. Decreased transfer factor but without increase in total lung capacity

14.38

1. A 29-year-old asthmatic who complains of acute exacerbation of his symptoms

2. A 42-year-old patient with restrictive lung defect whose symptoms are affected particularly on exercise

3. A 24-year-old student with a history of allergy whose response to the allergen is enhanced due to this pollutant

4. A 69-year-old allergic individual who has enhanced production of IgE antibody due to this pollutant

5. A 61-year-old man who has lung cancer due to exposure to this substance

Select the best match for each of the above

A. Polyaromatic hydrocarbons
B. Ozone
C. Sulphur dioxide
D. Nitrogen dioxide
E. Particulate matter less than 10 μm in diameter

Q14.39

The following statements are correct

A. Air pollutants are one of the causes of the dramatic increase in asthma and other allergic diseases
B. Nitrogen dioxide enhances the nasal and lung airway responses to inhaled allergens in those with established allergic disease
C. Asthmatics are advised to increase their anti-inflammatory medication (i.e. inhaled sodium cromoglicate/ nedocromil or inhaled corticosteroids) during periods of poor air quality
D. In Europe 70% of the particulates present in urban air result from the combustion of diesel fuel
E. Levels of NO_2 can be lower in poorly ventilated kitchens where gas is used for cooking

Q14.40

An 18-year-old girl complains of facial pain and a yellowish discharge from her nose. On examination she has tenderness over both maxillary sinuses. The following statements about this condition are correct

A. Co-amoxiclav is preferred to amoxicillin
B. It is a frequent finding in aspirin intolerant subjects
C. Xylometazoline helps to relieve symptoms
D. Fluticasone propionate nasal spray relieves symptoms
E. It is usually caused by *Streptococcus pneumoniae*

Q14.41

1. An 18-year-old patient complains of nasal irritation, sneezing, watery rhinorrhoea, itching of the eyes, ears and throat. Symptoms are worst in late summer

2. A 37-year-old cat owner complains of sneezing and watery rhinorrhoea. He has never had symptoms that affect the eye or the throat

3. A 29-year-old patient complains of sneezing and watery rhinorrhoea. The patient is also intolerant to aspirin and NSAIDs

4. A 33-year-old patient complains of watery rhinorrhoea and sneezing. No extrinsic allergic cause can be identified either from history or on skin testing. The nasal secretions lack eosinophilic granulocytes

Select the best match for each of the above

A. Vasomotor rhinitis
B. Seasonal rhinitis
C. Perennial allergic rhinitis
D. Perennial non-allergic rhinitis with eosinophilia
E. Nasal polyps

Q14.42

1. A 59-year-old smoker is very breathless at rest. He has pursed lip breathing. Arterial tensions of oxygen and carbon dioxide are relatively normal. There is no cor pulmonale

2. A 67-year-old smoker does not appear to be breathless but is cyanosed. Blood gases reveal arterial hypoxaemia and carbon dioxide retention. Haematocrit is 57%

3. A 36-year-old patient develops breathlessness. He has never smoked and has radiographic features of basal emphysema

4. A 57-year-old smoker has central cyanosis. More recently he is more breathless and has had ankle oedema. He also complains of upper abdominal discomfort. He has a greatly elevated jugular venous pressure, left parasternal heave, loud pulmonary second sound, and ascites

5. A 26-year-old patient suffers from persistent halitosis, recurrent febrile episodes with malaise and episodes of pneumonia. The sputum is foul-smelling, thick and khaki-coloured. On examination he has clubbing of the finger nails and coarse crackles at the bases of both lungs

Select the best match for each of the above

A. Bronchiectasis
B. Pink puffer
C. α_1-Antitrypsin deficiency
D. Chronic cor pulmonale
E. Chronic bronchitis

Q14.43

A 45-year-old previously healthy patient has an irritating productive cough together with discomfort behind the sternum. There is associated tightness of the chest, wheezing and shortness of breath. The patient improves spontaneously in 8 days without becoming seriously ill. The following statements about this condition are correct

A. The aetiology of this condition is rarely viral
B. *Haemophilus influenzae* is a likely aetiology in smokers
C. *Streptococcus pneumoniae* is a likely aetiology in chronic obstructive pulmonary disease
D. In previously healthy adults the disease improves spontaneously without the patient becoming seriously ill
E. Amoxicillin 250 mg three times daily has been clearly shown to hasten recovery in healthy individuals

Q14.44

A 58-year-old smoker complains of cough with expectoration for 4 months in the year for the past 3 years. Symptoms are worsened by cold, foggy weather. During acute exacerbations he becomes cyanosed and accessory muscles of respiration in the neck contract. He has tricuspid incompetence, elevated jugular venous pressure, ascites and upper abdominal discomfort. The following statements about this condition are correct

A. Lung function tests show evidence of restrictive disease
B. Sputum examination is unnecessary in the ordinary case as *Strep. pneumoniae* and *Haemophilus influenzae* are the only common organisms to produce acute exacerbations
C. In advanced cases the ECG shows features of left ventricular hypertrophy
D. Venesection is recommended if the packed cell volume is greater than 55%
E. Continuous administration of oxygen to achieve an oxygen saturation greater than 90% for a large proportion of the day and night has been shown to improve survival
F. In symptomatic patients with chronic obstructive pulmonary disease, a trial of corticosteroids is always indicated

Q14.45

A 45-year-old man has a body mass index of 42. His wife complains that he snores at night, and he often wakes at night complaining of unrefreshing sleep and headaches, and even sounding drunk. The following statements are correct

A. Inhaled steroids decrease the rate of progression
B. Arterial oxygen saturation will fall significantly in a cyclical manner
C. The diagnosis is confirmed if the patient has more than 15 episodes of this abnormality in any 1 hour of sleep
D. Continuous positive airway pressure (CPAP) delivered by a mask at night improves symptoms
E. In mild cases, intermittent chemotherapy with ciprofloxacin 50 mg twice daily may be the only therapy needed

Q14.46

1. A 16-year-old boy has a history of nasal polyps and spontaneous pneumothorax. He complains of cough with sputum production. He has a history of steatorrhoea. A 1 mm cube of saccharin placed on the inferior turbinate takes 45 minutes to taste. Sweat sodium concentration is 70 mmol/L. Sputum examination reveals *Pseudomonas aeruginosa*

2. A 28-year-old patient complains of cough with greenish-yellow sputum. He has had this condition for several years. His heart is on the right side and he has been told that his liver is on the left side. A 1 mm cube of saccharin placed on the inferior turbinate takes 40 minutes to taste

3. A 48-year-old patient complains of cough with greenish-yellow sputum. He developed this condition about 4 years

ago but he also has a 10-year history of chronic sinus infection. Sinus X-rays reveal concomitant purulent rhinosinusitis. A 1 mm cube of saccharin placed on the inferior turbinate takes 50 minutes to taste. Investigations for infertility reveal azoospermia

4. A 23-year-old patient has a history of recurrent cough with copious sputum production. CT reveals that the left lower lung has dilated and thickened bronchi. A 1 mm cube of saccharin placed on the inferior turbinate takes 20 minutes to taste

Select the best match for each of the above

A. Allergic bronchopulmonary aspergillosis
B. Young's syndrome
C. Kartagener's syndrome
D. Gene mutation of the long arm of chromosome 7
E. Pulmonary sequestration

Q14.47

1. A 48-year-old patient with emphysema with a life expectancy of <1 year

2. A 42-year-old patient with bilateral pulmonary fibrosis with a life expectancy of <18 months

3. A 62-year-old patient with chronic obstructive pulmonary disease and a life expectancy of 26 months

4. A patient with ventricular septal defect and a right-to-left shunt with a life expectancy of 13 months

5. A 27-year-old patient with α_1-antitrypsin deficiency with a life expectancy of 12 months

6. A 43-year-old patient with bilateral bronchiectasis with purulent sputum with a life expectancy of 10 months

Respiratory disease

Select the best match for each of the above

A. Transplantation is not indicated
B. Single lung transplantation is usually undertaken
C. Bilateral lung transplantation
D. Heart–lung transplantation
E. Heart transplantation

Select the best option for each of the above

A. Prednisolone 40 mg daily with salmeterol
B. As-required short-acting bronchodilators
C. Inhaled steroids up to 800 μg/daily
D. Add regular long-acting β_2-agonist
E. Hospital admission
F. Broad-spectrum antibiotic therapy

Q14.48

A 42-year-old patient is newly diagnosed with bronchial asthma. The following may precipitate an asthmatic attack

A. Aminophylline
B. Indometacin
C. Salbutamol
D. Atenolol
E. Exercise

Q14.49

1. A 23-year-old patient with bronchial asthma has symptoms once a month. His peak expiratory flow rate is 100% predicted

2. A 32-year-old patient who has exacerbations of asthma three or four times a week and is able to do her job as a clerk every day. Her peak expiratory flow rate is 90% predicted

3 A 47-year-old patient develops symptoms daily. She is limited in doing her job as a postal clerk. Her peak expiratory flow rate is 80% predicted

4. A 42-year-old asthmatic whose wheeze is deteriorating and whose peak expiratory flow rate is 40% predicted

5. A 28-year-old student who has symptoms daily and whose symptoms are not controlled by 2000 μg/daily of inhaled corticosteroids. Her peak expiratory flow rate is 70% predicted

Q14.50

The accident and emergency department physician sees the 39-year-old asthmatic for the first time. She complains of worsening shortness of breath in the past hour. The following features suggest a life-threatening asthmatic attack

A. P_aCO_2 of 7 kPa
B. P_aO_2 of 7 kPa
C. PEFR of 125 L/min
D. Blood pressure of 80/60 mmHg
E. Pulse oximetry 90% saturation

Q14.51

1. A 42-year-old asthmatic is on therapy with long-acting β_2-adrenoreceptor antagonists

2. A 23-year-old swimming coach is on nedocromil sodium aerosol 4 mg twice a day

3. A 35-year-old asthmatic has been taking 1000 μg twice a day of inhaled beclometasone dipropionate

4. A 45-year-old asthmatic has been prescribed zafirlukast for her aspirin-intolerant asthma

5. A 55-year-old asthmatic has been prescribed omalizumab for his asthma

Select the best match for each of the above

A. Cysteinyl leukotriene receptor antagonist
B. Tablets of this medication are less effective than when the drug is inhaled

C. This drug acts by preventing activation of eosinophils and epithelial cells by blocking a specific chloride channel

D. Blocks the interaction of IgE with mast cells and basophils

E. Subcapsular cataract formation may occur

Q14.52

1. A 23-year-old student develops pneumonia following influenza

2. An 85-year-old woman in hospital following surgery for hip fracture develops pneumonia

3. A 30-year-old man who has been smoking from the age of 17 develops virulent pneumonia

4. A 45-year-old heart transplant patient who is being treated with ciclosporin, mycophenolate and prednisolone develops pneumonia

5. A 62-year-old man with oesophageal obstruction develops pneumonia

Select the most likely causative organism for each of the above

A. Anaerobes

B. Cytomegalovirus infection

C. *Streptococcus pneumoniae*

D. Invasive pneumococcal disease

E. Gram-negative organisms

Q14.53

A 17-year-old boy lives in a boarding school. He develops headaches and malaise initially. Five days later he develops a cough and examination of the chest reveals occasional crackles. Chest X-ray shows consolidation in one lobe of the lung. White cell count is not raised and cold agglutinins are found. Complications that this patient may have include

A. Myocarditis

B. Erythema multiforme

C. Haemolytic anaemia

D. Meningoencephalitis

E. Thrombocytosis

Q14.54

A 28-year-old AIDS patient develops high fever, breathlessness and cough. Chest X-ray shows consolidation. Causes of shadowing on the chest X-ray include

A. Kaposi's sarcoma

B. *Mycobacterium tuberculosis*

C. *Mycobacterium avium-intracellulare*

D. *Cryptococcus* sp.

E. Non-specific interstitial pneumonitis

Q14.55

1. A 45-year-old patient presents with systemic severe symptoms of pneumonia. Chest X-ray shows irregular opacities in both lungs, particularly in the mid-zones. The patient responds to sulfadiazine therapy

2. A 17-year-old patient has a history of cystic fibrosis. He develops pneumonia which responds to ticarcillin and gentamicin

3. A 57-year-old patient with chronic bronchitis develops pneumonia confined to one lobe. The patient has yellow-green sputum and responds well to oral cefaclor therapy

4. A 35-year-old owner of parrots develops malaise, cough and muscular pains. The patient has hepatosplenomegaly. Chest X-ray shows segmental pneumonia. The patient responds to treatment with tetracycline

5. A 42-year-old patient with disseminated AIDS has a CD4 lymphocyte count of 90/mm^3. The patient has consolidation

which responds to a combination of rifampicin, ethambutol and clofazimine

Select the most likely organism in each of the above

A. *Mycobacterium avium-intracellulare*
B. *Nocardia asteroides*
C. *Pseudomonas aeruginosa*
D. *Haemophilus influenzae*
E. *Chlamydia psittaci*

Q14.56

A 58-year-old man from the Indian subcontinent presents with gradual onset of vague ill-health, loss of weight and, more recently low-grade fever. He has hepatosplenomegaly. The chest X-ray shows a number of shadows 2 mm in diameter throughout the lung. The following statements are correct

A. This condition is universally fatal without treatment
B. Occasionally this condition presents as symptoms of meningitis
C. The chest X-ray may be entirely normal in this condition
D. The Mantoux test may be negative in this condition
E. When diagnosis cannot be confirmed, starting chemotherapy in a susceptible patient with pyrexia of unknown origin is acceptable

Q14.57

1. A 29-year-old woman on anti-tuberculosis treatment complains that her urine, tears and sweat have a new pink hue

2. A 49-year-old man on anti-tuberculosis treatment complains of tingling in both feet. Neurological examination and nerve conduction studies confirm neuropathy

3. A 42-year-old man on anti-tuberculosis treatment complains of a painful and swollen knee. Aspiration of the joint reveals negatively birefringent crystals

4. A 23-year-old patient on anti-tuberculosis treatment complains of a diminution in his perception of the colour green. On examination he has a reduction in visual acuity and a central scotoma

5. A 68-year-old woman with azotaemia is on anti-tuberculosis therapy and she complains of dizziness and vertigo. Examination reveals an impairment in the vestibular nerve

Select the best match for each of the above

A. Streptomycin
B. Isoniazid
C. Ethambutol
D. Rifampicin
E. Pyrazinamide

Q14.58

A 42-year-old patient has a cough and tuberculosis is suspected. Definitive diagnosis can be made with the following tests

A. Polymerase chain reaction
B. Sputum stained with Ziehl–Neelsen stain for acid and alcohol-fast bacilli
C. ELISA
D. Complement fixation tests
E. CT scan of chest

Q14.59

1. A 70-kg man with pulmonary tuberculosis

2. A 75-kg athlete with tuberculous osteomyelitis of the tibia

3. An 80-kg male with tuberculous meningitis

4. A 75-kg HIV-infected patient with pulmonary tuberculosis

5. A 45-kg woman who has fever and axillary lymph-node enlargement. Lymph node biopsy reveals tuberculomas

Select the best option for each of the above

A. Nine months' treatment with once-daily rifampicin 600 mg and isoniazid 300 mg. Initial 2 months with pyrazinamide 2 g/daily

B. Six months' treatment with once-daily rifampicin 600 mg and isoniazid 300 mg. Initial 2 months with pyrazinamide 2 g/daily

C. Six months' treatment with once-daily rifampicin 450 mg and isoniazid 300 mg. Initial 2 months with daily pyrazinamide 1.5 g/daily

D. Twelve months' treatment with once-daily rifampicin 600 mg and isoniazid 300 mg. Initial 2 months with pyrazinamide 2 g/daily

E. Supervised treatment with once-daily rifampicin 600 mg, isoniazid 300 mg, pyrazinamide 2 g and ethambutol 25 mg/kg

Q14.60

A medical student wants to know about the utility of the BCG vaccination. The following statements about BCG are correct

A. It has protective efficacy of about 95%

B. It is given only to individuals who are tuberculin-positive

C. It results in a positive Mantoux test

D. It is particularly effective in preventing tuberculous meningitis

E. It is particularly effective in preventing miliary tuberculosis

Q14.61

A 28-year-old West Indian woman presents with fatigue, weight loss and cough. Her chest X-ray shows bilateral hilar adenopathy. The differential diagnosis includes

A. Lymphoma
B. Pulmonary tuberculosis
C. Carcinoma of the bronchus
D. Sarcoidosis
E. Pneumococcal pneumonia

Q14.62

A 31-year-old West Indian woman presents with fatigue, weight loss, and progressive shortness of breath on exertion. The chest X-ray shows a mottling in the mid-zones proceeding to generalized fine nodular shadows. The principal differential diagnoses are

A. Tuberculosis
B. Pneumoconiosis
C. Cryptogenic fibrosing alveolitis
D. Sarcoidosis
E. Alveolar cell carcinoma

Q14.63

A 27-year-old surgeon with known sarcoidosis complains of misting of vision, pain and a red eye. He has a list of ocular manifestations of sarcoidosis and would like to confirm the accuracy of his information. The following manifestations in his list are correct

A. Conjunctival lesions
B. Retinal lesions
C. Anterior uveitis
D. Posterior uveitis
E. Asymptomatic uveitis

Q14.64

A 44-year-old obstetrician has recently been diagnosed as having sarcoidosis. His chest X-ray shows bilateral hilar adenopathy. He would like to avoid steroids and wishes to know the indications for steroid therapy. The following are indications for steroid therapy

A. Asymptomatic bilateral hilar adenopathy with normal lung function tests
B. Hypercalcaemia
C. Abnormal lung function tests not improving spontaneously for the last 7 months
D. Bilateral uveitis
E. Myocardial involvement

Q14.65

A 44-year-old obstetrician has recently been diagnosed as having sarcoidosis. His chest X-ray shows bilateral hilar adenopathy. He would like to know about the prognosis of sarcoidosis. The following statements are correct

A. Black Americans tend to have a more benign variant of the disease
B. Myocardial sarcoidosis is the most common cause of fatality
C. Chest X-ray provides a guide for prognosis
D. Lung function tests are useful to monitor progression
E. Reduction of serum angiotensin-converting enzyme during treatment reflects the resolution of the disease

Q14.66

A 58-year-old woman has long-standing rheumatoid arthritis. Her son, who is a medical student, requests information about lung involvement in this condition. The following are features of rheumatoid arthritis

A. Inflammation of the cricoarytenoid joints
B. Obliterative bronchiolitis
C. Pleural effusion
D. Fibrosing alveolitis
E. Cryptogenic organizing pneumonia

Q14.67

A 45-year-old woman has a 9-month history of progressive shortness of breath. On examination she is cyanosed, has finger clubbing, and fine bilateral end-inspiratory crackles can be heard on auscultation. High-resolution CT scan shows peripheral reticular and ground-glass opacification in the basal regions. The following statements about this condition are correct

A. Blood gases typically show elevated arterial carbon dioxide
B. FEV_1 is reduced whereas FVC is normal
C. Carbon monoxide expiratory gas transfer is reduced
D. Chest X-ray shows irregular reticulonodular shadowing
E. Rheumatoid factor is characteristically absent

Q14.68

1. A 29-year-old farmer has been forking hay in the morning. Late in the afternoon he develops malaise, cough, fever and shortness of breath

2. A 37-year-old pigeon handler complains of malaise, cough and shortness of breath

3. A 44-year-old malt worker who is involved in turning germinating barley complains of dyspnoea, cough and malaise

4. A 47-year-old factory worker complains of shortness of breath and cough. The humidifiers in the factory's air conditioning system are contaminated

5. A 47-year-old mushroom grower who is involved in turning mushroom compost complains of dyspnoea and cough

Select the most appropriate antigen for each of the above

A. *Micropolyspora faeni*
B. Proteins present in the bloom on the feathers
C. *Aspergillus clavatus*
D. *Naegleria gruberi*
E. Thermophilic actinomycetes

Q14.69

1. A 42-year-old man with high blood pressure develops asthma when treated with this anti-hypertensive

2. A 39-year-old patient with congestive heart failure and non-sustained ventricular tachycardia is treated with medication for prevention of sustained ventricular tachycardia. He develops pulmonary fibrosis

3. A 47-year-old patient on treatment for diabetes and hypertension develops pulmonary eosinophilia

4. A 52-year-old woman develops systemic lupus erythematosus-like syndrome when treated with this medication for controlling her blood pressure

Select the best match for each of the above

A. Hydralazine
B. Thiazide diuretics
C. Chlorpropamide
D. Insulin
E. Atenolol
F. Amiodarone
G. Bleomycin
H. Quinidine

Q14.70

1. A 67-year-old retired coal miner has black sputum and shortness of breath.

His chest X-ray shows several fibrotic round masses in the upper lobes with necrotic central cavities

2. A 48-year-old stonemason's chest X-ray shows distinctive calcification around the lymph nodes ('eggshell' calcification)

3. A 23-year-old worker in a cotton mill develops tightness in the chest and cough within the first hour of work on Monday morning, after a weekend break

4. A 37-year-old industrial worker develops progressive shortness of breath with pulmonary fibrosis. The systemic illness resembles sarcoidosis

5. A 78-year-old retired power-station worker develops progressive dyspnoea. Examination reveals finger clubbing and bi-basal end-inspiratory crackles

6. A 75-year-old smoker who formerly worked in a ship-building yard and who has a history of pleural plaques develops haemoptysis. CT scan does not detect pulmonary fibrosis

7. A 58-year-old man who works in a navy ship-building yard develops persistent chest wall pain

Select the most likely option for each of the above

A. Asbestosis
B. Silicosis
C. Berylliosis
D. Mesothelioma
E. Simple pneumoconiosis
F. Byssinosis
G. Progressive massive fibrosis
H. Adenocarcinoma of the bronchus

Q14.71

1. Accounts for approximately 40% of all carcinomas. Most present as obstructive lesions of the bronchus leading to

infection. It occasionally cavitates (10%) at presentation but widespread metastases occur relatively late. The cells are usually well differentiated but occasionally anaplastic. Local spread is common

2. Accounts for 25% of all tumours. It is a less well-differentiated tumour that metastasizes early

3. Accounts for approximately 10% of all bronchial carcinomas and frequently arises in or around scar tissue. It is the most common bronchial carcinoma associated with asbestos and is proportionally more common in non-smokers, in women, in the elderly, and in the Far East. It arises peripherally from mucous glands in the small bronchi and often produces a subpleural mass. Invasion of the pleura and the mediastinal lymph nodes is common, as are metastases to the brain and bones

4. Accounts for only 1–2% of lung tumours and occurs either as a peripheral solitary nodule or as diffuse nodular lesions of multicentric origin. Occasionally this tumour is associated with expectoration of very large volumes of mucoid sputum

5. Accounts for 20–30% of all lung cancers. It arises from endocrine cells (Kulchitsky cells). These cells are members of the APUD system, which explains why many polypeptide hormones are secreted by these tumours. Some of these polypeptides act in an autocrine fashion: they feed back on the cells and cause cell growth. Although the tumour is rapidly growing and highly malignant, it is the only one of the bronchial carcinomas that responds to chemotherapy

Select the best match for each of the above

A. Small-cell carcinoma
B. Alveolar cell carcinoma
C. Adenocarcinoma
D. Large-cell carcinoma
E. Squamous or epidermoid carcinoma

Q14.72

1. A 48-year-old smoker with squamous-cell carcinoma develops joint stiffness and severe pain in the ankles and wrists. It is associated with clubbing of fingers. X-ray shows proliferative periostitis at the distal ends of long bones, which have an onion skin appearance

2. A 58-year-old smoker with squamous-cell carcinoma develops ataxia of gait. The patient has dysmetria, dyssynergia and dysdiadochokinesia

3. A 52-year-old smoker with squamous-cell carcinoma develops proximal muscle weakness. Weakness tends to improve after a few minutes' muscular contraction, and absent reflexes return (cf. myasthenia)

4. A 38-year-old smoker with squamous-cell carcinoma develops severe pain in the shoulder and down the inner surface of the arm. The patient has miosis, partial ptosis, enophthalmos and slight elevation of the lower lid

5. A 49-year-old smoker with squamous-cell carcinoma develops early morning headache, facial congestion, and oedema involving the upper limbs. The jugular veins are distended as are the veins on the chest which form a collateral circulation with veins arising from the abdominal wall

Select the best match for each of the above

A. Superior vena caval syndrome
B. Subacute cerebellar degeneration

C. Friedreich's ataxia

D. Eaton–Lambert syndrome

E. Pancoast's tumour

F. Hypertrophic pulmonary osteoarthropathy

G. Rheumatoid arthritis

H. Guillain–Barré syndrome

Q14.73

A 47-year-old smoker is diagnosed with bronchogenic carcinoma. The house officer wishes to know the relative merits of the various investigations. The following statements are correct

A. By the time lung cancer is causing symptoms it will almost always be visible on chest X-rays

B. CT is particulary useful for identifying disease in the mediastinum

C. MRI is particulary useful for the diagnosis of primary lung tumours

D. Widening and loss of the sharp angle of the carina observed during fibreoptic bronchoscopy almost always indicates the presence of enlarged malignant mediastinal lymph nodes

E. During fibreoptic bronchoscopy, if the tumour is found to involve the first 2 cm of the right main bronchus, then the tumour is inoperable

Q14.74

A 67-year-old patient has been losing weight. Chest X-ray shows multiple round shadows about 2 cm in diameter. Typical sites for the primary tumour include

A. Prostate

B. Breast

C. Bone

D. Cervix

E. Ovary

Q14.75

A 48-year-old airline pilot has a routine chest X-ray. She is asymptomatic. The chest X-ray shows a solitary round shadow. The differential diagnosis includes

A. Primary bronchial carcinoma

B. Tuberculoma

C. Benign tumour of the lung

D. Hydatid cyst

E. Metastatic renal cell carcinoma

Q14.76

A 38-year-old mother of two presents with progressive and severe shortness of breath. The chest X-ray shows bilateral lymphadenopathy together with streaky basal shadowing fanning out over both lung fields. The lesions which can cause this clinical picture include

A. Hydatid cyst

B. Benign tumour of the lung

C. Carcinoma of the stomach

D. Carcinoma of the pancreas

E. Carcinoma of the breast

Q14.77

Pleural fluid examination of a 49-year-old woman shows a protein content of 20 g/L and lactic dehydrogenase is 200 IU/L. The most likely causes for the pleural effusion include

A. Bacterial pneumonia

B. Tuberculosis

C. Meigs' syndrome

D. Acute pancreatitis

E. Heart failure

Q14.78

A 47-year-old woman's lung function tests are abnormal. On chest X-ray the left diaphragm is markedly elevated. On chest fluoroscopy, a sniff causes the left diaphragm to rise while the right diaphragm descends. Potential causes of this patient's condition include

A. Poliomyelitis
B. Herpes zoster
C. Tuberculosis
D. Post-cardiac bypass surgery
E. Subclavian vein puncture

Q14.79

A 58-year-old man complains of shortness of breath when lying down. He also has sleep apnoea, daytime headaches and somnolence. Respiratory rate is 30/min, and tidal volume is decreased. Vital capacity is substantially reduced when the patient is lying down and sniffing causes a paradoxical inward movement of the abdominal wall. Causes include

A. Guillain–Barré syndrome
B. Multiple sclerosis
C. Poliomyelitis
D. Quadriplegia due to a motor vehicle accident
E. Eaton–Lambert syndrome

Q14.80

A 28-year-old woman finds it difficult to breathe through the nose and prefers to keep her mouth open. She has had a thyroidectomy and has a hoarse voice. Correct statements regarding the anatomy of the respiratory system include

A. The nasal vestibule causes an increase in resistance to airflow when breathing through the nose rather than the mouth
B. The external branch of the superior laryngeal nerve can be injured during thryoidectomy
C. The left recurrent laryngeal nerve can be affected when the mediastinum

between the trachea and the oesphagus is affected by disease
D. The principal tensor of the vocal cords is the recurrent laryngeal nerve
E. The adenoids keep the airway open during breathing and occlude the airway during swallowing

Q14.81

A 68-year-old retired policeman has a stroke. On examination he is found to have aspiration pneumonia. Correct statements regarding his condition include

A. The left bronchus is more vertical than the right, and hence inhaled material is more likely to pass into it
B. Physical signs on the front of the chest on the right side are mainly due to lesions mainly of the lower lobe
C. The most usual sites for spillage are the apical and posterior segments of the right lower lobe
D. A substantial portion of the aspirated material generally leaks into the pleural cavity
E. The aspirated material usually stimulates the slow-twitch muscle fibres of the diaphragm

Q14.82

A 69-year-old smoker complains of shortness of breath. His bronchoscopy shows a large mass compressing the right main bronchus. The following are recognized features on the chest X-ray

A. The trachea will be deviated to the left
B. There will be gross elevation of the left hemi-diaphragm
C. Heart and apex beat will be deviated to the left
D. Compensatory emphysema of the left lung
E. Left-sided pleural effusion

Q14.83

The radiologist is reading all the chest X-rays done that day. One of the chest X-rays has several bilateral opacities which are 2 mm in size. Recognized causes of these findings include

A. Pulmonary oedema
B. Fibrosing alveolitis
C. Sarcoidosis
D. Pneumoconiosis
E. Bronchial asthma

Q14.84

A 55-year-old patient smokes about 40 cigarettes a day. She sees her general practitioner for a routine visit. The following statements about smoking cessation are correct

A. Simple advice and follow-up by the GP can motivate about half of patients to stop
B. Nicotine chewing gum is superior to verbal advice for smoking cessation
C. Over-the-counter nicotine patches are superior to placebo in helping smokers to stop
D. Nicotine patches can safely be used in those with heart disease
E. Bupropion should be avoided in smokers with heart disease

Q14.85

A 28-year-old pregnant woman has been smoking about 20 cigarettes a day since the age of 16. She does not drink alcohol and there is no history of abuse of illicit drugs. She is at increased risk of the following

A. Bladder cancer
B. A decrease in birthweight of her infant
C. Memory problems
D. Carcinoma of the oesophagus
E. Peripheral vascular disease

Q14.86

The following statements regarding the management of allergic rhinitis are correct

A. Pollen contact can be avoided completely
B. Terfenadine is the drug of choice in those whose ECG shows a long QT interval
C. Xylometazoline nasal spray is usually ineffective because of tachyphylaxis
D. Sodium cromoglicate when applied topically in a spray is of tremendous value in allergic rhinitis
E. The most effective treatment for rhinitis is to use small doses of topically administered corticosteroid preparations

Q14.87

Recognized manifestations of *Haemophilus influenzae* type b include

A. Rheumatoid arthritis
B. Meningitis
C. Septic arthritis
D. Acute epiglottitis
E. Osteomyelitis

Q14.88

A 27-year-old nursing student develops influenza. The following statements are correct

A. The most likely organism is *Haemophilus influenzae* type a
B. Influenza A causes localized outbreaks of a mild nature, unlike influenza B
C. A fourfold increase in complement-fixing antibody is usually necessary for making the diagnosis
D. Neuraminidase inhibitors are helpful in shortening the duration of symptoms
E. Protection by influenza vaccines is usually effective for 4–5 years

Respiratory disease

A14.1

C

About 10% of the patients with bronchogenic carcinoma have endocrine manifestations including ectopic ACTH syndrome, syndrome of inappropriate secretion of antidiuretic hormone, hypercalcaemia, and rarely hypoglycaemia, thyrotoxicosis, and gynaecomastia. Of these this patient has SIADH as evidenced by low serum sodium with normal renal function. Patients with SIADH often have CNS manifestations such as confusion.

Non-metastatic extrapulmonary manifestations of bronchial carcinoma (percentage of all cases)	
Metabolic (universal at some stage)	**Vascular and haematological** (rare)
Loss of weight	Thrombophlebitis migrans
Lassitude	Non-bacterial thrombotic endocarditis
Anorexia	Microcytic and normocytic anaemia
	Disseminated intravascular coagulopathy
Endocrine (10%) (usually small-cell carcinoma)	Thrombotic thrombocytopenic purpura
Ectopic adrenocorticotrophin syndrome	Haemolytic anaemia
Syndrome of inappropriate secretion of antidiuretic	
hormone (SIADH)	**Skeletal**
Hypercalcaemia (usually squamous cell	Clubbing (30%)
carcinoma)	Hypertrophic osteoarthropathy
Rarer: hypoglycaemia, thyrotoxicosis, gynaecomastia	(± gynaecomastia) (3%)
Neurological (2–16%)	**Cutaneous** (rare)
Encephalopathies – including subacute	Dermatomyositis
cerebellar degeneration	Acanthosis nigricans
Myelopathies – motor neurone disease	Herpes zoster
Neuropathies – peripheral sensorimotor neuropathy	
Muscular disorders – polymyopathy, myasthenic	
syndrome (Eaton–Lambert syndrome)	

A14.2

E

About 70% of all primary lung cancers, including virtually all small-cell lung cancers and most squamous cell carcinomas, arise in the hilar region.

A14.3

D

The only treatment of any curative value for non-small-cell cancer of the lung is surgery. An FEV_1 of less than 1.5 L is not compatible with an active life following pneumonectomy, although the surgery itself can be successfully accomplished.

High-dose radiotherapy is the treatment of choice if the tumour is inoperable for reasons such as poor lung function.

A14.4

C

'Pneumothorax' means air in the pleural space. It may be spontaneous or occur as a result of trauma to the chest. Spontaneous pneumothorax usually occurs in young males, the male-to-female ratio being 6:1. It is caused by the rupture of a pleural bleb, usually apical, and is thought to be due to congenital defects in the connective tissue of the alveolar walls. Both lungs are affected with equal frequency. Often these patients are tall and thin. In patients over 40 years of age, the usual cause is underlying chronic obstructive pulmonary disease (COPD). Rarer causes include bronchial asthma, carcinoma, a lung abscess breaking down and leading to bronchopleural fistula, and severe pulmonary fibrosis with cyst formation. The usual presenting features are sudden onset of unilateral pleuritic pain or progressively increasing breathlessness. If the pneumothorax enlarges, the patient becomes more breathless and may develop pallor and tachycardia. There may be few physical signs if the pneumothorax is small.

A14.5

B

A pulmonary metastasis may be detected as a solitary round shadow on chest X-ray in an asymptomatic patient. The most common primary tumour to do this is a renal cell carcinoma.

A14.6

C

This patient has miliary mottling on the chest X-ray and recognized causes include miliary tuberculosis, pneumoconiosis, sarcoidosis, fibrosing alveolitis, pulmonary oedema and pulmonary microlithiasis (rare). Pulmonary oedema is usually perihilar and accompanied by larger, fluffy shadows. The history of fever, night sweats and haemoptysis makes the diagnosis most likely to be miliary TB.

A14.7

D

The most common mediastinal mass is a retrosternal or intrathoracic thyroid,

which is nearly always an extension of the thyroid present in the neck. Enlargement of the thyroid by a colloid goitre or malignant disease and, rarely, in thyrotoxicosis causes displacement of the trachea and oesophagus to the opposite side. Symptoms of compression develop insidiously before producing the cardinal feature of dyspnoea. Very occasionally an intrathoracic thyroid may be the cause of dysphagia and, rarely, of hoarseness of the voice and vocal cord paralysis from stretching of the recurrent laryngeal nerve. The treatment is surgical removal.

A14.8

B

Emphysema has a radiological correlate in that patients who have lost more than 40% of their lung tissue will show hyperlucency of their lungs and in addition, the lung fields will be increased in area, because of air trapping.

A14.9

C

Catastrophic sudden severe (brittle) asthma is an unusual variant of asthma in which patients are at risk from sudden death in spite of the fact that their asthma may be well controlled between attacks. Severe life-threatening attacks may occur within hours or even minutes. Such patients need a carefully worked out management plan agreed by respiratory physician, primary care physician and patient, and require:

- emergency supplies of medications at home, in the car and at work
- oxygen and resuscitation equipment at home and at work
- nebulized β_2 agonists at home and at work

- self-injectable adrenaline (epinephrine): two EpiPens of 0.3 mg adrenaline (epinephrine) at home, at work and to be carried by patient at all times
- prednisolone 60 mg
- Medic Alert bracelet

The patient should attend the nearest hospital immediately. Admission to intensive care may be required.

A14.10

C

See answer to question 14.11.

A14.11

D

Legionella pneumophila breaks out among previously fit individuals staying in hotels, institutions or hospitals where the shower facilities or cooling systems have been contaminated with the organism. Sporadic cases occur in many parts of the world where the source of the infection is unknown; most cases involve middle-aged and elderly men who are smokers, but it is now being seen in children. The incubation period is 2–10 days. Males are affected twice as commonly as females. The infection may be mild, but the characteristic picture is of malaise, myalgia, headache and a fever with rigors and a pyrexia of up to 40°C. Half of the patients have gastrointestinal symptoms, with nausea, vomiting, diarrhoea and abdominal pain. Patients may be acutely ill, with mental confusion and other neurological signs. Haematuria occurs and occasionally renal failure. The patient is tachypnoeic with initially a dry cough that later may become productive and purulent. The chest X-ray usually shows lobar and then multilobar shadowing,

sometimes with a small pleural effusion. A strong presumptive diagnosis of *L. pneumophila* infection is possible in the majority of patients if they have three of the four following features: a) a prodromal virus-like illness; b) a dry cough, confusion or diarrhoea; c) lymphopenia without marked leucocytosis; and d) hyponatraemia. Diagnosis is confirmed by a fourfold increase in antibody titre in the blood, but the quickest way is by the direct immunofluorescent staining of the organism in the pleural fluid, sputum or bronchial washings. The organism is not seen on Gram staining. Culture on special media is possible but takes up to 3 weeks. A urinary antigen test is commercially available and is highly specific. Treatment is usually with one of the macrolides, clarithromycin now being the drug of choice. Ciprofloxacin is also effective and rifampicin can be used in addition in ill patients.

A14.12

B

Kaposi's sarcoma affecting HIV-infected homosexual men is now seen less often since the introduction of HAART. Intrathoracic involvement usually follows cutaneous manifestations and includes nodules or infiltrates in the lungs with lymph node enlargement and endobronchial lesions. Symptoms are those of progressive dyspnoea and cough. Chest X-ray appearances are non-specific. Bronchoscopy reveals multiple red or purple flat lesions which are not biopsied because of difficulty with histological diagnosis in crushed fragments and risk of haemorrhage. Treatment is with chemotherapy, vincristine 2 mg and bleomycin 10 mg/m² every 3 weeks.

A14.13

D

Counterimmunoelectrophoresis (CIE) for pneumococcal antigen of sputum, urine and serum is three to four times more sensitive than sputum or blood cultures for diagnosing pneumococcal pneumonia.

A14.14

B

In suspected pneumococcal pneumonia, when oral therapy is contraindicated, parenteral ampicillin or benzylpenicillin should be combined with clarithromycin. If *Staph. aureus* infection is suspected or is proven on culture, intravenous flucloxacillin ± sodium fusidate should be added. For severe cases requiring intensive care, parenteral antibiotics should be given with the combination of a broad-spectrum lactamase-stable beta-lactam antibiotic combined with clarithromycin.

A14.15

C

Fluoroquinolones are recommended for those intolerant of penicillins or macrolides.

A14.16

D

Pneumonia due to *Klebsiella* usually occurs in elderly people with a history of heart or lung disease, diabetes, alcohol excess or malignancy. The onset is often sudden, with severe systemic upset. The sputum is purulent, gelatinous or blood-stained. The upper lobes are more commonly affected and the consolidation is often extensive. There is often swelling of the infected lobe so that on the lateral chest X-ray there is bulging of the fissures. The organism can be found in the sputum or in the blood.

A14.17

D

The clinical features of lung abscess are those of persisting and worsening pneumonia associated with the production of large quantities of sputum, which is often foul-smelling owing to the growth of anaerobic organisms. There is usually a swinging fever. Fever, malaise and weight loss occur. The chest signs may be few but clubbing often develops if the condition is not rapidly cured. The patient is often anaemic with a high ESR.

A14.18

B

Patients who have any chest X-ray changes compatible with previous tuberculosis and who are about to undergo long-term treatment that has an immunosuppressive effect, such as renal dialysis or treatment with corticosteroids, should receive chemoprophylaxis with isoniazid 200–300 mg daily.

A14.19

B

Tuberculosis is spread from person to person and effective tracing of close contacts has helped to limit spread of the disease as well as to identify diseased individuals at an early stage. Screening procedures involve screening all close family members or other individuals who share the same kitchen and bathroom facilities. Occasionally, close contacts at work or school may also be screened.

Respiratory disease

Contacts who are ill should be thoroughly investigated for tuberculosis. If they are well, a chest X-ray is taken and a tuberculin test is performed.

A14.20

C

If the tuberculin test is negative in children and young adults (<35 years), it is repeated at 6 weeks, and if it remains negative then BCG is administered.

A14.21

D

Children under the age of 1 year who have a family member with tuberculosis are given chemoprophylaxis with a daily dose of isoniazid 5–10 mg/kg for 6 months together with immunization with a strain of BCG that is resistant to isoniazid.

A14.22

D

In children, a positive tuberculin test is usually taken as evidence of infection, and treatment is instituted.

A14.23

E

In adults, even if the tuberculin test is positive, provided the chest X-ray is negative nothing more need be done. In patients with HIV infection who have not had BCG chemoprophylaxis with isoniazid is given, reducing the relative risk of developing active TB by 40% in highly endemic areas.

A14.24

D

The association of bilateral symmetrical hilar lymphadenopathy with erythema nodosum occurs only in sarcoidosis.

A14.25

C

Uveoparotid fever is a syndrome of bilateral uveitis and parotid gland enlargement together with occasional development of facial nerve palsy and is sometimes seen with sarcoidosis. Keratoconjunctivitis sicca and lacrimal gland enlargement may also occur.

A14.26

B

Transbronchial biopsy is the most useful investigation in sarcoidosis. Positive results are seen in 90% of cases of pulmonary sarcoidosis with or without X-ray evidence of lung involvement. The test provides positive histological evidence of a granuloma in approximately one-half of patients with clinically extrapulmonary sarcoidosis in whom the chest X-ray is normal.

A14.27

D

Langerhans' cell histiocytosis (LCH) is a rare disease (a prevalence of 1 per 50 000) is characterized histologically by proliferation of LCH cells identified by the presence of Birbeck granules on electron-microscopy or the $CD1_a$ antigen on the surface of the cells. There is a wide variation in clinical presentation, from unifocal bone lesions in older children (which may regress spontaneously), to more disseminated disease in younger children (with a high mortality). Chest X-rays show multiple small cysts (honeycomb lung), fibrosis or widespread nodular shadows.

A14.28

B

Caplan's syndrome is due to a combination of dust inhalation and the disturbed immunity of rheumatoid arthritis. It occurs particularly in coal-worker's pneumoconiosis but it can occur in individuals exposed to other dusts, such as silica and asbestos. Typically the lesions appear as rounded nodules 0.5–5.0 cm in diameter, though sometimes they become incorporated into large areas of fibrosis that are indistinguishable radiologically from progressive massive fibrosis.

A14.29

C

Rheumatoid factor is always present in the serum in Caplan's syndrome.

A14.30

C

Wegener's granulomatosis is characterized by lesions involving the upper respiratory tract, the lungs and the kidneys. Often the disease starts with severe rhinorrhoea with subsequent nasal mucosal ulceration followed by cough, haemoptysis and pleuritic pain. Occasionally there may be involvement of the skin and nervous system. A chest X-ray usually shows single or multiple nodular masses or pneumonic infiltrates with cavitation. The most remarkable radiographic feature is the migratory pattern, with large lesions

clearing in one area and new lesions appearing in another. The typical histological changes are usually best seen in the kidneys, where there is a necrotizing glomerulonephritis.

A14.31

A

Churg–Strauss syndrome occurs in patients, usually male, in their fourth decade who have a triad of rhinitis and asthma, eosinophilia and systemic vasculitis. Occasionally Churg–Strauss syndrome may be revealed when oral steroids are withdrawn in patients being treated for asthma. The pathology of this condition is dominated by an eosinophilic infiltration with a characteristic high blood eosinophil count, vasculitis of small arteries and veins, and extravascular granulomas. Typically it involves the lungs, peripheral nerves and skin but kidney involvement is uncommon. Transient patchy pneumonia-like shadows may occur, but sometimes these can be massive and bilateral. Skin lesions include tender subcutaneous nodules as well as petechial or purpuric lesions. ANCA is usually positive. The disease responds well to corticosteroids.

A14.32

B

In allergic bronchopulmonary aspergillosis there are episodes of eosinophilic pneumonia throughout the year, particularly in late autumn and winter. The episodes present with a wheeze, cough, fever and malaise. They are associated with expectoration of firm sputum plugs containing the fungal mycelium, which results in the clearing of the pulmonary infiltrates on the chest

X-ray. The peripheral blood eosinophil count is usually raised, and total levels of IgE are usually extremely high (both that specific to *Aspergillus* and non-specific).

A14.33

E

Goodpasture's syndrome often starts with an upper respiratory tract infection followed by cough and intermittent haemoptysis, tiredness and eventually anaemia, though massive bleeding may occur. The chest X-ray shows transient blotchy shadows that are due to intrapulmonary haemorrhage. These features usually precede the development of an acute glomerulonephritis by several weeks or months. The course of the disease is variable: some spontaneously improve while others proceed to renal failure. The disease usually occurs in individuals over 16 years of age. It is due to a type II cytotoxic reaction driven by antibodies directed against the basement membrane of both kidney and lung. It has been proposed that there may be a shared antigen. ANCA may be positive.

A14.34

C

Single or combination chemotherapy in small-cell cancer has resulted in a fivefold increase in median survival from 2 to 10 months. A small number of patients enjoy several years of remission. Good results have been achieved with the combination of etoposide and cisplatin.

A14.35

1) B   2) D   3) C   4) E   5) A

Healthy lungs filter off most of the high-frequency component, which is mainly due to turbulent flow in the larynx. Normal breath sounds are harsher anteriorly over the upper lobes (particularly on the right) and described as vesicular. Vesicular sounds may be loud in a thin healthy subject or soft in patients with emphysema. Breath sounds are reduced or absent in a pneumothorax, over a pleural effusion, or when the bronchus to a lobe is obstructed by a carcinoma. Wheeze is usually heard during expiration and results from vibrations in the collapsible part of the airways when apposition occurs as a result of the flow-limiting mechanisms. Wheezes are heard in asthma and in chronic obstructive pulmonary disease, but are not invariably present. In the most severe cases of asthma a wheeze may not be heard, as the airflow may be insufficient to generate the sound. Wheezes may be monophonic (single large airway obstruction) or polyphonic (narrowing of many small airways). Crackles are brief crackling sounds are probably produced by opening of previously closed bronchioles, and their timing during breathing is of significance – early inspiratory crackles are associated with diffuse airflow limitation, whereas late inspiratory crackles are characteristically heard in pulmonary oedema, fibrosis of the lung and bronchiectasis. They may be described as fine or coarse. Pleural rub is a creaking or groaning sound that is usually well localized. It is indicative of inflammation and roughening of the pleural surfaces, which normally glide silently over one another. The first patient has bronchial asthma, the second has foreign body in trachea, the third has acute pulmonary oedema, the fourth patient has pleurisy and the fifth patient has a pleural effusion.

A14.36

1) A   **2)** C   **3)** C   **4)** B   **5)** C
6) C   **7)** F

The advent of rapid volumetric or 'spiral' scanning means that scans can be obtained rapidly (within seconds) during contrast injection. This is a useful technique for directly demonstrating pulmonary emboli within pulmonary vessels. Conventional CT is valuable in bronchial carcinoma staging to demonstrate mediastinal, pleural or chest wall invasion and to determine operability. High-resolution CT scanning (sampling lung parenchyma with 1–2 mm thickness scans at 10–20 mm intervals) allows assessment of diffuse lung parenchymal processes, particularly interstitial disease. It is valuable in the following situations. a) Detection of diffuse interstitial pulmonary involvement in any type of interstitial lung disease, including sarcoidosis, cryptogenic and extrinsic allergic alveolitis, occupational lung disease, and any other form of interstitial pulmonary fibrosis. b) Bronchiectasis. High-resolution CT has a sensitivity and specificity of greater than 90%. Inspiratory and expiratory scans may allow demonstration of air trapping in small airway disease. This technique has replaced bronchography. c) Distinguishing emphysema from interstitial lung disease or pulmonary vascular disease as a cause of a low gas transfer factor with otherwise normal lung function. d) Diagnosis of lymphangitis carcinomatosa. In the mediastinum, MRI is becoming the investigation of choice for assessing vascular and solid masses. The use of ECG-gating allows accurate images of the heart and aortic aneurysms to be obtained. The main strength of MRI in staging lung cancer is for assessing tumour invasion in the mediastinum, chest wall and particularly at the lung apex, by virtue of its ability to produce good images in the sagittal and coronal planes. Vascular structures can be clearly differentiated as flowing blood produces a signal void on MR.

A14.37

1) C   **2)** D   **3)** E

The forced expiratory volume in 1 second (FEV_1) expressed as a percentage of the forced vital capacity (FVC) is an excellent measure of airflow limitation. In normal subjects it is around 75%. With increasing airflow limitation the FEV_1 falls proportionately more than the FVC, so that the FEV_1/FVC ratio is reduced. In chronic airflow limitation (particularly in emphysema and asthma) the total lung capacity (TLC) is usually increased, yet there is nearly always some reduction in the FVC. Gas transfer is usually reduced in patients with severe degrees of emphysema and fibrosis. Overall gas transfer can be thought of as a relatively non-specific test of lung function but one that can be particularly used in the early detection and assessment of progress of diseases affecting the lung parenchyma (e.g. cryptogenic pulmonary fibrosis, sarcoidosis, asbestosis).

Respiratory disease

A14.38

1) C   2) B   3) D   4) E   5) A

Air pollutants and their health effects		
	Susceptible individuals	Mechanism of health effects
Sulphur dioxide (SO_2)	Asthmatics	Bronchoconstriction through neurogenic mechanism
Ozone (O_3)	All affected, particularly during exercise	Restrictive lung defect Airway inflammation Enhanced response to allergen
Nitrogen dioxide (NO_2)	Allergic individuals	Airway inflammation Enhanced response to allergen
Particulate matter (PM_{10})	Elderly Allergic individuals	Airway and alveolar inflammation Enhanced production selectively of the allergy antibody (IgE)

A14.39

1) F   2) T   3) T   4) T   5) F

Atmospheric air pollution, due to the burning of coal for energy and heat, has been a characteristic of urban living in developed countries for at least two centuries. It consists of black smoke and sulphur dioxide (SO_2). Air pollution of this type peaked in the 1950s in the UK, until legislation led to restrictions on coal burning. Such pollution continues to increase in newly industrialized countries (India, China) and continues in Eastern Europe and Russia. The combustion of petroleum and diesel oil in motor vehicles has led to new air pollution, consisting of primary pollutants such as the oxides of nitrogen (NO and NO_2), diesel particulates, polyaromatic hydrocarbons and the secondary pollutant ozone (O_3) generated by photochemical reactions in the atmosphere. Levels of NO_2 can be higher in poorly ventilated kitchens and living rooms where gas is used for cooking and in fires. In Europe 70% of the particulates present in urban air result from the combustion of diesel fuel. Very small particles (<2.5 mm, $PM_{2.5}$) remain airborne for long periods and are carried into rural areas. In the UK, ozone concentrations are highest in sunny rural areas. It has been proposed at various times that air pollutants are one of the causes of the dramatic increase in asthma and other allergic diseases. However, there is no current evidence that this is true. On the other hand, both NO_2 and ozone have been shown to enhance the nasal and lung airway responses to inhaled allergen, in those with established allergic disease. Asthmatics are advised not to exercise outdoors during periods of poor air quality and to increase their anti-inflammatory medication (i.e. inhaled sodium cromoglicate/nedocromil or inhaled corticosteroids).

A14.40

A) T   B) T   C) T   D) T   E) T

Sinusitis is an infection of the paranasal sinuses that is usually caused by *Streptococcus pneumoniae* and *Haemophilus influenzae*. Sinusitis is a frequent finding in aspirin intolerant subjects and in those with severe asthma. Treatment is with antibiotics. Many strains of *H. influenzae* are now resistant to amoxicillin, so co-amoxiclav or cefaclor is preferred. In addition, nasal treatment with decongestants such as xylometazoline or anti-inflammatory therapy with topical corticosteroids such as fluticasone propionate nasal spray should be given to reduce swelling of the mucosa and unblock the sinus openings.

A14.41

1) B   2) C   3) D   4) A

Seasonal rhinitis is often called 'hay fever' and is the most common of all allergic diseases. It is better described as seasonal allergic rhinitis. Nasal irritation, sneezing and watery rhinorrhoea are the most troublesome symptoms, but many also suffer from itching of the eyes and soft palate and occasionally even itching of the ears because of the common innervation of the pharyngeal mucosa and the ear. Patients with perennial rhinitis rarely have symptoms that affect the eyes or throat. Perennial allergic rhinitis can come from domestic pets (especially cats) and are proteins derived from urine or saliva spread over the surface of the animal as well as skin protein. No extrinsic allergic cause can be identified in perennial non-allergic rhinitis with eosinophilia, either from the history or on skin testing; but, as in patients with perennial allergic rhinitis, eosinophilic granulocytes are present in nasal secretions. Aspirin and NSAID intolerance is found in this group. Vasomotor rhinitis patients have no demonstrable allergy or eosinophilia in nasal secretions. They may be suffering from non-specific nasal hyperreactivity that is due to an imbalance of the autonomic nervous system innervating the erectile tissue (sinusoids) in the nasal mucosa.

A14.42

1) B   2) E   3) C   4) D   5) A

Clinical observations have led to the suggestion that there are two distinct types of chronic obstructive pulmonary disease (COPD) patient, types A and B:

- Type A is pink and puffing. Although the person is very breathless, arterial tensions of oxygen and carbon dioxide are relatively normal and there is no cor pulmonale. These individuals are thought to be suffering predominantly from emphysema with little bronchitis.

- Type B on the other hand, is blue and bloated. The person does not appear to be breathless, but has marked arterial hypoxaemia, carbon dioxide retention, secondary polycythaemia and cor pulmonale. These patients are thought to be suffering predominantly from chronic bronchitis.

Patients with advanced COPD may develop cor pulmonale which is defined as heart disease secondary to disease of the lung. It is characterized by pulmonary hypertension, right ventricular hypertrophy, and eventually right heart failure. On examination, the patient is centrally cyanosed (owing to the lung disease) and, when heart failure develops, the patient becomes more breathless and ankle oedema occurs. Initially a prominent parasternal heave may be felt that is due to right ventricular hypertrophy and a loud pulmonary second sound may be heard. In very severe pulmonary hypertension there is incompetence of the pulmonary valve. With right heart failure, tricuspid incompetence may develop with a greatly elevated jugular venous pressure (JVP), ascites and upper abdominal discomfort owing to swelling of the liver.

α_1-Antitrypsin inhibitor is an antiproteinase inhibitor produced in the

Respiratory disease

liver, secreted into the blood and which diffuses into the lung. Here it functions as an antiprotease that inhibits neutrophil elastase, a proteolytic enzyme capable of destroying alveolar wall connective tissue. Those who do develop breathlessness under the age of 40 years have radiographic evidence of basal emphysema and are usually, but not always, cigarette smokers.

Patients with mild bronchiectasis only produce yellow or green sputum after an infection. Localized areas of the lung may be particularly affected, when sputum production will depend on position. As the condition worsens, the patient suffers from persistent halitosis, recurrent febrile episodes with malaise, and episodes of pneumonia. Clubbing occurs, and coarse crackles can be heard over the infected areas, usually the bases of the lungs. When the condition is severe there is continuous production of foul-smelling, thick, khaki-coloured sputum. Haemoptysis, either as blood-stained sputum or as a massive haemorrhage, can occur. Breathlessness may result from airflow limitation.

A14.43

A) F   B) T   C) T   D) T   E) F

Acute bronchitis in previously healthy subjects is often viral. Bacterial infection with organisms such as *Streptococcus pneumoniae* and *Haemophilus influenzae* is a common sequel to viral infections, and is more likely to occur in individuals who are cigarette smokers and in those with chronic obstructive pulmonary disease (COPD). The illness begins with an irritating, unproductive cough, together with discomfort behind the sternum. This may be associated with tightness in the chest, wheezing and shortness of breath. The cough becomes productive, the

sputum being yellow or green. There is a mild fever and a neutrophil leucocytosis; wheeze with occasional crackles can be heard on auscultation. In otherwise healthy adults the disease improves spontaneously in 4–8 days without the patient becoming seriously ill. Treatment with antibiotics may be given (e.g. amoxicillin 250 mg three times daily), though it is not known whether this hastens recovery in otherwise healthy individuals.

A14.44

A) F   B) T   C) F   D) T   E) T   F) T

This patient has chronic cor pulmonale secondary to chronic bronchitis. Lung function tests show evidence of airflow limitation. Sputum examination is unnecessary in the ordinary case as *Strep. pneumoniae* or *Haemophilus influenzae* are the only common organisms to produce acute exacerbations. In advanced cor pulmonale the P wave is taller (P pulmonale) and there may be right bundle branch block (RSR' complex) and the changes of right ventricular hypertrophy. In symptomatic patients with chronic obstructive pulmonary disease (COPD), a trial of corticosteroids is always indicated, since a proportion of patients have a large, unsuspected, reversible element to their disease and airway function may improve considerably. The long-term value of regular inhaled corticosteroids in all patients with COPD has not been proven. Two controlled trials (chiefly in males) have indicated that life can be prolonged in patients with COPD and severe chronic hypoxia or cor pulmonale by the continuous administration of oxygen at 2 L/min via nasal prongs to achieve an oxygen saturation of greater than 90% for large proportions of the day and night. Venesection is recommended because it may be symptomatically helpful in the hypoxic patient, particularly if the PCV is above 0.55 L/L.

A14.45

A) F **B)** T **C)** T **D)** T **E)** F

Sleep apnoea occurs most often in overweight middle-aged men and affects 1–2% of the population. In many cases diagnosis can be made on the combination of a good history of the snore–silence–snore cycle reported by the patient's relatives, supported by non-invasive ear or finger oximetry performed at home. Characteristically, arterial oxygen saturation will fall significantly in a cyclical manner. The diagnosis of sleep apnoea/hypopnoea is confirmed if there are more than 15 apnoeas or hypopnoeas in any 1 hour of sleep. Management consists of correction of treatable factors with, if necessary, nasal continuous positive airway pressure (CPAP) delivered by a nasal mask during sleep. Such systems raise the pressure in the pharynx by about 1 kPa, keeping the pharyngeal walls apart. Steroids and antibiotics have not been shown to influence this condition.

A14.46

1) D **2)** C **3)** B **4)** E

All these patients have bronchiectasis because of mucociliary clearance defects. Mucociliary clearance is assessed by the ability of the nose to clear saccharin. A 1 mm cube of saccharin is placed on the inferior turbinate and the time to taste measured (normally less than 30 minutes). Causes of bronchiectasis due to mucociliary defects can be: a) genetic, such as Kartagener's syndrome with dextrocardia and situs inversus, and cystic fibrosis; b) acquired, such as Young's syndrome characterized by azoospermia and sinusitis. Pulmonary sequestration causes bronchiectasis but is not associated with a defect in mucociliary clearance and is characterized by recurrent lobar pneumonia confined to the same lobe, typically the left lower lung. CT scan will show a dilated lung with thickened bronchi.

A14.47

1) B **2)** B **3)** A **4)** D **5)** B **6)** C

Indications for lung or heart–lung transplantation are patients under 60 years with a life expectancy of less than 18 months, no underlying cancer and no serious systemic disease. The main diseases treated by transplantation are:

- pulmonary fibrosis
- primary pulmonary hypertension
- cystic fibrosis
- bronchiectasis
- emphysema – particularly α_1-antitrypsin inhibitor deficiency
- Eisenmenger's syndrome.

Donor selection includes age under 40 years, good cardiac and lung function, and chest measurements slightly smaller than those of the recipient. Matching for ABO blood group is essential, but rhesus blood group compatibility is not essential. Since donor material is limited, single lung transplantation is preferred to double lung or heart–lung transplantation and can be successfully undertaken in pulmonary fibrosis, pulmonary hypertension and emphysema. Bilateral lung transplantation is required in infective conditions to prevent spillover of bacteria from the diseased lung to a single lung transplant. Eisenmenger's syndrome requires heart–lung transplant.

A14.48

A) F   B) T   C) F   D) T   E) T

Aminophylline and salbutamol are used for treatment of asthma. NSAIDs, β-blockers and exercise can all precipitate asthma. Selective β_1-adrenergic blocking drugs such as atenolol may still induce attacks of asthma; their use in asthmatic patients for hypertension or angina should be questioned.

A14.49

1) B   2) B   3) C   4) A   5) D

The stepwise management of asthma

Step	PEFR	Treatment
1 Occasional symptoms, less frequent than daily	100% predicted	As-required bronchodilators If used more than once daily, move to step 2
2 Daily symptoms	≤80% predicted	Anti-inflammatory drugs Sodium cromoglicate or low-dose inhaled corticosteroids up to 800 µg If not controlled, move to step 3
3 Severe symptoms	50–80% predicted	High-dose inhaled corticosteroids up to 2000 µg daily
4 Severe symptoms uncontrolled with high-dose inhaled corticosteroids	50–80% predicted	Add regular long-acting β_2-agonists (e.g. salmeterol)
5 Severe symptoms deteriorating	≤50% predicted	Add prednisolone 40 mg daily
6 Severe symptoms deteriorating in spite of prednisolone	≤30% predicted	Hospital admission

Short-acting bronchodilator treatment taken at any step on as-required basis

A14.50

A) T   B) T   C) T   D) T   E) F

Features of life-threatening asthmatic attacks are:

- a silent chest, cyanosis or feeble respiratory effort
- exhaustion, confusion or coma
- bradycardia or hypotension
- PEFR <30% of predicted normal or best (approximately 150 L/min in adults).

Arterial blood gases should always be measured in asthmatic patients requiring admission to hospital. Pulse oximetry is useful in monitoring oxygen saturation during the admission and reduces the need for repeat arterial puncture. Features suggesting very severe life-threatening attacks are:

- a high P_aCO_2 >6 kPa
- severe hypoxaemia P_aO_2 <8 kPa irrespective of treatment with oxygen
- a low or falling arterial pH.

A14.51

1) B   2) C   3) E   4) A   5) D

The most widely used bronchodilator preparations contain β_2-adrenergic agonists that are selective for the respiratory tract and do not stimulate the β_1-adrenoceptors of the myocardium.

Tablets of β_2-adrenoceptor agonists are less effective than when the drug is inhaled. Sodium cromoglicate and nedocromil sodium prevent activation of many inflammatory cells, particularly mast cells, eosinophils and epithelial cells, but not lymphocytes, by blocking a specific chloride channel which in turn prevents calcium influx. These drugs are effective in patients with milder asthma. The unwanted effects of inhaled corticosteroids are oral candidiasis, which may develop in 5% of patients, and hoarseness due to the effect of corticosteroids on the laryngeal muscles. Subcapsular cataract formation can occur. Abnormalities of bone metabolism can be detected when inhaled steroids are taken in high doses (beclometasone or budesonide >800 µg daily). In children, inhaled steroids at doses greater than 400 µg daily have been shown to retard short-term growth. Omalizumab acts by blocking the interaction of IgE with mast cells and basophils. Montelukast and zafirlukast are cysteinyl leukotriene receptor antagonists (LTRAs) and are effective in a subpopulation of patients.

A14.52

1) C   2) E   3) D   4) B   5) A

The following are the common organisms which precipitate infection in different settings:

- *Streptococcus pneumoniae* – often follows viral infection with influenza or parainfluenza.
- Hospitalized 'ill' patients – often infected with Gram-negative organisms.
- Cigarette smoking (the strongest independent risk factor for invasive pneumococcal disease).
- Immunosuppression (e.g. AIDS or treatment with cytotoxic agents) –

organisms include *Pneumocystis carinii*, *Mycobacterium avium-intracellulare*, cytomegalovirus.
- Intravenous drug abuse – frequently associated with *Staphylococcus aureus* infection.
- Inhalation from oesophageal obstruction – often associated with infection with anaerobes.

A14.53

A) T   B) T   C) T   D) T   E) F

Mycoplasma pneumonia is relatively common and often occurs in patients in their teens and twenties, frequently among those living in boarding institutions. Generalized features such as headaches and malaise often precede the chest symptoms by 1–5 days. Cough may not be obvious initially and physical signs in the chest may be scanty. On chest X-ray, usually only one lobe is involved but sometimes there may be dramatic shadowing in both lungs. There is frequently no correlation between the X-ray appearances and the clinical state of the patient. The white blood cell count may not be raised. Cold agglutinins occur in half of the cases. The diagnosis is confirmed by a rising antibody titre.

Extrapulmonary complications can occur at any time during the illness and occasionally dominate the clinical picture. Most are rare but they include:

- myocarditis and pericarditis
- rashes and erythema multiforme
- haemolytic anaemia and thrombocytopenia
- myalgia and arthralgia
- meningoencephalitis and other neurological abnormalities
- gastrointestinal symptoms (e.g. vomiting, diarrhoea).

A14.54

A) T B) T C) T D) T E) T

Causes of shadowing on the chest X-ray in AIDS patients include:

- Cytomegalovirus
- *Mycobacterium avium-intracellulare*
- *Mycobacterium tuberculosis*
- *Legionella pneumophila*
- *Cryptococcus* sp.
- Pyogenic bacteria
- Kaposi's sarcoma
- Lymphoid interstitial pneumonia
- Non-specific interstitial pneumonitis
- *Pneumocystis carinii*

A14.55

1) B 2) C 3) D 4) E 5) A

Immunocompromised patients develop pneumonia with all the usual organisms and with a number of organisms which do not cause illness in healthy hosts – organisms include *Pneumocystis carinii*, *Mycobacterium avium-intracellulare*, *Mycobacterium avium-intracellulare* (MAI) causes lung disease in patients with AIDS primarily as part of disseminated disease when CD4 lymphocyte counts are £100/mm^3 with the pulmonary complications being of less significance than the extrapulmonary involvement. Therapeutic regimens include combinations of rifabutin or rifampicin, ethambutol and clofazimine. Clarithromycin and azithromycin may prove to be particularly efficacious. *Nocardia asteroides* produces a similar picture to *Actinomyces*, though of greater severity. The chest X-ray often shows irregular opacities in one or both lungs, particularly in the mid-zones. Treatment is with sulfadiazine in doses up to 9 g daily.

Pneumonia due to *Pseudomonas* is of considerable significance in patients with cystic fibrosis, since it correlates with a worsening clinical condition and mortality. It is also seen in patients with neutropenia following cytotoxic chemotherapy. The isolation of *P. aeruginosa* from sputum must be interpreted with care because the organism grows well on bacterial culture medium and may simply represent contamination from the upper airways. *Pseudomonas* and other Gram-negative infections respond well to treatment with the 4-quinolone antibiotic ciprofloxacin (200–400 mg i.v. over 30–60 minutes twice daily) or ceftazidime (2 g bolus i.v. 8-hourly). *H. influenzae* is frequently identified in the yellow-green sputum produced during exacerbation of chronic bronchitis. It is therefore not surprising that this organism may be the cause of pneumonia in people suffering from COPD. The pneumonia can be diffuse or confined to one lobe. There are no special features to separate it from other bacterial causes of pneumonia. It responds well to treatment with oral cefaclor 500 mg 8-hourly. *Chlamydia psittaci:* Typically the individual has been exposed to infected birds, especially parrots, but cases may occur without a history of contact. The incubation period is 1–2 weeks and the disease may pursue a very low-grade course over several months. Symptoms include malaise, high fever, cough and muscular pains. The liver and spleen are occasionally enlarged, and scanty 'rose spots' may be seen on the abdomen. The chest X-ray shows segmental or a diffuse pneumonia. Occasionally the illness presents with a high, swinging fever and dramatic prostration with photophobia and neck stiffness that can be confused with meningitis. The diagnosis is confirmed by the demonstration of a rising titre of complement-fixing antibody. Macrolides or tetracycline are the antibiotics of choice.

A14.56

A) T **B)** T **C)** T **D)** T **E)** T

Miliary tuberculosis is the result of acute diffuse dissemination of tubercle bacilli via the bloodstream. This form of disseminated tuberculosis is universally fatal without treatment. It may present in an entirely non-specific manner with the gradual onset of vague ill-health, loss of weight and then fever. Occasionally the disease presents as tuberculous meningitis. Usually there are no abnormal physical signs in the early stages, although eventually the spleen and liver become enlarged. The chest X-ray may be entirely normal in miliary tuberculosis as the tubercles are not visible until uniform miliary shadows 1–2 mm in diameter are seen throughout the lung; they have a hard outline. The lesions can increase in size up to 5–10 mm. The Mantoux test is positive but may be negative in 30–50% of people with very severe disease. Trans-bronchial biopsies are frequently positive before any abnormality is visible on the chest X-ray. Biopsy and culture of liver and bone marrow may be necessary in patients presenting with a pyrexia of unknown origin (PUO). A trial of antituberculous therapy can be used in individuals with a PUO. The fever should settle within 2 weeks of starting chemotherapy if it is due to tuberculosis. This approach is used in susceptible individuals when a diagnosis cannot be confirmed.

A14.57

1) D **2)** B **3)** E **4)** C **5)** A

Rifampicin stains body secretions pink and patients should be warned of the change in colour of their urine, tears and sweat. Isoniazid has very few unwanted effects. At high doses it may produce a polyneuropathy but this is extremely rare when the normal dose of 200–300 mg is given daily. Nevertheless, it is customary to prescribe pyridoxine 10 mg daily to prevent this effect. Pyrazinamide reduces the renal excretion of urate and may precipitate hyperuricaemic gout. Ethambutol can cause a dose-related optic retrobulbar neuritis that presents with colour blindness for green, reduction in visual acuity and a central scotoma (commoner at doses of 25 mg/kg). This usually reverses provided the drug is stopped when symptoms develop; patients should therefore be warned of its effects. All patients prescribed the drug should be seen by an ophthalmologist prior to treatment and doses of 15 mg/kg should be used. Streptomycin can cause irreversible damage to the vestibular nerve. It is more likely to occur in the elderly and in those with renal impairment.

A14.58

A) F **B)** F **C)** F **D)** F **E)** F

Definitive diagnosis requires that the sputum is cultured on Ogana or Lowenstein–Jensen medium or Baltec (Becton–Dickinson) medium. Radiolabelled DNA and RNA probes specific for various mycobacterial species can identify organisms in culture. The sensitivity of these methods has been enhanced by amplifying target DNA using the polymerase chain reaction. This allows direct testing of sputum and other fluids to provide a laboratory diagnosis within 48 hours. This is still not entirely reliable and should not be accepted as a final diagnosis, particularly in the difficult case when it is most likely to be used. ELISA techniques have been developed which have high specificities, but unfortunately low sensitivity.

A14.59

1) B   2) A   3) D   4) E   5) C

Six months' treatment with once-daily rifampicin 600 mg and isoniazid 300 mg is standard practice for patients with pulmonary and lymph node disease. (For those whose bodyweight is below 55 kg, rifampicin is reduced to 450 mg daily.) These are given as combination tablets and are taken 30 minutes before breakfast, since the absorption of rifampicin is influenced by food. This is supplemented for the first 2 months by pyrazinamide at a dose of 1.5 g (bodyweight <50 kg) or 2.0 g daily. Pyrazinamide is of particular value in treating mycobacteria present within macrophages, and for this reason it may have a very valuable effect on preventing subsequent relapse. Pyridoxine 10 mg daily is given to reduce the risk of isoniazid-induced neuropathy. Treatment of bone tuberculosis should be continued for a total of 9 months and of tuberculous meningitis for 1 year. The drugs used are the same as for pulmonary tuberculosis, with pyrazinamide prescribed for the first 2 months only and for drug-resistant disease. Treatment of TB in AIDS patients is with conventional therapy but four rather than three drugs and it should be supervised (directly observed therapy short course, DOTS).

A14.60

A) F   B) F   C) T   D) T   E) T

Vaccination with BCG (bacille Calmette–Guérin) has been given to schoolchildren in the UK since 1954. BCG is live attenuated vaccine derived from *Mycobacterium bovis* (a bovine strain of *M. tuberculosis*) that lost its virulence after growth in the laboratory for many passages. Early trials showed that it decreases the risk of developing tuberculosis by about 70%. BCG has been shown to be particularly effective in preventing miliary tuberculosis and tuberculous meningitis. In meta-analysis the protective efficacy is around 50%. However, the efficacy of BCG vaccination varies throughout the world from zero to 94% protection and appears to depend on latitude, being most beneficial in Norway, Sweden and Denmark (80–94%) and least so in the southern states of the USA and in India (0–20%). This lack of efficacy is thought to be related to a number of local factors including the frequency of infection with environmental mycobacteria (e.g. *M. fortuitum, M. kansasii*), which may induce a degree of protection similar to but not enhanced by BCG. BCG is given only to individuals who are tuberculin-negative; those with positive tests are further screened by a chest X-ray. The practice of BCG vaccination in the UK, thereby producing cellular immunity and a positive tuberculin test, means that the Mantoux test is of no value in clinical practice for diagnosis of active disease, although it is in the USA where BCG is not used.

A14.61

A) T   B) T   C) T   D) T   E) F

Bilateral hilar lymphadenopathy is a characteristic feature of sarcoidosis. It is often symptomless and simply detected on a routine chest X-ray. The differential diagnosis of the bilateral hilar lymphadenopathy includes: a) lymphoma – though it is rare for this to affect only the hilar lymph nodes; b) pulmonary tuberculosis – though it is rare for the hilar lymph nodes to be symmetrically enlarged;

c) carcinoma of the bronchus with malignant spread to the contralateral hilar lymph nodes – again it is rare for this to give rise to a typical symmetrical picture.

A 14.62

A) T **B)** T **C)** T **D)** T **E)** T

The combination of pulmonary infiltration and normal lung function tests is highly suggestive of sarcoidosis. The principal differential diagnoses are tuberculosis, pneumoconiosis, cryptogenic fibrosing alveolitis and alveolar cell carcinoma.

A 14.63

A) T **B)** T **C)** T **D)** T **E)** T

Anterior uveitis is common and may present with misting of vision, pain and a red eye, but posterior uveitis may present simply as progressive loss of vision. Although ocular sarcoidosis accounts for about 5% of uveitis presenting to ophthalmologists, evidence of asymptomatic uveitis may be found in up to 25% of patients with sarcoidosis. Conjunctivitis may occur and retinal lesions have also been reported.

A 14.64

A) F **B)** T **C)** T **D)** T **E)** T

Both the need to treat and the value of corticosteroid therapy are contested in many aspects of sarcoidosis. Hilar lymphadenopathy on its own with no evidence of chest X-ray involvement of the lungs or decrease in lung function tests does not require treatment. Persisting infiltration on the chest X-ray or abnormal lung function tests are unlikely to improve without corticosteroid treatment. Although there have been no controlled trials that have proved the efficacy of such treatment, it is difficult to withhold corticosteroids when there is continuing deterioration of the disease. Systemic prednisolone should be given for patients suffering from involvement of the eyes or persistent hypercalcaemia. Myocardial sarcoidosis and neurological manifestations are also treated with prednisolone.

A 14.65

A) F **B)** F **C)** T **D)** T **E)** F

Sarcoidosis is a much more severe disease in certain racial groups, particularly black Americans, in whom death rates of up to 10% have been recorded. It is probable that the disease is fatal in fewer than 5% of cases in the UK, most often as a result of respiratory failure and cor pulmonale but, rarely, from myocardial sarcoidosis and renal damage. The chest X-ray provides a guide to prognosis. The disease remits within 2 years in over two-thirds of patients with hilar lymphadenopathy alone, in approximately one-half with hilar lymphadenopathy plus chest X-ray evidence of pulmonary infiltration, but in only one-third of patients with X-ray evidence of infiltration without any demonstrable lymphadenopathy. Lung function tests are the most useful tests in monitoring progression. The serum angiotensin-converting enzyme (ACE) is useful in assessing the activity of the disease and therefore as a guide to treatment with corticosteroids. Reduction of serum ACE during treatment with corticosteroids has not, however, been proved to reflect resolution of the disease.

A 14.66

A) T **B)** T **C)** T **D)** T **E)** T

Pleural adhesions, thickening and effusion are the most common lesions. Several

Respiratory disease

forms of parenchymal disease can occur in patients with rheumatoid arthritis. These include fibrosing alveolitis, rheumatoid nodules, cryptogenic organizing pneumonia, and lymphoid interstitial pneumonia. The features of respiratory involvement in rheumatoid disease are illustrated in Figure 14.40 (p. 900 of the 5th edition of Kumar & Clark, 2002). Obliterative disease of the small bronchioles is rare.

A14.67

A) F   B) F   C) T   D) T   E) F

Cryptogenic fibrosing alveolitis (CFA), a relatively rare disorder, known in the US as idiopathic pulmonary fibrosis, causes diffuse fibrosis throughout the lung fields, usually in late middle age. The main features are progressive breathlessness and cyanosis, which eventually lead to respiratory failure, pulmonary hypertension and cor pulmonale. Gross finger clubbing occurs in two-thirds of cases and fine bilateral end-inspiratory crackles are heard on auscultation. Chest X-ray shows irregular reticulonodular shadowing, often maximal in the lower zones. High-resolution CT scan shows characteristic changes of peripheral reticular and ground-glass opacification, seen best in the basal regions but extending all over the lungs. Respiratory function tests show a restrictive ventilatory defect – the lung volumes are reduced, the FEV_1 and FVC ratio is normal to high (with both values being reduced), and carbon monoxide expiratory gas transfer is reduced. Peak flow rates may be normal. Blood gases show an arterial hypoxaemia caused by a combination of alveolar–capillary block and ventilation–perfusion mismatch with normal or low P_aCO_2 owing to hyperventilation. Antinuclear antibodies and rheumatoid factors are present in one-third of patients. The diagnosis of CFA is usually made in a patient presenting with the above signs and characteristic CT changes.

A14.68

1) E or A   2) B   3) C   4) D   5) E

Extrinsic allergic (bronchiolar) alveolitis – some causes		
Disease	Situation	Antigens
Farmer's lung	Forking mouldy hay or any other mouldy vegetable material	Thermophilic actinomycetes and *Micropolyspora faeni*
Bird fancier's lung	Handling pigeons, cleaning lofts or budgerigar cages	Proteins present in the 'bloom' on the feathers and in excreta
Maltworker's lung	Turning germinating barley	*Aspergillus clavatus*
Humidifier fever	Contaminated humidifying systems in air conditioners or humidifiers in factories (especially in printing works)	Possibly a variety of bacteria or amoeba (e.g. *Naegleria gruberi*)
Mushroom workers	Turning mushroom compost	Thermophilic actinomycetes

A14.69

1) E   2) F   3) C   4) A

Drug-induced respiratory disease

Disease	Drugs
Asthma ± rhinitis	Penicillins
	Sulphonamides
	Cephalosporins
	Aspirin
	NSAIDs
	Tartrazine
	Iodine-containing contrast media
	Non-selective β-adrenoceptor-blocking drugs (e.g. propranolol)
	Suxamethonium
	Thiopental
Diffuse lung injury infiltrate and/or fibrosis	Amiodarone
	Hexamethonium
	Nitrofurantoin
	Paraquat
	Continuous oxygen
	Cytotoxic agent (many, particularly busulfan, CCNU, bleomycin, methotrexate)
Pulmonary eosinophilia	Antibiotics
	Penicillin
	Tetracycline
	Sulphonamides
	NSAIDs
	Antidepressants
	Antiepileptic
	Phenytoin
	Carbamazepine
	Others
	Chlorpropamide
	Cytotoxic agents
Opportunistic pulmonary infections	Corticosteroids
	Azathioprine
	Other cytotoxic drugs
Respiratory depression	Sedatives
	Opiates
SLE-like syndrome including pulmonary infiltrates, effusions and fibrosis	Hydralazine
	Procainamide
	Isoniazid
	Phenytoin
	ACE inhibitors

CCNU, chloroethyl-cyclohexyl-nitrosourea (lomustine); NSAIDs, non-steroidal anti-inflammatory drugs; SLE, systemic lupus erythematosus

A14.70

1) G   2) B   3) F   4) C   5) A
6) H   7) D

In progressive massive fibrosis, patients develop round fibrotic masses several centimetres in diameter, almost invariably in the upper lobes and sometimes having necrotic central cavities. Silicosis is encountered in workers in foundries where sand used in moulds has to be removed from the metal casts (fettling), in sand blasting, and among stonemasons, pottery and ceramic workers. The chest X-ray appearances of silicosis include distinctive thin streaks of calcification which may be seen around the hilar lymph nodes ('eggshell' calcification). The diseases caused by asbestos include bilateral diffuse pleural thickening, asbestosis, mesothelioma and asbestos-related carcinoma. A synergistic relationship between asbestosis and cigarette smoking and the development of bronchial carcinoma, usually adenocarcinoma, exists; the risk is multiplied fivefold above the risk attributable to smoking. Asbestosis is defined as fibrosis of the lungs caused by asbestos dust, which may or may not be associated with fibrosis of the parietal or visceral layers of the pleura. It is a progressive disease characterized by breathlessness and accompanied by finger clubbing and bilateral basal end-inspiratory crackles. fibrosis, not detectable on chest X-ray, may be revealed on CT scan. Pleural effusions are the most common presentation of mesothelioma, typically with persistent chest wall pain, which should raise the index of suspicion even if the initial pleural fluid or biopsy samples are non-diagnostic. Byssinosis occurs world-wide but is declining rapidly in areas where the numbers of people employed in cotton mills are falling. The symptoms start on the first day back at work after a break (Monday sickness) with improvement as the week progresses. Tightness in the chest, cough and breathlessness occur within the first hour in dusty areas of the mill, particularly in the blowing and carding rooms where raw cotton is cleaned and the fibres are straightened. Beryllium–copper alloy has a high tensile strength and is resistant to metal fatigue, high temperature and corrosion. It is used in the aerospace industry, in atomic reactors and in many electrical devices. Although beryllium is inhaled into the lungs, it causes a systemic illness with a clinical picture similar to sarcoidosis. The major chronic problem is that of progressive dyspnoea with pulmonary fibrosis. However, strict control of levels in the working atmosphere have made the disease a rarity.

A14.71

1) E   2) D   3) C   4) B   5) A

A14.72

1) F   2) B   3) D   4) E   5) A

Carcinoma in the apex of the lung can erode the ribs and involve the lower part of the brachial plexus (C8, T1 and T2), causing severe pain in the shoulder and down the inner surface of the arm (Pancoast's tumour). The sympathetic ganglion can also be involved, producing Horner's syndrome. Superior vena caval obstruction causes early morning headache, facial congestion and oedema involving the upper limbs; the jugular veins are distended, as are the veins on the chest that form a collateral circulation with veins arising from the abdomen. Hypertrophic pulmonary osteoarthropathy (HPOA) occurs particularly in squamous-cell carcinomas

and adenocarcinomas. Symptoms include joint stiffness and severe pain in the wrists and ankles, sometimes associated with gynaecomastia. X-rays show a characteristic proliferative periostitis at the distal ends of long bones, which have an onion-skin appearance. HPOA is invariably associated with clubbing of the fingers. Eaton–Lambert syndrome, a rare non-metastatic manifestation of small-cell carcinoma of the bronchus, is due to defective acetylcholine release at the neuromuscular junction. Proximal muscle weakness, sometimes involving the ocular and bulbar muscles is found, with absent reflexes. Weakness tends to improve after a few minutes' muscular contraction, and absent reflexes return, (cf. myasthenia). Diagnosis is confirmed by EMG and repetitive stimulation of a motor nerve. Antibodies to P/Q-type voltage-gated calcium channels are found in most cases (90%). 3,4-diaminopyridine is used in treatment, with variable effect. One of the non-metastatic manifestations of bronchogenic carcinoma is cerebellar syndrome. The patient presents with typical features of cerebellar involvement as in case 2.

A14.73

A) T   B) T   C) F   D) F   E) T

By the time the lung cancer is causing symptoms, it will almost always be visible on chest X-rays. CT is particularly useful for identifying disease in the mediastinum, such as enlarged lymph nodes. MRI is not useful for the diagnosis of primary lung tumours but is very useful for staging as it provides better images of the mediastinum than CT. Fibreoptic bronchoscopy is used to define the bronchial anatomy and to obtain biopsy and cytological specimens. If the carcinoma involves the first 2 cm of either main bronchus, the tumour is inoperable as there would be insufficient resection margins for pneumonectomy. Widening and loss of the sharp angle of the carina indicates the presence of enlarged mediastinal lymph nodes, either malignant or reactive.

A14.74

A) T   B) T   C) T   D) T   E) T

Metastases in the lung are very common and usually present as round shadows (1.5–3.0 cm diameter). They may be detected on chest X-ray in patients already diagnosed as having carcinoma. Typical sites for the primary tumour include the kidney, prostate, breast, bone, gastrointestinal tract, cervix or ovary. Metastases nearly always develop in the parenchyma and are often relatively asymptomatic even when the chest X-ray shows extensive pulmonary metastases.

A14.75

A) T   B) T   C) T   D) T   E) T

A pulmonary metastasis may be detected as a solitary round shadow on chest X-ray in an asymptomatic patient. The most common primary tumour to do this is a renal cell carcinoma. The differential diagnosis includes primary bronchial carcinoma, tuberculoma, benign tumour of the lung and hydatid cyst.

A14.76

A) F   B) F   C) T   D) T   E) T

Carcinoma, particularly of the stomach, pancreas and breast, can involve mediastinal glands and spread along the lymphatics of both lungs (lymphangitis carcinomatosa), leading to progressive and severe breathlessness. On the chest X-ray, bilateral lymphadenopathy is seen together with streaky basal shadowing fanning out over both lung fields.

A14.77

A) F   B) F   C) T   D) F   E) T

Pleural fluid may be an exudate or a transduate. Effusions that are transudates can be bilateral, but are often larger on the right side. The protein content is less than 30 g/L and the lactic dehydrogenase is less than 200 IU/L. Causes include: heart failure, hypoproteinaemia (e.g. nephrotic syndrome), constrictive pericarditis, hypothyroidism, ovarian tumours producing right-sided pleural effusion – Meigs' syndrome. The protein content of exudates is >30 g/L and the lactic dehydrogenase is >200 IU/L. Causes include bacterial pneumonia (common), carcinoma of the bronchus and pulmonary infarction – fluid may be blood-stained (common), tuberculosis, connective-tissue disease, post-myocardial infarction syndrome (rare), acute pancreatitis (high amylase content) (rare), mesothelioma (rare), sarcoidosis (very rare), yellow-nail syndrome (effusion due to lymphoedema) (very rare) and familial Mediterranean fever (rare).

A14.78

A) T   B) T   C) T   D) T   E) T

Unilateral diaphragmatic paralysis is common and symptomless. The affected diaphragm is usually elevated and moves paradoxically on inspiration. The diagnosis is confirmed when a sniff causes the paralysed diaphragm to rise, the unaffected diaphragm to descend. Causes include surgery, carcinoma of the bronchus with involvement of the phrenic nerve, neurological, including poliomyelitis, herpes zoster, trauma to cervical spine, birth injury, subclavian vein puncture and infection: tuberculosis, syphilis, pneumonia.

A14.79

A) T   B) T   C) T   D) T   E) F

Bilateral diaphragmatic weakness or paralysis causes breathlessness in the supine position and is a cause of sleep apnoea leading to daytime headaches and somnolence. Tidal volume is decreased and respiratory rate increased. Vital capacity is substantially reduced when lying down, and sniffing causes a paradoxical inward movement of the abdominal wall best seen in the supine position. Causes include viral infections, multiple sclerosis, motor neurone disease, poliomyelitis, Guillain–Barré syndrome, quadriplegia after trauma, and rare muscle diseases. Treatment is either diaphragmatic pacing or night-time assisted ventilation.

A14.80

A) T   B) T   C) T   D) F   E) F

The nasal vestibule leads to the internal ostium which is the narrowest part of the nasal cavity. This causes a 50% increased resistance to airflow when breathing through the nose rather than through the mouth. There are numerous collections of lymphoid tissue arranged in a circular fashion around the nasopharynx; these include the adenoids. The tonsils lie between the anterior and posterior fauces, separating the mouth from the oropharynx. The larynx consists of a number of articulated cartilages, vocal cords, muscles and ligaments, all of which serve to keep the airway open during breathing and occlude it during swallowing. The main motor nerve to the larynx is the recurrent laryngeal nerve. The left recurrent laryngeal nerve leaves the vagus at the level of the aortic arch, hooking round it to run upwards through the mediastinum between the trachea and the oesophagus; it can be affected by disease in these areas. The principal tensor of the vocal cords is the external branch of the superior laryngeal nerve, which can be injured during thyroidectomy.

A14.81

A) F   B) F   C) T   D) F   E) F

The right main bronchus is more vertical than the left and, hence, inhaled material is more likely to pass into it. Because of the bronchial anatomy, the most usual sites for spillage are the apical and posterior segments of the right lower lobe. The upper lobe lies mainly in front of the lower lobe and therefore signs on the right side in the front of the chest found on physical examination are due to lesions mainly of the upper lobe or part of the middle lobe. In health, the pleurae are in apposition apart from a small quantity of lubricating fluid, so the pleural cavity is only a potential space. Fifty per cent of the muscle fibres are of the slow-twitch type with a low glycolytic capacity; they are relatively resistant to fatigue.

A14.82

A) F   B) F   C) F   D) T   E) F

Collapse of the whole right lung should cause the mediastinum to shift towards the right, that is, the trachea will be deviated to the right, the heart and apex beat will deviate to the right, there will be raised right diaphragm and compensatory emphysema of the left lung (see Fig. 14.12, p. 847 of the 5th edition of Kumar & Clark, 2002).

A 14.83

A) T   B) T   C) T   D) T   E) F

These findings are typical of miliary mottling which is the term describing numerous minute opacities 1–3 mm in size which have been described in pulmonary oedema, miliary tuberculosis, sarcoidosis, pneumoconiosis and fibrosing alveolitis.

A 14.84

A) T   B) F   C) T   D) F   E) F

Simple advice and follow-up can motivate some 50% of patients to stop. In smoking withdrawal clinics, success rates of 80% can be achieved in the first month, though only 15–20% of patients remain abstinent in the long term. Nicotine chewing gum has been advocated but is probably no better than verbal advice. Nicotine patches are available over the counter and are better than placebo in helping smokers to stop, though they must not be used by those suffering from heart disease. The introduction of amfebutamone/bupropion (a noradrenaline (norepinephrine) and dopamine reuptake inhibitor) may prove a significant step forward in providing pharmacological support to those who wish to give up their habit.

A 14.85

A) T   B) T   C) T   D) T   E) T

The dangers of cigarette smoking	
General	**Passive smoking**
Lung cancer	Risk of asthma, pneumonia and bronchitis in infants
COPD	of smoking parents
Carcinoma of the oesophagus	An increase in cough and breathlessness in
Ischaemic heart disease	smokers and non-smokers with COPD and asthma
Peripheral vascular disease	Increased cancer risk
Bladder cancer	
An increase in abnormal spermatozoa	
Memory problems	
Maternal smoking	
A decrease in birthweight of the infant	
An increase in fetal and neonatal mortality	
An increase in asthma	

A 14.86

A) F   B) F   C) F   D) F   E) T

Complete avoidance of pollen is impossible. Contact may be diminished by wearing sunglasses, driving with the car windows shut, avoiding walks in the countryside (particularly in the late afternoon when the number of pollen grains is highest at ground level), and keeping the bedroom window shut at night. These measures are rarely sufficient in themselves to control symptoms. Exposure to pollen is generally lower at the seaside, where sea breezes keep pollen grains inland. Fatal cardiac arrhythmias (torsades de points) have been described with terfenadine and astemizole and these drugs should be replaced with those that do not influence the ECG QT interval. Xylometazoline and oxymetazoline are widely used because they have a prolonged action and tachyphylaxis does not develop. Sodium cromoglicate applied topically in spray or powder form is of limited value in the treatment of allergic rhinitis, though along with nedocromil sodium, it is very effective in the management of allergic conjunctivitis. The most effective treatment for rhinitis is to use small doses of topically administered corticosteroid preparations (e.g. beclometasone spray twice daily or fluticasone propionate spray once daily).

A14.87

A) F   B) T   C) T   D) T   E) T

Haemophilus influenzae type b can cause life-threatening infection of the epiglottis, a condition that is rare over the age of 5 years. Other manifestations of *H. influenzae* type b (Hib) are meningitis, septic arthritis and osteomyelitis.

A14.88

A) F   B) F   C) T   D) T   E) F

The influenza virus belongs to the orthomyxovirus group and exists in two main forms, A and B. Influenza B is associated with localized outbreaks of milder nature, whereas influenza A is the cause of world-wide pandemics. Laboratory diagnosis is not usually necessary, but a definitive diagnosis can be established by demonstrating a fourfold increase in the complement-fixing antibody or the haemagglutinin antibody when measured before and after an interval of 1–2 weeks or demonstration of the virus in throat or nasal secretion. The recent introduction of neuraminidase inhibitors may prove helpful in shortening the duration of symptoms in patients with influenza. Protection by influenza vaccines is only effective in up to 70% of people and is of short duration, usually lasting for only a year. Routine vaccination is now recommended for all individuals over 65 years of age and also for younger people with chronic heart disease, chronic lung disease (including asthma), chronic renal failure, diabetes mellitus and those who are immunosuppressed.

Intensive care medicine **15**

Q 15.1

Blood gases of a patient in the intensive care unit are as follows: pH 7.30, Po_2 7.3 kPa (55 mmHg) and Pco_2 7.3 kPa (55 mmHg). The most likely cause of this picture is which one of the following?

A. Pulmonary oedema
B. Idiopathic pulmonary fibrosis
C. Severe pneumonia
D. Exacerbation of chronic obstructive pulmonary disease
E. Methaemoglobinaemia

Q 15.2

Mechanical ventilation is not indicated in which one of the following situations?

A. A 22-year-old patient with a head injury whose P_aO_2 is 6.9 kPa (52 mmHg) and P_aCO_2 is 7.3 kPa (50 mmHg)
B. A 45-year-old patient with acute myasthenia gravis whose vital capacity is 9 mL/kg
C. A 34-year-old man with Guillain–Barré syndrome whose vital capacity is 15 mL/kg
D. A 45-year-old asthmatic who is exhausted, unable to speak, and whose respiratory rate is >40/min following nebulized bronchodilator therapy
E. A 45-year-old patient with acute left ventricular failure with pulmonary oedema and whose P_aO_2 is 6.53 kPa (49 mmHg) on 28% oxgyen

Q 15.3

A 28-year-old woman with sepsis and multiorgan failure is beginning to recover from her illness. Initially the intensivist finds it difficult to wean her off respiratory support. Neurological examination reveals muscle wasting, the limbs are weak and flaccid and deep tendon reflexes are reduced or absent. Cranial nerves are spared. Nerve conduction studies indicate axonal degeneration and cerebrospinal fluid examination is normal. This patient most likely has

A. Guillain–Barré syndrome
B. Myasthenia gravis
C. Critical illness polyneuropathy
D. Polymyositis
E. Eaton–Lambert syndrome

Q 15.4

1. Tension of the myocardial fibres at the end of diastole just before the onset of ventricular contraction
2. The ability of the heart to perform independent of changes in preload and afterload
3. Myocardial wall tension developed during systolic ejection

Select the best match for each of the above

A. Afterload
B. Preload
C. Myocardial contractility

Intensive care medicine

Q15.5

1. A 55-year-old patient is seen in accident and emergency. Heart rate is 91 beats/minute, blood pressure is 120/80 mmHg, temperature is 38.2°C, respiratory rate is 22 breaths per minute

2. A 65-year-old patient is seen in accident and emergency. Heart rate is 91 beats/minute, blood pressure is 120/80 mmHg, temperature is 37°C, respiratory rate is 20 breaths per minute. Blood gases reveal metabolic acidosis

3. A 75-year-old patient is seen in accident and emergency. Heart rate is 91 beats/minute, blood pressure is 120/80 mmHg, temperature is 37.1°C, respiratory rate is 22 breaths per minute. Blood gases reveal respiratory acidosis

4. A 75-year-old patient is seen in accident and emergency. Heart rate is 91 beats/minute, blood pressure is 120/80 mmHg, temperature is 37.1°C, respiratory rate is 21 breaths per minute. Red blood cell 2,3-DPG concentration is decreased

Select the best match for each of the above

A. Oxyhaemoglobin dissociation curve moves to the left
B. Oxyhaemoglobin dissociation curve moves up
C. Oxyhaemoglobin dissociation curve moves down
D. Oxyhaemoglobin dissociation curve does not move
E. Oxyhaemoglobin dissociation curve moves to the right

Q15.6

1. A 58-year-old patient with an exacerbation of chronic obstructive pulmonary disease

2. A 45-year-old mountain climber in Nepal

3. A 16-year-old insulin-dependent diabetic with blood sugar of 24 mmol/L

4. A 52-year-old patient with severe pyloric stenosis

5. A 65-year-old patient after cardiac arrest

6. A 32-year-old patient with untreated chronic renal failure

7. A 28-year-old patient with newly diagnosed renal tubular acidosis

Select the best match for each of the above

A. pH of 7.26, P_aO_2 of 6.6 kPa (50 mmHg), P_aCO_2 of 7.9 kPa (60 mmHg), plasma HCO_3 is 25 mmol/L
B. pH of 7.5, P_aO_2 of 7.9 kPa (60 mmHg), P_aCO_2 of 2.6 kPa (20 mmHg), plasma HCO_3 is 25 mmol/L
C. pH of 7.24, P_aO_2 of 7.9 kPa (60 mmHg), P_aCO_2 of 2.6 kPa (20 mmHg), plasma HCO_3 is 18 mmol/L
D. pH of 7.51, P_aO_2 of 7.9 kPa (60 mmHg), P_aCO_2 of 6.6 kPa (50 mmHg), plasma bicarbonate is 32 mmol/L
E. pH of 7.20, P_aO_2 of 7.9 kPa (60 mmHg), P_aCO_2 of 2.6 kPa (20 mmHg), plasma HCO_3 is 18 mmol/L, elevated plasma lactate

Q15.7

1. A 45-year-old patient has had an ST elevation myocardial infarction in leads II, III and AVF. Blood pressure is 80/60 mmHg. His jugular venous pressure is elevated and his lungs are clear to auscultation

2. A 55-year-old patient has had an ST elevation myocardial infarction in leads V$_3$–V$_6$. Blood pressure is 80/60 mmHg. Signs include pulsus alternans, elevated jugular venous pressure, 'gallop rhythm' and bi-basal crackles

3. A 47-year-old patient had mitral valve replacement 4 years ago. He complains of fever, nausea and vomiting. On examination he has a bounding pulse, blood pressure is 80/40 mmHg. Swan–Ganz catheter shows the systemic vascular resistance is markedly reduced and cardiac output is high. Blood cultures are negative

4. A 67-year-old ice-skater develops cardiac arrest while skating. He is given a 'thump' on the chest followed by cardiopulmonary resuscitation. He is taken to the local accident and emergency department where he goes into atrial fibrillation. The doctor starts heparin and amiodarone. Eight hours later he is found to have a blood pressure of 80/50 mmHg, an elevated jugular venous pressure, pulsus paradoxus and muffled heart sounds. Kussmaul's sign is present

5. A 68-year-old patient returns to the critical care unit after surgery for cardiac transplantation. On examination he has a blood pressure of 90/40 mmHg, his peripheries are cold and clammy. His urine output is less than 10 mL/hour in the past 2 hours. Swan–Ganz catheter shows the systemic vascular resistance is markedly elevated, central venous pressure and pulmonary capillary wedge pressure are low

Select the best match for each of the above

A. Septic shock
B. Right ventricular infarction
C. Cardiogenic shock
D. Cardiac tamponade
E. Hypovolaemic shock

Q15.8

1. Noradrenaline (norepinephrine)
2. Adrenaline (epinephrine)
3. Dopamine
4. Dobutamine
5. Milrinone

Select the best match for each of the above

A. Phosphodiesterase inhibitor
B. Stimulates both α- and β-adrenergic receptors but at low doses β effects seem to predominate
C. This is predominantly an α-agonist
D. Acts on β receptors and α receptors as well as DA$_1$ and DA$_2$ receptors
E. This is predominantly a β-agonist

Q15.9

The circulating volume must be replaced quickly (in minutes not hours) to reduce tissue damage in the following situations

A. A 45-year-old patient has had an ST elevation myocardial infarction in leads II, III and AVF. Blood pressure is 80/60 mmHg. His jugular venous pressure is elevated and his lungs are clear to auscultation

B. A 55-year-old patient has had an ST elevation myocardial infarction in leads V$_3$–V$_6$. Blood pressure is 80/60 mmHg. Signs include pulsus alternans, elevated jugular venous pressure, 'gallop rhythm' and bi-basal crackles

C. A 47-year-old patient had mitral valve replacement 4 years ago. He now complains of fever, nausea and vomiting. On examination he has a bounding pulse, blood pressure is 80/40 mmHg. Swan–Ganz catheter shows the systemic vascular resistance is markedly reduced and cardiac output is high. Blood cultures are negative

D. A 67-year-old ice skater develops cardiac arrest while skating. He is given a 'thump' on the chest followed by cardiopulmonary resuscitation. He is taken to the local accident and emergency department where he goes into atrial fibrillation. The doctor starts heparin and amiodarone. Eight hours later he is found to have a blood pressure of 80/50 mmHg, an elevated jugular venous pressure, pulsus paradoxus and muffled heart sounds. Kussmaul's sign is present

E. A 68-year-old patient returns to the critical care unit after surgery for cardiac transplantation. On examination he has a blood pressure of 90/40 mmHg, his peripheries are cold and clammy. His urine output is less than 10 mL/hour in the past 2 hours. Swan–Ganz catheter shows the systemic vascular resistance is markedly elevated, central venous pressure and pulmonary capillary wedge pressure are low

Q15.10

A 48-year-old patient is in the operating room undergoing coronary artery bypass grafting. Following the surgery his blood pressure falls and he is noted to have massive quantities of blood in the chest-tube. He requires massive transfusions of blood to maintain his blood pressure. Complications which may be expected as result of his blood transfusions include

A. Hypercalcaemia
B. Hypokalaemia
C. Hypothermia
D. Metabolic alkalosis
E. Coagulopathy

Q15.11

The following therapies have been found to substantially improve mortality in septic shock

A. High-dose steroids
B. Tumour necrosis factor antibodies.
C. Nitric oxide synthase inhibition
D. Activated protein C
E. N-acetylcysteine

Q15.12

In the intensive care unit the physician decides to initiate BiPAP (bilevel positive airway pressure) in a patient. The following statements about BiPAP are correct

A. Both inspiratory and expiratory pressure levels and time are set independently
B. BiPAP can be triggered by patient
C. BiPAP reduces risk of ventilator-associated pneumonia
D. Spontaneous cough is hampered with this technique
E. Sedation can be avoided in these patients

Q15.13

A 22-year-old patient with severe burns is in the intensive care unit. On the fourth day she develops tachypnoea and cyanosis. Fine crackles are heard on both lung bases. Chest X-ray shows bilateral diffuse shadowing. The next day the patient has 'white-out' on both sides. P_aO_2 is 5.33 kPa (40 mmHg), P_aCO_2 is 4.0 kPa (30 mmHg). Pulmonary capillary wedge pressure is 14 mmHg. The following statements regarding this condition are correct

A. Colloidal solutions have been shown to improve mortality
B. Repeated position changes between the prone and supine positions may allow reductions in airway pressures and inspired oxygen fraction
C. Inhaled nitric oxide improves survival
D. Aerosolized prostacyclin (eproprostenol) improves survival
E. High-dose steroids improve outcome

Q15.14

The cardiac surgeon wants to know whether the patient is brain dead before harvesting a heart from a 24-year-old patient in the intensive care unit. The following diagnostic tests are used to confirm brain death

A. Absent knee jerks
B. Absent oculocephalic reflexes
C. Absent vestibulo-ocular reflexes to caloric tests
D. Absent gag reflex
E. Absent cough reflex in response to laryngeal or tracheal stimulation

Q15.15

The critical care team should be involved in the following instances

A. A 91-year-old man is brought to the accident and emergency department. His vital signs are heart rate of 98 beats per minute, blood pressure is 120/80 mmHg, core temperature is 38°C and respiratory rate is 18 breaths per minute
B. A 78-year-old woman is brought to the accident and emergency department. Her vital signs are heart rate of 98 beats per minute, blood pressure is 100/60 mmHg, core temperature is 39.1°C and respiratory rate is 16 breaths per minute

C. A 59-year-old woman is brought to the accident and emergency department. Her vital signs are heart rate of 126 beats per minute, blood pressure is 100/60 mmHg, core temperature is 37.1°C and respiratory rate is 19 breaths per minute
D. A 42-year-old man is brought to the accident and emergency department. His vital signs are heart rate of 58 beats per minute, blood pressure is 100/60 mmHg, core temperature is 34.6°C and respiratory rate is 20 breaths per minute
E. A 73-year-old woman weighing 70 kg is in the rehabilitation ward. Her vital signs are heart rate of 97 beats per minute, blood pressure is 120/60 mmHg, core temperature is 37.1°C and respiratory rate is 16 breaths per minute. Her urine output in the past 3 hours is 30 mL
F. A 47-year-old man is brought to the accident and emergency department. His vital signs are heart rate of 98 beats per minute, blood pressure is 100/60 mmHg, core temperature is 37.1°C and respiratory rate is 32 breaths per minute
G. A 71-year-old man is brought to the accident and emergency department. His vital signs are heart rate of 98 beats per minute, blood pressure is 120/80 mmHg, core temperature is 38°C and respiratory rate is 18 breaths per minute. He is administered supplemental oxygen and his oxygen saturation is 84%

Intensive care medicine

Q15.16

Neuroendocrine responses to shock include

A. Release of catecholamines from adrenal medulla
B. Release of renin by the juxtaglomerular apparatus
C. Release of adrenocorticotrophic hormone
D. Release of vasopressin
E. Release of insulin
F. Release of glucagon

Q15.17

The following statements are correct

A. When the heart rate increases the duration of systole remains essentially unchanged
B. As the end-diastolic volume of the ventricle increases, tension in myocardial fibres is decreased and stroke volume falls
C. Decreasing the afterload can decrease the stroke volume achieved at a given preload
D. Right ventricular afterload is normally negligible
E. In the normal heart diastole becomes prolonged at rates greater than 160 beats/minute

Q15.18

The following are correct

A. An 18-year-old asthmatic is being treated. Oxygen saturation is 93%. A modest fall in arterial oxygen (provided the oxygen saturation does not change) is easily tolerated
B. A 52-year-old patient with chronic obstructive pulmonary disease is being treated. Oxygen saturation is 93%. Increasing the arterial oxygen saturation in this patient by administering 28% oxygen through a mask will substantially increase the oxygen content
C. The oxygen saturation, in a 56-year-old patient with chronic obstructive pulmonary disease, is 86%. Administering 28% oxygen can lead to a useful increase in oxygen saturation
D. In a 2-year-old child with Fallot's tetralogy, increasing the arterial oxygen content in this patient by administering 28% oxygen through a mask will substantially increase the oxygen content
E. A 55-year-old patient with a completely collapsed left lung has arterial hypoxaemia. Increasing the arterial oxygen content in this patient by administering 28% oxygen through a mask will substantially increase the oxygen content

A15.1

D

Type II or 'ventilatory failure' occurs when alveolar ventilation is insufficient to excrete the volume of carbon dioxide being produced by tissue metabolism. Inadequate alveolar ventilation is due to reduced ventilatory effort, inability to overcome an increased resistance to ventilation, failure to compensate for an increase in deadspace and/or carbon dioxide production, or a combination of these factors. The most common cause is chronic obstructive pulmonary disease (COPD). Other causes include chest-wall deformities, respiratory muscle weakness (e.g. Guillain–Barré syndrome) and depression of the respiratory centre (e.g. overdose).

A15.2

C

Indications for mechanical ventilation are as follows:

Acute respiratory failure, with signs of severe respiratory distress (e.g. respiratory rate >40/min, inability to speak, patient exhausted) persisting despite maximal therapy. Confusion, restlessness, agitation, a decreased conscious level, a rising P_aCO_2 (>8 kPa) and extreme hypoxaemia (<8 kPa), despite oxygen therapy, are further indications.

Acute ventilatory failure due, for example, to myasthenia gravis or Guillain–Barré syndrome. Mechanical ventilation should usually be instituted when the vital capacity has fallen to 10 mL/kg or less. This will avoid complications such as atelectasis and infection as well as preventing respiratory arrest. The tidal volume and respiratory rate are relatively insensitive in the above

conditions and change late in the course of the disease. A high P_aCO_2 (particularly if rising) is an indication for urgent artificial ventilation.

Other indications include:

- Prophylactic postoperative ventilation in high-risk patients

- Head injury – to avoid hypoxia and hypercarbia which increase cerebral blood flow and intracranial pressure, hyperventilation to reduce intracranial pressure

- Trauma – chest injury and lung contusion

- Severe left ventricular failure with pulmonary oedema

- Coma with breathing difficulties, e.g. following drug overdose.

A15.3

C

Critical illness polyneuropathy has most often been described in association with persistent sepsis and multiple organ failure. Clinically the initial manifestation is often difficulty in weaning the patient from respiratory support. There is muscle wasting, the limbs are weak and flaccid, and deep tendon reflexes are reduced or absent. Cranial nerves are relatively spared. Nerve conduction studies confirm axonal damage. The cerebrospinal fluid (CSF) protein concentration is normal or minimally elevated. These findings differentiate critical illness neuropathy from Guillain–Barré syndrome, in which nerve conduction studies show evidence of demyelination and CSF protein is usually high. With resolution of the underlying critical illness, recovery can be expected after 1–6 months, although weaning from respiratory support and rehabilitation are likely to be prolonged. Critical illness can also be complicated by various myopathies, including a severe quadriplegic myopathy, which have been particularly associated with the administration of steroids and muscle relaxants to mechanically ventilated patients with acute, severe asthma. Often the most severely ill patients will have a combined neuropathy and myopathy.

A15.4

1) B   2) C   3) A

Preload is defined as the tension of the myocardial fibres at the end of diastole, just before the onset of ventricular contraction, and is therefore related to the degree of stretch of the fibres. Myocardial contractility refers to the ability of the heart to perform work, independent of changes in preload and afterload.
Afterload is defined as the myocardial wall tension developed during systolic ejection. In the case of the left ventricle, the resistance imposed by the aortic valve, the peripheral vascular resistance and the elasticity of the major blood vessels are important determinants of afterload.

A15.5

1) E   2) E   3) E   4) A

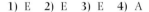

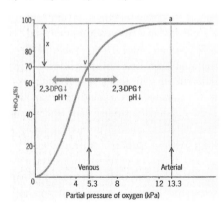

A15.6

1) A   2) B   3) C   4) D   5) E
6) C   7) C

Respiratory acidosis is caused by retention of carbon dioxide. The P_aCO_2 and $[H^+]$ rise. A chronically raised P_aCO_2 is compensated by renal retention of bicarbonate and the $[H^+]$ returns towards normal. A constant arterial bicarbonate concentration is then usually established within 5 days. This represents a primary respiratory acidosis with a compensatory metabolic alkalosis. Common causes of respiratory acidosis include ventilatory failure and chronic obstructive pulmonary disease (COPD) (type II respiratory failure where there is a high P_aCO_2 and a low P_aO_2). In respiratory alkalosis the reverse occurs and there is a fall in P_aCO_2 and $[H^+]$, often with a small reduction in bicarbonate concentration. A respiratory alkalosis is often produced, intentionally or unintentionally, when patients are mechanically ventilated; it may also be seen with hypoxaemic (type I) respiratory failure, spontaneous hyperventilation and in those living at high altitudes. Metabolic acidosis may be due to excessive acid production, most commonly lactic acid as a consequence of anaerobic metabolism during an episode of shock or following cardiac arrest. A metabolic acidosis may also develop in chronic renal failure or in diabetic ketoacidosis. It can also follow the loss of bicarbonate from the gut, for example, or from the kidney in renal tubular acidosis. Respiratory compensation for a metabolic acidosis is usually slightly delayed because the blood–brain barrier initially prevents the respiratory centre from sensing the increased blood $[H^+]$. Following this short delay, however, the patient hyperventilates and 'blows off' carbon dioxide to produce a compensatory respiratory alkalosis. There is a limit to this respiratory compensation, since in practice values for $P_a\text{CO}_2$ less than about 1.4 kPa (11 mmHg) are never achieved. It should also be noted that respiratory compensation cannot occur if the patient's ventilation is controlled or if the respiratory centre is depressed, for example by drugs or head injury. Metabolic alkalosis can be caused by loss of acid, for example from the stomach with nasogastric suction, or in high intestinal obstruction, or excessive administration of absorbable alkali. Overzealous treatment with intravenous sodium bicarbonate is frequently implicated. Respiratory compensation for a metabolic alkalosis is often slight, and it is rare to encounter a $P_a\text{CO}_2$ above 6.5 kPa (50 mmHg), even with severe alkalosis.

A15.7

1) B   2) C   3) A   4) D   5) E

Haemodynamic changes in shock

Hypovolaemic shock
Low central venous pressure (CVP) and pulmonary artery occlusion pressure (PAOP)
Low cardiac output
Increased systemic vascular resistance

Pulmonary embolism
Low cardiac output
High CVP, high pulmonary artery pressure but low PAOP
Increased systemic vascular resistance

Cardiogenic shock
Signs of myocardial failure
Increased systemic vascular resistance
CVP and PAOP high (except when hypovolaemic)

Anaphylaxis
Low systemic vascular resistance
Low CVP and PAOP
High cardiac output

Cardiac tamponade
Parallel increases in CVP and PAOP
Low cardiac output
Increased systemic vascular resistance

Septic shock
Low systemic vascular resistance
Low CVP and PAOP
Cardiac output usually high
Myocardial depression – low ejection fraction
Stroke volume maintained by ventricular dilatation
Cardiac output increased by tachycardia

A15.8

1) C   2) B   3) D   4) E   5) A

Adrenaline (epinephrine) stimulates both α- and β-adrenergic receptors, but at low doses β effects predominate. Noradrenaline (norepinephrine) is predominantly an α-adrenergic agonist. Dopamine is a natural precursor of adrenaline (epinephrine) which acts on β receptors and α receptors, as well as dopaminergic DA_1 and DA_2 receptors. Dobutamine is closely related to dopamine and has predominantly $β_1$ activity. Phosphodiesterase inhibitors include amrinone, milrinone, enoximone.

A15.9

A) T   B) F   C) T   D) F   E) T

Volume replacement is obviously essential in hypovolaemic shock but is also required in anaphylactic and septic shock because of vasodilatation, sequestration of blood and loss of circulating volume because of capillary leak. Patients with severe cardiac failure, in whom ventricular filling pressures may be markedly elevated, often benefit from measures to reduce preload (and afterload) – such as the administration of diuretics and vasodilators. The circulating volume must be replaced quickly (in minutes not hours) to reduce tissue damage and prevent acute renal failure.

A15.10

A) F   B) F   C) T   D) T   E) T

Special problems arise when large volumes of stored blood are transfused rapidly. These include:

Temperature changes. Bank blood is stored at 4°C and transfusion may result in hypothermia, peripheral venoconstriction (which slows the rate of the infusion) and arrhythmias. If possible blood should therefore be warmed during massive transfusion and in those at risk of hypothermia (e.g. during prolonged major surgery with open body cavity).

Coagulopathy. Stored blood has virtually no effective platelets and is deficient in clotting factors. Large transfusions can therefore produce a coagulation defect. This may need to be treated by replacing clotting factors with fresh frozen plasma and administering platelet concentrates.

Metabolic acidosis/alkalosis. Stored blood is preserved in citrate/phosphate/dextrose (CPD) solution, and metabolic acidosis attributable solely to blood transfusion is rare and in any case seldom requires correction. A metabolic alkalosis often develops 24–48 hours after a large blood transfusion, probably mainly owing to metabolism of the citrate.

Hypocalcaemia. Stored blood is anticoagulated with citrate, which binds calcium ions. This can reduce total body ionized calcium levels and cause myocardial depression.

Hyperkalaemia. Plasma potassium levels rise progressively as blood is stored. However, hyperkalaemia is rarely a problem as rewarming of the blood increases red cell metabolism – the sodium pump becomes active and potassium levels fall.

A15.11

A) F   B) F   C) F   D) T   E) F

Although all the therapeutic strategies have been tested in randomized controlled phase II or phase III trials in human sepsis, none of them has demonstrably improved mortality except activated protein C which has been shown to reduce mortality significantly in severe sepsis.

A15.12

A) T   B) T   C) T   D) F   E) T

With BiPAP, inspiratory and expiratory pressure levels and times are set independently and unrestricted spontaneous respiration is possible throughout the respiratory cycle. BiPAP can also be patient triggered. There is a reduced risk of ventilator-associated pneumonia and improved patient comfort, with preservation of airway defence mechanisms, speech and swallowing. Spontaneous coughing and expectoration are not hampered and sedation may be avoided. Institution of non-invasive respiratory support can rest the respiratory muscles, reduce respiratory acidosis and breathlessness, improve clearance of secretions and re-expand collapsed lung segments. The intubation rate, length of ICU and hospital stay and, in some categories of patient, mortality may all be reduced.

A15.13

A) F   **B)** T   **C)** F   **D)** F   **E)** F

Acute lung injury (ALI) and acute respiratory distress syndrome (ARDS) are diagnosed in an appropriate clinical setting with one or more recognized risk factors. ALI/ARDS can be defined as follows: a) respiratory distress; b) stiff lungs (reduced pulmonary compliance resulting in high inflation pressures); c) chest radiograph: new bilateral, diffuse, patchy or homogeneous pulmonary infiltrates; d) cardiac: no apparent cardiogenic cause of pulmonary oedema (pulmonary artery occlusion pressure <18 mmHg if measured or no clinical evidence of left atrial hypertension); e) profound gas exchange abnormalities: ALI – arterial oxygen tension/fractional inspired oxygen (P_aO_2/F_IO_2) ratio <40 kPa (<300 mmHg); ARDS – P_aO_2/F_IO_2 <26.6 kPa (<200 mmHg) (in both cases despite normal arterial carbon dioxide tension and regardless of positive end-expiratory pressure). The criterion for arterial oxygen tension/fractional inspired oxygen is arbitrary and the value of differentiating ALI from ARDS has been questioned; f) a cause other than primary pneumonia. In patients with ALI/ARDS, however, colloids are unlikely to be retained within the vascular compartment; once they enter the interstitial space, the transvascular oncotic gradient is lost and the main determinants of interstitial oedema formation become the microvascular hydrostatic pressure and lymphatic drainage. There is therefore some controversy concerning the relative merits of colloids or crystalloids for volume replacement in patients likely to develop ALI/ARDS, or in whom the condition is established. Repeated position changes between prone and supine may allow reductions in airway pressures and the inspired oxygen fraction. The response to prone positioning is, however, variable and it remains uncertain whether this strategy improves outcome. When nitric oxide is inhaled, it can improve $\dot{V}/\dot{Q}$ matching by increasing perfusion of ventilated lung units, as well as reducing pulmonary hypertension. It has been shown to improve oxygenation in so-called responders with ALI/ARDS but so far has not been shown to increase survival. As with inhaled NO, the response to aerosolized prostacyclin is variable and although it has been shown to improve oxygenation its effect on outcome has yet to be established. Administration of high-dose steroids to patients with established ALI/ARDS does not appear to improve outcome, and current evidence suggests that prophylactic administration to those at risk is of no value.

A15.14

A) F   **B)** T   **C)** T   **D)** T   **E)** T

All brainstem reflexes are absent in brain death. The following tests should not be performed in the presence of seizures or abnormal postures. a) Oculocephalic reflexes should be absent: when the head is rotated from side to side, the eyes move with the head and therefore remain stationary relative to the orbit. In a comatose patient whose brainstem is intact, the eyes will rotate relative to the orbit (i.e. doll's eye movements will be present). b) The pupils are fixed and unresponsive to bright light. Both direct and consensual light reflexes are absent. The size of the pupils is irrelevant, although most often they will be dilated. c) Corneal reflexes are absent. d) There are no vestibulo-ocular reflexes on caloric testing. e) There is no motor response within the cranial nerve territory to

Intensive care medicine

painful stimuli applied centrally or peripherally. Spinal reflexes may be present. f) There is no gag or cough reflex in response to pharyngeal, laryngeal or tracheal stimulation. g) Spontaneous respiration is absent. The patient should be ventilated with 5% CO_2 in 95% O_2 for 10 minutes and then disconnected from the ventilator for a further 10 minutes. Oxygenation is maintained by insufflation with 100% oxygen via a catheter placed in the endotracheal tube. The patient is observed for any signs of spontaneous respiratory efforts. A blood gas sample should be obtained during this period to ensure that the P_aco_2 is sufficiently high to stimulate spontaneous respiration (>6.7 kPa (50 mmHg)). The examination should be performed and repeated by two senior doctors.

A15.15

A) F   B) T   C) T   D) T   E) T
F) T   G) T

Guidance for involving a Medical Emergency or 'Patient at Risk' team should be activated if the following criteria are fulfilled and the patient is being actively treated: heart rate below 40 b.p.m., heart rate above 120 b.p.m., systolic blood pressure above 200 mmHg, systolic blood pressure below 80 mmHg, urine output less than 0.5 mL/kg/h for 2 consecutive hours, respiratory rate above 30 breaths per minute, respiratory rate below 8 breaths per minute, oxygen saturation less than 90% while receiving supplemental oxygen, Glasgow coma score less than 8, core temperature greater than 39°C and core temperature less than 35°C.

A15.16

A) T   B) T   C) T   D) T   E) T   F) T

Hypotension stimulates the baroreceptors, and to a lesser extent the chemoreceptors, causing increased sympathetic nervous activity. Later this is augmented by the release of catecholamines from the adrenal medulla. The resulting vasoconstriction, together with increased myocardial contractility and heart rate, help to restore blood pressure and cardiac output. Reduction in perfusion of the renal cortex stimulates the juxtaglomerular apparatus to release renin. There is release of pituitary hormones such as adrenocorticotrophic hormone (ACTH), vasopressin (antidiuretic hormone, ADH) and endogenous opioid peptides. There is release of cortisol which causes fluid retention and antagonizes insulin.There is release of glucagon which raises the blood sugar level.

A15.17

A) T   B) F   C) F   D) T   E) F

When heart rate increases, the duration of systole remains essentially unchanged, whereas diastole, and thus the time available for ventricular filling, becomes progressively shorter, and the stroke volume eventually falls. In the normal heart this occurs at rates greater than about 160 beats per minute. As the end-diastolic volume of the ventricle increases, tension in the myocardial fibres is increased and stroke volume rises. Decreasing the afterload can increase the stroke volume achieved at a given preload, while reducing myocardial oxygen consumption. Right ventricular afterload is normally negligible because the resistance of the pulmonary circulation is very low.

A15.18

A) T B) F C) T D) F E) F

The sigmoid shape of the curve in the figure accompanying Answer 15.5 (above) is important clinically for a number of reasons. a) Modest falls in the partial pressure of oxygen in the arterial blood (P_aO_2) may be tolerated (since oxygen content is relatively unaffected) provided that the percentage saturation remains above 90%. b) Increasing the P_aO_2 to above normal has only a minimal effect on oxygen content unless hyberbaric oxygen is administered (when the amount of oxygen in solution in plasma becomes significant). d) Once on the steep 'slippery slope' of the curve (percentage saturation below about 90%), a small decrease in P_aO_2 can cause large falls in oxygen content, while increasing P_aO_2 only slightly, e.g. by administering 28% oxygen to a patient with chronic obstructive pulmonary disease (COPD), can lead to a useful increase in oxygen saturation and content. In certain congenital cardiac lesions, such as Fallot's tetralogy and when a segment of lung is completely unventilated, a considerable amount of blood bypasses the lungs and causes arterial hypoxaemia. This hypoxaemia cannot be corrected by administering oxygen to increase the P_aO_2, because blood leaving normal alveoli is already fully saturated and further increases in PO_2 will not significantly affect its oxygen content.

A 28-year-old woman's jaundice is exacerbated by the initiation of oral contraceptives containing oestrogen. The defective enzyme is

A. HMG-CoA reductase
B. Alcohol dehydrogenase
C. UDP glucuronosyl transferase
D. Cytochrome p450 enzymes
E. Glucose-6-phosphate dehydrogenase

Q16.2

A 29-year-old Nigerian man develops malaria and is treated with primaquine. He develops severe haemolysis and methaemoglobinaemia. The deficient enzyme is

A. HMG-CoA reductase
B. Alcohol dehydrogenase
C. UDP glucuronosyl transferase
D. Cytochrome p450 enzymes
E. Glucose-6-phosphate dehydrogenase

Q16.3

Type 2 statistical errors can be avoided by

A. Increasing the odds ratio
B. Estimating the number of subjects needed to examine specific levels of difference
C. Requiring a higher level of probability (e.g. $p < 0.01$)
D. Increasing the correlation coefficient
E. Requiring a lower level of probability

Q16.4

Most cases of adult self-poisoning are

A. Münchausen's syndrome by proxy
B. For financial gain
C. For sexual gain
D. A 'cry-for-help'
E. Carefully premeditated attempts to commit suicide

Q16.5

A 78-year-old woman is started on verapamil therapy. Select the most likely adverse effect of this drug in this patient

A. Confusion
B Constipation
C. Glucose intolerance
D. Euphoria
E. Urinary incontinence

Q16.6

An 'intention-to-treat' analysis is one

A. That includes only those patients who have completed the study
B. That includes only patients who intend to participate in the study before randomization
C. That includes all the patients from randomization
D. That aims to determine whether one treatment is better than another
E. That aims to determine whether two (or possibly more) treatments produce similar benefits

Q16.7

A 27-year-old nursing student is in the emergency room following an overdose of paracetamol. She ingested the pills about 4 hours ago. Select the best option for treatment

A. Gastric lavage
B. Syrup of ipecacuanha
C. Single-dose activated charcoal
D. Multiple-dose activated charcoal
E. N-acetylcysteine

Q16.8

A 38-year-old psychiatric patient took an overdose of lithium several hours ago. She now has clinical features of poisoning (drowsiness, hypertonia and convulsions) and high plasma levels of lithium. Select the best option for treatment

A. Gastric lavage
B. Syrup of ipecacuanha
C. Single-dose activated charcoal
D. Forced alkaline diuresis
E. Haemodialysis

Q16.9

1. A 42-year-old patient is having a CT scan. She has been administered dye during a prior study without any complications. On this occasion, on injection of the dye, she develops bronchospasm, nausea and dizziness, and she vomits and collapses. During intubation by the cardiac arrest team the anaesthesiologist notes that she has severe laryngeal oedema

2. A 35-year-old woman has hypertension during her pregnancy and is started on alpha-methyldopa. Two weeks later she is noted to be pale and breathless. Blood smear shows several schizocytes and helmet cells. Coombs' test is positive

3. A 58-year-old patient with Graves' disease is being treated with propylthiouracil. Several days after initiating therapy the patient is noted to have fever, urticaria, arthropathy, lymphadenopathy and proteinuria. Blood smear shows eosinophilia

4. A 28-year-old patient has been advised to apply antibiotic ointment for her skin lesion. Her skin lesion gets worse and the dermatologist diagnoses contact dermatitis

5. A 45-year-old patient with acute myocardial infarction is administered aspirin. Soon afterwards he develops flushing, urticaria and bronchospasm

6. A 45-year-old patient with acute myocardial infarction is administered morphine for pain. Soon afterwards he develops itching, bronchospasm and hypotension

Select the best match for each of the above

A. Pseudoallergic reaction
B. Due to the formation of hapten–protein complexes which trigger a lymphocytic cellular immune reaction
C. Caused by the formation of antigen–antibody complexes which lodge in the small blood vessels, supplying various organs
D. Caused by the interaction of drug and a circulating or membrane-bound protein to cause production of circulating antibody of the IgG and IgM class with subsequent complement activation
E. Involves the recognition of the drug (or drug–protein complex) by IgE molecules on the surface of the mast cells and subsequent degranulation with release of antihistamine and other inflammatory mediators

Q16.10

1. A 28-year-old asthmatic on theophylline develops cardiac arrhythmias when this medication is initiated

2. A 45-year-old patient on digoxin for atrial fibrillation develops heart block when this medication is initiated

3. A 57-year-old patient with coronary artery disease on beta-blockers develops asystole when this medication is started

4. A 25-year-old patient with manic depression is on lithium. She develops convusions when this medication is initiated

5. A 45-year-old cardiac transplant patient is on azathioprine. He develops bone marrow failure when this medication is initiated

Select the best match for each of the above

A. Allopurinol
B. Verapamil
C. Thiazide diuretics
D. Quinidine
E. Warfarin
F. Erythromycin

Q16.11

1. ACE inhibitors
2. Amiodarone
3. Carbamazepine
4. Chloramphenicol
5. Non-steroidal anti-inflammatory drugs (NSAIDs)
6. Phenytoin
7. Diethylstilbestrol
8. Tetracylines

Select the common fetal adverse effect of each of the above drugs in pregnancy

A. Neural tube defects
B. Vaginal carcinoma in the offspring
C. Cleft palate
D. Damage to bones and teeth
E. Grey baby syndrome
F. Delayed closure of ductus arteriosus
G. Renal damage and oligohydramnios
H. Neonatal goitre

Q16.12

1. The average of a distribution of values that are grouped symmetrically around a central tendency

2. The middle value in a sample. It is used, particularly, where the values in a sample are asymmetrically distributed around a central tendency

3. The interval, in a distribution of values, that contains more values than any other

4. The probability of a sample mean being a certain distance from the population mean

5. The degree of association between the variables

6. Erroneous rejection of the null hypothesis – in this situation the null hypothesis is actually true, although we believe it to have been false

7. The basic assumption that there is no difference between two variables in one (or more) groups, e.g. in the analysis of a prospective, randomized, placebo-controlled trial this assumption asserts that there is no difference between the results in patients treated with placebo and those on the active treatment

8. Erroneous acceptance of the null hypothesis when there is, indeed, a difference

Select the best match for each of the above

A. Mode
B. Mean
C. Median
D. Correlation coefficient
E. Null hypothesis
F. Confidence interval
G. Type 1 error
H. Type 2 error

C. Vitamin K_1
D. Oxygen
E. Oxygen, sodium nitrite, sodium thiosulphate
F. Ethanol and fomepizole
G. N-acetylcysteine
H. Dimercaprol
I. Desferrioxamine
J. Sodium calcium edetate
K. Naloxone
L. Penicillamine

Q16.13

1. A 42-year-old woman has taken an overdose of temazepam
2. A 34-year-old factory worker has taken an overdose of ethylene glycol
3. A 48-year-old patient with prosthetic heart valves has taken an overdose of coumadin. Her INR is 9.2
4. A 26-year-old student with long-standing anaemia has taken an overdose of ferrous sulphate tablets
5. A 28-year-old nursing student has taken an overdose of paracetamol
6. A 37-year-old chemist has taken an overdose of cyanide
7. A 27-year-old anaesthetist has taken an overdose of morphine
8. An oil executive locked himself up in his garage with the car engine running and inhaled directly from the exhaust
9. A 33-year-old hypertensive took an overdose of atenolol. Heart rate was 36 beats/minute, blood pressure was normal
10. A 16-year-old schoolboy drank methanol from the school laboratory

Select the best antidote for each of the above

A. Glucagon and atropine
B. Flumazenil

Q16.14

1. A 42-year-old woman has taken an overdose of temazepam
2. A 28-year-old nursing student has taken a large overdose of paracetamol
3. A 37-year-old chemist has taken an overdose of cyanide
4. A 27-year-old anaesthetist has taken an overdose of cocaine
5. A 16-year-old schoolboy drank methanol from the school laboratory
6. A 58-year-old patient with rheumatoid arthritis has taken an overdose of aspirin and plasma salicylate concentrations are moderately elevated
7. A 23-year-old man has taken an overdose of organophosphorus insecticide
8. A 32-year-old chronic asthmatic took an overdose of theophylline about 10 hours ago
9. A 48-year-old patient with depression has taken an overdose of tricyclic antidepressants

Select the best match for each of the above

A. Reversible inhibition of cytochrome oxidase a_3
B. Irreversible inhibition of cytochrome oxidase a_3
C. Respiratory alkalosis

Drug therapy and poisoning

D. Widening of QRS complex on the ECG
E. Ataxia, dysarthria and nystagmus
F. Aortic dissection
G. Reduced visual acuity and metabolic acidosis
H. Inhibition of acetyl cholinesterase
I. Stimulation of acetyl cholinesterase
J. Depletion of liver glutathione stores
K. Activation of sodium/potassium ATPase

16.15

1. A 28-year-old man in North Africa is bitten by a scorpion

2. An 18-year-old student eats mackerel kept out of his refrigerator for over a day

3. A 42-year-old executive eats shellfish. Within 45 minutes he develops paraesthesia in mouth, lips and extremities. As the day progresses he develops dysphonia, dysphagia, muscle weakness and paralysis

4. A 22-year-old British tourist going to India wants to know about the most important cause of snake-bite mortality in the area he is going to visit

5. A 19-year-old is bitten by a sea snake while swimming

Select the best match for each of the above

A. Cause cholinergic and adrenergic symptoms
B. Contaminated with neurotoxins
C. Contain high concentrations of histamine
D. Myalgia, myoglobinuria
E. Russell's viper

16.16

A 22-year-old woman has hepatic failure. Problems with drug overdose may occur with

A. Verapamil
B. Lidocaine (lignocaine)
C. Isosorbide dinitrate
D. Propranolol
E. Morphine

16.17

A 58-year-old man is on warfarin therapy for a prosthetic heart valve. His general practitioner starts him on new medication and he develops uncontrollable bleeding. The following could have precipitated this bleeding

A. Cimetidine
B. Erythromycin
C. Ciprofloxacin
D. Imidazoles
E. Sulphonamides

16.18

A 27-year-old patient with epilepsy is currently on phenytoin. The following could precipitate phenytoin-induced ataxia

A. Oral contraceptive pill
B. Penicillin
C. Cimetidine
D. Isoniazid
E. Allopurinol

16.19

Drugs which inhibit the cytochrome p450 enzymes include

A. Alcohol
B. Griseofulvin
C. Phenytoin
D. Rifampicin
E. Ciprofloxacin

Q16.20

A 42-year-old patient who is an alcoholic now has liver failure. The metabolism of the following drugs is reduced in liver failure so that serious toxicity can occur

A. Opiate analgesics
B. NSAIDs
C. Anticoagulants
D. Anticonvulsants
E. Theophylline

Q16.21

A 37-year-old diabetic patient has chronic renal failure. The concentration of the following drugs can increase with azotemia causing toxicity

A. Diazepam
B. Digoxin
C. Lithium
D. Aminoglycoside antibiotics
E. Paracetamol

Q16.22

A 42-year-old man is known to be a slow acetylator of drugs. The following statements are correct

A. He is more likely to develop relapse with isoniazid because of inadequate plasma concentrations
B. He is more likely to develop polyneuropathy with isoniazid

C. He is is more likely to develop systemic lupus erythematosus with procainamide
D. He is less likely to develop systemic lupus erythematosus with hydralazine
E. Inhibition of phenytoin metabolism is less likely to occur when prescribed concurrently with isoniazid

Q16.23

A 45-year-old woman is newly diagnosed as having acute porphyria. The following drugs are safe and do not precipitate acute porphyria

A. Barbiturates
B. Diuretics
C. ACE inhibitors
D. Methyldopa
E. Erythromycin

Q16.24

A 21-year-old woman is admitted for a drug overdose. On examination she has constricted pupils. The following drugs are known to cause pupillary constriction

A. Tricyclic antidepressants
B. Amfetamines
C. Cocaine
D. Anticholinergic drugs
E. Organophosphorus insecticides

A16.1

C

Gilbert's syndrome is exacerbated by oestrogens and improved by low doses of barbiturates, which induce the defective enzyme UDP glucuronosyl transferase.

A16.2

E

Glucose-6-phosphate-dehydrogenase (G6PD) deficiency is a fairly common X-linked recessive disorder. Individuals with this trait are less able to synthesize NADPH in response to oxidative stress and are susceptible to red cell haemolysis and methaemoglobinaemia when challenged with certain oxidizing drugs as well as broad beans. Antimalarial drugs, particularly primaquine, can produce severe haemolysis resulting in renal failure.

A16.3

B

Statisticians call erroneous rejection of the null hypothesis a type 1 error. In this situation the null hypothesis is actually true, although we believe it to have been false. Erroneous acceptance of the null hypothesis when there is, indeed, a difference is known as a type 2 error. Type 1 errors can be reduced by requiring a higher level of probability (e.g. $p < 0.01$) but can never be absolutely excluded. Type 2 errors are usually the result of too few participants in the study and can be avoided by estimating the number of subjects needed to examine specific levels of difference. Such estimates are known as 'power calculations'.

A16.4

D

In adults, self-poisoning is commonly a 'cry for help'. Those involved are most often females under the age of 35 who are in good physical health. They take an overdose in circumstances where they are likely to be found, or in the presence of others. In those older than 55 years of age, men predominate and the overdose is usually taken in the course of a depressive illness or because of poor physical health. A third of patients admitted with an overdose state that they are unaware of the toxic effects of the substance involved; the majority take whatever drug is easily available at home.

A16.5

B

In the elderly, verapamil can result in chronic constipation.

A16.6

C

There are two ways to look at the outcome(s) of a clinical trial. One is to include only those patients who completed the study ('per protocol' analysis) and the other is to include all patients from the time of randomization ('intention-to-treat' analysis). Ideally there should be no difference, but in reality the results of a per protocol analysis are usually more advantageous to a treatment than an intention-to-treat analysis. The reason is that the intention-to-treat analysis will take account of patients who have withdrawn from the trial because of intolerance to the treatment or adverse reactions. It is therefore a much more robust approach.

A16.7

E

Management of paracetamol poisoning depends on the time of presentation and includes the following: a) admit the patient. b) Take blood for urgent estimation of the plasma paracetamol concentration as soon as 4 hours or more have elapsed since ingestion. Check INR, plasma creatinine and ALT. c) Assess whether the patient is at increased risk of liver damage. d) Give treatment (see p. 986–987 and Box 16.8 of Kumar & Clark, 5th edition, 2002) if needed. e) If the plasma paracetamol concentration is not available within 8 hours of the overdose, and if >150 mg/kg paracetamol has been ingested, treatment should be started at once and stopped if the plasma paracetamol concentration subsequently indicates that treatment is not required. Check INR, plasma creatinine and ALT on the completion of treatment and before discharge.

A16.8

E

Haemodialysis is of little value in patients who ingest poisons with large volumes of distribution, e.g. tricyclic antidepressants, because the plasma contains only a small proportion of the total amount of drug in the body. Haemodialysis is indicated in patients with severe clinical features and high plasma concentrations of ethanol, ethylene glycol, isopropanol, lithium, methanol or salicylate.

A16.9

1) E   2) D   3) C   4) B   5) A   6) A

Anaphylactic reactions (type I hypersensitivity) are more common in patients with a history of anaphylaxis with drugs (penicillin, radio-opaque contrast media, local anaesthetics and streptomycin), foods (such as nuts) or insect stings and in atopic individuals with a history of asthma and eczema. Typically anaphylaxis occurs on the second or third exposure to the drug, and may occur following administration of only very small amounts. The mechanism involves recognition of the drug (or a drug–protein complex) by IgE molecules on the surface of mast cells and subsequent degranulation with release of histamine and other inflammatory mediators. Type II reactions occur because of interaction of the drug and a circulating or membrane-bound protein to cause production of a circulating antibody of the IgG or IgM class with subsequent complement activation. The most common target for this type of immune-mediated damage is the haematological system resulting in Coombs-positive haemolytic anaemia (e.g. with methyldopa and penicillin) or thrombocytopenia (e.g. with quinine). Type III (Arthus, serum sickness or immune complex) reaction used to occur most commonly following injection of foreign serum to treat infectious diseases (e.g. antitetanus serum). It also occurs with antibiotics such as penicillins, streptomycin and sulphonamides as well as with the antithyroid drugs propylthiouracil and carbimazole. It is thought to be caused by the formation of antibody–antigen complexes which lodge in the small blood vessels of the skin, kidney and joints, and may mimic systemic lupus erythematosus, in which such complexes are also found. The classic clinical presentation occurs several days after starting therapy and includes fever, urticaria, arthropathy, lymphadenopathy and proteinuria. Eosinophilia is a common and diagnostically useful feature. The typical example of a type IV reaction is the

Drug therapy and poisoning

contact dermatitis which is sometimes produced following application of antibiotic or other topical therapy on the skin. It is thought to be due to the formation of hapten–protein complexes which trigger a lymphocytic cellular immune reaction. Pseudoallergic reactions mimic those detailed above, but are not thought to involve immune recognition. They are due to release of immunological mediators by other mechanisms. They typically occur on first-time exposure to the drug rather than after previous sensitization. Examples of this type of reaction include: a) itching, bronchospasm and vasodilatation following treatment with intravenous morphine; b) flushing, urticaria, bronchospasm and even circulatory shock caused by aspirin.

A16.10

1) F   2) B   3) B   4) C   5) A

Some potentially serious drug interactions

Drug	Interacting drug	Problem caused
Theophylline	Cimetidine	Convulsions
	Erythromycin	Arrhythmias
	Ciprofloxacin	
Digoxin	Amiodarone	Arrhythmias
	Verapamil	Heart block
	Quinidine	
	Diuretics	
Beta-blockers	Verapamil	Bradycardia,
	Diltiazem	asystole
Lithium	Thiazide diuretics	Ataxia, convulsions
Azathioprine Mercaptopurine	Allopurinol	Bone marrow failure

A16.11

1) G   2) H   3) A   4) E   5) F   6) A or C   7) B   8) D

Common adverse effects of drugs in pregnancy

Drug	Effect
ACE inhibitors	Renal damage and oligohydramnios
Retinoic acid derivatives	Multiple gross abnormalities (up to 2 years after stopping)
Alcohol	Fetal alcohol syndrome and growth retardation Withdrawal syndrome in newborn
Aminoglycosides	Vestibular damage (esp. streptomycin)
Amiodarone	Neonatal goitre
Warfarin	Bone abnormalities and neonatal haemorrhage
Sedatives, tranquillizers and hypnotics	Sedation or apnoea in neonate
Beta-blockers	May cause growth retardation
Carbamazepine	Neural tube defects (may be reduced with folate supplementation)
Carbimazole	Neonatal hypothyroidism
Chloramphenicol	Grey baby syndrome
Glucocorticoids	Neonatal adrenal suppression in high doses
Cytotoxic drugs	Most are potently teratogenic
NSAIDs	Delayed closure of ductus arteriosus
Opiate analgesics	Neonatal depression and withdrawal syndrome
Phenytoin	Hare lip, cleft palate and cardiac abnormalities; neural tube defects
Antimalarial drugs	Methaemoglobinaemia and haemolysis in neonate
Diethylstilbestrol	Vaginal carcinoma in offspring
Tetracyclines	Damage to bones and teeth
Valproate	Neural tube defects

NSAIDs, non-steroidal anti-inflammatory drugs

1) B   2) C   3) A   4) F   5) D
6) G   7) E   8) H

The 'average' value (or 'central tendency' in statistical parlance) may be expressed as the mean, median or mode depending on the circumstances. a) The *mean* is the average of a distribution of values that are grouped symmetrically around a central tendency. b) The median is the middle value in a sample. It is used, particularly, where the values in a sample are asymmetrically distributed around a central tendency. c) The mode is the interval, in a distribution of values, that contains more values than any other. The average value of a sample, on its own, is of only modest interest. Of equal (and often greater) relevance is the confidence we can place on this sample average truly reflecting the average value of the population from which it has been drawn. This is most often expressed as a confidence interval which expresses the probability of a sample mean being a certain distance from the population mean. d) The degree of correlation between two variables can be investigated by estimating the correlation coefficient. This coefficient (often abbreviated to 'r') measures the degree of association between the variables and may range from 1 to -1. If $r = 1$ then there is complete and direct concordance between the two variables; if $r = -1$ there is complete but inverse concordance; and where $r = 0$ there is no concordance. Standard statistical tables enable the investigator to determine the probability that r is due to chance.

Much of statistics is concerned with testing hypotheses. The basic assumption – known as the 'null hypothesis' – is that there is no difference between two variables in one (or more) groups. The reason for this confusing terminology is that statistical techniques are designed to assess the extent by which a zero difference might be due to the play of chance (or to sampling error). In the analysis of a prospective, randomized, placebo-controlled trial the null hypothesis asserts that there is no difference between the results in patients treated with placebo and those on the active treatment. Statistical tests are used to determine the probability that the observed difference is due to chance. Where this is less than 1 in 20 ($p < 0.05$) it is described as 'statistically significant'. Again, as with correlations, the 1 in 20 rule is arbitrary and is a convention that has been widely adopted. When the results of a statistical test indicate rejection of the null hypothesis, and that the probability of the results being due to chance is less than 1 in 20 ($p < 0.05$) it means that 95 times out of 100 we are correct in our decision; but that 5 times out of 100 we will be wrong. Statisticians call erroneous rejection of the null hypothesis a type 1 error. In this situation the null hypothesis is actually true, although we believe it to have been false. Erroneous acceptance of the null hypothesis when there is, indeed, a difference is known as a type 2 error.

A16.13

1) B   2) F   3) C   4) I   5) G
6) E   7) K   8) D   9) A   10) F

Antidotes of value in poisoning	
Poison	**Antidote**
Anticoagulants (oral)	Vitamin K_1
Arsenic	DMSA
	Dimercaprol (BAL)
Benzodiazepines	Flumazenil
β-Adrenoceptor blocking drugs	Atropine
	Glucagon
Carbon monoxide	Oxygen
Cyanide	Oxygen
	Dicobalt edetate
	Hydroxocobalamin
	Sodium nitrite
	Sodium thiosulphate
Digoxin	Digoxin-specific antibody fragments
Ethylene glycol	Ethanol
	Fomepizole
Iron salts	Desferrioxamine
Lead (inorganic)	Sodium calcium edetate
	DMSA
Methaemoglobinaemia	Methylthioninium chloride (methylene blue)
Methanol	Ethanol
	Fomepizole
Mercury (inorganic)	DMPS
	Dimercaprol (BAL)
	Penicillamine
Opioids	Naloxone
Organophosphorus insecticides	Atropine
	Pralidoxime
Paracetamol	N-acetylcysteine or methionine
Thallium	Berlin (Prussian) blue

DMSA, dimercaptosuccinic acid (succimer); DMPS, dimercaptopropanesulphonate (unithiol)

A16.14

1) E   2) J   3) A   4) F   5) G   6) C
7) H   8) K   9) D

Organophosphorus insecticides inhibit acetyl cholinesterase causing accumulation of acetylcholine at central and peripheral cholinergic nerve endings, including neuromuscular junctions. In paracetamol overdose, large amounts of paracetamol are metabolized by oxidation because of saturation of the sulphate conjugation pathway. Liver glutathione stores become depleted so that the liver is unable to deactivate the toxic metabolite. After initial euphoria, cocaine produces agitation, tachycardia, hypertension, sweating, hallucinations, convulsions, metabolic acidosis, hyperthermia, rhabdomyolysis, and ventricular arrhythmias. Dissection of the aorta, myocarditis, myocardial infarction, dilated cardiomyopathy, subarachnoid haemorrhage and cerebral haemorrhage also occur. Cyanide reversibly inhibits cytochrome oxidase a_3 so that cellular respiration ceases. Salicylates stimulate the respiratory centre, increase the depth and rate of respiration, and induce a respiratory alkalosis. Benzodiazepines produce drowsiness, ataxia, dysarthria and nystagmus. Coma and respiratory depression develop in severe intoxication. Methanol causes inebriation and drowsiness. After a latent period coma supervenes. Blurred vision and diminished visual acuity occur. The presence of dilated pupils that are unreactive to light suggests that permanent blindness is likely to ensue. In theophylline toxicity hypokalaemia probably results from activation of Na^+/K^+-ATPase. In tricyclic antidepressant overdose the ECG will often show a wide QRS interval and there is a reasonable correlation between the width of the QRS complex and the severity of poisoning.

A16.15

1) A 2) C 3) B 4) E 5) D

Scorpion venoms stimulate the release of acetylcholine and catecholamines causing both cholinergic and adrenergic symptoms. Scrombrotoxic fish poisoning is due to the action of bacteria such as *Proteus morgani* and *Klebsiella pneumoniae* in decomposing the flesh of fish such as tuna, mackerel, bonito and skipjack if the fish are stored at insufficiently low temperatures. The spoiled fish can contain excessively high concentrations of histamine (muscle histidine is broken down by the bacteria to histamine), though the precise role of histamine in the pathogenesis of the clinical syndrome is uncertain. Russell's viper is the most important cause of snake-bite mortality in India, Pakistan and Burma. Sea snakes' bites result in muscle involvement, myalgia and myoglobinuria, which can lead to acute renal failure. Cardiac and respiratory paralysis may occur. Paralytic shell fish poisoning is uncommon and is caused by bivalve molluscs being contaminated with neurotoxins, including saxitoxin, produced by the toxic dinoflagellates *Gonyaulax catenella* and *Gonyaulax tamarensis*. Symptoms develop within 30 minutes of ingestion. The illness is characterized by paraesthesiae of the mouth, lips, face and extremities and is often accompanied by nausea, vomiting and diarrhoea. In more severe cases, dysphonia, dysphagia, muscle weakness, paralysis, ataxia and respiratory depression occur.

A16.16

A) T B) T C) T D) T E) T

Drugs which have extensive pre-systemic (first-pass) metabolism include: a) verapamil; b) propranolol; c) lidocaine (lignocaine); d) glyceryl trinitrate; e) isosorbide dinitrate; f) morphine; g) pethidine; h) clomethiazole. There is a risk of overdose with these drugs in patients with hepatic failure.

A16.17

A) T B) T C) T D) T E) T

Drug	Interacting drug	Problem caused
Warfarin	Cimetidine Erythromycin Ciprofloxacin Imidazoles Sulphonamides	Uncontrolled bleeding

A16.18

A) F B) F C) T D) T E) F

Drug	Interacting drug	Problem caused
Phenytoin	Cimetidine Isoniazid Sulphonamides Imidazoles	Ataxia
	Oral contraceptive pill	Reduced effect

A16.19

A) F B) F C) F D) F E) T

Serious drug interactions are often due to drugs which inhibit liver p450 enzymes. There are a limited number of such drugs, which include cimetidine, erythromycin, ciprofloxacin and sodium valproate. Not all these drugs will inhibit all p450 isoenzymes, and therefore such interactions are not entirely predictable.

A16.20

A) T B) F C) T D) T E) T

Metabolism of many drugs is largely dependent on normal hepatic function and extreme caution must be taken in prescribing to patients with liver failure. In particular reduced metabolism of opiate analgesics, anticoagulants, anticonvulsant drugs and theophylline may cause serious toxicity.

A16.21

A) F B) T C) T D) T E) F

The major route of excretion for most drugs is via the kidneys. In drugs which are not subject to hepatic metabolism, renal excretion is the main factor which determines the concentration of active drug circulating in the plasma. Particular care must be taken with drugs with a low therapeutic ratio which are principally excreted by the kidneys, such as digoxin, lithium and aminoglycoside antibiotics.

A16.22

A) F B) T C) T D) F E) F

The best-known genetic cause of altered drug handling is acetylator phenotype. Certain drugs are metabolized by acetylation in the liver and individuals can be classified as slow acetylators or fast acetylators. Those who acetylate slowly will have higher plasma concentrations of drug for any given dose and will tend to develop adverse effects more readily. The antituberculous drug isoniazid will cause a polyneuropathy more commonly in patients with slow acetylator status; inhibition of metabolism of the anticonvulsant phenytoin when prescribed concurrently with isoniazid is also more common in slow acetylators. Rapid acetylators may, conversely, be more likely to relapse because of inadequate plasma concentrations of isoniazid. Systemic lupus erythematosus is more likely to develop with procainamide and hydralazine in slow acetylators.

A16.23

A) F B) F C) F D) F E) F

All these drugs may precipitate acute porphyria.

Commonly used drugs which may precipitate acute porphyria – a complete list is given in the *British National Formulary*

Barbiturates
Anticonvulsants
Benzodiazepines
Oral hypoglycaemics
Tricyclic antidepressants
Diuretics
ACE inhibitors
Flucloxacillin
Cephalosporins
Erythromycin
Sulphonamides
Methyldopa
Metoclopramide
Sex steroids
Theophylline
Antihistamines
Calcium-channel blockers

A16.24

A) F B) F C) F D) F E) T

Features	Likely poisons
Constricted pupils	Opioids Organophosphorus insecticides Nerve agents
Dilated pupils	Tricyclic antidepressants Amfetamines Cocaine Anticholinergic drugs

Q 17.1

A 27-year-old fisherman falls from a trawler while sailing in the Atlantic and is airlifted to his local hospital. He feels icy to touch. Which one of the following ECG changes is pathgnomonic of his condition?

A. Prolongation of PR, QT and QRS complexes – all present together
B. 'J' waves – rounded waves above the isoelectric line immediately after the QRS complex
C. PR depression
D. Notched P wave
E. Notched T wave

Q 17.2

A 28-year-old doctor from the UK is on his first expedition to the Himalayas. He is expected to climb up to 4000 m. The best prophylaxis for acute mountain sickness is which one of the following?

A. Thiazide diuretic
B. Chloroquine
C. Acetazolamide (a carbonic anhydrase inhibitor)
D. Acclimatizing by ascending gradually
E. Proton pump blocker

Q 17.3

A 25-year-old medical student from the University of Aberdeen medical school liked to 'moonlight' as a deep sea diver on the oil rigs in the North Sea. When she appeared to the surface from her most recent underwater expedition she developed irritation of the skin and joint pain. She had skin mottling. Select the best option for treatment

A. Oxygen only
B. Hyperbaric oxygen and recompression in a pressure chamber
C. Thiazide diuretic
D. Clonidine
E. Acetazolamide

Q 17.4

A 45-year-old radiation oncologist is accidentally contaminated with radioiodine. The best treatment is which one of the following?

A. Observe the patient and treat symptomatically
B. Carbimazole
C. L-thyroxine
D. Propranolol
E. Potassium iodide

Q 17.5

A 55-year-old rock singer who has been exposed for many years to sound frequencies of 2–6 kHz now complains of hearing loss. The likely cause for her deafness is damage of the

A. Stapedius muscle
B. Ossicles in the middle ear
C. Ossicles causing otosclerosis
D. Hair cells in the organs of Corti
E. Facial nerve as it crosses the auditory channel

Environmental medicine

Q17.6

A 22-year-old man on his first sea voyage develops nausea, sweating, dizziness and profuse vomiting accompanied by an irresistible desire to stop moving. Which one of the following medications is of some value in preventing these clinical features?

A. Propranolol
B. Cinnarizine
C. Paracetamol
D. Codeine
E. Thiazide diuretic

Q17.7

A 72-year-old Canadian man with diabetes enjoys his alcohol. He goes on his dream safari in Africa. Three days after arrival he complains of headache, nausea, vomiting and weakness. He is confused. His core temperature is 41°C. Head CT is normal. The complications of this condition include

A. Hypovolaemia
B. Intravascular coagulation
C. Rhabdomyolysis
D. Renal failure
E. Hepatic failure

Q17.8

A 22-year-old man drowns in a swimming pool. He has been underwater for about 15 minutes. The following statements are correct

A. He is most likely to have brain damage since he has been under water for a prolonged period and hence resuscitation should not be attempted
B. Despite the absence of a pulse and a fixed dilated pupil, resuscitation should be attempted
C. All patients who are resuscitated successfully should be subsequently admitted to hospital
D. The prognosis is poor if the patient remains in a coma for 30 minutes after resuscitation
E. The management of drowning depends on whether it is saltwater or freshwater drowning

A 17.1

B

Ventricular arrhythmias (tachycardia/ fibrillation) or asystole is the usual cause of death in hypothermia. 'J' waves – rounded waves above the isoelectric line immediately after the QRS complex – are pathognomonic of hypothermia. Prolongation of PR and QT intervals and QRS complex occurs.

A 17.2

D

Prophylactic treatment with acetazolamide, a carbonic anhydrase inhibitor and a respiratory stimulant is of some value in preventing acute mountain sickness. Acclimatizing, i.e. ascending gradually, is the best prophylaxis.

A 17.3

B

Treatment of decompression sickness is with oxygen. All but the mildest forms of decompression sickness (i.e. skin mottling alone) require recompression in a pressure chamber.

A 17.4

E

Radioiodine contamination should be treated immediately with potassium iodide 133 mg per day. This will block 90% of radioiodine absorption by the thyroid if given immediately before exposure.

A 17.5

D

Repeated prolonged exposure to loud noise, particularly between 2 and 6 kHz, causes first temporary and later permanent hearing loss by physically destroying hair cells in the organ of Corti and, eventually, auditory neurones. This is a common occupational problem, not only in industry and the armed forces, but also in the home (electric drills and sanders), in sport (motor racing), and in entertainment (pop stars, disc jockeys and their audiences).

A 17.6

B

Prophylactic antihistamines or vestibular sedatives (hyoscine or cinnarizine) are of some value in motion sickness.

A 17.7

A) T   B) T   C) T   D) T   E) T

The complications of heat stroke include hypovolaemia (shock), intravascular coagulation, cerebral oedema, rhabdomyolysis, and renal and hepatic failure.

A17.8

A) F   B) T   C) T   D) T   E) F

In practice there is little difference between saltwater and freshwater drowning. In both, severe hypoxaemia develops rapidly after water aspiration. Patients can survive for up to 30 minutes under water without suffering brain damage – and for longer if the water temperature is near 0°C. This is probably related to the protective role of the diving reflex – submersion causes reflex slowing of the pulse and vasoconstriction. In addition, hypothermia decreases oxygen consumption.

Cardiopulmonary resuscitation (CPR) should be started immediately. Resuscitation should always be attempted, even in the absence of a pulse and the presence of fixed dilated pupils. Patients frequently make a dramatic recovery. All patients should be subsequently admitted to hospital for intensive monitoring. Survivors are liable to develop acute respiratory distress syndrome (ARDS). Severe metabolic acidosis develops in the majority of survivors. Prognosis is good if patients regain consciousness promptly but poor if they remain in coma for 30 minutes after resuscitation.

Q18.1

The mother of a 15-year-old boy is concerned that her son may have not attained puberty because there is family history of delayed development. Which one of the following is the best indicator of the onset of puberty in boys?

A. A fall in luteinizing hormone and follicle-stimulating hormone levels
B. A testicular volume of >5 mL
C. A rising serum oestrogen
D. Enlargement of epididymis
E. Undescended testis

Q18.2

A 45-year-old man presents with headaches. On examination his blood pressure is elevated, urinary potassium is 35 mmol/24 h and serum potassium is 3.0 mmol/L. The most likely cause for this clinical picture is which one of the following?

A. Renal artery stenosis
B. Phaeochromocytoma
C. Conn's syndrome
D. Idiopathic adrenal hyperplasia
E. Cushing's syndrome

Q18.3

A 24-year-old patient presents with anxiety, sweating, tremor and palpitations. On examination his heart rate is 110 beats/minute and blood pressure is elevated. He is treated with a beta-blocker which causes the blood pressure to increase by 30 mmHg and heart rate is 140 beats/minute. The most likely cause for his symptoms is which one of the following?

A. Hypoaldosteronism
B. Secondary hyperaldosteronism
C. Renal artery stenosis
D. Conn's syndrome
E. Pheochromocytoma

Q18.4

A 28-year-old pregnant nurse presents with weight loss, increased appetite, irritability, heat intolerance and palpitations. Clinical examination reveals tachycardia, full pulse and warm, vasodilated peripheries. The thyroid is not enlarged. Serum thyroid-stimulating hormone <0.05 mU/L (normal 0.3–3.5 mU/L), increased total T_4, increased free T_4, and increased free T_3. The best therapeutic option is which one of the following?

A. Radioactive iodine
B. Radioactive iodine with propranolol
C. Carbimazole
D. Total thyroidectomy
E. ACE-inhibitor

Endocrine disease

Q18.5

A 42-year-old man is diagnosed as having localized papillary carcinoma of the thyroid. The primary therapeutic option is which one of the following?

A. Radioiodine thyroid scan
B. Total or near-total thyroidectomy
C. Suppressive doses of levothyroxine (thyroxine)
D. Carbimazole
E. Propranolol

Q18.6

A 35-year-old man has weight gain, thin skin, bruising, hypertension, dorsal fat pad, central obesity and proximal myopathy. Which one of the following tests suggests a pituitary-dependent cause for these clinical features?

A. Solitary adrenal adenoma on CT of abdomen
B. Hyperkalaemia
C. An exaggerated adrenocorticotrophic hormone and cortisol response to exogenous corticotropin-releasing hormone
D. High-dose dexamethasone test
E. Low levels of adrenocorticotrophic hormone

Q18.7

A 57-year-old woman presents with paraesthesia, circumoral numbness, cramps, anxiety and tetany. She also has vitiligo. Signs include Chvostek's sign and Trousseau's sign. The most likey cause for this clinical picture is which one of the following?

A. Renal failure
B. Idiopathic hypoparathyroidism
C. DiGeorge syndrome
D. Pseudo-hypoparathyroidism
E. Pseudo-pseudohypoparathyroidism

Q18.8

A 9-year-old girl develops hirsutism. She has no signs of puberty. 17-Hydroxyprogesterone levels are increased, basal adrenocorticotrophic hormone levels are raised and urinary pregnanetriol excretion is increased. The most likely explanation for the clinical picture is which one of the following?

A. Ectopic pregnancy
B. Cushing's syndrome
C. Polycystic ovarian disease
D. Congenital adrenal hyperplasia
E. Nelson's syndrome

Q18.9

A 35-year-old woman presents with increased thirst. Investigations reveal 24-h urinary output of 2 L, high plasma osmolality, high plasma sodium, failure of urinary concentration with fluid deprivation and restoration of urinary concentration with vasopressin. This clinical picture is most likely to be due to which one of the following?

A. Cranial diabetes insipidus
B. Diabetes mellitus
C. Hypokalaemia
D. Primary polydispsia
E. Nephrogenic diabetes insipidus

Q18.10

A 25-year-old woman complains of intolerance to cold, weight gain, deep voice and constipation. On examination the hair is dry, the skin is thick, the heart rate is 50 beats per minute and ankle jerks are delayed. Serum thyroid-stimulating hormone 20 mU/L, low total T_4, low free T_4 and low T_3. There is associated pernicious anaemia and vitiligo. Which one of the following conditions is most likely to cause this clinical picture?

A. Hashimoto's thyroiditis
B. Postpartum thyroiditis
C. Iodine deficiency
D. Dyshormonogenesis
E. Atrophic hypothyroidism

Q18.11

A 22-year-old woman presents with excessive hair on the upper lip. She has noticed it initially during menarche and over the years it has got worse requiring frequent removal of hair. Associated there is acne and oligomenorrhoea. The physician suspects that she has polycystic ovarian disease but would like to exclude congenital adrenal hyperplasia. Which one of the following tests would be the best indicator of congenital adrenal hyperplasia?

A. Elevated serum androstenedione
B. Elevated serum dehydroepiandrosterone
C. Elevated 17-α-hydroxyprogesterone
D. Luteinizing hormone hypersecretion
E. Mild hyperprolactinaemia

Q18.12

A 24-year-old man complains of decreased libido, decreased potency and galactorrhoea. Prolactin level is 2000 mU/L and MRI shows a 4 mm pituitary tumour. The best therapeutic option is which one of the following?

A. Radiotherapy
B. Radiotherapy with cyclophosphamide
C. Bromocriptine
D. Trans-sphenoidal surgery with radiotherapy
E. Bromocriptine plus radiotherapy

Q18.13

A 34-year-old man presents with a history of tiredness, headaches, excessive sweating, a change in appearance and increased size of gloves and shoes. There is a visual field defect. MRI reveals a 5 mm pituitary adenoma and the IGF-1 level is raised. The most appropriate first-line therapy is which one of the following?

A. External radiotherapy
B. Trans-sphenoidal surgery
C. Octreotide
D. Bromocriptine
E. Transfrontal surgery

Q18.14

1. Adrenocorticotrophic hormone
2. Luteinizing hormone
3. Follicle-stimulating hormone
4. Parathyroid hormone
5. Thyrotrophin-releasing hormone
6. Vasopressin
7. Angiotensin-II
8. Insulin
9. Insulin-like growth factor-1

Select the 'second messenger' for each of the above hormones

A. Tyrosine kinase and other intracellular kinases
B. Calcium phospholipid system
C. Cyclic AMP

Q18.15

1. Chlorpromazine
2. Amiodarone
3. Ketoconazole
4. Diuretics

5. ACE inhibitors

6. Anticonvulsants

Select the best match for each of the above

A. Hypoaldosteronism

B. Secondary aldosteronism

C. Hypoadrenalism

D. Bind to TBG – decrease total T_4

E. Hypothyroidism

F. Increase prolactin causing galactorrhoea

Q18.16

1. Stimulates testosterone production from Leydig cells of the testis

2. Stimulates the Sertoli cells in the seminiferous tubules to produce the mature sperm

3. Stimulates ovarian androgen production by ovarian theca cells

4. Stimulates follicular development and aromatase activity in the ovarian granulosa cells

5. Stimulates the release of inhibin from ovarian stromal cells

6. Feedback inhibition of follicle-stimulating hormone release

7. Causes uterine endometrial proliferation in preparation for possible implantation

8. Maintains corpus luteum function

Select the best match for each of the above

A. Human chorionic gonadotrophin

B. Oestrogen and progesterone

C. Inhibin A and B

D. Follicle-stimulating hormone

E. Sex hormone binding globulin

F. Luteinizing hormone

G. Prolactin

Q18.17

1. An 8-year-old girl has fully developed breasts and nipples, vaginal and vulval growth and pubic hair development. Other features are café-au-lait spots and polyostotic fibrotic dysplasia

2. A 3-year-old girl has early breast development. There are no other secondary sexual characteristics. There is no evidence of ovarian follicular development

3. A 6-year-old girl has early development of pubic hair without any of the other changes of puberty

4. A 17-year-old boy presents with hypogonadism. On examination he has loss of sense of smell. Studies reveal isolated GnRH deficiency

5. An 18-year-old boy presents with poor sexual development. Clinical examination shows small, pea-size, but firm testes, gynaecomastia and signs of androgen deficiency. Chromosomal studies reveal a 47XXY picture

6. A 19-year-old girl has short stature, a webbed neck, coarctation of the aorta, streak gonads. Chromosomal studies show a 45X picture

7. A 19-year-old boy has cryptorchidism, impaired conversion of testosterone to dihydrotestosterone and chromosomal studies reveal a 46XY picture

Select the best match for each of the above

A. Sheehan's syndrome

B. Forbes–Albright syndrome

C. Premature thelarche

D. Premature adrenarche

E. Klinefelter's syndrome

F. Kallman's syndrome

G. 5α-Reductase deficiency

H. Turner's syndrome

Q18.18

1. Serum TSH <0.05 mU/L (normal 0.3–3.5 mU/L), increased total T_4, increased free T_4, and increased free T_3

2. Serum TSH 20 mU/L, low total T_4, low free T_4, low T_3

3. Low normal TSH, low total T_4, low free T_4, and normal T_3

4. Serum TSH <0.05 mU/L, normal total T_4, normal free T_4, increased T_3

5. Serum TSH 9 mU/L, normal total T_4, normal free T_4, normal T_3

Select the best match for each of the above

A. Compensated euthyroidism
B. Primary hypothyroidism
C. T_3 toxicosis
D. TSH deficiency
E. Thyrotoxicosis

Q18.19

The following statements about hormone physiology are correct

A. The secretion of gonadotrophins is normally pulsatile
B. The effect of T_3 and T_4 on the pituitary and hypothalamus is known as a 'positive feedback' system
C. Growth hormone secretion is stimulated by somatostatin
D. Thyroid-stimulating hormone release is partially inhibited by somatostatin
E. The posterior pituitary acts merely as a storage organ
F. Secretion of growth hormone is inhibited during sleep

Q18.20

A 58-year-old cigarette smoker and alcoholic with ischaemic cardiomyopathy, micronodular cirrhosis and peptic ulcer presents with cough and haemoptysis. Sputum cytology reveals bronchogenic carcinoma. He is currently on aspirin, cimetidine, captopril, digoxin and spironolactone. On examination he has gynaecomastia. Factors which could have caused his gynaecomastia include

A. Bronchogenic carcinoma
B. Digoxin
C. Spironolactone
D. Captopril
E. Cirrhosis
F. Cimetidine

Q18.21

A 22-year-old woman presents with excessive hair on her upper lip. She first noticed it during menarche and over the years it has got worse, requiring frequent shaving. There is associated acne and oligomenorrhoea. Ovarian ultrasound shows a thickened capsule, multiple 3–5 mm cysts and a hyperechogenic stroma. Testosterone levels are normal but sex hormone binding globulins are low and estradiol levels are normal. The following statements about this condition are correct

A. It is unclear whether the basic defect in this condition is in the ovary, adrenals or pituitary
B. This condition is associated with insulin resistance
C. Spironolactone has been used to treat hirsutism
D. Finasteride is effective in reducing hirsutism
E. Oestrogens are not useful in improving hirsutism

Endocrine disease

Q18.22

A 24-year-old woman complains of decreased libido, amenorrhoea and galactorrhoea. Likely causes for this clinical picture include

A. Hypothyroidism
B. Polycystic ovarian disease
C. Stalk compression due to pituitary adenoma
D. Prolactinoma
E. Oestrogen contraceptive pill

Q18.23

The following statements about the development of the reproductive organs are correct

A. Up to 20 weeks' gestation the sexes share a common development, with a primitive genital tract including Wolffian and Müllerian ducts
B. In the presence of a Y chromosome the potential testis develops while the ovary regresses
C. In the absence of a Y chromosome the potential ovary develops and related ducts form a uterus and the upper vagina
D. Testosterone causes atrophy of the Müllerian duct
E. Testosterone and dihydrotestosterone influence the Wolffian duct to differentiate into an epididymis, vas deferens, seminal vesicles and prostate

Q18.24

A 29-year-old man presents with weakness, tiredness, weight loss and anorexia. On examination there is a dull slaty pigmentation of the mouth, opposite the molars, and of the palmar creases and face. The patient has a postural decrease in systolic blood pressure although supine blood pressure is normal. The following are features of this disease

A. Random cortisol levels >550 nmol/L
B. Cortisol levels do not increase with short ACTH stimulation
C. Hyponatraemia, hyperkalaemia and a high urea
D. Reduced serum aldosterone with high plasma renin activity
E. Hypercalcaemia

Q18.25

A 69-year-old patient presents with nausea and vomiting. Laboratory tests reveal that serum calcium is 4 mmol/L. These features are usually associated with

A. Malignant disease
B. Hyperparathyroidism
C. Renal failure
D. Vitamin D therapy
E. Cushing's disease

Q18.26

A 45-year-old woman presents with confusion and irritability. Serum sodium 120 mmol/L, low plasma osmolality, urine osmolality higher than plasma osmolality, urinary sodium 34 mmol/L, normal renal and adrenal function. This clinical picture can be caused by

A. Alcohol withdrawal
B. Small-cell carcinoma of the lung
C. Pneumonia
D. Meningitis
E. Phenothiazines

A18.1

B

In constitutional pubertal delay, pubertal development, bone age and stature are in parallel. A family history may confirm that other family members experienced the same delayed development, which is common in boys but very rare in girls. In boys, a testicular volume >5 mL indicates the onset of puberty. A rising serum testosterone is an earlier clue.

A18.2

C

Conn's syndrome is caused by excess aldosterone production leading to sodium retention, potassium loss and the combination of hypokalaemia and hypertension.

A18.3

E

Phaeochromocytomas, tumours of the sympathetic nervous system, are very rare (less than 1 in 1000 cases of hypertension). Ninety per cent arise in the adrenal, while 10% occur elsewhere in the sympathetic chain. The clinical features are those of catecholamine excess and are frequently, but not necessarily, intermittent. Tumours should be removed if this is possible; 5-year survival is about 95% where not malignant. Medical preoperative and perioperative treatment is vital and includes complete alpha- and beta-blockade with phenoxybenzamine (20–80 mg daily initially in divided doses), then propranolol (120–240 mg daily), plus transfusion of whole blood to re-expand the contracted plasma volume. The alpha-blockade must precede the beta-blockade, as worsened hypertension may

otherwise result. Labetolol is not recommended.

A18.4

C

Three possibilities are available for the treatment of hyperthyroidism/thyrotoxicosis: antithyroid drugs (e.g. carbimazole), radioiodine, and surgery. Practices and beliefs differ widely within and between countries. Treatment also depends on patient preference and local expertise. Radioiodine is now more widely used in the UK, as has previously happened elsewhere, although it is absolutely contraindicated in pregnancy and while breast-feeding. Thyroidectomy should be performed only in patients who have previously been rendered euthyroid. Carbimazole is the antithyroid drug most often used in the UK, and propylthiouracil is also used.

A18.5

B

The primary treatment in papillary carcinoma of the thyroid is surgical, normally total or near-total thyroidectomy for local disease. Regional, or more extensive, neck dissection is needed where there is local nodal spread or involvement of local structures.

A18.6

C

An exaggerated adrenocorticotrophic hormone (ACTH) and cortisol response to exogenous corticotropin-releasing hormone (CRH) suggests pituitary-dependent Cushing's disease, as ectopic sources rarely respond.

Endocrine disease

A18.7

B

Hypocalcaemia may be due to deficiencies of calcium homeostatic mechanisms, secondary to high phosphate levels or other causes of hypocalcaemia. All forms of hypoparathyroidism, except transient surgical effects, are uncommon. Renal failure is the most common cause of hypocalcaemia. Hypocalcaemia after thyroid or parathyroid surgery is common but usually transient – fewer than 1% of thyroidectomies leave permanent damage. Idiopathic hypoparathyroidism is one of the rarer autoimmune disorders, often accompanied by vitiligo, cutaneous moniliasis and other autoimmune disease. The DiGeorge syndrome is a familial condition where the hypoparathyroidism is associated with intellectual impairment, cataracts and calcified basal ganglia, and occasionally with specific autoimmune disease. Pseudo-hypoparathyroidism is a syndrome of end-organ resistance to parathyroid hormone (PTH) owing to a mutation in the $G_{s\alpha}$-protein which is coupled to the PTH receptor. It is associated with short stature, short metacarpals, subcutaneous calcification and sometimes by intellectual impairment. Variable degrees of resistance involving other G-protein-linked hormone receptors may also be seen (thyroid-stimulating hormone, luteinizing hormone, follicle-stimulating hormone). Pseudo-pseudo-hypoparathyroidism describes the phenotypic defects but without any abnormalities of calcium metabolism. These individuals may share the same gene defect as pseudo-hypoparathyroidism and occur in the same families.

A18.8

D

Hirsutism developing before puberty is suggestive of congenital adrenal hyperplasia. Biochemistry reveals increased 17-hydroxyprogesterone levels, increased urinary pregnanetriol excretion and raised basal adrenocorticotrophic hormone levels.

A18.9

A

In normal subjects, plasma osmolality remains normal while urine osmolality rises above 700 mOsm/kg. In diabetes insipidus (DI), plasma osmolality rises while the urine remains dilute, only concentrating after exogenous vasopressin is given (in 'cranial' DI) or not concentrating after vasopressin if nephrogenic DI is present. This test can give equivocal results and measurement of vasopressin during the test is helpful.

A18.10

E

Atrophic (autoimmune) hypothyroidism is the most common cause of hypothyroidism and is associated with antithyroid autoantibodies leading to lymphoid infiltration of the gland and eventual atrophy and fibrosis. It is six times more common in females and the incidence increases with age. The condition is associated with other autoimmune disease such as pernicious anaemia, vitiligo and other endocrine deficiencies.

A18.11

C

17-α-Hydroxyprogesterone is elevated in classical congenital adrenal hyperplasia (CAH).

A18.12

C

Definitive therapy will depend upon the size of the tumour, the patient's wishes, including desire for fertility, and local expertise and facilities. In most cases a dopamine agonist will be the first, and usually only, therapy. Prolactinomas usually shrink in size on a dopamine agonist; in macroadenomas any pituitary mass effects commonly resolve and in most cases it is simply sufficient to continue successful dopamine agonist therapy in the long term. Prolactin should therefore always be measured before surgery on a pituitary mass. Microprolactinomas may not recur after several years of dopamine agonist therapy in a substantial minority of cases, but in the majority hyperprolactinaemia will recur if treatment is stopped.

A18.13

B

Trans-sphenoidal surgery is generally agreed to be the appropriate first-line therapy for acromegalic pituitary tumours. It will result in clinical remission in a majority of cases (60–80%) with pituitary microadenoma, but in only 50% of those with macroadenoma. Transfrontal surgery is rarely required except for massive macroadenomas.

A18.14

1) C   2) C   3) C   4) C   5) B
6) B   7) B   8) A   9) A

Common 'second messengers' involved in these cascades include: cyclic AMP (for adrenocorticotrophic hormone (ACTH), luteinizing hormone (LH), follicle-stimulating hormone (FSH) and parathyroid hormone (PTH)); a calcium-phospholipid system (for thyrotrophin-releasing hormone (TRH), vasopressin and angiotensin II); tyrosine kinase and other intracellular kinases (for insulin and insulin-like growth factor-1 (IGF-1)) and membrane-bound phosphoinositide pathways.

A18.15

1) E   2) F   3) C   4) B   5) A   6) D

Drugs and endocrine disease

Drug*	Effect
Drugs inducing endocrine disease	
Chlorpromazine	
Metoclopramide (dopamine agonists)	Increase prolactin, causing galactorrhoea
Oestrogens	
Iodine	
Amiodarone	Hyperthyroidism
Lithium	
Amiodarone	Hypothyroidism
Chlorpropamide	Inappropriate ADH secretion
Ketoconazole	
Metyrapone, aminoglutethimide	Hypoadrenalism
Drugs simulating endocrine disease	
Sympathomimetics	
Amfetamines	Mimic thyrotoxicosis or phaeochromocytoma
Liquorice	
Carbenoxolone	Increase mineralocorticoid activity; mimic aldosteronism
Purgatives	Hypokalaemia
Diuretics	Secondary aldosteronism
ACE inhibitors	Hypoaldosteronism
Drugs affecting hormone binding proteins	
Anticonvulsants	Bind to TBG – decrease total T_4
Oestrogens	Raise TBG and CBG – increase total T_4/cortisol
Exogenous hormones or stimulating agents	
Use, abuse or misuse, by patient or doctor, of the following:	
Steroids	Cushing's syndrome
	Diabetes
Thyroxine	Thyrotoxicosis factitia
Vitamin D preparations	
Milk and alkali preparations	Hypercalcaemia
Insulin	
Sulphonylureas	Hypoglycaemia

*Drugs causing gynaecomastia are listed in Table 18.15 of Kumar & Clark, 5th edition, 2002.
Amiodarone may cause both hypo- or hyperthyroidism
ADH, antidiuretic hormone; TBG, thyroxine-binding globulin; CBG, corticosteroid-binding globulin

A18.16

1) F 2) D 3) F 4) D 5) D
6) C 7) B 8) A

Luteinizing hormone (LH) stimulates testosterone production from Leydig cells of the testis. Follicle-stimulating hormone (FSH) stimulates the Sertoli cells in the seminiferous tubules to produce mature sperm and the inhibins A and B. Inhibin causes feedback on the pituitary to decrease FSH secretion. LH stimulates ovarian androgen production by the ovarian theca cells. FSH stimulates follicular development and aromatase activity (an enzyme required to convert ovarian androgens to oestrogens) in the ovarian granulosa cells. FSH also stimulates release of inhibin from ovarian stromal cells which inhibits FSH release. Oestrogen initially and then progesterone cause uterine endometrial proliferation in preparation for possible implantation. If implantation and pregnancy follow, human chorionic gonadotrophin (HCG) production from the corpus luteum maintains corpus luteum function until 10–12 weeks of gestation, by which time the placenta will be making sufficient oestrogen and progesterone to support itself.

A18.17

1) B 2) C 3) D 4) F 5) E
6) H 7) G

Forbes–Albright syndrome usually occurs in girls, and manifestations include precocity, polyostotic fibrous dysplasia and skin pigmentation (café-au-lait).

Premature thelarche is early breast development alone, usually transient, at age 2–4 years. It may regress or persist until puberty. There is no evidence of follicular development. Premature adrenarche is early development of pubic hair without significant other changes, usually after age 5 years and most commonly in girls. Klinefelter's syndrome (seminiferous tubule dysgenesis), a chromosomal disorder (47XXY) affecting 1 in 1000 males, involves both loss of Leydig cells and seminiferous tubular dysgenesis. Patients usually present with poor sexual development, small or undescended testes, gynaecomastia or infertility. They are occasionally mentally retarded. Clinical examination shows small pea-size but firm testes, usually gynaecomastia and often signs of androgen deficiency. Confirmation is by chromosomal analysis. Kallman's syndrome is due to isolated GnRH deficiency. It is often associated with decreased or absent sense of smell (anosmia), and sometimes with other bony (cleft-palate), renal and cerebral abnormalities (e.g. colour blindness). It is often familial and is usually X-linked; one sex-linked form is due to an abnormality of a cell adhesion molecule. Turner's syndrome is seen with women with 45X chromosome. Typically these patients have short stature, a web neck, coarctation of the aorta and streak gonads. 5α-reductase deficiency is seen in males with a normal chromosomal pattern. There is impaired conversion of testosterone to dihydrotestosterone and the patient may have ambiguous genitalia or is cryptorchid or both.

A18.18

1) E   2) B   3) D   4) C   5) A

Characteristics of thyroid function tests in common thyroid disorders (the clinically most informative tests in each situation are shown in bold)				
	TSH (0.3–3.5 mU/L)	Total T$_4$ (60–160 mmol/L)	Free T$_4$ (10–25 pmol/L)	T$_3$ (1.2–3.1 nmol/L)
Thyrotoxicosis	**Suppressed (< 0.05 mU/L)**	Increased	**Increased**	Increased
Primary hypothyroidism	**Increased (> 10 mU/L)**	Low/low-normal	Low/low-normal	Normal or low
TSH deficiency	Low-normal or subnormal	Low/low-normal	**Low/low-normal**	Normal or low
T$_3$ toxicosis	Suppressed (< 0.05 mU/L)	Normal	Normal	**Increased**
Compensated euthyroidism	**Slightly increased (5–10 mU/L)**	Normal	**Normal**	Normal

A18.19

A) T   B) F   C) F   D) T   E) T   F) F

The 'negative feedback' system, referring to the effect of T$_3$ and T$_4$ on the pituitary and hypothalamus, represents the most common mechanism for regulation of circulating hormone levels. The secretion of the gonadotrophins, luteinizing hormone (LH) and follicle-stimulating hormone (FSH), is normally pulsatile, with major pulses released every 1–2 hours depending on the phase of the menstrual cycle. Secretion of growth hormone (GH) and prolactin is increased during sleep, especially the rapid eye movement (REM) phase. The posterior pituitary acts merely as a storage organ. Antidiuretic hormone (ADH, vasopressin) and oxytocin, both nonapeptides, are synthesized in the supraoptic and paraventricular nuclei in the anterior hypothalamus. They are then transported along the axon and stored in the posterior pituitary. Growth hormone release is stimulated by growth hormone-releasing hormone (GHRH) but inhibited by somatostatin (growth hormone release inhibitory hormone, GHRIH). Thyroid-stimulating hormone (TSH) release is stimulated by TRH but partially inhibited by somatostatin.

A18.20

A) T   B) T   C) T   D) F   E) T   F) T

Causes of gynaecomastia	
Physiological	**Drugs**
Neonatal	Oestrogenic
Pubertal	oestrogens
Old age	digitalis
Hyperthyroidism	cannabis
Liver disease	diamorphine
Oestrogen-producing	Anti-androgens
tumours (testis,	spironolactone
adrenal)	cimetidine
HCG-producing	cyproterone
tumours	Others
(testis, lung)	gonadotrophins
Starvation/refeeding	cytotoxics
Carcinoma of breast	

A18.21

A) T B) T C) T D) T E) F

Polycystic ovary syndrome (PCOS), originally known in its severe form as the Stein–Leventhal syndrome, is characterized by multiple small cysts within the ovary and by excess androgen production from the ovaries and to a lesser extent from the adrenals, although whether the basic defect is in the ovary, adrenal or pituitary remains unknown. The precise levels of androgens in blood vary widely from patient to patient. Oestrogens are used to treat hirsutism. Oestrogens (e.g. oral contraceptives) suppress ovarian androgen production and reduce free androgens by increasing sex hormone binding globulin (SHBG) levels. Combined pills, which contain a non-androgenic progestogen (e.g. Dianette or Marvelon), have an advantage over older combined pills, will result in a slow improvement in hirsutism in a majority of cases and should normally be used first unless there is a contraindication. Spironolactone (200 mg daily) also has antiandrogen activity and can cause useful improvements in hirsutism in selected cases. Finasteride (5 mg daily), a 5-alpha-reductase inhibitor which prevents the formation of dihydrotestosterone in the skin, has also been shown to be effective in hirsutism but long-term experience is still awaited.

A18.22

A) T B) T C) T D) T E) T

Hyperprolactinaemia has many causes. Common pathological causes include prolactinoma, co-secretion of prolactin in acromegaly, stalk compression due to pituitary adenomas and other pituitary masses, polycystic ovary syndrome, hypothyroidism and 'idiopathic' hyperprolactinaemia; rarer causes are oestrogen therapy (e.g. the oral contraceptive pill), renal failure, liver failure, postictal and chest wall injury. Dopamine antagonist drugs are a common iatrogenic cause (metoclopramide, domperidone and most other antiemetics except cyclizine, opiates). Physiological hyperprolactinaemia occurs in pregnancy, lactation and severe stress, as well as during sleep and coitus.

A18.23

A) F B) T C) T D) F E) T

Up to 8 weeks of gestation the sexes share a common development, with a primitive genital tract including the Wolffian and Müllerian ducts. There are additionally a primitive perineum and primitive gonads. In the presence of a Y chromosome the potential testis develops while the ovary regresses. In the absence of a Y chromosome, the potential ovary develops and related ducts form a uterus and the upper vagina. Production of Müllerian inhibitory factor from the early 'testis' produces atrophy of the Müllerian duct, while, under the influence of testosterone and dihydrotestosterone, the Wolffian duct differentiates into an epididymis, vas deferens, seminal vesicles and prostate.

Endocrine disease

A18.24

A) F   B) T   C) T   D) T   E) T

In Addison's disease single cortisol measurements are of little value, although a random cortisol below 100 nmol/L during the day is highly suggestive, and a random cortisol >550 nmol/L makes the diagnosis unlikely (but not impossible). Electrolytes and urea classically show hyponatraemia, hyperkalaemia and a high urea, but they can be normal. Serum aldosterone is reduced with high plasma renin activity. Hypercalcaemia and anaemia (after rehydration) are sometimes seen. They resolve on treatment, but are occasionally the first clue to the diagnosis.

A18.25

A) T   B) T   C) F   D) T   E) F

Severe hypercalcaemia (>3 mmol/L) is usually associated with malignant disease, hyperparathyroidism or vitamin D therapy. It is very occasionally seen in end-stage renal failure as a result of tertiary hyperparathyroidism.

A18.26

A) T   B) T   C) T   D) T   E) T

Common causes of the syndrome of inappropriate ADH secretion (SIADH)

Tumours	Metabolic causes
Small-cell carcinoma of lung	Alcohol withdrawal
Prostate	Porphyria
Thymus	**Drugs**
Pancreas	Chlorpropamide
Lymphomas	Carbamazepine
	Cyclophosphamide
Pulmonary lesions	Vincristine
Pneumonia	Phenothiazines
Tuberculosis	
Lung abscess	

CNS causes
Meningitis
Tumours
Head injury
Subdural haematoma
Cerebral abscess
SLE vasculitis

Q19.1

The glucose uptake in this organ is obligatory and is not dependent on insulin. It is a major consumer of glucose and its requirement is 1 mg/kg bodyweight per minute or 100 g daily in a 70 kg man.

A. Liver
B. Muscle
C. Fat
D. Kidney
E. Brain

Q19.2

The process by which liver combines 3-carbon molecules derived from breakdown of fat (glycerol), muscle glycogen (lactate) and protein (e.g. alanine) into the 6-carbon glucose molecule

A. Glycogenolysis
B. Lipolysis
C. Glycolysis
D. Gluconeogenesis
E. Triglyceride synthesis

Q19.3

A middle-aged alcoholic man presents with a bullous eruption. He has a family history of porphyria. Urine examination reveals increased levels of urinary uroporphyrin. This is due to an abnormality of which one of the following?

A. Protoporphyrinogen oxidase
B. Hepatic uroporphyrinogen decarboxylase
C. Porphobilinogen deaminase
D. δ-ALA synthetase
E. Haemoglobin oxidase

Q19.4

A 32-year-old woman has a history of depression. After an alcoholic binge she develops abdominal pain, nausea and vomiting. On examination she has hypertension, tachycardia and polyneuropathy. Urinary examination reveals excess porphobilinogen. This is due to an abnormality in which one of the following enzymes?

A. Protoporphyrinogen oxidase
B. Hepatic uroporphyrinogen oxidase
C. Porphobilinogen deaminase
D. Delta ALA synthetase
E. Haemoglobin oxidase

Diabetes mellitus and other disorders of metabolism

Q19.5

A 28-year-old insulin-dependent diabetic is found unconscious, at home, by his wife. She calls for an ambulance but in the interim she uses his bedside blood test and finds that his blood sugars are extremely low. Select the best option for what she can administer next

A. Intravenous 5% glucose
B. Intramuscular glucagon
C. Intravenous 50% glucose
D. Oral glucose
E. Oral Lucozade

Q19.6

A 35-year-old Jewish patient complains of pain in the left hypochondrium. On examination he has pigmentation in sun-exposed areas of his skin and hepatosplenomegaly including a massive spleen. Lab investigations include anaemia and hypersplenism. There is also a history of repeated fractures of the bone. Which one of the following deficiencies is responsible for this clinical picture?

A. Cystathione synthetase
B. Phosphorylase
C. Phenylalanine hydroxylase
D. Homogentisic acid oxidase
E. Glucocerebrosidase

Q19.7

A 65-year-old diabetic patient presents in a coma. Na 155 mmol/L, K 5 mmol/L, Cl 110 mmol/L, HCO_3 30 mmol/L, urea 15 mmol/L, glucose 50 mmol/L and arterial pH 7.35. His calculated plasma osmolality is

A. 300 mOsm/kg
B. 328 mOsm/kg
C. 385 mOsm/kg
D. 350 mOsm/kg
E. 285 mOsm/Kg

Q19.8

A 22-year-old presents with a coma. His labs are as follows: Na 140 mmol/L, K 5 mmol/L, Cl 100 mmol/L, HCO_3 5 mmol/L, urea 8 mmol/L, arterial pH 7.0 and blood glucose 30 mmol/L. The anion gap is

A. 17
B. 40
C. 20
D. 30
E. Less than 17

Q19.9

A 57-year-old diabetic patient on metformin presents in a coma. Blood glucose is 9 mmol/L, Na 140 mmol/L, K 5 mmol/L, Cl 100 mmol/L, HCO_3 5 mmol/L. There is no ketosis. Which one of the following is the best option for treatment?

A. Intravenous insulin and 5% dextrose
B. Rehydration and infusion of 1.26% bicarbonate
C. Ion exchange resin
D. Salbutamol
E. Hypertonic saline

Q19.10

A 38-year-old patient has incomplete erection secondary to longstanding diabetes. There is no history of angina and no previous myocardial infarction. The best option for treatment is which one of the following?

A. Insertion of alprostadil into the urethra
B. Intravcavernosal injection of alprostadil
C. Papaverine
D. Moxisylyte (thymoxamine)
E. Sildenafil citrate

Q19.11

After the diagnosis of diabetes, the earliest functional abnormality in diabetic nephropathy is

A. Decreased glomerular filtration rate
B. Rising plasma creatinine
C. Decrease in the size of the kidney with a decreased glomerular filtration rate
D. Persistent proteinuria
E. Renal hypertrophy associated with a raised glomerular filtration rate

Q19.12

1. Enables basal non-insulin-stimulated glucose uptake into many cells
2. Transports glucose into the beta-cell: a prerequisite for glucose sensing
3. Enables non-insulin-mediated glucose uptake into brain neurones
4. Enables much of the peripheral action of insulin. It is the channel through which glucose is taken up into muscle and adipose tissue cells following stimulation of the insulin receptor

Select the best match for each of the above among a family of specialized glucose-transporter (GLUT) proteins

A. GLUT-2
B. GLUT-1
C. GLUT-3
D. GLUT-4

2. A 23-year-old patient has had maturity-onset diabetes from birth. She had a low birthweight. There has been little deterioration of hyperglycaemia with age. Microvascular complications are rare. It has been localized to the small arm of chromosome 7

3. A 22-year-old patient was diagnosed with maturity-onset diabetes 3 years ago. Hyperglycaemia is progressive and microvascular complications are frequent. It is localized to the long arm of chromosome 12

4. A 22-year-old patient has maturity-onset diabetes but progression is unclear. There are few data about microvascular complications. There is pancreatic agenesis in homozygotes. It is localized to the long arm of chromosome 13

5. A 24-year-old patient has maturity-onset diabetes but progression is unclear. There are few data about microvascular complications. Other features include renal cysts, proteinuria and renal failure. It is localized to the long arm of chromosome 17

Select the best match for each of the above

A. Hepatic nuclear factor-4a
B. Glucokinase
C. Hepatic nuclear factor-1b
D. Hepatic nuclear factor-1a
E. Insulin-promoter factor-1

Q19.13

1. A 19-year-old boy was diagnosed with maturity-onset diabetes a year ago. The hyperglycaemia is progressive, microvascular complications are frequent and there are no non-diabetes related features. It has been localized to the long arm of chromosome 20

Q19.14

1. Tolbutamide
2. Acarbose
3. Glibenclamide
4. Rosiglitazone
5. Gliclazide
6. Metformin

Diabetes mellitus and other disorders of metabolism

Select the mechanism of action of each of the above

A. α-Glucosidase inhibitor

B. Reduces insulin resistance by interaction with peroxisome proliferator-activated receptor gamma

C. Reduces gluconeogenesis, thus suppressing hepatic glucose output, and it increases insulin sensitivity

D. Promotes insulin secretion in response to glucose and other secretagogues

Q19.15

1. An 83-year-old diabetic

2. A 65-year-old diabetic whose body mass index is 45

3. A 35-year-old patient with diabetic ketoacidosis

4. A 45-year-old diabetic whose body mass index is 22 and who has renal impairment

5. A 60-year-old diabetic who has been adhering to diet and oral therapy and now has HbA_{1c} 11%

Select the best option for each of the above

A. Insulin

B. Metformin

C. Tolbutamide

D. Gliclazide

E. Glibenclamide

Q19.16

1. An 18 year-old diabetic whose blood glucose before breakfast is persistently too high

2. A 23-year-old diabetic whose blood glucose before lunch is persistently too high

3. A 21-year-old diabetic whose blood glucose before lunch is persistently too low

4. A 24-year-old diabetic whose blood glucose before the evening meal is persistently too high

5. A 29-year-old diabetic whose blood glucose before going to bed is persistently too low

Select the best option for each of the above

A. Increase morning long-acting insulin or lunch short-acting insulin

B. Reduce evening short-acting insulin

C. Increase morning short-acting insulin

D. Reduce morning short-acting insulin or increase mid-morning snack

E. Increase evening long-acting insulin

F. Reduce evening long-acting insulin

Q19.17

1. Coronary artery disease

2. Peripheral vascular disease

3. Stroke

4. Diabetic retinopathy

5. Diabetic nephropathy

6. Diabetic neuropathy

Select the best match for each of the above complications of diabetes mellitus

A. Microvascular disease

B. Macrovascular disease

Q19.18

1. A 57-year-old diabetic on fundoscopy has dot haemorrhages, blot haemorrhages and hard exudates

2. A 38-year-old diabetic has cotton-wool spots, venous beading, venous loops and intraretinal microvascular abnormalities

3. A 48-year-old diabetic has new blood vessels, subhyaloid haemorrhages and vitreous haemorrhage

4. A 49-year-old diabetic has retinal fibrosis and traction retinal detachment

5. A 38-year-old diabetic has hard exudates encroaching on the macula

Select the best match for each of the above

A. Non-urgent referral to the ophthalmologist
B. Urgent referral to the ophthalmologist
C. Annual screening only

Q 19.19

1. A 49-year-old diabetic has dot haemorrhages
2. A 67-year-old diabetic has blot haemorrhages
3. A 57-year-old diabetic has hard exudates
4. A 43-year-old diabetic has cotton-wool spots

Select the best match for each of the above

A. Exudation of fluid rich in lipids and proteins
B. Leakage of blood into the deeper layers of retina
C. Capillary microaneurysms
D. Oedema resulting from retinal infarcts
E. New vessel formation

Q 19.20

1. Colestyramine
2. Gemfibrozil
3. Simvastatin
4. Nicotinic acid
5. Omega-3 marine triglycerides

Select the mechanism of action of each of the above

A. Limits substrate availability for hepatic triglyceride synthesis, modulates LDL/ligand interaction, promotes action of lipoprotein lipase and stimulates reverse transport of cholesterol

B. Reduces hepatic VLDL secretion
C. Binds bile acids in the gut preventing enterohepatic circulation
D. Inhibits the rate-limiting step in the synthesis of cholesterol
E. Inhibits lipid synthesis in the liver by reducing free fatty acid concentrations owing to an inhibitory effect on lipolysis in fat tissue

Q 19.21

1. Colestyramine
2. Gemfibrozil
3. Simvastatin
4. Nicotinic acid
5. Omega-3 marine triglycerides

Select the expected lipid lowering effect of each of the above

A. 30–40% reduction in LDL cholesterol, little effect on triglycerides or HDL
B. Reduction of LDL by 10–15% and triglycerides by 25–35%, HDL concentrations increase by 0–15%
C. Reduce LDL and triglycerides by 5–10%, modest HDL increase
D. Reduces triglycerides in severe hypertriglyceridaemia, no favourable change in other lipids and may aggravate hypercholesterolaemia in a few patients
E. 8–15% reduction in LDL, little or no effect on HDL cholesterol and 5–15% rise in triglyceride concentration

Q 19.22

1. A middle-aged adult who develops muscle cramps and myoglobinuria after exercise
2. A 23-year-old patient with Marfan-like features, mental handicap and homocystine is excreted in urine

3. A 22-year-old patient with whitish hair, pink-white skin, grey-blue eyes, nystagmus, photophobia and strabismus

4. A 19-year-old patient with brain damage, mental retardation and epilepsy. Phenolpyruvate and its derivatives are excreted in urine

5. A 24-year-old patient with deposition of blackish-brown pigment in cartilages

Select the enzyme defect for each of the above

A. Cystathionine synthetase
B. Phosphorylase
C. Phenylalanine hydroxylase
D. Homogentisic acid oxidase
E. Tyrosinase

Q19.23

1. A 62-year-old woman with multiple myeloma presents with shortness of breath. Echocardiography shows thickening of the ventricular walls and low voltage complexes are seen on the ECG

2. A 42-year-old man has a family history of amyloidosis and he presents with peripheral sensorimotor neuropathy

3. A 63-year-old woman with longstanding rheumatoid arthritis presents with proteinuria. Renal biopsy reveals amyloidosis

4. A 43-year-old patient with Down's syndrome has longstanding premature dementia

5. A patient with chronic renal failure on long-term haemodialysis develops carpal tunnel syndrome due to deposition of amyloid

Select the best match for each of the above

A. AA amyloidosis
B. β_2-Microglobulin
C. Deposits of A4 protein
D. Immunoglobulin light chain-associated (AL) amyloid
E. Transthyretin-associated (ATTR) protein

Q19.24

The following patients are diabetic according to the World Health Organization diagnostic criteria of 1999

A. An 18-year-old girl who has thirst, polyuria and polydipsia. Glycosuria is present and a single plasma glucose is 7 mmol/L (126 mg/dL)

B. A 19-year-old army recruit who has no symptoms undergoes routine screening tests. Fasting venous plasma glucose on two different occasions is 8 mmol/L (140 mg/dL) and 7.9 mmol/L (135 mg/dL)

C. An asymptomatic pilot of a commercial airline as a part of an annual examination has two random venous samples where plasma glucose is 11.2 mmol/L and 11.1 mmol/L (200 mg/dL and 210 mg/dL)

D. A 28-year-old man whose fasting venous plasma glucose is 6 mmol/L and level 2 h after 75 g glucose is load is 10 mmol/L

E. A 23-year-old woman who is 6 months pregnant. Fasting venous plasma glucose is 7.1 mmol/L and levels 2 h after 75 g glucose load is 12 mol/L

Q19.25

A 35-year-old diabetic (compared to the general population) is

A. Twice as likely to have a stroke
B. Three to five times as likely to have myocardial infarction
C. Fifty times as likely to have amputation of the foot for gangrene
D. Likely to lose her premenopausal protection from coronary artery disease
E. At risk of excess mortality from diabetic nephropathy rather than cardiovascular disease

Q19.26

A 26-year-old diabetic on twice-daily mixed insulin has nocturnal hypoglycaemia but awakes with high blood glucose. The problem may be helped by

A. Injecting more insulin at night
B. Checking that a bedtime snack is taken regularly
C. Separating the evening dose and taking the intermediate insulin at bedtime rather than before supper
D. Reducing the dose of soluble insulin before supper
E. Changing the multiple injection regimen with soluble insulin to a rapid-acting insulin analogue

Q19.27

Intensive control of blood sugar in type 2 diabetes results in

A. A reduction in overall risk of microvascular disease but causes a deterioration in albuminuria
B. A reduction in the need for laser treatment but exacerbates microvascular disease

C. A reduction in albuminuria
D. A reduction in cardiovascular risk
E. An increase in the level of glycosylated haemoglobin

Q19.28

An 18-year-old insulin-dependent diabetic wishes to work. He can pursue the following occupations

A. Taxi driver
B. Heavy goods vehicle driver
C. Commercial pilot
D. Nurse
E. Police constable

Q19.29

A 17-year-old insulin-dependent diabetic presents with nausea, vomiting and abdominal pain. He is confused, hyperventilating and is dehydrated. Initial blood tests reveal Na 140 mmol/L, K 5 mmol/L, Cl 100 mmol/L, HCO_3 5 mmol/L, urea 8 mmol/L, arterial pH 7.0 and blood glucose 30 mmol/L. The following processes could have contributed to his clinical condition

A. Accelerated production of hepatic glucose
B. Reduction in peripheral uptake of glucose
C. Osmotic diuresis
D. Rapid lipolysis
E. Breakdown of free fatty acids to fatty acyl-CoA

Diabetes mellitus and other disorders of metabolism

Q19.30

A 45-year-old diabetic has retinopathy and renal failure due to nephropathy. The following plans for further management are correct

A. Aggressive treatment of blood pressure with a target below 135/85 mmHg
B. Aggressive management of blood sugar with chlorpropamide or glibenclamide
C. Drastic increases in insulin doses may be required
D. Frequent ophthalmologist supervision
E. Long-term antibiotic treatment to prevent infections

Q19.31

A 52-year-old diabetic seeks advice on foot care. The following advice is appropriate

A. Inspect feet daily
B. Check shoes inside and out for sharp bodies/areas before wearing
C. Use lace-up shoes with plenty of room for the toes
D. Keep feet away from sources of heat (hot sand, hot-water bottles, radiators, fires)
E. Check the bath temperature before stepping in

Q19.32

A 45-year-old insulin-dependent diabetic is undergoing amputation of her right leg. The following statements are correct

A. Long-acting insulin should be continued and in addition soluble insulin should be initiated
B. Long-acting insulin should be stopped the day before surgery and soluble insulin should be substituted
C. An infusion of glucose, insulin and potassium is given during surgery

D. Preferably diabetic patients should be at the end of the theatre list
E. Postoperatively the patient should be given an infusion of glucose, insulin and potassium until she is able to eat

Q19.33

A 22-year-old diabetic is pregnant and her HbA_{1c} is around 12 throughout her pregnancy. There is an increased risk of

A. Stillbirth
B. Fetal macrosomia
C. Hydramnios
D. Pre-eclampsia
E. Gestational diabetes

Q19.34

A 23-year-old diabetic has recurrent ketoacidosis. The following could have resulted in unstable glycaemic control

A. Poorly controlled hypertension
B. Thyrotoxicosis
C. Urinary tract infection
D. Hypogonadism
E. Tuberculosis

Q19.35

A 42-year-old nurse presents with confusion, diplopia, palpitations and grand mal seizures. Her blood glucose is low and her symptoms respond to 50% dextrose. After an overnight fast she has low glucose and elevated insulin levels. The following tests would rule out factitious hypoglycaemia

A. A prolonged 72-hour supervised fast
B. Measurement of C-peptide levels
C. Plasma chromatography for sulphonylurea
D. Fructose tolerance test
E. Glucose tolerance test

A19.1

E

The brain is the major consumer of glucose. Its requirement is 1 mg/kg bodyweight per minute, or 100 g daily in a 70 kg man. Glucose uptake by the brain is obligatory and is not dependent on insulin, and the glucose used is oxidized to carbon dioxide and water. Other tissues, such as muscle and fat, are facultative glucose consumers.

A19.2

D

The liver combines 3-carbon molecules derived from breakdown of fat (glycerol), muscle glycogen (lactate) and protein (e.g. alanine) into the 6-carbon glucose molecule by the process of gluconeogenesis.

A19.3

B

Porphyria cutanea tarda (cutaneous hepatic porphyria), which has a genetic predisposition, presents with a bullous eruption on exposure to sunlight; the eruption heals with scarring. Alcohol is the most common aetiological agent. There is an abnormality in hepatic uroporphyrinogen decarboxylase. Evidence of biochemical or clinical liver disease may also be present.

A19.4

C

Acute intermittent porphyria is an autosomal dominant disorder. Presentation is in early adult life, usually around the age of 30 years, and women

are affected more than men. It may be precipitated by alcohol and drugs such as barbiturates and oral contraceptives, but a wide range of lipid-soluble drugs have also been incriminated. The abnormality lies at the level of porphobilinogen deaminase in the haem biosynthetic pathway.

A19.5

B

The diagnosis of severe hypoglycaemia resulting in confusion or coma is simple and can usually be made on clinical grounds, backed by a bedside blood test. Unconscious patients should be given intramuscular glucagon (1 mg). Glucagon acts by mobilizing hepatic glycogen, and works almost as rapidly as glucose. It is simple to administer and can be given at home by relatives. It does not work after a prolonged fast. Oral glucose is given to replenish glycogen reserves once the patient revives.

A19.6

E

Gaucher's disease is the most prevalent lysosomal storage disease and is due to a deficiency in glucocerebrosidase, a specialized lysosomal acid β-glucosidase. This results in accumulation of glucosylceramide in the lysosomes of the reticuloendothelial system, particularly the liver, bone marrow and spleen. Several mutations have been characterized in the glucocerebrosidase gene, the most common being a single base change causing the substitution of arginine for serine; this is seen in 70% of Jewish patients. The typical Gaucher cell, a glucocerebroside-containing reticuloendothelial histiocyte, is found in the bone marrow. There are three clinical

Diabetes mellitus and other disorders of metabolism

types, the most common presenting in adult life with an insidious onset of hepatosplenomegaly. There is a high incidence in Ashkenazi Jews (1 in 3000 births), and patients have a characteristic pigmentation on exposed parts, particularly the forehead and hands. The clinical spectrum is variable, with patients developing anaemia, evidence of hypersplenism and pathological fractures that are due to bone involvement. Nevertheless, many have a normal life span.

A19.7

C

Osmolality is calculated from the formula $2(Na + K) + glucose + urea$. Therefore, $2(155+5) + 50 + 15 = 385$ mOsm/kg.

A19.8

B

The normal anion gap is less than 17. It is calculated as $(Na^+ + K^+) - (Cl^- + HCO_3^-)$. The anion gap in the above example is 40.

A19.9

B

Lactic acidosis may occur in diabetic patients on biguanide therapy. The risk in patients taking metformin is extremely low provided that the therapeutic dose is not exceeded and the drug is withheld in patients with advanced hepatic or renal dysfunction. Patients present in severe metabolic acidosis with a large anion gap (calculated as $(Na^+ + K^+) - (Cl^- + HCO_3^-)$, normally less than 17 mmol/L), usually without significant hyperglycaemia or ketosis. Treatment is by rehydration and infusion of isotonic 1.26% bicarbonate.

A19.10

E

A therapeutic trial of sildenafil citrate, a phosphodiesterase type-5 inhibitor, which enhances the effects of nitric oxide on smooth muscle and increases penile blood flow, is warranted in most impotent diabetic patients who do not suffer from angina or previous myocardial infarction (contraindications). Patients can be trained by a clinician or impotence nurse specialist in the intracavernosal injection of alprostadil to cause erection. Papaverine (smooth muscle relaxant) and phentolamine and moxisylyte (thymoxamine) (alpha-adrenoceptor blockers) are sometimes also used.

A19.11

E

The earliest functional abnormality in the diabetic kidney is renal hypertrophy associated with a raised glomerular filtration rate. This appears soon after diagnosis and is related to poor glycaemic control.

A19.12

1) B   2) A   3) C   4) D

Cell membranes are not inherently permeable to glucose. A family of specialized glucose-transporter (GLUT) proteins carry glucose through the membrane into cells:

- GLUT-1 – enables basal non-insulin-stimulated glucose uptake into many cells

- GLUT-2 – transports glucose into the beta-cell: a prerequisite for glucose sensing

- GLUT-3 – enables non-insulin-mediated glucose uptake into brain neurones
- GLUT-4 – enables much of the peripheral action of insulin. It is the channel through which glucose is taken up into muscle and adipose tissue cells following stimulation of the insulin receptor.

A19.13

1) A   2) B   3) D   4) E   5) C

Maturity-onset diabetes of the young (MODY)					
	HNF-4a (MODY 1)	Glucokinase (MODY 2)	HNF-1a (MODY 3)	IPF-1 (MODY 4)	HNF-1b (MODY5)
Chromosomal location	20q	7p	12q	13q	17q
Proportion of all MODY cases	5%	15%	65%	<1% (MODY)	1%
Clinical features	Onset in teens/ twenties Progressive hyperglycaemia	Present from birth Little deterioration with age	Onset in teens/ twenties Progressive hyperglycaemia	?Early adulthood Progression unclear currently	?Early adulthood Progression unclear currently
Microvascular complications	Frequent	Rare	Frequent	Few data	Frequent
Non-diabetes-related features	None	Reduced birthweight	Low renal threshold for glucose and aminoaciduria	Pancreatic agenesis in homozygotes	Renal cysts Proteinuria Renal failure

The glucokinase gene is intimately involved in the glucose-sensing mechanism within the pancreatic beta-cell. The hepatic nuclear factor (HNF) genes and the insulin promoter factor-1 (IPF-1) gene control nuclear transcription in the beta-cell where they regulate its development and function. Abnormal nuclear transcription genes may cause pancreatic agenesis or more subtle progressive pancreatic damage

A19.14

1) D   2) A   3) D   4) B   5) D   6) C

The principal action of sulphonylureas is to promote insulin secretion in response to glucose and other secretagogues. The mechanism of action of metformin remains unclear but it reduces gluconeogenesis, thus suppressing hepatic glucose output, and it increases insulin sensitivity. Acarbose is a sham sugar that competitively inhibits alpha-glucosidase enzymes situated on the brush border of the intestine. As a result, dietary carbohydrate is poorly absorbed, and the postprandial rise in blood glucose is reduced. The thiazolidinediones (more conveniently known as the 'glitazones') reduce insulin resistance by interaction with peroxisome proliferator-activated receptor-gamma (PPAR-gamma) a nuclear receptor which regulates genes involved in lipid metabolism and insulin action.

Diabetes mellitus and other disorders of metabolism

A19.15

1) C   2) B   3) A   4) D   5) A

Tolbutamide is the safest drug in the very elderly because of its short duration of action. Gliclazide has a fairly long biological half life and is largely metabolized by the liver and can be used in renal impairment. Metformin is usually reserved for patients in middle or old age, particularly for the overweight since it does not promote weight gain. It may be given in combination with sulphonylureas when a single agent has proved to be ineffective. Insulin is useful in diabetic ketoacidosis and should be considered in patients with type 2 diabetes if oral hypoglycaemic agents fail to provide adequate control of blood glucose.

A19.16

1) E   2) C   3) D   4) A   5) B

Guide to adjusting insulin dosage according to blood glucose test results		
	Blood glucose persistently too high	Blood glucose persistently too low
Before breakfast	Increase evening long-acting insulin	Reduce evening long-acting insulin
Before lunch	Increase morning short-acting insulin	Reduce morning short-acting insulin or increase mid-morning snack
Before evening meal	Increase morning long-acting insulin or lunch short-acting insulin	Reduce morning long-acting insulin or lunch short-acting insulin or Increase mid-afternoon snack
Before bed	Increase evening short-acting insulin	Reduce evening short-acting insulin

A19.17

1) B   2) B   3) B   4) A   5) A   6) A

Diabetes is usually irreversible and, although patients can have a reasonably normal lifestyle, its late complications result in reduced life expectancy and major health costs. These include macrovascular disease, leading to an increased prevalence of coronary artery disease, peripheral vascular disease and stroke, and microvascular damage causing diabetic retinopathy and nephropathy, and contributing to diabetic neuropathy.

A19.18

1) C   2) A   3) B   4) B   5) A

	Fundoscopy/photography findings	Action needed
Background retinopathy	Microaneurysms (dot haemorrhages) Blot haemorrhages Hard exudates	Annual screening only
Pre-proliferative retinopathy	Cotton-wool spots Venous beading Venous loops Intraretinal microvascular abnormalities	Non-urgent referral to an ophthalmologist
Proliferative retinopathy	New blood vessel formation Preretinal (subhyaloid) haemorrhage Vitreous haemorrhage	Urgent referral to an ophthalmologist
Advanced retinopathy	Retinal fibrosis Traction retinal detachment	Urgent referral to an ophthalmologist – but much vision already lost

A19.19

1) C   2) B   3) A   4) D

In background retinopathy the first abnormality visible through the ophthalmoscope is the appearance of dot 'haemorrhages', which are actually due to capillary microaneurysms. Leakage of blood into the deeper layers of the retina produces the characteristic 'blot' haemorrhage, while exudation of fluid rich in lipids and protein give rise to hard exudates. These have a bright yellowish white colour and are often irregular in outline with a sharply defined margin. Progressive retinal ischaemia will, in some patients, cause background retinopathy to progress to pre-proliferative, sight-threatening retinopathy. The earliest sign is the appearance of 'cotton-wool spots', representing oedema resulting from retinal infarcts.

A19.20

1) C   2) A   3) D   4) E   5) B

Drugs used in the management of hyperlipidaemia	
Drug	Mechanism of action
Fibric acid derivatives e.g. Gemfibrozil Bezafibrate Fenofibrate Ciprofibrate	Complex and not fully understood 1. Limit substrate availability for hepatic triglyceride synthesis 2. Modulate LDL/ligand interaction 3. Promote action of lipoprotein lipase 4. Stimulate reverse transport of cholesterol
Cholesterol-binding resins e.g. Colestyramine Colestipol	Anion exchange resins Bind bile acids in the gut, preventing enterohepatic circulation This promotes liver to convert cholesterol to bile acids Also stimulates formation of hepatic LDL receptors which take up more cholesterol from the circulation
HMG-CoA reductase inhibitors ('statins') e.g. Simvastatin Pravastatin Atorvastatin Fluvastatin	Inhibit the rate-limiting step in cholesterol synthesis
Nicotinic acid and derivatives e.g. Nicotinic acid Acipimox	Unclear Probably inhibit lipid synthesis in the liver by reducing free fatty acid concentrations owing to an inhibitory effect on lipolysis in fat tissue
ω-3 marine triglycerides	Reduce hepatic VLDL secretion

VLDL, very low-density lipoprotein; LDL, low-density lipoprotein

A19.21

1) F   2) C   3) A   4) D   5) E

Drugs used in the management of hyperlipidaemia	
Drug	Expected lipid-lowering effect
Fibric acid derivatives e.g. Gemfibrozil Bezafibrate Fenofibrate Ciprofibrate	Reduction of LDL cholesterol by 10–15% and triglycerides by 25–35% HDL cholesterol concentrations increase by 0–15% (newer agents often have greater beneficial effect on HDL)
Cholesterol-binding resins e.g. Colestyramine Colestipol	8–15% reduction in LDL Little or no effect on HDL cholesterol 5–15% rise in triglyceride concentration
HMG-CoA reductase inhibitors ('statins') e.g. Simvastatin Pravastatin Atorvastatin Fluvastatin	30–40% reduction in LDL cholesterol Moderate reduction in triglycerides or moderate elevation of HDL cholesterol
Nicotinic acid and derivatives e.g. Nicotinic acid Acipimox	Reduce LDL and triglycerides by 5–10% Modest HDL increase
ω-3 marine triglycerides	Reduce triglycerides in severe hypertriglyceridaemia No favourable change in other lipids, and may aggravate hypercholesterolaemia in a few patients

LDL, low-density lipoprotein; HDL, high-density lipoprotein

A19.22

1) B   2) A   3) E   4) C   5) D

The first patient has type V glycogen storage disease and the defect is in muscle phosphorylase. Typically adults develop muscle cramps and myoglobinuria after exercise. These patients have a normal life span and should avoid exercise. The second patient has type 1 homocystinuria which is due to a defect in cystathionine synthetase. Features include Marfan-like features, mental defect, thrombotic episodes and homocystine is excreted in the urine. The third patient has albinism where the defect is in the enzyme tyrosinase. It is seen in 1 in 13 000 individuals and is characterized by amelanosis, whitish hair, pale-white skin and grey-blue eyes. The fourth patient has phenylketonuria where the effect is in the enzyme phenylalanine hydroxylase. The incidence is 1 in 20 000 and is characterized by brain damage with mental retardation and epilepsy. The urine contains phenylpyruvate and its derivatives. The treatment is a diet low in phenylalanine in the first few months of

Diabetes mellitus and other disorders of metabolism

life to prevent damage. The prognosis is good but there remains some intellectual impairment. The fifth patient has alkaptonuria due a defect in the enzyme homogentisic acid oxidase. The incidence is 1 in 100 000. In these patients homogentisic acid polymerizes to produce a black-brown product that is deposited in cartilage and other tissues (ochronosis). These patients do not require treatment and prognosis is good.

A19.23

1) D 2) E 3) A 4) C 5) B

AL amyloidosis is a plasma cell dyscrasia, related to multiple myeloma, in which clonal plasma cells in the bone marrow produce immunoglobulins that are amyloidogenic. Familial amyloidoses are autosomally dominant transmitted diseases where the mutant protein forms amyloid fibrils, starting usually in middle age. The most common form is due to a mutant – transthyretin – which is a tetrameric protein with four identical subunits. AA (reactive or secondary) amyloidosis depends on the nature of the disorder. Chronic inflammatory disorders include rheumatoid arthritis, inflammatory bowel disease, and untreated familial Mediterranean fever. In developing countries it is still associated with infectious diseases such as tuberculosis, bronchiectasis and osteomyelitis. Intracerebral and cerebrovascular amyloid deposits are seen in Alzheimer's disease. Amyloid deposits are frequently found in the elderly, particularly cerebral deposits of A4 protein. This is also seen in Down's syndrome.

Carpal tunnel syndrome due to β_2-microglobulin deposition as amyloid fibrils is seen in patients on long-term haemodialysis.

A19.24

A) F B) T C) T D) F E) T

The glucose tolerance test – WHO criteria			
	Normal	Impaired glucose tolerance	Diabetes mellitus
Fasting	Less than 7.0 mmol/L	Less than 7.0 mmol/L	More than 7.0 mmol/L
2 h after glucose	Less than 7.8 mmol/L	Between 7.8 and 11.0 mmol/L	11.1 mmol/L or more

The diagnosis of diabetes is usually simple. Blood glucose is so closely controlled by the body that even small deviations become important.

- In symptomatic patients, a single elevated plasma glucose ≥11 mmol/L, measured by a reliable method, indicates diabetes.

- In asymptomatic or mildly symptomatic patients, the diagnosis is made on:
  (a) two fasting venous plasma glucose levels above 7.0 mmol/L (126 mg/dL); OR
  (b) two random values ≥11.1 mmol/L (200 mg/dL) in venous plasma.
- A glucose tolerance test is only needed for borderline cases.

A19.25

A) T   B) T   C) T   D) T   E) F

Time has proved that insulin-treated patients still have a considerably reduced life expectancy. Those diagnosed before the age of 20 years in older studies had only a 50–60% chance of living past the age of 50 years, although there are indications of a steady improvement in survival. The excess deaths in early-onset patients are mainly related to diabetic nephropathy, but there is also a considerable excess cardiovascular mortality. Heart disease, peripheral vascular disease and stroke are the major causes of death in patients over the age of 50 years. The excess risk to diabetics compared with the general population increases as one moves down the body: a) stroke is twice as likely; b) myocardial infarction is 3–5 times as likely and women with diabetes lose their premenopausal protection from coronary artery disease; c) amputation of a foot for gangrene is 50 times as likely.

A19.26

A) F   B) T   C) T   D) T   E) T

Basal insulin requirements fall during the night but increase again from about 4 a.m. onwards, at a time when levels of injected insulin are falling. As a result many patients awake with high blood glucose levels, but find that injecting more insulin at night increases the risk of hypoglycaemia in the early hours of the morning. The problem may be helped by: a) checking that a bedtime snack is taken regularly; b) for patients taking twice-daily mixed insulin to separate their evening dose and take the intermediate insulin at bedtime rather than before supper; c) reducing the dose of soluble insulin before supper, since the effects of this persist well into the night; d) changing patients on a multiple injection regimen with soluble insulin to a rapid-acting insulin analogue. The new longer-acting insulin analogues with a flatter profile of action overnight may also prove of value.

A19.27

A) F   B) F   C) T   D) F   E) F

The UK Prospective Diabetic Study (UKPDS) compared standard and intensive treatment in a large prospective controlled trial of type 2 diabetes patients. There was a 25% overall reduction in microvascular disease end points, a 33% reduction in albuminuria and a 30% reduction in the need for laser treatment for retinopathy in the more intensively treated patients. There appeared to be little difference in outcome between the tools used to achieve good metabolic control (metformin, sulphonlyurea or insulin). A proportion of the total patients in the UKPDS were further randomized into standard and intensive blood pressure control groups. Cardiovascular risk was very considerably reduced in the intensive blood pressure treatment arm.

A19.28

A) F   B) F   C) F   D) T   E) F

On a practical level patients need to inform the driving and vehicle licensing authority and their insurance companies after diagnosis. They would also be wise to inform their family, friends and employers in case unexpected hypoglycaemia occurs. Insulin treatment can be undertaken by people in most walks of life; a few jobs are unsuitable. These include driving heavy goods or public service vehicles, working at heights, piloting aircraft or working close to dangerous machinery in motion.

Certain professions such as the police and the armed forces are barred to all diabetic patients.

A19.29

A) T B) T C) T D) T E) T

In the absence of insulin, hepatic glucose production accelerates, and peripheral uptake by tissues such as muscle is reduced. Rising glucose levels lead to an osmotic diuresis, loss of fluid and electrolytes, and dehydration. Plasma osmolality rises and renal perfusion falls. In parallel, rapid lipolysis occurs, leading to elevated circulating free fatty-acid levels. The free fatty acids are broken down to fatty acyl-CoA within the liver cells, and this in turn is converted to ketone bodies within the mitochondria. Accumulation of ketone bodies produces a metabolic acidosis. Vomiting leads to further loss of fluid and electrolytes. The excess ketones are excreted in the urine but also appear in the breath, producing a distinctive smell similar to that of acetone. Respiratory compensation for the acidosis leads to hyperventilation, graphically described as 'air hunger'. Progressive dehydration impairs renal excretion of hydrogen ions and ketones, aggravating the acidosis.

A19.30

A) T B) F C) F D) T E) F

The management of diabetic nephropathy is similar to that of other causes of renal failure, with the following provisos: a) aggressive treatment of blood pressure with a target below 135/85 mmHg has been shown to slow the rate of deterioration of renal failure considerably. Angiotensin-converting enzyme inhibitors are the drugs of choice. Recent evidence suggests that these drugs should be considered in normotensive patients with persistent microalbuminuria. b) Oral hypoglycaemic agents partially excreted via the kidney (e.g. chlorpropamide) must be avoided. c) Insulin sensitivity increases and drastic reductions in dosage may be needed. d) Associated diabetic retinopathy tends to progress rapidly, and frequent ophthalmic supervision is essential.

A19.31

A) T B) T C) T D) T E) T

Principles of diabetic foot care

Inspect feet daily

Seek early advice for any damage

Check shoes inside and out for sharp bodies/areas before wearing

Use lace-up shoes with plenty of room for the toes

Keep feet away from sources of heat (hot sand, hot-water bottles, radiators, fires)

Check the bath temperature before stepping in

A19.32

A) F B) T C) T D) F E) T

The procedure for insulin-treated patients is simple: a) long-acting and/or intermediate insulin should be stopped the day before surgery, with soluble insulin substituted; b) whenever possible, diabetic patients should be first on the morning theatre list; c) an infusion of glucose, insulin and potassium is given during surgery. The insulin can be mixed into the glucose solution or administered separately by syringe pump. A standard combination is 16 U of soluble insulin with 10 mmol of KCl in 500 mL of 10% glucose, infused at 100 mL/h NS. d) Postoperatively, the infusion is maintained until the patient is able to eat. Other fluids needed in the perioperative period must be given through a separate intravenous line and must not interrupt the glucose/ insulin/potassium infusion. Glucose levels are checked every 2–4 hours and potassium levels are monitored. The amount of insulin and potassium in each infusion bag is adjusted either upwards or downwards according to the results of regular monitoring of the blood glucose and serum potassium concentrations.

A19.33

A) T   B) T   C) T   D) T   E) F

Poorly controlled diabetes is associated with stillbirth, mechanical problems in the birth canal owing to fetal macrosomia, hydramnios, and pre-eclampsia.

A19.34

A) F   B) T   C) T   D) F   E) T

Unsuspected infections, including urinary tract infections and tuberculosis, may be present. Thyrotoxicosis can also manifest as unstable glycaemic control.

A19.35

A) F   B) T   C) T   D) F   E) F

Factitious hypoglycaemia is a relatively common variant of self-induced disease and is much more common than an insulinoma. Hypoglycaemia is produced by surreptitious self-administration of insulin or sulphonylureas. Many patients in this category have been extensively investigated for an insulinoma. Measurement of C-peptide levels during hypoglycaemia should identify patients who are injecting insulin; sulphonylurea abuse can be detected by chromatography of plasma or urine.

Q20.1

A patient has a stroke as a result of which there is reduced fluency of speech with comprehension relatively preserved. The patient makes great efforts to initiate speech. Language is reduced to a few disjointed words and there is a failure to construct sentences

Select the area of damage

A. Non-dominant hemisphere
B. Medial surfaces of both temporal lobes and their brainstem connections – the hippocampi, fornices and mammillary bodies
C. Left posterior temporal/inferior parietal area
D. Left temporo-parietal damage
E. Left frontal lobe

Q20.2

A 49-year-old woman has tingling and pain in the right hand at night. On examination she has weakness of the thenar muscles, wasting of the abductor pollicis brevis, sensory loss in the palm and radial three-and-a-half fingers. This is due to the compression of which one of the following?

A. Radial nerve
B. Posterior interosseous nerve
C. Median nerve
D. Ulnar nerve
E. Common peroneal nerve

Q20.3

A 52-year-old lorry driver living in the UK is admitted with a seizure which occurred while he was playing basketball. At weekends his recreations includes driving his motorbike on his farm. He would like to know about his eligibility to go back to work and other restrictions regarding driving. Which one of the following statements is correct?

A. He can go back to driving his car immediately but not his motorcycle
B. He must refrain from riding his motorcycle or driving his car for 1 year from the date of seizure
C. He cannot drive his car for 1 year from the date of seizure but can ride his motorcycle on discharge
D. He must refrain from driving his lorry for 1 year from the date of the attack before a driving licence may be issued
E. He must refrain from riding his motorcycle or driving his car for 12 weeks from the date of seizure

Q20.4

A 21-year-old nursing student loses consciousness while helping out with a blood donation. She has never seen blood before. While unconscious her heart rate is 50 beats/minute. The senior nurse, who is there quickly, elevates her feet and within minutes she recovers although she is a little drowsy. The most likely aetiology for her syncope is which one of the following?

A. Drop attack
B. Transient ischaemic attack
C. Complete heart block
D. Vasovagal syncope
E. Pseudoseizure

A. Parkinson's disease
B. Multiple sclerosis
C. Hyperthyroidism
D. Anxiety
E. Idiopathic

Q20.5

On examination of a patient the neurologist notes that light touch is preserved but pain and temperature sensation is impaired. The most likely aetiology for this clinical picture is which one of the following?

A. Alcoholic neuropathy
B. Root compression due to spinal tumour
C. Syringomyelia
D. Tabes dorsalis
E. Parietal cortex lesion

Q20.6

A 48-year-old patient complains of numbness on the right side and weakness on the left. On examination there is loss of pain and temperature on the right side and upper motor neurone signs on the left side. The aetiology of this clinical picture is which one of the following?

A. Pure spinothalamic lesion
B. Hemisection of the cord
C. Multiple sclerosis of the pons
D. Thalamic infarct
E. Parietal cortex lesions

Q20.7

A 47-year-old man has tremor made worse by action. He also has titubation and nystagmus. The most likely cause of his tremor is which one of the following?

Q20.8

A patient has a stroke as a result of which language is fluent but the words themselves are incorrect. This varies from the insertion of a few incorrect or nonexistent words into fluent speech to a profuse outpouring of jargon. Select the area of damage

A. Non-dominant hemisphere
B. Medial surfaces of both temporal lobes and their brainstem connections – the hippocampi, fornices and mammillary bodies
C. Left posterior temporal/inferior parietal area
D. Left temporo-parietal damage
E. Left frontal lobe

Q20.9

A 23-year-old plumber presents with high fever, headache, mood change and drowsiness over several hours. In the emergency department he has seizures. MR imaging reveals oedema in the temporal lobes. EEG shows slow wave changes. CSF shows raised cell count. The patient should receive immediate treatment with intravenous (select the best option)

A. Benzylpenicillin
B. Aciclovir
C. Cefotaxime
D. Benzylpenicillin and chloramphenicol
E. Chloramphenicol

Neurological disease

Q20.10

A 55-year-old man presents with lightning pains in his arms. On examination he is ataxic, deep tendon reflexes are absent, and there is sensory loss and muscle wasting. He has Charcot joints. The most likely diagnosis is which one of the following?

A. Vitamin B$_{12}$ deficiency
B. Folic acid deficiency
C. Tabes dorsalis
D. Friedreich's ataxia
E. Diabetic neuropathy

Q20.11

A patient has a stroke as a result of which she has difficulty in naming familiar objects. Select the area of damage

A. Non-dominant hemisphere
B. Medial surfaces of both temporal lobes and their brainstem connections – the hippocampi, fornices and mammillary bodies
C. Left posterior temporal/inferior parietal area
D. Left temporo-parietal damage
E. Left frontal lobe

Q20.12

A patient who is right-handed has a stroke as a result of which he is unable to put on his clothing correctly. Select the area of damage

A. Non-dominant hemisphere
B. Medial surfaces of both temporal lobes and their brainstem connections – the hippocampi, fornices and mammillary bodies
C. Left posterior temporal/inferior parietal area
D. Left temporo-parietal damage
E. Left frontal lobe

Q20.13

A patient has a stroke as a result of which there is a disorder of memory. This is characterized by poor recall of more recent events with the relative preservation of distant memories. Select the area of damage

A. Non-dominant hemisphere
B. Medial surfaces of both temporal lobes and their brainstem connections – the hippocampi, fornices and mammillary bodies
C. Left posterior temporal/inferior parietal area
D. Left temporo-parietal damage
E. Left frontal lobe

Q20.14

A 29-year-old woman presents to the accident and emergency department with headaches and projectile vomiting. Fundal examinations reveals that the margins of the optic disc are blurred and the physiological cup is dilated. The most likely aetiology of this condition is which one of the following?

A. Migraine
B. Cluster headaches
C. Refractive error causing eye strain
D. Raised intracranial pressure
E. Pancoast's syndrome

Q20.15

The neurologist flashes a light into the patient's right eye as a result of which the right pupil constricts. She also notes that the contralateral pupil constricts. Select the best option for the changes noted by the neurologist

A. Afferent fibres in each optic nerve, which pass through both lateral geniculate bodies, also relay to the convergence centre. This centre receives 1a spindle afferent fibres from the extraocular muscles – principally medial recti – which are innervated by the third nerve. The efferent route is from the convergence centre to the Edinger–Westphal nucleus, ciliary ganglion and pupils

B. Afferent fibres in each optic nerve (some crossing in the chiasm) pass to both lateral geniculate bodies and relay to the Edinger–Westphal nuclei via the pretectal nucleus. Efferent (parasympathetic) fibres from each Edinger–Westphal nucleus pass via the third nerve to the ciliary ganglion and thence to the pupil

C. Afferent fibres in each optic nerve (some crossing in the chiasm) pass to both lateral geniculate bodies and relay to the Edinger–Westphal nuclei via the pretectal nucleus. The efferent route is from the convergence centre to the Edinger–Westphal nucleus, ciliary ganglion and pupils

D. Afferent fibres in each optic nerve, which pass through both lateral geniculate bodies, also relay to the convergence centre. This centre receives 1a spindle afferent fibres from the extraocular muscles – principally medial recti – which are innervated by the third nerve. Efferent (parasympathetic) fibres from each Edinger–Westphal nucleus pass via the third nerve to the ciliary ganglion and thence to the pupil

E. Afferent (parasympathetic) fibres from each Edinger–Westphal nucleus pass via the third nerve to the ciliary ganglion and thence to the pupil. Efferent fibres in each optic nerve, which pass through both lateral geniculate bodies, also relay to the convergence centre

Q20.16

The neurologist asks the patient to fix his eyes on a near object. She notices that the patient's eyes converge and there is bilateral pupillary constriction. Select the best option for the pathway of the reflex

A. Afferent fibres in each optic nerve (some crossing in the chiasm) pass to both lateral geniculate bodies and relay to the Edinger–Westphal nuclei via the pretectal nucleus. Efferent (parasympathetic) fibres from each Edinger–Westphal nucleus pass via the third nerve to the ciliary ganglion and thence to the pupil

B. Afferent fibres in each optic nerve (some crossing in the chiasm) pass to both lateral geniculate bodies and relay to the Edinger–Westphal nuclei via the pretectal nucleus. The efferent route is from the convergence centre to the Edinger–Westphal nucleus, ciliary ganglion and pupils

C. Afferent fibres in each optic nerve, which pass through both lateral geniculate bodies, also relay to the convergence centre. This centre receives 1a spindle afferent fibres from the extraocular muscles – principally medial recti – which are innervated by the third nerve. Efferent (parasympathetic) fibres from each Edinger–Westphal nucleus pass via the third nerve to the ciliary ganglion and thence to the pupil

D. Afferent (parasympathetic) fibres from each Edinger–Westphal nucleus pass via the third nerve to the ciliary ganglion and thence to the pupil. Efferent fibres in each optic nerve, which pass through both lateral geniculate bodies, also relay to the convergence centre

Neurological disease

E. Afferent fibres in each optic nerve, which pass through both lateral geniculate bodies, also relay to the convergence centre. This centre receives 1a spindle afferent fibres from the extraocular muscles – principally medial recti – which are innervated by the third nerve. The efferent route is from the convergence centre to the Edinger–Westphal nucleus, ciliary ganglion and pupils

Q20.17

A 35-year-old woman with multiple sclerosis has a past history of left retrobulbar neuritis. She is diagnosed as having a relative afferent pupillary defect (RAPD). Which one of the following best correlates with her diagnosis?

A. The left pupil is unreactive to light. The consensual reflex is also absent

B. The left pupil is unreactive to light. When light is shone into the intact right eye, only the right pupil constricts. When the light source is then swung to the previously affected left eye, its pupil dilates, relative to its previous state

C. The left pupil is reactive to light whereas the right pupil is unreactive to light. When light is shone into the intact right eye, only the left pupil constricts. When the light source is then swung to the previously affected left eye, its pupil dilates, relative to its previous state

D. Light shone in the left eye causes both left and right pupils to constrict. When light is shone into the intact right eye, both pupils again constrict. When the light source is then swung to the previously affected left eye, its pupil dilates, relative to its previous state

E. Light shone in the left eye causes both left and right pupils to constrict. The consensual reflex is absent

Q20.18

A 42-year-old man has constriction of the right pupil with relative ptosis and enophthalmos on the same side. The patient also has loss of sweating over the entire right half of the head, arm and upper trunk. Select the best option for the cause of these symptoms

A. Apical bronchial neoplasm
B. Cervical sympathectomy
C. Pontine glioma
D. Carotid artery occlusion in the neck
E. Cervical rib

Q20.19

A 44-year-old businessman has a small, irregular pupil. The pupil does not respond to light but constricts on convergence. Select the best option for the site of lesion

A. Denervation in the ciliary ganglion
B. Fibres in the nasocilary nerve pass to the dilator pupillae muscle
C. Neural tissue of the brainstem surrounding the aqueduct of Sylvius
D. Bilateral occipital lobe damage
E. Infarction of one optic pole alone

Q20.20

A 67-year-old patient has a history of axial rigidity, frequent falls and dementia. On examination she is unable to move the eyes vertically or laterally. The most likely diagnosis is which one of the following?

A. Shy–Drager syndrome
B. Olivo-ponto-cerebellar degeneration
C. Progressive supranuclear palsy
D. Wilson's disease
E. Athetoid cerebral palsy

Q20.21

On attempted left lateral gaze the patient's right eye fails to adduct. The left eye develops coarse nystagmus on abduction. On attempted right lateral gaze the patient's left eye fails to adduct. Also the right eye develops coarse nystagmus in abduction. This sign is pathognomonic of which one of the following?

A. Pontine glioma
B. Pinealoma
C. Progressive supranuclear palsy
D. Myasthenia gravis
E. Multiple sclerosis

Q20.22

A 59-year-old patient has complete ptosis on the right side. The eye is facing down and out. The pupil is normal and reactive to light. When the patient makes an attempt to converge and look downwards the conjuctival vessels of the right eye are seen to twist clockwise. This clinical picture is most likely to correlate with which one of the following investigations

A. CT head scan showing aneursmal dilatation of the posterior communicating artery
B. CT head scan showing coning of the temporal lobe
C. Glycosylated haemoglobin of 12
D. CT head scan showing a midbrain tumour
E. CT head scan showing midbrain infarction

Q20.23

A 32-year-old woman has sensory loss on the right side of the face, tongue and buccal mucosa. The right corneal reflex is absent. The muscles on the right side of the face are weak and she has nerve deafness on the right side. The most likely

cause of her clinical picture is which one of the following?

A. Thrombosis of the cavernous sinus
B. Aneurysm of the internal carotid artery
C. Syringobulbia
D. Acoustic neuroma in the cerebellopontine angle
E. Trigeminal neuralgia

Q20.24

A 32-year-old man complains of a band of pain around the thorax which is worse on coughing and straining. There is weakness in both legs and numbness which commenced in the feet and is currently just below the level of the band of pain around the thorax. He has retention of urine and constipation. On examination the upper level of his numbness is at the level of the 6th thoracic spine and there is spasticity in both legs. Select the best option for the management of this condition

A. Contrast myelography
B. MR of spine
C. Lumbar puncture
D. CT head scan
E. Sputum for acid fast bacilli

Q20.25

A 28-year-old man complains of pain in both hands while coughing or on exertion. The patient has also noticed that while smoking he does not feel burns in his fingers but can feel objects. In addition he has difficulty in walking. On examination there are areas of loss of pain and temperature sensation but light touch is intact. There is a loss of upper limb reflexes, wasting of the small muscles of the hand, and paraparesis with spasticity in both lower limbs. The most likely explanation for this clinical picture is which one of the following?

417

A. Anterior spinal artery occlusion
B. Vitamin B_{12} deficiency
C. Acute transverse myelitis
D. Cervical syrinx
E. Radiation myelopathy

20.26

A 65-year-old man presents with sudden onset of violently swinging movements of the right arm. CT reveals intracerebral haemorrhage. The most likely site for the haemorrhage is which one of the following?

A. Right caudate nucleus
B. Left caudate nucleus
C. Left subthalamic nucleus
D. Right subthalamic nucleus
E. Left motor cortex

20.27

A 14-year-old boy has a right middle ear infection. He has pain on the right side of the face, together with sensory loss on the right side of the face and tongue. The patient also has a convergent squint with diplopia maximal on looking towards the right. The right eye cannot be abducted beyond the midline. Select one of the following

A. Thrombosis of the cavernous sinus
B. Aneurysm of the internal carotid artery
C. Gradenigo's syndrome
D. Acoustic neuroma in the cerebellopontine angle
E. Trigeminal neuralgia

20.28

A 35-year-old man wakes up with pain behind his right ear and notices weakness of the right side of his face. On examination there is loss of taste on the anterior two-thirds of the tongue. The most likely diagnosis is which one of the following?

A. Hemifacial spasm
B. Myokymia
C. Bell's palsy
D. Dystrophia myotonica
E. Myasthenia gravis

20.29

A 28-year-old physician has sudden unprovoked attacks of vertigo with vomiting and loss of balance which last from minutes to hours. Tinnitus and deafness accompany an attack. The most likely diagnosis is which one of the following?

A. Temporal lobe epilepsy
B. Cerebellopontine angle
C. Ménière's disease
D. Vestibular neuronitis
E. Benign positional vertigo

20.30

A 65-year-old man complains of difficulty in swallowing, hoarseness of voice and nasal regurgitation. There is visible weakness of elevation of the palate, depression of palatal sensation and loss of the gag reflex. The most likely explanation for this clinical picture is which one of the following?

A. Myasthenia gravis
B. Bulbar palsy caused by disease of lower cranial nerves
C. Parkinson's disease
D. Oesophageal spasm
E. Glossopharyngeal neuralgia

Q20.31

A 58-year-old man complains of hoarseness of voice and there is a failure of the forceful, explosive part of voluntary and reflex coughing. On examination there is no visible weakness of the palate. ENT examination reveals right palatal paralysis. The most likely cause is which one of the following?

A. Aneurysm of the aorta
B. Surgery in the neck
C. Pseudobulbar palsy
D. Parkinson's disease
E. Cerebellar disease

Q20.32

A 66-year-old woman presents with a right-sided weakness. CT shows subarachnoid haemorrhage. She recovers completely. The best next option for management is which one of the following?

A. Rehabilitation
B. Aspirin 75 mg PO once a day long term
C. Urgent referral for angiography
D. Beta-blockers
E. Immediate carotid endarterectomy

Q20.33

The body of a 67-year-old man, following a vague warning, becomes rigid for a minute. He utters a cry and falls. He bites his tongue and is incontinent of urine. This is soon followed by a generalized convulsion with frothing at the mouth and rhythmic jerking of muscle. This lasts for a few minutes. This period is followed by drowsiness and he is brought to the accident and emergency department. Which one of the following drugs is ineffective in preventing recurrent attacks of this condition?

A. Carbamazepine
B. Ethosuximide
C. Phenobarbital
D. Phenytoin
E. Valproate

Q20.34

A 14-year-old girl has a history of several episodes where all activity stops, she stares and pales slightly for a few seconds. The eyelids twitch and soon thereafter she resumes normal activity. EEG during one of these attacks shows 3 Hz spike-and-wave pattern. The most effective drug for this condition is which one of the following?

A. Carbamazepine
B. Valproate
C. Phenobarbital
D. Primidone
E. Phenytoin

Q20.35

1. A 42-year-old woman complains of recurrent headaches lasting hours or days – band-like, generalized head pains, with a history going back for several years. She vaguely ascribes it to muscle tension. She has a history of depression

2. A 38-year-old man has headache that is present on waking. It is made worse by coughing, straining or sneezing. These episodes are often accompanied by vomiting

3. A 66-year-old man complains of patches of exquisite tenderness overlying superficial scalp arteries

4. A 22-year-old teacher complains of a single episode of severe headache accompanied by vomiting. Examination reveals neck stiffness

5. A 44-year-old woman complains of headache. On examination her blood pressure is 220/110 mmHg

Select the best match for each of the above

A. High blood pressure alone
B. Subarachnoid haemorrhage
C. Malignant hypertension with arterial damage and brain swelling
D. Eyestrain from underlying refractive error
E. Posterior fossa mass
F. Giant cell arteritis
G. Chronic benign recurrent headache

20.36

1. The toes of the shoes catch level ground and become scuffed. The pace shortens but the narrow base of the gait is maintained. The patient has clonus

2. The gait is shuffling with a narrow base. A stoop is apparent and the arm swing is diminished. The gait is hurried with small rapid steps. There is particular difficulty in initiating movement and turning quickly. When the patient is stopped he takes small backwards steps involuntarily

3. The stance is broad-based, unstable and tremulous. The patient veers to one side

4. The gait is broad-based, high-stepping or stamping. When the patient closes his eyes while standing he becomes unstable

5. Leg movement is normal when sitting or lying but initiation and organization of walking fail

Select the best match for each of the above

A. Sensory ataxia
B. Frontal lobe disease
C. Disease of lateral cerebellar lobes
D. Spasticity
E. Parkinson's disease

20.37

1. Paracentral scotoma
2. Monoocular field loss
3. Bitemporal hemianopia
4. Homonymous hemianopia
5. Homonymous quandrantanopia

Select the best match for each of the above

A. Parietal lesion
B. Temporal lesion
C. Occipital cortex
D. Chiasmal lesion
E. Retinal lesion
F. Optic nerve lesion

20.38

1. A 31-year-old woman has a fine pendular, jelly-like nystagmus
2. A 42-year-old man has a down-beat jerk nystagmus
3. Ice-cold water in the left ear causes nystagmus with fast movement to the right
4. Warm water in the left ear causes nystagmus with fast movement to the right
5. Warm water in the right ear causes nystagmus with fast movement to the right

Select the best match for each of the above

A. Normal caloric test
B. Abnormal caloric test
C. Multiple sclerosis
D. Meningioma around the foramen magnum

Q20.39

1. Flexion at the elbow when the biceps tendon is struck

2. Extension of the elbow when the triceps tendon is struck

3. Extension at the knee when the patellar tendon is struck

4. Plantarflexion of the foot when the Achilles tendon is struck

5. Flexion and supination of the forearm upon striking the styloid process of the radius

Select the spinal level for each of the above tendon reflexes

A. C3–4
B. C5–6
C. C7
D. L1–2
E. L3–4
F. S1
G. S2, 3, 4
H. T12

Q20.40

1. A 79-year-old man who has paucity of movement, stiffness and rest tremor

2. A 42-year-old man with an inherited dementia and progressive jerky movements

3. A 57-year-old man with wild, flinging limb movements

4. A 43-year-old patient who has vertigo, vomiting and ataxia of gait

5. A 53-year-old patient who has sensory loss and neglect of one side, apraxia and subtle disorders of sensation

Select the best match for each of the above

A. Parietal cortex lesions
B. Lesions of floccuonodular region of the cerebellum extending to the roof of the fourth ventricle

C. Infarct of the subthalamic nucleus
D. Damage to GABA, enkephalin neurones in the indirect pathway from the striatum to the lateral globus pallidus
E. Loss of dopamine activity in the striatum
F. Temporal lobe
G. Lateral cerebellar lobes

Q20.41

1. Bladder wall relaxation

2. Contraction of internal sphincter

3. Contraction of external sphincter

4. Orgasm

5. Engorgement of penis

Select the nerve supply for each of the above

A. Sympathetic T12–L2
B. Parasympathetic S2–4
C. Pudendal nerves
D. Inguinal nerve
E. Coccygeal nerve

Q20.42

1. A 28-year-old motorcyclist, following a road traffic accident, is brought to the accident and emergency department. Cyclical eye opening is present. She has no purposeful movements and does not respond to painful stimuli. Respiratory function is normal. EEG shows polymorphic delta waves with slow alpha waves

2. A 23-year-old nursery school teacher is brought into accident and emergency. On examination there are no purposeful limb movements. Cyclical eye opening is present. Eye movement is preserved in the vertical plane and he is able to blink volitionally. He responds to painful stimuli by withdrawal. EEG is normal

Neurological disease

3. A 45-year-old woman is found unconscious. Cyclical eye opening is absent. There is no purposeful movement. Perception of pain is absent. Respiratory muscle is depressed. EEG shows polymorphic delta waves

4. A 52-year-old patient is unconscious and is on a ventilator. Cyclical eye opening is absent. There is only reflex spinal movement. There is no motor function and perception of pain is absent. Respiratory function is absent when attempts are made to wean the patient of the ventilator. EEG shows occasional theta waves only

Select the best match for each of the above

A. Patient is malingering
B. Brainstem death
C. Coma
D. Locked-in syndrome
E. Vegetative state

Q20.43

1. A 52-year-old woman with an intracerebral bleed is noted to have alternating hyperpnoea and apnoea

2. A 47-year-old man has deep, sighing hyperventilation

3. A 42-year-old woman has sustained, rapid, deep breathing. It is episodic, i.e. it switches abruptly on and off

4. A 29-year-old woman in a critical care unit has shallow, halting irregular respiration

5. A 67-year-old patient in a stupor has vomiting, hiccups and excessive yawning

Select the best match for each of the above

A. Lower brainstem lesion
B. Damage to the medullary centre and frequently precedes death

C. Pontine lesions
D. Sign of incipient coning
E. Diabetic ketoacidosis

Q20.44

1. A 29-year-old patient is unconscious following a motor vehicle accident. He has dilatation of one pupil which is fixed to light

2. A 45-year-old patient who is unconscious has bilateral mid-point reactive pupils (i.e. normal pupils)

3. A 49-year-old unconscious patient who has bilateral light-fixed dilated pupils

4. A 57-year-old patient who is unconscious and has bilateral pinpoint pupils which are fixed to light

Select the best match for each of the above

A. Cardinal sign of brainstem death.
B. Pontine haemorrhage
C. Metabolic coma
D. Herniation of the uncus of the temporal lobe
E. Horner's syndrome
F. Holmes–Adie syndrome

Q20.45

1. A 45-year-old man has a broad-based gait, cerebellar signs, vestibular paralysis, amnesia with confabulation, nystagmus and bilateral lateral rectus palsy

2. A 77-year-old woman has numbness and tingling of the fingers and toes. On examination there are absent ankle jerks, exaggerated knee jerks, extensor plantar responses and distal sensory loss of vibration and pain. Bone marrow shows a megaloblastic picture and the blood smear shows macrocytes

3. A 58-year-old patient has progressive variable loss of sensation, distal limb wasting and weakness. The legs resemble inverted champagne bottles

4. A 22-year-old man has fatigue of the proximal limb muscles, extraocular muscles and speech. Reflexes are preserved. On injection of edrophonium, weakness improves within seconds but the improvement lasts only for 3 minutes

5. A 67-year-old chronic smoker has proximal muscle weakness and absent reflexes. Weakness tends to improve after a few minutes of muscular contraction and also absent reflexes return

6. A 7-year-old boy has difficulty in running and in rising to an erect positon from the floor (he uses his hands to climb up his legs). The calves are hypertrophied but weak.

7. A 34-year-old man has progressive distal muscle weakness with ptosis, weakness and thinning of the face and sternomastoids. Myotonia is present. Other features are cataracts, frontal baldness, mild intellectual impairment and hypogonadism

8. A patient is easily fatigued, has severe cramps on exercise and myoglobinuria. Venous lactate does not increase despite ischaemic exercise

Select the best match for each of the above

A. Defective chloride ion membrane conductance

B. Absence of the gene product for dystrophin

C. Lack of skeletal muscle myophosphorylase

D. Antibodies to P/Q type voltage gated calcium channels

E. Antibodies to serum acetylcholine receptors

F. Thiamin deficiency

G. Pyridoxine deficiency

H. Vitamin B_{12} deficiency

I. Mutations of the peripheral myelin protein gene

Q20.46

1. A 65-year-old woman presents with a transient history of vomiting, diplopia and vertigo. She is also dysarthric and has ataxia for a few minutes after that. She completely recovers within a few minutes

2. A 67-year-old patient has a stroke. On examination, on the right side he has numbness of the face, double vision, nystagmus, ataxia and Horner's syndrome, ninth and tenth nerve lesion. On the left side there is mild hemiparesis and loss of pain and temperature sensation

3. A 58-year-old patient with hypercholesterolaemia has a sudden transient loss of vision in the right eye

4. A 44-year-old man has paralysis of the right third cranial nerve with hemiplegia on the left side. Upward gaze is paralysed

Select the best match for each of the above

A. Transient ischaemic attack due to involvement of the right internal carotid artery

B. Transient ischaemic attack due to involvement of the left internal carotid artery

C. Transient ischaemic attack due to involvement of the vertebrobasilar system

D. Thrombosis of the right posterior inferior cerebellar artery

E. Thrombosis of the left posterior inferior cerebellar artery

F. Weber's syndrome

Neurological disease

Q20.47

1. A 23-year-old woman complains of unilateral headache and photophobia. Examination is normal. The CSF is crystal clear, mononuclear cells 4 mm³, no polymorphs, protein 0.3 g/L, CSF glucose is 60 g/dL and blood glucose is 120 g/dL

2. A 19-year-old student presents with fever, headache, nausea, vomiting. On examination there is neck stiffness. CSF is clear, mononuclear cells 50 mm³, no polymorphs, protein is 0.5 g/L and glucose is 70 g/dL, whereas blood glucose is 120 g/dL

3. A 33-year-old footballer presents with fever, headache, vomiting and photophobia. On examination there is neck stiffness. CSF is purulent, mononuclear cells 40 mm³, polymorph cells 300 mm³, protein 2 g/L, glucose is 40 mg/dL, whereas blood glucose is 160 mg/dL

4. A 43-year-old executive from Bangladesh presents with fever, headache, nausea and vomiting. On examination there is neck stiffness, CSF is turbid, mononuclear cells 200 mm³, polymorph cells 200/mm³, protein 3 g/L, glucose is 45 mg/dL, whereas blood glucose is 140 mg/dL

Select the best option

A. Tuberculous meningitis
B. Pyogenic meningitis
C. Migraine
D. Viral meningitis

Q20.48

1. An 87-year-old man living in a nursing home has had a vague change in his personality over the years. In additon he is apathetic and his intellect seems to have deteriorated. More recently he has

developed an expressive aphasia and on examination he has right hemiparesis. He complains of headaches, and fundus examination reveals papilloedema

2. A 67-year-old woman has had difficulties with her vision and episodes of tingling in the left limbs. On examination there is a left homonymous field defect. Subsequently she has cortical sensory loss in the left limbs and left hemiparesis

3. A 29-year-old patient with von Recklinghausen's disease presents with a 3-year history of deafness on the left side, vertigo, numbness and weakness of the left side of the face. More recently, he has become unsteady on his feet and on examination he has cerebellar ataxia on the left side

Select the best match for each of the above

A. Right frontal meningioma
B. Left frontal meningioma
C. Right parietal lobe glioma
D. Left parietal glioma
E. Left eighth nerve sheath neurofibroma
F. Right eighth nerve sheath neurofibroma

Q20.49

1. A 42-year-old woman has multiple pale brown patches on her body. She also has multipe subcutaneous soft tumours which have been increasing in number throughout her life

2. A 17-year-old boy has a history of epilepsy and mental retardation. On examination he has reddish nodules on his cheeks. Examination of the retina shows phakomas

3. A 22-year-old patient with epilepsy has an extensive port-wine naevus on the right side of the face in the distribution of the fifth cranial nerve

4. A 14 year-old boy presents with ataxia. On examination he has polycythaemia, retinal and cerebellar haemangiomas

5. A 24-year-old man has had progressive difficulty in walking since the age of 12. On examination he has ataxia of gait, nystagmus, dysarthria, absent lower limb joint and position sense, absent lower limb deep tendon reflexes, and pes cavus

Select the best match for each of the above

A. von Hippel–Lindau syndrome
B. Sturge–Weber syndrome
C. Neurofibromatosis 1
D. Neurofibromatosis 2
E. The expression of protein fraxatin is decreased
F. Tuberous sclerosis

Q20.50

A patient presents with double vision. On examination of the right eye there is a convergent squint with diplopia maximal on looking towards the right. The right eye cannot be abducted beyond the midline. The left eye is normal. Recognized causes of these features include

A. Pontine glioma
B. Multiple sclerosis
C. Diabetes mellitus
D. Raised intracranial pressure
E. Nasopharyngeal carcinoma

Q20.51

A 25-year-old patient complains of hearing loss on the right side. The examiner places a vibrating 256 Hz tuning fork adjacent to the right external auditory meatus and then places it on the right mastoid process. The latter manoeuvre improves the perception of sound. The causes of this clinical feature include

A. Middle ear infection
B. Ménière's disease
C. Acoustic neuroma
D. Multiple sclerosis
E. Gentamicin toxicity

Q20.52

A 58-year-old man develops an acute stroke. The following are characteristic of a pyramidal (upper motor neurone) lesion

A. When both upper limbs are held outstretched, palms uppermost, the affected limb drifts downwards and medially
B. In the upper limbs the flexors are weaker than the extensors
C. The increase in tone affects all muscle groups on the side affected but is detectable most easily in stronger muscles
D. The abdominal reflex is abolished
E. The tendon reflexes in the affected limbs become exaggerated and clonus is often evident

Q20.53

Efferent fibres pass from the cerebellum to the

A. Proprioceptive organs in joints and muscles
B. Vestibular nuclei
C. Basal ganglia
D. Corticospinal system
E. Olivary nuclei

Neurological disease

Q20.54

A 24-year-old medical student has tremor (8–12 Hz) when her arms are outstretched. This tremor can be increased with

A. Anxiety
B. Hyperthyroidism
C. Lithium
D. Sodium valproate
E. Sympathomimetics

Q20.55

The neurologist is examining a person referred to him for weakness. On examination the patient has muscle weakness and wasting. Fasciculations are seen. The tone is decreased. Examples of this lesion include

A. Bell's palsy
B. Motor neurone disease
C. Poliomyelitis
D. Spinal root involvement due to cervical disc protrusion
E. Mononeuritis multiplex

Q20.56

The neurologist is performing an examination. She notes that when the neck is flexed the patient complains of an electric-shock-like sensation which radiates down the trunk and limbs. This indicates a cervical cord lesion due to

A. Multiple sclerosis
B. Cervical spondylotic myelopathy
C. Subacute combined degeneration of the cord
D. Radiation myelopathy
E. Cord compression

Q20.57

A 42-year-old patient complains of weakness in both legs. The tone is increased in both legs and is characterized by changing resistance to passive movement. The tendon reflexes in both the legs are exaggerated and clonus is evident. These clinical features can be caused by

A. Parasagittal meningioma
B. Motor neurone disease
C. Spinal cord compression
D. Multiple sclerosis
E. Myelitis due to varicella zoster virus

Q20.58

The following statements about physiology of pain are correct

A. The gate theory of pain proposes that the entry of afferent impulses is monitored by the cells of the substantia gelatinosa
B. Pain perception is mediated by free nerve endings
C. Sensory impulses enter the spinal cord via the ventral spinal roots
D. Acupuncture achieves analgesia by a gating effect on large myelinated nerve fibres
E. Calcium-channel blockers (nifedipine) improve sympathetically mediated pain

Q20.59

The value of computed tomography in the diagnosis of neurological conditions includes the following

A. It is useful in detecting lesions under 1 cm diameter
B. It is useful in imaging multiple sclerosis plaques

C. It very sensitive in detecting posterior fossa lesions
D. It images the spinal cord without contrast
E. It is useful in imaging isodense subdural haematomas

Q20.60

A 65-year-old patient presents with weakness of the right side of the body and aphasia which occurred suddenly about an hour ago. Blood pressure is 170/100 mmHg and heart rate is 100 beats/minute regular. CT excludes haemorrhagic stroke. The following statements about the management of this condition are correct

A. Aspirin is contraindicated because it increases the risk of intracerebral haemorrhage
B. Warfarin should be started to reduce the risk of future strokes
C. Intravenous tissue plasminogen activator should be avoided in this patient
D. The blood pressure should be rapidly lowered to reduce the risk of future stroke
E. Lumbar puncture must be done

Q20.61

A 32-year-old patient with epilepsy would like to know which of the following side-effects are associated with chronic phenytoin therapy

A. Gum hypertrophy
B. Hypertrichosis
C. Osteomalacia
D. Folate deficiency
E. Encephalopathy

Q20.62

A 79-year-old man complains that his limbs and joints feel stiff and ache and that fine movements are difficult. He has difficulty in rising from a chair and with getting into and out of bed. His writing has become small and spidery, with a tendency to fall off at the end of a line. He has a mask-like facies, a rest tremor that is increased by emotion with pill rolling movements between thumb and finger and increased muscle tone in opposing muscle groups. The following statements regarding this condition are correct

A. There is no laboratory test to confirm the diagnosis of this condition
B. Remissions are rare
C. Selegiline, a monoamine oxidase B inhibitor, will alter the course of this condition
D. Levodopa and/or dopaminergic agents produce striking initial symptomatic improvement in the great majority of patients, but do not alter the natural progression of the condition
E. The drug of choice for depression in this condition is a combination of type A MAO inhibitor phenelzine and levodopa

Q20.63

A 67-year-old woman with Parkinson's disease on levodopa for about 5 years now complains of episodes of immobility and frequent falls. These episodes alternate with dystonic movements and chorea. She has also noticed recently that the action of the levodopa wears off sooner than before and she often has dyskinesia before her next dose. Approaches to treatment of these complications include

Neurological disease

A. Stereotactic neurosurgery
B. Shortening the interval between levodopa doses and increasing each dose
C. Subcutaneous metered infusion of apomorphine
D. Entacapone
E. Periods of drug withdrawal

20.64

A 39-year-old woman with schizophrenia has been on long-term phenothiazines. As a result of her medication she may develop the following disorders of movement

A. Benign essential tremor
B. Restless, repetitive and irresistable need to move
C. Acute dystonic reactions
D. Mouthing and lip-smacking grimaces of the neck
E. Benign essential myoclonus

20.65

A 39-year-old man has jerky, quasi-purposive, fidgety movements which are flitting in nature. He also has dementia. The following statements about this condition are correct

A. The diagnosis is Sydenham's chorea
B. The patient is likely to have CAG expansions of 40–55 repeats on the short arm of chromosome 4
C. The involuntary movements may be reduced by phenothiazines
D. The dementia and chorea steadily progress over time
E. Imaging shows hypertrophy of the caudate nucleus

20.66

A 29-year-old woman has dystonia which commenced in childhood. It has spread to all parts of her body affecting both gait and posture. Correct statements about this condition include

A. Cognitive function is considerably affected
B. Spontaneous remissions are common
C. It is inherited as an autosomal recessive disorder
D. The diagnosis is Gilles de la Tourette syndrome
E. Stereotactic thalmotomy is curative

20.67

A 39-year-old woman complains of blurring of vision of the right eye which developed over several hours. She says that it is like looking through frosted glass in that eye. She has mild pain in the eye. She had a similar episode 3 years ago from which she recovered fully. On examination with an ophthalmoscope the eye is completely normal. The following statements about this condition are correct

A. MRI of the brain and spinal cord is the first-line investigation
B. Peripheral blood and urine tests are very helpful in the diagnosis
C. A delayed visual-evoked response can provide evidence of a previous optic nerve lesion
D. Corticosteroids influence the long-term outcome of the condition
E. Beta-interferon reduces the relapse rate of this condition

Q20.68

A 39-year-old woman presents with a history of fever, rigors, headache, photophobia and vomiting. On examination she has a petechial rash, neck stiffness and a positive Kernig's sign. The following statements about the management of this condition are correct

A. Lumbar puncture must be performed as soon as possible to make the diagnosis
B. Parenteral antibiotics should be administered after blood cultures are carried out
C. Prednisolone should be given to prevent septicaemic shock
D. The local public health authorities must be notified
E. Optimal care reduces the mortality to <1%

Q20.69

A 22-year-old doctor has a 1-year history of recurrent splitting left-sided headaches accompanied by nausea and vomiting. The headaches are preceded by vague weakness on that side and images of jagged lines. He is irritable during this period and prefers to lie down in a dark room. Future attacks can be prevented by

A. Paracetamol given round the clock
B. Subcutaneous sumatriptan
C. Pizotifen
D. Propranolol
E. Amitriptyline

Q20.70

A 72-year-old man presents with jaw pain which is worse on eating. Opening the mouth and protruding the tongue is difficult. ESR is 100 mm/1st hour. The following statements are correct

A. Immediate high doses of steroids should be started even before biopsy
B. The diagnosis should be established immediately by superficial temporal lobe biopsy
C. High-dose steroids should be given life-long
D. Risk of visual loss occurs in 25% of untreated patients
E. Extradural cranial arteries are involved

Q20.71

A 29-year-old motorcyclist has a head injury. Local complications of skull fracture include

A. Extradural haematoma
B. Subdural haematoma
C. CSF rhinorrhoea
D. CSF otorrhoea
E. Risk of meningitis

Q20.72

Following head trauma the major mechanisms of brain injury include

A. Shearing and rotational stress on the decelerating brain, at sites distant from the impact, causing axonal and neuronal damage
B. Axonal and neuronal damage from direct trauma
C. Brain oedema
D. Raised intracranial pressure
E. Brain hypoxia
F. Brain ischaemia

Neurological disease

Q20.73

A 22-year-old boxer is recovering consciousness from a traumatic head injury. Late sequelae include

A. Cognitive impairment
B. Epilepsy
C. Cognitive impairment with extrapyramidal and pyramidal signs
D. Benign paroxysmal positional vertigo
E. Hydrocephalus

Q20.74

A 32-year-old woman has difficulty in swallowing, nasal regurgitation of fluids, a choking sensation and difficulty speaking. On examination her tongue is wasted and has fasciculations and the palate is weak and spastic. Eye movements are unaffected. There are no cerebellar or extrapyramidal signs. She is orientated in person, place and time. The following statements about this patient's condition are correct

A. There are no specific tests; diagnosis is clinical
B. Remissions are common
C. Death is often due to bronchopneumonia
D. Patients usually survive for a decade or longer
E. Riluzole has been shown to slow progression slightly

Q20.75

A child is initially noted to have delayed milestones. Later he is noted to have mental retardation, spasticity in both lower limbs and scissor gait. Factors which have been held responsible in this condition include

A. Hypoxia in utero and/or during birth
B. Status epilepticus
C. Kernicterus
D. Neonatal cerebral infarction
E. Trauma during parturition

Q20.76

A 53-year-old man has tingling and pain in the right hand at night. On examination he has weakness of the thenar muscles, wasting of the abductor pollicis brevis, sensory loss in the palm and radial three-and-a-half fingers. This condition is sometimes seen in

A. Hyperthyroidism
B. Diabetes insipidus
C. Pregnancy
D. Acromegaly
E. Rheumatoid arthritis

Q20.77

A 46-year-old woman has involvement of the right ulnar nerve, left median nerve, right radial nerve and left lateral popliteal nerve. This clinical picture occurs in

A. Diabetes mellitus
B. Leprosy
C. Vasculitis
D. HIV infection
E. Meralgia paraesthetica

Q20.78

A 47-year-old man complains of weakness of distal limbs and muscles and numbness in both legs. Over a period of weeks this progresses with ascending weakness, areflexia and sensory loss. Correct statements about this condition include

A. Nerve conduction is typically normal in the common demyelinating form

B. CSF protein is typically depressed with cell count and sugar level being normal

C. High-dose gamma-globulin reduces the duration and severity of the paralysis

D. *Campylobacter jejuni* is known to cause severe forms of this condition

E. Corticosteroids substantially improve prognosis

Neurological disease

A20.1

E

In Broca's aphasia (expressive aphasia, anterior aphasia) a lesion in the left frontal lobe causes reduced fluency of speech with comprehension relatively preserved. The patient makes great efforts to initiate speech. Language is reduced to a few disjointed words and there is failure to construct sentences. Patients who recover from this form of aphasia say that they knew what they wanted to say, but could not get the words out.

A20.2

C

Carpal tunnel syndrome is the common condition of median nerve compression at the wrist.

A20.3

B

It is illegal to drive a motor vehicle if any form of seizure or any episode of unexplained loss of consciousness has occurred during the previous year. There is some variation between different countries. In the UK those who have suffered from epilepsy cannot legally hold a Group 1 driving licence (for a car or motorcycle) unless they satisfy the following legal criteria, whether on or off treatment. The regulations state: a) a person who has suffered an epileptic attack while awake must refrain from driving for 1 year from the date of the attack before a driving licence may be issued; b) a person who has suffered a single epileptic attack while asleep must also refrain from driving for 1 year from the date of that attack, unless they have had attacks exclusively while asleep over a period of 3 years and no awake attacks, i.e. attacks occurring exclusively in sleep must be shown to have occurred over a 3-year period. c) In any event, the driving of a vehicle by such a person should not be likely to cause danger to the public. For UK Group 2 drivers (vocational and for truck drivers) regulations are stricter. Persons with previous seizures must meet *all* these three criteria: a) they must have been free of attacks for at least 10 years; b) they must not have taken anticonvulsants during this 10 years; c) they do not have any continuing liability to seizures.

A20.4

D

Sudden reflex bradycardia with vasodilatation both peripheral and splanchnic leads to loss of consciousness – a fainting attack. This is simple syncope (also known as neurocardiogenic syncope), a common response to prolonged standing, fear, venesection or pain. Syncope almost never occurs in the recumbent posture. The subject falls to the ground and is unconscious for less than 2 minutes. Recovery is rapid. Jerking movements can occur. Incontinence of urine is exceptional. This is the simple faint that over half the population experience at some time, particularly in childhood, in youth or in pregnancy.

A20.5

C

Pure spinothalamic lesions cause isolated contralateral loss of pain and temperature sensation below the level of the lesion. This is called dissociated sensory loss – pain and temperature are dissociated from light touch, which remains preserved. This is seen typically in syringomyelia where a cavity occupies the central spinal cord.

A20.6

B

Involvement of one spinothalamic tract (contralateral loss of pain and temperature) together with one corticospinal tract (ipsilateral pyramidal signs) is known as the Brown–Séquard syndrome of hemisection of the cord. The patient complains of numbness on one side and weakness on the other.

A20.7

B

Tremor exacerbated by action, with past pointing and accompanying slowness and incoordination of rapid alternating movement (dysdiadochokinesis), occur in cerebellar lobe disease and with lesions of cerebellar connections. Titubation (head tremor) and nystagmus may be present. Multiple sclerosis is a common cause of cerebellar dysfunction.

A20.8

D

In Wernicke's aphasia (receptive aphasia, posterior aphasia) left temporo-parietal damage leaves language that is fluent but the words themselves are incorrect. This varies from insertion of a few incorrect or nonexistent words into fluent speech to a profuse outpouring of jargon (that is, rubbish with wholly nonexistent words). Severe jargon aphasia may be so bizarre as to be confused with psychotic behaviour. Patients who have recovered from Wernicke's aphasia say that when aphasic they found speech, both their own and others', like a wholly unintelligible foreign language. They could neither stop themselves nor understand themselves or those around them.

A20.9

B

Suspected herpes simplex encephalitis is treated immediately with intravenous aciclovir, the active form of which inhibits DNA synthesis. Phosphorylation of aciclovir is dependent upon viral thymidine kinase; the drug is thus specific for herpesvirus infections.

A20.10

C

The elements of tabes dorsalis are: a) lightning pains; b) ataxia, stamping gait, reflex and sensory loss, muscle wasting; c) neuropathic joints (Charcot joints); d) Argyll Robertson pupils; e) ptosis and optic atrophy.

A20.11

C

Nominal aphasia (anomic aphasia or amnestic aphasia) describes difficulty naming familiar objects. Naming difficulty is an early sign in all types of aphasia. A left posterior temporal/inferior parietal lesion causes a severe, isolated form.

A20.12

A

Disorders in right-handed patients with right hemisphere lesions are often difficult to recognize. They comprise abnormalities of perception of internal and external space. Examples are losing the way in familiar surroundings, failing to put on clothing correctly (dressing apraxia), or failure to draw simple shapes – constructional apraxia.

Neurological disease

A20.13

B

Disorders of memory follow damage to the medial surfaces of both temporal lobes and their brainstem connections – the hippocampi, fornices and mammillary bodies. Bilateral lesions are necessary to cause amnesia. It is characteristic of all organic disorders of memory that more recent events are recalled poorly, in contrast to the relative preservation of distant memories.

A20.14

D

Causes of optic disc swelling (papilloedema)	
Raised intracranial pressure Brain tumour, abscess, haematoma, intracranial haemorrhage and SAH, idiopathic intracranial hypertension, hydrocephalus, encephalitis	**Venous occlusion** Cavernous sinus thrombosis Central retinal vein thrombosis/occlusion Orbital mass lesions
Optic nerve disease Optic neuritis (e.g. multiple sclerosis) Hereditary optic neuropathy Ischaemic optic neuropathy (e.g. giant cell arteritis) Toxic optic neuropathy (e.g. methanol ingestion Hypervitaminosis A	**Retinal vascular disease** Malignant hypertension Vasculitis (e.g. SLE) **Metabolic causes** Hypercapnia, chronic hypoxia, hypocalcaemia **Disc infiltration** Leukaemia, sarcoidosis, optic nerve glioma

SAH, subarachnoid haemorrhage: SLE, systemic lupus erythematosus

A20.15

B

In the light reflex afferent fibres in each optic nerve (some crossing in the chiasm) pass to both lateral geniculate bodies and relay to the Edinger–Westphal nuclei via the pretectal nucleus. Efferent (parasympathetic) fibres from each Edinger–Westphal nucleus pass via the third nerve to the ciliary ganglion and thence to the pupil. Light constricts the pupil being illuminated (direct reflex) and, by the consensual reflex, the contralateral pupil.

A20.16

E

In the convergence reflex fixation on a near object requires convergence of the ocular axes and is accompanied by pupillary constriction. Afferent fibres in each optic nerve, which pass through both lateral geniculate bodies, also relay to the convergence centre. This centre receives 1a spindle afferent fibres from the extraocular muscles – principally medial recti – which are innervated by the third nerve. The efferent route is from the convergence centre to the Edinger–Westphal nucleus, ciliary ganglion and pupils. Voluntary or reflex fixation on a near object is thus accompanied by appropriate convergence and pupillary constriction.

A20.17

D

After previous left retrobulbar neuritis: a) light shone in the left eye causes both left and right pupils to constrict; b) when light is shone into the intact right eye, both pupils again constrict (i.e. right direct and consensual reflexes are intact); c) when the light source is then swung to the previously affected left eye, its pupil dilates, relative to its previous state. The finding of a left RAPD by the swinging light test, showing that the consensual reflex is stronger than the direct, indicates residual damage in the afferent pupillary fibres of the left optic nerve.

A20.18

C

Causes of Horner's syndrome

Hemisphere and brainstem	Sympathetic chain in neck
Massive cerebral infarction	Following thryoid/laryngeal surgery
Pontine glioma	Carotid artery occlusion and dissection
Lateral medullary syndrome	Neoplastic infiltration
'Coning' of the temporal lobe	Cervical sympathectomy
Cervical cord	**Miscellaneous**
Syringomyelia	Congenital
Cord tumours	Migrainous neuralgia (usually transient)
T1 root	Isolated and of unknown cause
Bronchial neoplasm (apical)	
Apical tuberculosis	
Cervical rib	
Brachial plexus trauma	

Horner's syndrome is a collection of signs – of unilateral pupillary constriction with slight relative ptosis and enophthalmos – which indicate a lesion of the sympathetic pathway on the same side. The conjunctival vessels are slightly injected. Causes of Horner's syndrome are shown in the table. There is loss of sweating of the same side of the face or body, the extent depending upon the level of the lesion. Central lesions affect sweating over the entire half of the head, arm and upper trunk.

A20.19

C

The Argyll Robertson pupil is a small, irregular (3 mm or less) pupil which is fixed to light but constricts on convergence. The lesion is in the brainstem in neural tissue surrounding the aqueduct of Sylvius. The Argyll Robertson pupil is (almost) diagnostic of neurosyphilis. Similar changes are occasionally seen in diabetes mellitus. Myotonic pupil (Holmes–Adie pupil) is a dilated pupil seen most commonly in young women. It is usually unilateral, and the pupil is often irregular. There is no reaction (or a very slow reaction) to bright light and also incomplete constriction to convergence. The condition is due to denervation in the ciliary ganglion, of unknown cause.

A20.20

C

Progressive supranuclear palsy (Steele–Richardson–Olzewski syndrome) is the most common parkinson-plus disorder, and consists of parkinsonism, axial rigidity, falls, dementia, and inability to move the eyes vertically or laterally. Other examples are multiple system atrophies,

Neurological disease

such as olivo-ponto-cerebellar degeneration and primary autonomic failure (Shy–Drager syndrome). These conditions tend to be progressive, unresponsive to levodopa and cause death within a decade.

A20.21

E

Internuclear ophthalmoplegia (INO) is one of the more common complex brainstem oculomotor signs and is seen commonly in multiple sclerosis. When present bilaterally, INO is almost pathognomonic of this disease. Unilateral lesions are also caused by small brainstem infarcts. In a right INO there is a lesion of the right medial longitudinal fasciculus (MLF). On attempted left lateral gaze the right eye fails to ADduct. The left eye develops coarse nystagmus in ABduction. The side of the lesion is on the side of impaired adduction, not on the side of the (obvious, unilateral) nystagmus.

A20.22

C

Typically in complete third cranial nerve palsy the affected pupil is fixed and dilated. Sparing of the pupil means that parasympathetic fibres which run in a discrete bundle on the superior surface of the nerve remain undamaged, and so the pupil is of normal size and reacts normally. In diabetes, infarction of the third nerve usually spares the pupil. A glycosylated haemoglobin of 12 suggests poorly controlled diabetes mellitus (normal 3.7–5.1%) making this the best option.

A20.23

D

At the cerebellopontine angle, the trigeminal nerve is compressed by: a) acoustic neuroma; b) meningioma; c) secondary neoplasm. As these lesions enlarge, the neighbouring seventh and eighth nerves become involved, producing facial weakness and deafness.

A20.24

B

Cord compression is a medical emergency. It is sometimes difficult to distinguish chronic progressive cord compression from other (medical) causes of worsening paraparesis and tetraparesis on clinical grounds alone: the principal reason for this is that pain at the site of compression and a sensory level can be absent. Early recognition of cord compression is vital. MR identifies most lesions and has entirely replaced contrast myelography.

A20.25

D

Patients with classical syringomyelia associated with the Arnold–Chiari malformation usually develop symptoms at the age of 20–30. Upper limb pain exacerbated by exertion or coughing is typical. Spinothalamic sensory loss (pain and temperature) leads to painless upper limb burns, and trophic changes. Difficulty in walking with paraparesis develops. The following are typical signs of a cervical syrinx: a) areas of 'dissociated' sensory loss, i.e. spinothalamic loss without loss of light touch. Bizarre patterns are seen. b) Loss of upper limb reflexes. c) Muscle wasting in the hand and forearm. d)

Spastic paraparesis – initially mild and symptomless. e) Neuropathic joints, trophic skin changes (scars, nail dystrophy) and ulcers. f) Brainstem signs – as the syrinx extends into the brainstem (syringobulbia), there is tongue atrophy and fasciculation, bulbar palsy, nystagmus, Horner's syndrome, hearing loss and impairment of facial sensation.

A20.26

C

Hemiballismus is violent swinging movements of one side caused usually by infarction or haemorrhage in the contralateral subthalamic nucleus.

A20.27

C

At the apex of the petrous temporal bone, spreading infection from the middle ear, or a secondary tumour, damages the nerve. The combination of a fifth nerve lesion with pain and a sixth nerve lesion is called Gradenigo's syndrome.

A20.28

C

The seventh (facial) nerve is largely motor in function. In Bell's palsy the patient notices marked unilateral facial weakness, sometimes with loss of taste on the anterior two-thirds of the tongue. Pain behind the ear is common at onset. Diagnosis is made on clinical grounds. No other cranial nerves are involved.

A20.29

C

Ménière's disease is characterized by recurrent attacks of the three symptoms – vertigo, tinnitus and deafness. Sudden, unprovoked attacks of vertigo with vomiting and loss of balance last from minutes to hours. Tinnitus and deafness accompany an attack but may be overshadowed by the degree of vertigo. Vestibular neuronitis is characterized by an acute attack of isolated severe vertigo with nystagmus, often with vomiting, but without loss of hearing. Positional vertigo is vertigo precipitated by head movements, usually into a particular position. It may occur when turning in bed or on sitting up.

A20.30

B

'Bulbar palsy' is a general term describing palatal, pharyngeal and tongue weakness of lower motor neurone (LMN) type. The patient complains of difficulty in swallowing, hoarseness, nasal regurgitation and choking (particularly with fluids) – a dangerous situation. Bilateral combined lesions of the ninth and tenth nerves cause visible weakness of elevation of the palate, depression of palatal sensation and loss of the gag reflex. The vagal recurrent laryngeal branches are involved. The cough is depressed and the vocal cords paralysed.

Neurological disease

A20.31

B

This patient has right recurrent laryngeal nerve palsy. The left recurrent laryngeal nerve loops beneath the aorta making aneurysm of the aorta an unlikely cause. The other conditions do not cause recurrent laryngeal nerve palsy.

A20.32

C

All surviving subarachnoid haemorrhage (SAH) cases should be discussed urgently with a specialist centre for a decision about angiography and possible surgery. Nearly half the cases of SAH are either dead or moribund before they reach hospital. Of the remainder, a further 10–20% die in the early weeks in hospital from rebleeding. Delay in diagnosis of minor SAH without coma (or mistaking the sudden headache for migraine) contributes to this mortality.

A20.33

B

Ethosuximide has been shown to be ineffective in preventing tonic–clonic seizures whereas the others have demonstrated efficacy.

A20.34

B

Valproate and ethosuximide have been found to be effective in petit mal epilepsy whereas the others listed either worsen seizures or are ineffective in this condition.

A20.35

1) G   2) E   3) F   4) B   5) C

Chronic (benign) and recurrent headaches: almost all recurring headaches lasting hours or days – band-like, generalized head pains, with a history going back for several years or months – are vaguely ascribed to muscle tension and/or migraine. Malignant hypertension, with arterial damage and brain swelling, occasionally causes headache. Headaches are not caused by high blood pressure alone. Eyestrain from underlying refractive error is not itself a cause of headache, though new prescription lenses sometimes provoke pain. Any headache, however mild, that is present on waking and made worse by coughing, straining or sneezing may well be due to a mass lesion. Vomiting often accompanies pressure headaches. Such headaches are caused early, over weeks, by posterior fossa masses. Patches of exquisite tenderness overlying superficial scalp arteries are caused by giant cell arteritis. A single episode of severe headache may be caused by subarachnoid haemorrhage.

A20.36

1) D   2) E   3) C   4) A   5) B

Spasticity, particularly in extensor muscles, with or without pyramidal weakness, causes stiffness and jerkiness of walking. The toes of shoes catch level ground, and become scuffed. The pace shortens but a narrow base is maintained. Clonus may be noticed as involuntary extensor rhythmic jerking of the legs. In Parkinson's disease there is muscular rigidity throughout leg extensors and flexors. While power is preserved, the gait slows. The pace shortens to a shuffle; the base remains narrow. Falls occur. A stoop becomes apparent and arm swinging is diminished. The gait becomes festinant (hurried) in small rapid steps. There is particular difficulty initiating movement and turning quickly. Retropulsion describes small backwards steps, taken involuntarily when a patient is stopped or is halted. In disease of the lateral cerebellar lobes the stance becomes broad-based, unstable and tremulous. Ataxia describes this state of imperfect control. The gait tends to veer towards the side of the more affected cerebellar lobe. In sensory ataxia, broad-based, high-stepping, or stamping gait develops. This ataxia is made worse by removal of additional sensory input, such as in darkness. When the patient closes the eyes while standing, he becomes unstable. With frontal lobe disease (e.g. tumour, hydrocephalus, infarction), there is disorganization of walking as an acquired skill. Leg movement is normal when sitting or lying but initiation and organization of walking fail. This is apraxia of gait – a failure of the skilled movement of walking.

A20.37

1) E   2) F   3) D   4) C   5) B or A

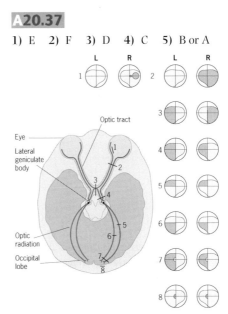

The visual pathway
1. Paracentral scotoma–retinal lesion.
2. Mononuclear field loss–optic nerve lesion.
3. Bitemporal hemianopia–chiasmal lesion.
4. Homonymous hemianopia–optic tract lesion.
5. Homonymous quadrantanopia–temporal lesion.
6. Homonymous quadrantanopia–parietal lesion.
7. Homonymous hemianopia–occipital cortex or optic radiation.
8. Homonymous hemianopia–occipital pole lesion.
Dark grey = lesion; light grey = normal field.

A20.38

1) C   2) D   3) A   4) B   5) A

In the normal caloric test: a) ice-cold water in the left ear causes nystagmus with fast movement to the right; b) warm water in the left ear causes nystagmus with the fast movement to the left. A fine pendular, jelly-like nystagmus is a sign of a multiple sclerosis (MS) brainstem plaque, or brainstem glioma. Down-beat jerk nystagmus is caused by lesions around the foramen magnum.

Neurological disease

A20.39

1) B 2) C 3) E 4) F 5) B

Spinal level	Reflex
C5–6	Supinator
C5–6	Biceps
C7	Triceps
L3–4	Knee
S1	Ankle

A20.40

1) E 2) D 3) C 4) B 5) A

Parkinson's disease is characterized by slowness, stiffness and rest tremor. Degeneration in SN*c* causes loss of dopamine activity in the striatum. Dopamine is excitatory for synapse A and inhibitory for synapse B. Through the direct pathway there is reduced activity at synapse F, leading to increased inhibitory output (G) and decreased cortical activity (H). Huntington's disease is an inherited dementia with progressive jerky movements (chorea). Chorea may result from damage to neurones (GABA, enkephalin) in the indirect pathway from striatum to GP*l*, reducing activity at synapse C. In turn, there is increased inhibition of subthalamic neurones at D, reduced stimulation at E and decreased inhibition of VA/VL at G. Cortical activity at H increases. Hemiballismus describes wild, flinging limb movements usually caused by a small infarct in the subthalamic nucleus (SThN). This reduces excitatory activity at synapse E, resulting in a reduction of inhibition at G with increased activity of thalamo-cortical neurones and increased activity at H (see Fig. 20.9, p. 1146 of the 5th edition of Kumar & Clark, 2002).

Midline cerebellar vermis lesions have a dramatic effect on the equilibrium of the trunk and axial musculature. This truncal ataxia means difficulty in standing and sitting unsupported, with a rolling, broad, ataxic gait. Lesions of the flocculonodular region of the cerebellum cause vertigo, vomiting and ataxia of gait if they extend to the roof of the fourth ventricle. In parietal cortex lesions sensory loss, neglect of one side, apraxia and subtle disorders of sensation occur. Pain is not a feature of destructive cortical lesions. Irritative phenomena (e.g. partial sensory seizures from a glioma) arising in the parietal cortex cause tingling sensations in a limb, or elsewhere.

A20.41

1) A 2) A 3) C 4) A 5) B

Sympathetic T12–L2 is the nerve supply for bladder wall relaxation, internal sphincter contraction, orgasm and ejaculation. Parasympathetic S2–4 nerve supply includes bladder wall contraction, internal sphincter relaxation, penis and clitoris erection/engorgement. Pudendal nerves supply the external sphincter.

A20.42

1) E   2) D   3) C   4) B

Differentiation of forms of unresponsiveness				
Condition	Vegetative state	Locked-in syndrome	Coma	Brainstem death
Self-awareness	Absent	Present	Absent	Absent
Cyclical eye opening	Present	Present	Absent	Absent
Glasgow Coma Scale	E4, M1–4, VI	E4, M1, V1	E1–2, M1–4, V1–2	E1, M1–2, V1
Motor function	No purposeful movement	Eye movement preserved in the vertical plane and able to blink volitionally	No purposeful movement	None or only reflex spinal movement
Pain perception	No/little	Yes	No/little	No
Respiration function	Normal	Normal	Depressed or varied	Absent
EEG activity	Delta theta; or slow alpha	Usually normal	Delta or theta, sometimes silent	Electrocerebral silence or theta
Cerebral metabolism	Reduced by 50% or more	Minimally or moderately reduced	Reduced by 50% or more	Greatly reduced or absent
Prognosis	Depends on cause and length	Depends on cause; recovery unlikely	Recovery, vegetative state, or death within 2–4 weeks	No recovery

Modified from Working Group of Royal College of Physicians (1996) The permanent vegetative state. *Journal of the Royal College of Physicians of London* **30**: 119–121.

A20.43

1) D   2) E   3) C   4) B   5) A

Cheyne–Stokes respiration (periodic respiration) is alternating hyperpnoea and apnoea. In primary neurological disease this points to bilateral cerebral dysfunction, usually deep in the hemispheres or in the upper brainstem, and is a sign of incipient coning. This respiratory pattern also occurs in metabolic comas, if there is CO_2 retention from pulmonary disease, with chronic hypoxia at high altitude above 3500 m and in normal people during sleep.

Kussmaul (acidotic) respiration is deep, sighing hyperventilation seen principally in diabetic ketoacidosis and uraemia. Central neurogenic (pontine) hyperventilation describes sustained, rapid, deep breathing seen with pontine lesions. It may be episodic, i.e. switch abruptly on and off. Ataxic respiration is shallow, halting, irregular respiration that occurs when the medullary respiratory centre is damaged. It frequently precedes death. Vomiting, hiccup and excessive yawning often indicate a lower brainstem lesion in a stuporose patient.

Neurological disease

1) D   2) C   3) A   4) B

Dilatation of one pupil, which becomes fixed to light, indicates herniation of the uncus of the temporal lobe (coning) which compresses the third nerve. This is a neurosurgical emergency. Horner's syndrome (ipsilateral pupillary constriction and ptosis) occurs with lesions of the hypothalamus and also, rarely, in coning. Bilateral mid-point reactive pupils (i.e. normal pupils) are characteristic in metabolic comas and following most CNS-depressant drugs except opiates. Bilateral light-fixed, dilated pupils are a cardinal sign of brainstem death. They also occur in deep coma of any cause, but particularly in coma due to barbiturate intoxication or hypothermia. Bilateral pinpoint, light-fixed pupils occur with pontine lesions (e.g. a pontine haemorrhage) that interrupt sympathetic pathways, and with opiate drugs. Bilateral mid-position light-fixed or slightly dilated light-fixed pupils (4–6 mm), which are sometimes irregular, are seen when brainstem damage interrupts the light reflex.

1) F   2) H   3) I   4) E   5) D
6) B   7) A   8) C

Thiamin deficiency leads to an amnestic syndrome (Wernicke–Korsakoff psychosis). It comprises a typical triad of ocular signs, ataxia and a confusional state because of ischaemic damage in the brainstem and its connections. Combined spinal cord and peripheral nerve damage is due to vitamin B_{12} deficiency. The patient complains initially of numbness and tingling of fingers and toes. There is combined distal sensory loss, particularly posterior column, absent ankle jerks (neuropathy), with cord disease – exaggerated knee jerks, extensor plantar responses. Macrocytosis with megaloblastic changes in bone marrow are usual but not invariable in subacute combined degeneration of the cord. Charcot–Marie–Tooth (CMT) disease also called peroneal muscular atrophy describes a common clinical phenotype – of distal limb wasting and weakness that slowly progresses over many years, mostly in the legs, with variable loss of sensation and reflexes. In advanced disease, distal wasting is so marked that the legs are said to resemble inverted champagne bottles. Many genetic variants of the CMT phenotype are recognized including involvement of the peripheral myelin gene in the commonest type. In myasthenia gravis, antibodies to postsynaptic membrane acetylcholine receptor protein cause blocking of neuromuscular transmission. In Lambert–Eaton myasthenic–myopathic syndrome (LEMS), antibodies to muscle calcium-channel components are found. In myotonias, defective chloride ion membrane conductance is associated with delayed muscle relaxation. In McArdle's syndrome, myophosphorylase deficiency produces weakness after exercise. Duchenne muscular dystrophy (DMD) is inherited as an X-linked recessive disorder, though one-third of cases are spontaneous mutants. DMD occurs in 1 in 3000 male infants. The DMD locus has been localized to the Xp21 region of the X chromosome; there is absence of the gene product – the protein dystrophin, which is a rod-shaped cytoskeletal muscle protein. DMD is usually obvious by the fourth year, and often causes death by 20. The boy with DMD is noticed to have difficulty in running and in rising to an erect position from the floor, when he has to use the hands to climb up his legs (Gowers's sign). There is initially a proximal limb weakness with pseudohypertrophy of the calves. The myocardium is affected. The boy becomes severely disabled by the age of 10.

A20.46

1) C   2) D   3) A   4) F

Features of transient ischaemic attacks

Anterior circulation	Posterior circulation
Carotid system	**Vertebrobasilar system**
Amaurosis fugax	Diplopia, vertigo, vomiting
Aphasia	Choking and dysarthria
Hemiparesis	Ataxia
Hemisensory loss	Hemisensory loss
Hemianopic visual loss	Hemianopic visual loss
	Transient global amnesia
	Tetraparesis
	Loss of consciousness (rare)

Transient ischaemic attacks (TIAs) cause sudden loss of function, usually within seconds, and last for minutes or hours (but by definition <24 hours). The site of damage is often suggested by the type of attack. The clinical features of the principal forms of TIA are given in the table. A TIA causing an episode of amaurosis fugax (sudden transient loss of vision in one eye) is often the first clinical evidence of internal carotid artery stenosis, which may herald a hemiparesis. The lateral medullary syndrome, also called posterior inferior cerebellar artery (PICA) thrombosis, or Wallenberg's syndrome, is the most widely recognized syndrome of brainstem infarction. Weber's syndrome is ipsilateral third nerve paralysis with a contralateral hemiplegia due to a lesion in one half of the midbrain. Paralysis of upward gaze is usually present.

A20.47

1) C   2) D   3) B   4) A

Typical CSF changes in meningitis

	Normal	Viral	Pyogenic	Tuberculosis
Appearance	Crystal-clear	Clear/turbid	Turbid/purulent	Turbid/viscous
Mononuclear cells	< 5 mm³	10–100 mm³	< 50 mm³	100–300 mm³
Polymorph cells	Nil	Nil*	200–300/mm³	0–200/mm³
Protein	0.2–0.4 g/L	0.4–0.8 g/L	0.5–2.0 g/L	0.5–3.0 g/L
Glucose	$^2/_3$ > $^1/_2$ blood glucose	> $^1/_2$ blood glucose	< $^1/_2$ blood glucose	< $^1/_2$ blood glucose

*Some polymorph cells may be seen in the early stages of viral meningitis and encephalitis

A20.48

1) B   2) C   3) E

The hallmark of a direct effect of a mass is local progressive deterioration of function. Tumours can occur anywhere within the brain. Three examples are given. a) A left frontal meningioma caused a frontal lobe syndrome over several years – a vague disturbance of personality, apathy and impairment of intellect. Expressive aphasia was followed by a progressive right hemiparesis as the corticospinal pathways became involved. As the mass enlarged further, pressure headaches and papilloedema developed. b) A right parietal lobe glioma caused a left homonymous field defect (optic radiation). Cortical sensory loss in the left limbs and left hemiparesis followed over 3 months. Partial seizures (episodes of tingling of the left limbs) developed. c) A left eighth nerve sheath neurofibroma (an acoustic neuroma or Schwannoma) growing in the cerebellopontine angle over 3 years caused progressive perceptive deafness (VIII), vertigo (VIII), numbness of the left side of the face (V) and facial weakness (VII), followed by cerebellar ataxia on the same side. Papilloedema is a late sequel.

A20.49

1) C   2) F   3) B   4) A   5) E

In peripheral neurofibromatosis (NF1) skin neurofibromas present as subcutaneous, soft, sometimes pedunculated, tumours. They increase in numbers throughout life. Multiple café-au-lait patches – pale brown macules 1–20 cm in diameter – develop. Isolated patches are common in the normal population; more than five patches is suggestive of neurofibromatosis. In central neurofibromatosis (NF2) many neural tumours occur: a) eighth-nerve sheath neurofibroma; b) spinal cord and nerve root neurofibroma (acoustic neuroma often bilateral); c) meningioma; d) glioma (including optic nerve glioma); e) plexiform neuroma (massive cutaneous overgrowth); f) cutaneous neurofibroma – these are few. Tuberous sclerosis is a rare autosomal dominant condition. It comprises adenoma sebaceum, epilepsy and mental retardation (often severe). Adenoma sebaceum are reddish nodules (angiofibromas) which develop on the cheeks in childhood. Other lesions include shagreen patches, amelanotic naevi, retinal phakomas (glial masses), renal tumours, glial overgrowth in brain and gliomas. Sturge–Weber syndrome is an extensive port-wine naevus on one side of the face (usually in the distribution of a division of the fifth nerve) and a leptomeningeal angioma. Epilepsy is common. Familial occurrence is exceptional. In von Hippel–Lindau syndrome retinal and cerebellar haemangioblastomas develop or, less commonly, haemangioblastomas of the cord and cerebrum. Most patients with Friedreich's ataxia are homozygous for the GAA triplet expansion in the Friedreich's ataxia gene. This gene, mapped to chromosome 9q13, encodes a mitochondrial protein of unknown function. Impaired mitochondrial ATP is likely to be involved. The expression of this protein, fraxatin, is decreased in Friedreich's patients.

A20.50

A) T   B) T   C) T   D) T   E) T

The abducens nerve supplies the lateral rectus muscle which causes the eye to ABduct. In a sixth nerve lesion there is a convergent squint with diplopia maximal on looking to the side of the lesion. The eye cannot be ABducted beyond the midline. There are many causes of a sixth nerve lesion, as the nerve has a long intracranial course. The nerve can be involved within the brainstem (e.g. multiple sclerosis or pontine glioma). In raised intracranial pressure it is compressed against the tip of the petrous temporal bone. The nerve sheath may be infiltrated by tumours, particularly nasopharyngeal carcinoma. An isolated sixth nerve palsy due to infarction occurs in diabetes mellitus. A sixth nerve lesion is a common sequel of head trauma.

A20.51

A) F   B) T   C) T   D) T   E) T

In sensorineural deafness, perception improves when the base of the vibrating tuning fork is placed on the mastoid process: sound is conducted directly to the ossicles through the bone.

Causes of sensorineural deafness	
End organ	Advancing age
	Occupational acoustic trauma
	Ménière's disease
	Drugs (e.g. gentamicin, neomycin)
Eighth nerve lesions	Acoustic neuroma
	Cranial trauma
	Inflammatory lesions:
	Tuberculous meningitis
	Sarcoidosis
	Neurosyphilis
	Carcinomatous meningitis
Brainstem lesions (rare)	Multiple sclerosis
	Infarction

A20.52

A) T   B) F   C) T   D) T   E) T

With a pyramidal (upper motor neurone, UMN) lesion, when both upper limbs are held outstretched, palms uppermost, the affected limb drifts downwards and medially. The forearm tends to pronate and the fingers flex slightly. This upper limb sign is often first to occur, sometimes before weakness or reflex changes become obvious. In the upper limb flexors remain stronger than extensors, while in the lower limb extensors remain stronger than flexors. In the upper arm the weaker movements are thus shoulder abduction and elbow extension; in the forearm and hand, wrist and finger extensors and abductors are weaker than their antagonists. This increase in tone affects all muscle groups on the side affected but is detectable most easily in stronger muscles. The tone itself is characterized by changing resistance to passive movement; the change is sudden – the clasp-knife effect. The tendon reflexes in the affected limbs become exaggerated and clonus is often evident. The normal flexor plantar response becomes extensor (a positive Babinski). In a severe lesion (e.g. the internal capsule infarct) this extensor response can be elicited from a wide area of the affected limb. The abdominal (and cremasteric reflexes) are abolished on the affected side.

A20.53

A) F   B) T   C) T   D) T   E) F

Efferent fibres pass from the cerebellum to: a) each red nucleus; b) vestibular nuclei; c) basal ganglia; d) corticospinal system. The cerebellum receives afferent fibres from: a) proprioceptive organs in joints and muscles; b) vestibular nuclei; c) basal ganglia; d) the corticospinal system; e) olivary nuclei.

A20.54

A) T   B) T   C) T   D) T   E) T

Everyone has a physiological tremor (often barely perceptible) of the outstretched hands at 8–12 Hz. This is increased with anxiety, hyperthyroidism and certain drugs (sympathomimetics, sodium valproate, lithium) or in mercury poisoning. A coarse, postural tremor is seen in chronic alcohol abusers and in benign essential tremor (usually at 5–8 Hz). Postural tremor does not worsen on movement, though it may become more obvious.

Neurological disease

A20.55

A) T   B) T   C) T   D) T   E) T

Examples of lower motor neurone lesions at various levels are: a) cranial nerve nuclei and anterior horn cell – Bell's palsy, motor neurone disease, poliomyelitis; b) spinal root – cervical and lumbar disc protrusion, neuralgic amyotrophy; c) peripheral (or cranial) nerve – nerve trauma or entrapment, mononeuritis multiplex.

A20.56

A) T   B) T   C) T   D) T   E) T

Lhermitte's phenomenon is an electric-shock-like sensation which radiates down the trunk and limbs when the neck is flexed. This indicates a cervical cord lesion. Lhermitte's sign is common in acute exacerbations of multiple sclerosis. It also occurs in cervical spondylotic myelopathy, subacute combined degeneration of the cord, radiation myelopathy, and occasionally in cord compression.

A20.57

A) T   B) T   C) T   D) T   E) T

Causes of spastic paraparesis include: a) parasagittal meningioma; b) motor neurone disease; c) spinal cord compression; d) multiple sclerosis; e) myelitis.

Causes of a spastic paraparesis

Spinal lesions
Spinal cord compression
Multiple sclerosis
Myelitis (e.g. varicella zoster virus)
Motor neurone disease
Subacute combined degeneration of the cord
Syringomyelia
Syphilis
Familial or sporadic paraparesis
Vascular disease of the cord
Non-metastatic manifestation of malignancy
Tropical spastic paraparesis (HTLV-1)
HIV-associated myelopathy

Cerebral lesions*
Parasagittal cortical lesions:
  Meningioma
  Venous sinus thrombosis
Hydrocephalus
Multiple cerebral infarction

*All are rare causes of a paraparesis
HTLV-1, human T-cell leukaemia virus

A20.58

A) T   B) T   C) F   D) T   E) T

Pain perception is mediated by free nerve endings, the terminations of finely myelinated A-delta and of non-myelinated C fibres. Sensory impulses enter the cord via dorsal spinal roots. Within it, impulses ascend either in each dorsal (posterior) column or in each spinothalamic tract. Gate theory proposes that the entry of afferent impulses is monitored by the cells of the substantia gelatinosa. Acupuncture achieves analgesia by a gating effect on large myelinated nerve fibres. Calcium-channel blockers (nifedipine) improve sympathetically mediated pain, as occurs in, for example, Raynaud's disease.

A20.59

A) F   B) F   C) F   D) F   E) F

Limitations of computed tomography (CT) include: a) lesions under 1 cm diameter may be missed; b) lesions with attenuation close to that of bone may be missed if near the skull; c) lesions with attenuation similar to that of brain are poorly imaged (e.g. multiple sclerosis plaques, isodense subdural haematoma); d) CT images sometimes miss lesions within the posterior fossa; e) the spinal cord is not imaged directly by CT (contrast is necessary); f) results are poor when patients cannot cooperate – a general anaesthetic is occasionally required. The principal advantages of MRI over CT are: a) MR images distinguish clearly between white matter and grey matter in the brain; b) spinal cord and nerve roots are imaged directly; c) imaging the pituitary; d) the resolution of MRI is greater than CT (lesions around 0.5 cm are seen); e) no radiation is involved; f) magnetic resonance angiography (MRA) images blood vessels without the need for contrast.

A20.60

A) F   B) F   C) F   D) F   E) F

Aspirin 300 mg daily should be given as soon as a diagnosis of ischaemic stroke or thromboembolic transient ischaemic attack is confirmed, reducing to 75 mg after several days. Immediate thrombolytic agents, such as intravenous tissue plasminogen activator (alteplase), are promising in the early treatment of ischaemic (non-haemorrhagic) stroke though not yet in general use in the UK. They must be given within 3 hours to be effective, presenting a logistic problem in many clinical settings. The transient hypertension often seen after acute stroke usually does not require treatment with hypotensive drugs provided the diastolic pressure does not remain consistently higher than 100 mmHg. If hypertension is sustained it needs treatment, but the pressure must be lowered slowly to avoid a sudden fall in cerebral perfusion pressure. Heparin and warfarin should be given when there is atrial fibrillation, other paroxysmal dysrhythmias or when there are certain cardiac valve lesions (uninfected) or cardiomyopathies. All patients on anticoagulants must be aware of the small risks of cerebral (and other) haemorrhage. The drugs are potentially dangerous in the 2 weeks following cerebral infarction because of the risk of provoking cerebral haemorrhage. Lumbar puncture is indicated only in unusual circumstances, such as when blood syphilitic serology is positive.

A20.61

A) T   B) T   C) T   D) T   E) T

Chronic phenytoin causes gum hypertrophy, hypertrichosis, osteomalacia, folate deficiency, polyneuropathy and encephalopathy.

A20.62

A) T   B) T   C) F   D) T   E) F

There is no laboratory test for Parkinson's disease. Diagnosis consists of recognizing the clinical pattern. Conventional imaging (MR) is unhelpful. PET scanning is used in research. Idiopathic Parkinson's disease must be distinguished from other akinetic–rigid syndromes. While no drugs alter the course of Parkinson's disease, levodopa and/or dopaminergic agonists produce striking initial symptomatic

Neurological disease

improvement. Selegiline, a monoamine oxidase B inhibitor, may delay the need for levodopa therapy by some months. Antioxidants are also used with this aim, but their value is unproven. Levodopa therapy does not alter the natural progression of Parkinson's disease. Depression is common in Parkinson's disease as symptoms worsen. SSRIs are the drugs of choice. Tricyclic antidepressants (e.g. amitriptyline) have extrapyramidal side-effects. Type A monoamine oxidase inhibitors (e.g. phenelzine) are absolutely contraindicated with levodopa.

A20.63

1) F B) T C) T D) T E) T

After several years of therapy, levodopa gradually becomes ineffective, even with increasing doses. As treatment continues, episodes of immobility develop (freezing). Falls are common. Fluctuation in response to levodopa also appears, its effect apparently turning on and off, causing freezing alternating with dopa-induced dyskinesias, chorea and dystonic movements. Levodopa's duration of action shrinks, with dyskinesia becoming prominent several hours after the dose (end-of-dose dyskinesia). The patient begins to suffer not only from Parkinson's disease but also from a chronic levodopa-induced syndrome. Approaches to treatment of these complications include: a) shortening the interval between levodopa doses and increasing each dose; b) selegiline, a type B monoamine oxidase inhibitor, inhibits catabolism of dopamine in the brain. This sometimes smoothes out the response to levodopa. c) Dopaminergic agonists (such as apomorphine) are added, or replace levodopa. d) Entacapone, a catechol-O-methyl transferase inhibitor, is used. e) Drug holidays – periods of drug withdrawal – are occasionally helpful. They require close supervision since severe relapse may follow levodopa withdrawal.

A20.64

A) F B) T C) T D) T E) F

Neuroleptic drugs (i.e. phenothiazines and butyrophenones) produce varieties of movement disorder. They include: a) akathisia, which is a restless, repetitive and irresistible need to move. b) Acute dystonic reactions sometimes follow, dramatically and unpredictably, single doses of neuroleptics, and related drugs widely used as antiemetics and vestibular sedatives (such as prochlorperazine and metoclopramide). Spasmodic torticollis, trismus and oculogyric crises (i.e. episodes of sustained upward gaze) occur. Both the offending drug, and all drugs from the same group, should be avoided subsequently. c) Chronic tardive dyskinesias are mouthing and lip-smacking grimaces of the face and neck. These disabling disorders tend to occur several years after commencing neuroleptic therapy and may be made temporarily worse when the dose of the drug is reduced. Resolution seldom occurs when the drug can be stopped.

A20.65

A) F B) T C) T D) T E) F

In Huntington's disease mutation has been identified in the distal short arm of chromosome 4 (4p16.3) with a variable expansion of a CAG-repeat sequence located in exon 1 of a large gene containing 67 exons. The majority of adult Huntington cases have CAG expansions of 40–55 repeats, while expansions of greater than 70 repeats are associated with onset of the disease in childhood. This results in translation of an extended glutamine sequence in huntingtin, the protein product of the gene. Huntingtin is expressed throughout the body. Its function is unclear. Imaging in Huntington's, if it is possible with the chorea, shows caudate nucleus atrophy. There is steady progression of both dementia and chorea. No treatment arrests the disease, although phenothiazines (e.g. sulpiride) may reduce chorea, by causing drug-induced parkinsonism. Sydenham's chorea is a postinfective chorea occurring largely in children and young adults.

A20.66

A) F   B) F   C) F   D) F   E) F

In primary torsion dystonia (PTD), dystonia affecting gait and posture commences in childhood and progresses, spreading to all parts of the body over one to four decades. Cognitive function is not impaired. Spontaneous remissions very occasionally occur. This rare disease is usually inherited as an autosomal dominant. A PTD gene has been located on chromosome 9 (9q34); this is a deletion of three base pairs encoding an ATP-binding protein torsin A.

A20.67

A) T   B) F   C) T   D) F   E) T

In multiple sclerosis blurring of vision in one eye develops over hours or days, varying between a sensation of looking through frosted glass to severe unilateral visual loss, but rarely complete blindness. Mild ocular pain is usual. Recovery occurs, typically within 1 or 2 months. The optic disc appearance depends upon the site of the plaque within the optic nerve. When

the lesion is in the nerve head there is disc swelling. If the lesion is several millimetres behind the disc there are often no ophthalmoscopic features – 'the doctor sees nothing and the patient sees nothing'. This is retrobulbar neuritis. MRI of brain and spinal cord is the first-line investigation. Multiple plaques are visible, principally in the periventricular region, brainstem, and cervical cord. Lesions are rarely visible on CT. Peripheral blood and urine tests are unhelpful. Delay in visual-evoked responses (VER) follows optic neuropathy (ON). As some ON attacks are subclinical, a delayed VER can provide evidence of a previous optic nerve lesion. This provides valuable evidence of a second CNS lesion in, for example, an undiagnosed and apparently solitary spinal cord lesion. Short courses of corticosteroids for several days, are used widely in relapses and do sometimes reduce their severity. They do not influence long-term outcome. Beta-interferon (both interferon beta 1b and 1a) by self-administered injection is available in relapsing and remitting disease. This reduces the relapse rate by a third and prevents an increase in lesions seen on MRI over time. Long-term outcome is unclear.

A20.68

A) F   B) F   C) F   D) T   E) F

When meningococcal meningitis is diagnosed clinically by the petechial rash, immediate parenteral antibiotic treatment should be given before any investigations. In this acute illness, minutes save lives. The condition is lethal, and even with optimal care mortality is around 15%. Lumbar puncture is usually contraindicated if the clinical diagnosis is meningococcal disease, because coning of

Neurological disease

the cerebellar tonsils may follow – the organism is found by blood culture. Meningococcal infection should be notified to local public health authorities, and advice sought about immunization and prophylaxis of contacts with rifampicin. MenC, a meningococcal C conjugate vaccine, is available and is part of routine childhood UK immunization. Reported cases have reduced. This vaccine should be given to case contacts.

A20.69

A) F   B) F   C) T   D) T   E) T

When drugs are necessary to prevent migraine, the following are helpful: a) pizotifen (a 5-HT antagonist) 0.5 mg at night for several days, increasing to 1.5 mg at night – common side-effects are slight weight gain and drowsiness; b) propranolol 10 mg three times daily, increasing to 40–80 mg three times daily; c) methysergide (a 5-HT antagonist) 2–6 mg daily – an occasional side-effect is periaortitis which precludes use for longer than 6 months; d) amitriptyline 10–30 mg at night is sometimes helpful; e) sodium valproate, verapamil, nifedipine and naproxen are also used.

A20.70

A) T   B) T   C) F   D) T   E) T

Giant cell arteritis (GCA) is a granulomatous arteritis of unknown aetiology occurring chiefly over the age of 60. It affects extradural arteries. Immediate high doses of steroids (prednisolone, initially 60–100 mg daily) should be started in a patient with typical features, even before biopsy. The dose is reduced as the ESR falls. A frequent feature of treated GCA is that headache subsides within hours of the first large steroid dose. Opinions differ about the need for long-term steroids. The diagnosis should be established immediately by superficial temporal artery biopsy because of the risk of blindness. Visual loss owing to arterial inflammation and occlusion occurs in 25% of cases of untreated GCA.

A20.71

A) T   B) T   C) T   D) T   E) T

Principal local complications of skull fracture are: a) meningeal artery rupture – causing extradural haematoma; b) dural vein tears – causing subdural haematoma; c) or CSF rhinorrhoea/otorrhoea with the risk of meningitis.

A20.72

A) T   B) T   C) T   D) T   E) T   F) T

Mechanisms of traumatic brain injury (TBI) are complex and interrelated: a) axonal and neuronal damage – shearing and rotational stresses on decelerating brain, often at sites distant from impact (*contrecoup* effect); b) axonal and neuronal damage from direct trauma; c) brain oedema; d) raised intracranial pressure; e) brain hypoxia; f) brain ischaemia.

A20.73

A) T   B) T   C) T   D) T   E) T

Late sequelae of traumatic brain injury include: a) incomplete and prolonged recovery – e.g. cognitive impairment, hemiparesis; b) post-traumatic epilepsy; c) chronic traumatic encephalopathy – this follows repeated (and often minor) injuries. This 'punch drunk' syndrome is cognitive impairment with extrapyramidal and pyramidal signs. It is seen principally in professional boxers. d) The post-traumatic (post-concussional) syndrome describes the vague complaints of headache, dizziness and malaise that follow even minor head injuries. Litigation is frequently an issue. Depression is prominent. Symptoms may be prolonged; e) benign paroxysmal positional vertigo; f) chronic subdural haematoma; g) hydrocephalus .

A20.74

A) T   B) F   C) T   D) F   E) T

There are no specific tests for motor neurone disease; diagnosis is clinical – and usually motor neurone disease is an easily identifiable condition. Remission is unknown. The disease progresses, spreading gradually, and causes death, often from bronchopneumonia. Survival for more than 3 years is unusual. No treatment has been shown to influence outcome, although riluzole, a sodium-channel blocker that inhibits glutamate release, has been shown to slow progression slightly, particularly in patients with disease of bulbar onset.

A20.75

A) T   B) T   C) T   D) T   E) T

The precise cause of damage in an individual child with cerebral palsy may be difficult to determine. The following are responsible: a) hypoxia in utero and/or during parturition; b) neonatal cerebral haemorrhage and/or infarction; c) trauma, neonatal or during parturition; d) prolonged seizures – status epilepticus or hypoglycaemia; e) kernicterus.

A20.76

A) F   B) F   C) T   D) T   E) T

Many cases of carpal tunnel syndrome are idiopathic, but this entrapment neuropathy is sometimes seen in: a) hypothyroidism; b) diabetes mellitus; c) pregnancy and obesity; d) rheumatoid arthritis; e) acromegaly.

A20.77

A) T   B) T   C) T   D) T   E) F

Multifocal neuropathy or mononeuritis multiplex occurs in: a) diabetes mellitus; b) leprosy (commonest cause world-wide); c) vasculitis; d) sarcoidosis; e) amyloidosis; f) malignancy; g) neurofibromatosis; h) HIV infection; i) Guillain–Barré syndrome (typically polyneuropathy); j) idiopathic multifocal motor neuropathy. Diagnosis is largely clinical, supported by electrical studies.

A20.78

A) F   B) F   C) T   D) T   E) F

Campylobacter jejuni and cytomegalovirus infections are well-recognized causes of severe Guillain-Barré syndrome (GBS). Diagnosis is established on clinical grounds and confirmed by nerve conduction studies; these show slowing of conduction in the common demyelinating form, prolonged distal motor latency and/or conduction block. CSF protein is typically raised to 1–3 g/L. The cell count and sugar level remain normal. High-dosage intravenous γ-globulin reduces the duration and severity of paralysis. Corticosteroids were used for many years but have been shown to be of no value.

Psychological medicine

Q21.1

A 38-year-old artist presents with a history of excessive energy and elevated mood. She talks fast and is unable to sleep. This is the first time she has had these symptoms. The psychiatrist who sees her diagnoses that she has a severe manifestation of her illness. The best management of her condition is which one of the following?

A. Beta blockers
B. Lithium only
C. Haloperidol
D. Haloperidol for 2–3 months with lithium
E. Haloperidol lifelong with lithium
F. Haloperidol for 2–3 weeks with lithium

Q21.2

A 68-year-old hypertensive has a history of repeated transient ischaemic attacks with brief impairment of consciousness. Progressively the patient has had an impaired ability to carry out motor activities, despite intact motor function. There has been a failure to recognize or identify objects despite intact sensory function, and he has had increased difficulty with names and in understanding what is being said. The most likely diagnosis is which one of the following?

A. Alzheimer's disease
B. Multi-infarct dementia
C. Dementia with Lewy bodies
D. Pick's disease
E. Acute psychosis

Q21.3

A 45-year-old man with a 20-year history of drinking about 15 units of alcohol every day decides to stop drinking. He makes a clean break and stops suddenly. Three days later his wife brings him to the accident and emergency department because he is agitated and disorientated. He says he can see small animals or insects coming menacingly towards him. He has marked tremor, sweating, tachycardia, tachypnoea and pyrexia. The most likely diagnosis is which one of the following?

A. Pneumonia with meningitis
B. Unmasking of underlying paranoid schizophrenia
C. Delirium tremens
D. Catatonic schizophrenia
E. That he is most likely abusing intravenous drugs in addition to alcohol

Q21.4

A 22-year-old drug addict initially experienced increased sweating, running nose and restlessness. Now he has aches and pains, muscular twitching, abdominal cramps, vomiting and diarrhoea and is agitated. His blood pressure is elevated. The most likely cause of his symptoms is which one of the following?

A. Glue sniffing
B. The effects of cannabis
C. Dependence on benzodiazepines
D. Opiate withdrawal
E. Misuse of amphetamines

Q21.5

A 45-year-old man on long-term lithium therapy presents with drowsiness, nausea, vomiting, blurred vision, a coarse tremor, ataxia and dysarthria. On examination his blood pressure is elevated. The most likely cause of his clinical picture is which one of the following?

A. Recurrence of his mania
B. A manifestation of resolving mania
C. The symptoms suggest associated catatonic schizophrenia
D. Lithium level of 4 mmol/L
E. Hypertensive encephalopathy

Q21.6

1. The patient believes that his thoughts are being planted in his mind by someone else

2. The patient complains that his thoughts are being taken away from him without his control

3. A recurrent, persistent thought impulse, image or musical theme enters the patient's mind despite the individual's effort to resist it

4. A repetitive and purposeful action that is performed in a stereotyped way

5. A patient, on being offered a glass of wine, believes that this indicates that he is Jesus Christ

Select the best match for each of the above

A. Mood change
B. Disorder of the stream of thought
C. Disorder of the form of thought
D. Thought content
E. Abnormal belief

Q21.7

1. Misperceptions of external stimuli
2. A perception in the absence of a stimulus
3. A change in self-awareness so that the person feels unreal or detached from their body
4. An unpleasant feeling that the external environment has become unreal and/or remote
5. A sudden familiarity with a situation or event as having been encountered before when it is in fact novel
6. Failure to recognize a situation or event that has been encountered before

Select the best match for each of the above

A. Déjà vu
B. Jamais vu
C. Derealization
D. Depersonalization
E. Hallucination
F. Illusion

Q21.8

1. Despite being told that a close relative has died, the patient continues to behave as though the relative were still alive

2. Attribution to another person of thoughts that are in fact one's own

3. The exclusion from awareness of memories, emotions and/or impulses that would cause anxiety or distress if allowed to enter consciousness

4. A 23-year-old patient with severe congestive heart failure and leukaemia becomes child-like and highly dependent on her parents

5. Transfer of emotion from a situation with which it is properly associated to another that gives less distress

Select the best match for each of the above

A. Sublimation
B. Repression
C. Regression
D. Projection
E. Identification
F. Displacement
G. Denial

Q21.9

1. A 22-year-old patient with atypical facial pain

2. A 42-year-old man with tension headaches

3. A 35-year-old patient with irritable bowel syndrome with constipation as the dominant symptom

4. A 23-year-old patient with irritable bowel syndrome with diarrhoea as the dominant symptom

5. An 18-year-old girl with severe headache, irritability, breast tenderness and abdominal discomfort just before menstruation (symptoms diminish or disappear after the period starts)

Select the best option for treatment of each of the above

A. Selective serotonin reuptake inhibitors
B. Dosulepin (dothiepin)
C. Amitryptyline
D. Angiotensin-converting enzyme inhibitors
E. Steroids

Q21.10

1. A 39-year-old man is unable to recall a long period of his life and even denies knowledge of that period including his identity at that time

2. A 39-year-old woman who left her home town and has been living in another country has no recollection of her past and when found by her relatives denies any memory of her whereabouts during this wandering

3. A 58-year-old surgeon who has clinical features of dementia including memory loss. His dementia improves with behaviour therapy, electroconvulsive therapy and SSRIs

4. A 41-year-old woman, who is unable to recall long periods of her life, is administered intravenous midazolam – this produces a dramatic but short-lived recollection of the past

5. A 52-year-old architect feels the world looks grey, no longer has a zest for life and has no interest in his work

Select the best match for each of the above

A. Anhedonia
B. Dissociative amnesia
C. Depressive pseudodementia
D. Dissociative pseudodementia
E. Fugue
F. Abreaction

Q21.11

1. Dosulepin (dothiepin)
2. Venlafaxine
3. Nefazodone
4. Mirtazapine
5. Reboxetine
6. Moclobemide
7. Phenelzine

Select the mechanism of action of each of the above

A. Selective noradrenaline (norepinephrine) reuptake inhibitor (NaRI)
B. Monoamine oxidase inhibitor (MAOI)
C. Reversible inhibitor of monoamine oxidase A (RIMA)
D. Tricyclic antidepressant
E. Blocks both serotonin and noradrenaline (norepinephrine) reuptake (sNaRI)
F. $5\text{-}HT_2$ receptor antagonist and α_2-adrenergic blocker (NaSSA)
G. $5\text{-}HT_2$ receptor antagonist with weak sNARI activity

Q21.12

1. Feeling sad, tearful, melancholic or low in spirits
2. Thought block where the mind goes blank
3. The patient's thoughts rapidly jump from one topic to another so that one train of thought is not completed before another appears
4. An internal feeling of exasperation or anger
5. When the patient experiences their thoughts being understood by others without talking

A. Mood change
B. Disorder of the stream of thought
C. Disorder of the form of thought
D. Thought content
E. Abnormal belief

Q21.13

1. A 29-year-old man fears being away from home. He avoids travelling, walking down a road and even going to shops
2. A 33-year-old man fears travelling in a small elevator alone
3. A 42-year-old woman fears spiders
4. A 22-year-old woman has repeated sudden attacks of anxiety during which she has trouble taking a deep breath, and suffers palpitations, chest discomfort, a choking sensation and dizziness

Select the best match for each of the above

A. Claustrophobia
B. Arachnodactyly
C. Arachnophobia
D. Panic disorder
E. Benzodiazepine withdrawal syndrome
F. Agoraphobia

Q21.14

1. Absence of any thought and the patient reports their mind is empty
2. A feeling of constant, excessive worry, apprehension, tension or inner restlessness
3. A feeling of high spirits, exuberant happiness, vitality or ecstasy
4. Persistent and inappropriate repetition of the same thoughts or actions
5. Speech which is loud, rapid and difficult to interrupt

Select the best match for each of the above

A. Mood change
B. Disorder of the stream of thought
C. Disorder of the form of thought
D. Thought content
E. Abnormal belief

Q21.15

A 38-year-old woman has a history of fatigue which is made worse on minimal exertion. Associated symptoms include poor concentration, impaired registration of memory, irritability, hypersomnia and muscular pain. Management of this condition includes

A. Stopping late night caffeine
B. Cognitive behaviour therapy to change coping strategies
C. Supervised and graded exercise therapy
D. Antidepressants
E. Calcium-channel blockers

Q21.16

Poor response to lithium is associated with

A. A positive family history of mania
B. Unstable premorbid personality
C. A rapid cycling illness
D. The presence of tremors
E. Weight gain

Q21.17

A 29-year-old surgeon presents because she is a perfectionist. She is intolerant of shortcomings in both herself and others. She takes pride in her high standards but this trait is now so marked that it dominates other aspects of her personality. She is now anxious and repeatedly washes her hands at home after meals as if she were scrubbing up ready for the operating theatre. The following statements about this patient's condition are correct

A. This condition can follow head trauma
B. There is hyperactivity of the orbitofrontal cortex
C. Serotonin reuptake inhibitors should be avoided in this condition
D. Two-thirds of such patients improve within a year
E. The prognosis is worse when the personality is anankastic

Q21.18

A 45-year-old man with a 20-year history of drinking about 15 units of alcohol every day decides to stop drinking. He stopped drinking about a month ago and now would like to know which drugs can be used for prevention of alcohol dependence. These include

A. Diazepam
B. Clomethiazole
C. Naltrexone
D. Acamprosate
E. Disulfiram

Q21.19

A 24-year-old medical student breaks up with his girlfriend. Soon afterwards he hears voices commenting on his behaviour. He believes that his thoughts and feelings are controlled by others. Usually he is quite a placid person but now he is aggressive and he believes that others are out to get him. The following medications are used in the management of this condition

A. Chlorpromazine
B. Haloperidol
C. Clozapine
D. Risperidone
E. Olanzapine

Q21.20

An 18-year-old girl presents with a history of weight loss, induced by avoidance of fatty foods, vomiting and exercise. She also has a history of binge eating and amenorrhoea. Indicators of poor outcome include

A. Higher social class
B. A long initial illness
C. Bulimia
D. Difficulty in relationships
E. The presence of lanugo hair

Q21.21

A 48-year-old hypertensive and diabetic with a history of myocardial infarction and peripheral vascular disease on treatment for congestive heart failure presents with sexual dysfunction. The following could have contributed to his sexual dysfunction

A. Aspirin
B. ACE inhibitors
C. Carvedilol
D. Spironolactone
E. Clonidine
F. Diabetes mellitus
G. Peripheral vascular disease

Psychological medicine

A21.1

F

Severe mania is best treated with a combination of lithium and a neuroleptic such as haloperidol, allowing the neuroleptic to be withdrawn after the first 2 or 3 weeks. First attacks of mania usually require treatment for up to 3 months.

A21.2

B

Vascular or multi-infarct dementia is the second most common cause of dementia and is distinguished from Alzheimer's disease by its history of onset, clinical features and subsequent course. There is usually a history of transient ischaemic attacks with brief impairment of consciousness, fleeting pareses or visual loss. The dementia may follow a succession of acute cerebrovascular accidents or, less commonly, a single major stroke.

A21.3

C

Delirium tremens is the most serious withdrawal state and occurs 1–3 days after alcohol cessation, so is commonly seen a day or two after admission to hospital. Patients are disorientated, agitated, and have a marked tremor and visual hallucinations (e.g. insects or small animals coming menacingly towards them). Signs include sweating, tachycardia, tachypnoea and pyrexia.

A21.4

D

Opiate withdrawal syndrome	
Yawning Rhinorrhoea Lacrimation Pupillary dilatation Sweating Piloerection Restlessness	12–16 hours after last dose of opiate
Muscular twitches Aches and pains Abdominal cramps Vomiting Diarrhoea Hypertension Insomnia Anorexia Agitation Profuse sweating Weight loss	24–72 hours after last dose of opiate

The opiate withdrawal syndrome consists of a constellation of signs and symptoms (see table) that reaches peak intensity on the second or third day after the last dose of the opiate. These rapidly subside over the next 7 days.

A21.5

D

Lithium toxicity begins to occur when the serum concentration exceeds 1.5 mmol/L. Symptoms include drowsiness, nausea, vomiting, blurred vision, a coarse tremor, ataxia and dysarthria. Toxicity is more likely when the patient is dehydrated or with a drug interaction increasing concentrations.

A21.6

1) C **2)** C **3)** D **4)** D **5)** E

Thought insertion occurs when a patient's thought is perceived as being planted in their mind by someone else. Thought withdrawal occurs when a patient experiences their thoughts being taken away from them, without their control. An obsessional rumination is a recurrent, persistent thought, impulse, image or musical theme that enters the mind despite the individual's effort to resist it. The individual recognizes that the obsessional thought is their own, but it is usually unpleasant and often 'out of character', such as the thought that the patient has accidentally killed someone while driving their car. Common obsessions concern dirt, contamination and orderliness. A compulsion is a repetitive and seemingly purposeful action performed in a stereotyped way, referred to as a compulsive ritual. Compulsions are accompanied by a subjective sense that they must be carried out (or the patient will be overwhelmed by either anxiety or a superstitious belief that something bad will occur) and by an urge to resist. Compulsive rituals are used to counteract ruminations, so patients repetitively wash their hands to diminish the fear of contamination with dirt. Primary delusions are rare and appear suddenly and with full conviction but without any preceding mental events. For example, a patient on being offered a glass of wine suddenly believes that this indicates that he is Jesus Christ.

A21.7

1) F **2)** E **3)** D **4)** C **5)** A **6)** B

Illusions are misperceptions of external stimuli and are most likely to occur when the general level of sensory stimulation is reduced. Hallucinations are perceptions in the absence of a stimulus. Healthy people occasionally experience hallucinations, such as in normal grief, or during the transition between sleeping and waking (hypnagogic and hypnapompic). Hallucinations can be elementary (e.g. bangs, whistles) or complex (e.g. faces, voices, music), and may affect any of the perceptions: auditory, visual, tactile, gustatory, olfactory or of deep sensation. Depersonalization is a change in self-awareness such that the person feels unreal or detached from their body. The individual is aware, however, of the subjective nature of this alteration. Derealization is the unpleasant feeling that the external environment has become unreal and/or remote; patients may describe themselves as though they are in a dream-like state. Both this and depersonalization can occur in healthy people when they are tired, after sensory deprivation and when using hallucinogenic drugs. They also occur in anxiety disorders, schizophrenia and temporal lobe epilepsy. Déjà vu is a sudden familiarity with a situation or event as having been encountered before when it is in fact novel. Jamais vu is the reverse experience when there is failure to recognize a situation or event that has been encountered before. Déjà vu experiences occur in healthy people as well as in extreme anxiety states. Both types of experience can occur in temporal lobe epilepsy.

Psychological medicine

A21.8

1) G **2)** D **3)** B **4)** C **5)** F

Denial is similar to repression and occurs when patients behave as though unaware of something that they might be expected to know. One example would be a patient who, despite being told that a close relative has died, continues to behave as though the relative were still alive. Displacement involves the transferring of emotion from a situation or object with which it is properly associated to another that gives less distress. Identification refers to the unconscious process of taking on some of the characteristics or behaviours of another person, often to reduce the pain of separation or loss. Projection involves the attribution to another person of thoughts or feelings that are in fact one's own. Regression is the adoption of primitive patterns of behaviour appropriate to an earlier stage of development. It can be seen in ill people who become child-like and highly dependent. Repression is the exclusion from awareness of memories, emotions and/or impulses that would cause anxiety or distress if allowed to enter consciousness. Sublimation refers to the unconscious diversion of unacceptable behaviours into acceptable ones.

A21.9

1) B **2)** C **3)** A **4)** C **5)** A

The antidepressant dosulepin (dothiepin) is an effective treatment in half of patients with atypical facial pain, and this effect seems to be independent of dosulepin's effect on mood. Another tricyclic antidepressant, amitriptyline, is more effective than a selective serotonin reuptake inhibitor (SSRI) in tension headaches, which might be related to its independent analgesic effect. Amitriptyline has the added bonus of increasing slow wave sleep, which may be why it is more effective than NSAIDs in chronic widespread pain. There is some preliminary evidence that tricyclics are superior to SSRIs in chronic pain syndromes. In irritable bowel syndrome when indicated, the choice of antidepressant should be determined by the effects of these drugs on bowel transit times, with tricyclic antidepressants normally slowing and selective serotonin reuptake inhibitors (SSRIs) normally speeding up transit times. Several studies have now demonstrated that SSRIs are effective treatments for the premenstrual dysphoric syndrome.

A21.10

1) B **2)** E **3)** C **4)** F **5)** A

Dissociative amnesia commences suddenly. Patients are unable to recall long periods of their lives and may even deny any knowledge of their previous life or personal identity. In a dissociative fugue, patients not only lose their memory but wander away from their usual surroundings, and, when found, deny all memory of their whereabouts during this wandering. The differential diagnosis of a fugue state includes postictal automatism, depressive illness and alcohol abuse. Dissociative pseudodementia involves memory loss and behaviour that initially suggest severe and generalized dementia. A differential diagnosis is depressive pseudodementia Abreaction brought about by hypnosis or by intravenous injections of small amounts of midazolam may produce a dramatic, if short-lived, recovery. In the abreactive state, the patient is encouraged to relive the stressful events that provoked the disorder and to express the accompanying emotions; i.e. to abreact. Such an approach has been useful in the treatment of acute dissociative states in wartime, but appears to be of much less value in civilian life. Patients who describe the world as looking grey, themselves as lacking a zest for living and devoid of pleasure and interest in life are said to have anhedonia.

A21.11

1) D   2) E   3) G   4) F   5) A
6) C   7) B

Dosulepin (dothiepin), imipramine and amitriptyline are the three most commonly used tricyclic antidepressants in the UK, but many related compounds have been introduced, some having fewer autonomic and cardiotoxic effects (e.g. lofepramine). Venlafaxine is a potent blocker of both serotonin and noradrenaline (norepinephrine) reuptake (SNaRI). Nefazodone is a potent $5\text{-}HT_2$ receptor antagonist, with weak SNaRI activity. Mirtazapine is a $5\text{-}HT_2$ and $5\text{-}HT_3$ receptor antagonist and a potent α_2-adrenergic blocker. Reboxetine is a selective noradrenaline (norepinephrine) reuptake inhibitor (NaRI). Phenelzine acts by irreversibly inhibiting the intracellular enzymes monoamine oxidase A and B leading to an increase of noradrenaline (norepinephrine), dopamine and 5-hydroxytryptamine in the brain. Moclobemide is a reversible inhibitor of monoamine oxidase A (RIMA).

A21.12

1) A   2) B   3) C   4) A   5) C

In 'flight of ideas' the patient's thoughts rapidly jump from one topic to another, such that one train of thought is not completed before another appears. It is often produced by clang associations (the use of two or more words with a similar sound: 'sun, son, song'), punning, rhyming, and responding to distracting cues in the immediate surroundings. Flight of ideas is characteristic of mania and often accompanies pressure of speech.Thought broadcast is when the patient experiences their thoughts as being understood by others without talking, as though their thoughts are literally being broadcast to all around them. Irritability can be either expressed (as in a temper or impatience) or an internal feeling of exasperation or anger, seen in both mania and depressive illness, especially in men. Thought block occurs in schizophrenia. There is an abrupt and complete interruption of the stream of thought, so the mind goes blank.

A21.13

1) F   2) A   3) C   4) D

Agoraphobia menas 'fear of the market place'. This common phobia (4% prevalence) presents as a fear of being away from home, with avoidance of travelling, walking down a road, and shops being common presentations. Claustrophobia, is a fear of enclosed spaces. Panic disorder is diagnosed when the patient has repeated sudden attacks of overwhelming anxiety, accompanied by severe physical symptoms, usually related to both hyperventilation and sympathetic nervous system activity. The phobia of spiders is known as arachnophobia. Arachnodactyly is long spidery fingers seen in Marfan's syndrome.

Psychological medicine

A21.14

1) B   2) A   3) A   4) D   5) B

Anxiety is a feeling of constant, inappropriate or excessive worry, fear, apprehension, tension or inner restlessness, seen in anxiety and depressive disorders and drug withdrawal. Elation is a feeling of high spirits, exuberant happiness, vitality and even ecstasy, seen in mania and acute drug intoxication. Pressure of speech occurs in mania and can be recognized by loudness, rapidity, and difficulty in interrupting speech. Poverty of speech is the opposite experience, when there appears to be an absence of any thought and patients reports their minds to be empty. It occurs in depressive illness. An obsessional rumination is a recurrent, persistent thought, impulse, image or musical theme that enters the mind despite the individual's effort to resist it. The individual recognizes that the obsessional thought is their own, but it is usually unpleasant and often 'out of character', such as the thought that the patient has accidentally killed someone while driving their car. Common obsessions concern dirt, contamination, and orderliness.

A21.15

A) T   B) T   C) T   D) T   E) F

This patient has chronic fatigue syndrome or myalgic encephalomyelitis. The first principle is the identification and treatment of maintaining factors (e.g. dysfunctional beliefs and behaviours, mood and sleep disorders). A) Communication: i) explanation of ill-health, including diagnosis and causes; ii) education about management (including self-help leaflets). B) Stopping drugs (e.g. caffeine causing insomnia, analgesics causing dependence). C)

Rehabilitative therapies: i) cognitive behaviour therapy (to challenge unhelpful beliefs and change coping strategies); ii) supervised and graded exercise therapy (to reduce inactivity and improve fitness). E) Pharmacotherapies: i) specific antidepressants for mood disorders, analgesia and sleep disturbance; ii) symptomatic medicines (e.g. appropriate analgesia, taken only when necessary).

A21.16

A) F   B) T   C) T   D) F   E) F

Poor responses to lithium are associated with a negative family history, an unstable premorbid personality, and a rapid cycling illness. Tremors and weight gain are a side-effect of lithium therapy.

A21.17

A) T   B) T   C) F   D) T   E) T

Obsessive–compulsive disorder (OCD) is characterized by obsessional ruminations and compulsive rituals. The obsessions and compulsions are so persistent and intrusive that they greatly impede a patient's functioning and cause considerable distress. There is a constant need to check that things have been done correctly, and no amount of reassurance can remove the small amount of doubt that persists. OCD can follow head trauma. Hyperactivity of the orbitofrontal cortex has been a consistent finding in brain imaging research on OCD patients. Serotonin function is probably abnormal in patients with OCD. Serotonin reuptake inhibitors are effective drugs. Two-thirds of cases improve within a year. The remainder run a fluctuating or persistent course. The prognosis is worse when the personality is anankastic and the OCD is primary and severe.

A 21.18

A) F **B)** F **C)** T **D)** T **E)** T

Drugs which have been used for prevention of alcohol dependence include the following: a) naltrexone, the opioid antagonist (50 mg per day), reduces the risk of relapse into heavy drinking and the frequency of drinking; b) acamprosate (1–2 g per day) is a drug that affects several receptors including those for GABA, noradrenaline (norepinephrine) and serotonin. There is good evidence that it reduces drinking frequency. Neither drug seems particularly helpful in maintaining abstinence. Both drug effects are enhanced by combining them with counselling. c) Drugs such as disulfiram react with alcohol to cause unpleasant acetaldehyde intoxication and histamine release. A daily maintenance dose means that the patient must wait until the disulfiram is eliminated from the body before drinking safely. There is mixed evidence of efficacy.

A 21.19

A) T **B)** T **C)** T **D)** T **E)** T

The best results in schizophrenia are obtained by combining drug and social treatments. Neuroleptic drugs act by blocking the D_1 and D_2 groups of dopamine receptors. Such drugs are most effective against acute, positive symptoms and are least effective in the management of chronic, negative symptoms. Complete control of positive symptoms can take up to 3 months and premature discontinuation of treatment can result in relapse. Phenothiazines are the group of neuroleptics used most extensively. Chlorpromazine (100–1000 mg daily) is the drug of choice when a more sedating drug is required. Trifluoperazine is used when sedation is undesirable. Fluphenazine decanoate is used as a long-term prophylactic to prevent relapse, as a depot injection. The butyrophenones (e.g. haloperidol 2–30 mg daily) are also powerful antipsychotics, used in the treatment of acute schizophrenia and mania. Clozapine is used in patients with intractable schizophrenia who have failed to respond to at least two conventional antipsychotic drugs. This drug is a dibenzodiazepine with a relative high affinity for D_1 compared with D_2 dopamine receptors, muscarinic and α-adrenergic receptors. It also blocks 5-HT_2 and 5-HT_1 receptors. Clozapine has been shown to exercise a dramatic therapeutic effect on both intractable positive and negative symptoms. Neither risperidone nor olanzapine seem as specific a treatment for intractable chronic schizophrenia as clozapine.

A 21.20

A) F **B)** T **C)** T **D)** T **E)** F

In anorexia nervosa indicators of a poor outcome include: a) a long initial illness; b) severe weight loss; c) older age at onset; d) bulimia, vomiting or purging; e) personality difficulties; f) difficulties in relationships.

A21.21

A) F B) F C) T D) T E) T
F) T G) T

Medical conditions affecting sexual performance

Endocrine
Diabetes mellitus
Hyperthyroidism
Hypothyroidism

Cardiovascular
Angina pectoris
Previous myocardial
infarction
Disorders of peripheral
circulation

Hepatic
Cirrhosis, particularly
alcohol-related

Renal
Renal failure

Neurological
Neuropathy
Spinal cord lesions

Musculoskeletal
Arthritis

Respiratory
Asthma
COPD

Psychiatric
Depressive illness
Substance misuse

Drugs affecting sexual arousal

Male arousal	Female arousal
Alcohol	Alcohol
Benzodiazepines	CNS depressants
Neuroleptics	Antidepressants (SSRIs)
Cimetidine	Oral combined contraceptives
Opiate analgesics	Methyldopa
Methyldopa	Clonidine
Clonidine	
Spironolactone	
Antihistamines	
Metoclopramide	
Diuretics	
Beta-blockers	
Cannabis	

Alcohol increases the desire but diminishes the performance

Q22.1

A 38-year-old woman presents with muscle weakness and a heliotrope (purple) discoloration of the eyelids and periorbital oedema. On examination she has scaly, purple-red raised vasculitic patches over the extensor surface of joints and knuckles. The nail fold is ragged with dilated capillaries. Which one of the following is the most likely diagnosis?

A. Scleroderma
B. Discoid lupus erythematosus
C. Rheumatoid arthritis
D. Systemic lupus erythematosus
E. Dermatomyositis

Q22.2

A 64-year-old policeman with varicose veins presents with a long-standing ulcer on the lower leg. On examination it is reddish-brown and indurated. There is scarring white atrophy with telangiectasia. The best treatment is which one of the following?

A. Vascular reconstruction
B. Correctly fitting boots
C. High-compression bandaging with leg elevation
D. Bed rest to keep pressure off bony areas
E. A course of steroid therapy

Q22.3

A 38-year-old woman presents with muscle weakness and a heliotrope (purple) discoloration of the eyelids and periorbital oedema. On examination she has scaly, purple-red raised vasculitic patches over the extensor surface of joints and knuckles. The nail fold is ragged with dilated capillaries. Which one of the following tests is not diagnostic in this condition?

A. History
B. Clinical appearance
C. Skin biopsy
D. Muscle biopsy
E. EMG

Q22.4

A 27-year-old woman presents with fixed erythematous, scaly, atrophic plaques on the face and sun-exposed area. Telangiectasia, hypopigmentation and follicular plugging are apparent. Examination of the scalp reveals scarring alopecia and the mouth has erythematous patches. She also suffers from Raynaud's phenomenon and serum ANF is positive. Skin biopsy shows dense patchy, dermal lymphocyte infiltrate which is centered around appendages. The epidermal basal layer is damaged and hyperkeratosis is also present. The most likely diagnosis is which one of the following?

Skin disease

A. Basal cell carcinoma

B. Squamous cell carcinoma

C. Discoid lupus erythematosus

D. Plaque like psoriasis

E. Scleroderma

Q22.5

A 42-year-old patient presents with an annular rash that is in concentric rings – target lesions. The rash is on the palms and soles and around the mouth. The most common identifiable cause of this condition is which one of the following?

A. Mycoplasma

B. Anticonvulsants

C. Systemic lupus erythematosus

D. Herpes simplex

E. Sulphonamides

Q22.6

A 7-year-old girl presents with an erythematous rash which was followed by a non-itchy skin angio-oedema (but no urticaria). She has a family history of sudden death due to choking and stridor. The most effective treatment in an acute setting for this patient is which one of the following?

A. Adrenaline (epinephrine)

B. Steroids

C. C1 esterase inhibitor concentrates with fresh frozen plasma

D. Stanozolol

E. Danazol

Q22.7

In early spring a 17-year-old girl presents to her GP with a rash on the back. Initially there was a large solitary patch with peripheral scaling. Now she has oval pink macules which are arranged along the dermatomal lines giving a 'Christmas tree' appearance. The most likely diagnosis is which one of the following?

A. Tinea corporis

B. Pediculosis corporis

C. Pityriasis versicolor

D. Nummular eczema

E. Pityriasis rosea

Q22.8

A 24-year-old woman presents with an intensely itchy rash on the flexors of the wrist and lower legs. The rash is also present on the scalp. On examination it consists of small, purple flat-topped polygonal papules. The most likely diagnosis is which one of the following?

A. Granuloma annulare

B. Urticarial vasculitis

C. Lichen planus

D. Pityriasis rosea

E. Erythema multiforme

Q22.9

A 19-year-old girl recently underwent cardiac transplantation and is on immunosuppressive therapy. She develops a rash on the chest and back. The rash is characterized by pustules and inflammatory papules – it appears as pustular folliculitis. The most likely diagnosis is which one of the following?

A. Oil acne

B. Follicular occlusion triad

C. Acne fulminans

D. Steroid-induced acne

E. Seborrhoeic eczema

Q22.10

A 43-year-old woman presents with facial flushing, which is exacerbated by alcohol, hot drinks and sunlight. On examination she has inflammatory papules and pustules on the nose, forehead and cheeks. There are no comedones but there is telangiectasia, and inflammation of the margins of the eyelids. Which one of the following should be avoided in this condition?

A. Long-term topical metronidazole
B. Topical steroids
C. Oral tetracycline
D. Oral metronidazole
E. Oral isotretinoin

Q22.11

A 68-year-old man presents with malaise and fever. He complains that his skin itches and feels 'tight'. On examination he has 'red skin' and skin biopsy shows clonal expansion of T cells. The most likely diagnosis is which one of the following?

A. Psoriasis
B. Atopic eczema
C. Photodermatitis
D. Sézary syndrome
E. Seborrhoeic dermatitis

Q22.12

A 12-year-old child presents with multiple small translucent papules which appear like fluid-filled vesicles. Many of the lesions have a central depression or punctum. The most likely diagnosis is which one of the following?

A. Common warts
B. Plantar warts
C. Filiform warts
D. Molluscum contagiosum
E. Plane warts

Q22.13

A 29-year-old Caucasian male presents with reddish-brown scaly macules on the trunk. He is asymptomatic. Skin scrapings reveal mycelia. The most likely diagnosis is

A. Candida albicans
B. Pityrosporum folliculitis
C. Pityriasis versicolor
D. Tinea corporis
E. Norwegian scabies

Q22.14

A 9-year-old schoolgirl presents with itching and excoriation of the scalp. In addition there are erythematous papules on the neck. Examination of the hair reveals nits tightly bound to the hair shaft. The most likely diagnosis is which one of the following?

A. Scabies
B. Norwegian scabies
C. Pediculosis capitis
D. Atopic eczema
E. Tinea capitis

Q22.15

A 12-year girl presents with itching which is worse at night. On examination there are itchy red papules between the web spaces of her fingers and toes. Skin scrapings of a lesion examined with a potassium hydroxide preparation under the microscope reveal mites and eggs. The most likely organism is which one of the following?

A. Pityrosporum orbiculare
B. Pitryrosporum ovale
C. Sarcoptes scabiei
D. Malassezia furfur
E. Candida albicans

Skin disease

Q22.16

A 6-year-old child presents with itchy erythematous scaly patches on the front of the elbows and ankles, behind the knees and around the neck. The most likely diagnosis is which one of the following?

A. Psoriasis
B. *Candida albicans*
C. Erysipeloid
D. Atopic eczema
E. Shingles

Q22.17

A 68-year-old patient with Parkinson's disease presents with an erythematous scaling along the sides of the nose, in the eyebrows, around the eyes and extending into the scalp (which shows marked dandruff). The most likely aetiology is which one of the following?

A. *Pityrosporum orbiculare*
B. *Pityrosporum ovale*
C. *Sarcoptes scabiei*
D. *Corynebacterium minutissimum*
E. *Candida albicans*

Q22.18

A 19-year-old boy presents with thickened, slow-growing, yellow nails and cough with expectoration. CT shows bronchiectasis and pleural effusion. This condition is most likely to be due to which one of the following?

A. Koilonychia
B. Hypoalbuminaemia
C. Severe illness
D. Disorder of the lymphatic system
E. Psoriasis

Q22.19

A 25-year-old man presents with multiple inflammatory papules, plaques and nodules. He also complains of nasal stuffiness. On examination there is loss of eyebrows and some anaesthesia. Biopsy shows acid-fast bacilli. The most likely diagnosis is which one of the following?

A. Lupus vulgaris
B. Tuberculosis verrucosa cutis
C. Scrofuloderma
D. Tuberculoid leprosy
E. Lepromatous leprosy

Q22.20

A 33-year-old woman presents with a few hypopigmented plaques with an erythematous rim. The lesions are markedly anaesthetic, dry and hairless. Nerves are enlarged and palpable. Biopsy shows a perineural granulomatous infiltrate with scant acid-fast bacilli. The most likely diagnosis is which one of the following?

A. Tuberculides
B. Tuberculosis verrucosa cutis
C. Bazin's disease
D. Tuberculoid leprosy
E. Lepromatous leprosy

Q22.21

1. A layer consisting predominantly of adipose tissue as well as blood vessels and nerves. It provides insulation and acts as a lipid store

2. This layer is of mesodermal origin and contains blood vessels and lymphatic vessels, nerves, muscle, appendages (such as sweat glands, sebaceous glands and hair follicles) and a variety of immune cells such as mast cells and lymphocytes

3. It consists of stratified epithelium of ectodermal origin that arises from dividing basal keratinocytes

4. It arises from a downgrowth of epidermal keratinocytes into the dermis

5. This is a complex proteinaceous structure consisting of type IV and VII collagen, hemidesmosomal proteins, integrins and laminin

Select the best match for each of the above

A. Hair
B. Subcutaneous layer
C. Dermis
D. Basement membrane zone
E. Epidermis

Q22.22

1. A 7-year-old child presents with weeping exudative areas with a typical honey-coloured crust on the surface

2. A 53-year-old man presents with a hot, tender area of confluent erythema of the skin of the lower leg. It has been spreading in an upward direction. The patient is unwell and has a high temperature

3. A 23-year-old patient with HIV presents with chronic well-demarcated, deeply ulcerative lesions with an exudative crust

4. A 17-year-old diabetic presents with painful red swellings

5. An 18-year-old woman presents with a painful, discharging chronic inflammation of the skin of the axilla, groin and natal cleft

Select the best match for each of the above

A. Folliculitis
B. Furuncles
C. Cellulitis
D. Erythrasma
E. Ecthyma
F. Impetigo

G. Pitted keratolysis
H. Hidradenitis suppurativa

Q22.23

1. A 41-year-old woman presents with mouth ulcers which are followed by painful blisters on the trunk. These blisters extend on gentle sliding pressure. Antibodies against desmoglein 3 are present

2. A 68-year-old woman presents with large tense bullae on the limbs, hands and feet. The mouth is not involved. Antibodies against 180 kDa hemidesmosomal protein are present

3. A 26-year-old man presents with small, intensely itchy blisters on the elbows, extensor aspects of forearm, scalp and buttocks. The tops of the blisters are scratched off and crusted lesions are seen. Antibodies to gliadin and reticulin are present

4. A 12-year-old boy presents with circular clusters of large blisters. The mouth is involved

5. A 14-year-old girl with a family history of blisters presents with intermittent blistering of the hands and feet especially in hot weather. The teeth and nails are normal and scarring is absent

Select the best match for each of the above

A. Dermatitis herpetiformis
B. Pemiphigus vulgaris
C. Bullous pemiphigoid
D. Linear IgA disease
E. Epidermolysis bullosa

Skin disease

Q22.24

1. A 73-year-old farmer presents with a small ulcer on his face. It started as a papule and grew slowly before it ulcerated. On examination telangiectasia are present over the tumour and it has a 'jelly-like' edge

2. A 67-year-old farmer presents with an ulcer on the ear. It started as a nodule and grew very rapidly

3. A 45-year-old surfer who has been surfing since his teens presents with a change in the size, shape and colour of a mole. On examination it has an irregular border, colour variegation and is 6 mm in diameter

4. A 29-year-old patient with HIV infection presents with slow-growing purple tumour on the lower leg

5. A 43-year-old woman presents with scaly patches and plaques on the buttocks. Skin biopsy shows invasion by atypical lymphocytes. T-cell receptor gene rearrangement studies show that there is often monoclonal expansion of lymphocytes in the skin

Select the best match for each of the above

A. Basal cell carcinoma
B. Squamous cell carcinoma
C. Malignant melanoma
D. Kaposi's sarcoma
E. Cutaneous T cell lymphoma

Q22.25

1. A 22-year-old patient has skin which is hyperextensible but recoils normally after stretching. It is known to injure easily and healing occurs slowly with scarring like tissue paper. The joints are hypermobile

2. A 43-year-old patient presents with yellowish and papular skin on the sides of the neck. Retinal examination reveals angioid streaks

3. A 29-year-old man has tall stature and long thin digits. There is a history of frequent dislocation of the joints

4. A 22-year-old woman has well-demarcated macules of complete pigment loss. There is no history of previous inflammation. The lesions are on the face and hands

5. A 23-year-old African man has several small (2–4 mm) asymptomatic porcelain-white macules in sun-exposed areas. The borders are sharply defined and angular. Sensation is intact

Select the best match for each of the above

A. Marfan's syndrome
B. Pseudoxanthoma elasticum
C. Ehlers–Danlos syndrome
D. Vitiligo
E. Post-inflammatory hypopigmentation
F. Oculocutaneous albinism
G. Idiopathic guttate hypomelanosis
H. Leprosy

Q22.26

1. A 10-year-old boy has small brown macules after sun exposure. They fade in the winter months

2. A 22-year-old woman has several brown macules which persist in the winter months

3. A 32-year-old woman on oral contraceptives presents with brown macules symmetrically over the cheeks and forehead

4. A 19-year-old man has brown macules of the lips and perioral region. He also has a history of benign colonic polyps

5. A 7-year-old child has multiple pigmented macules which tend to become red, itchy and urticated if they are rubbed

Select the best match for each of the above

A. Chloasma
B. Lentigos
C. Skin biopsy shows mast cells
D. Freckles
E. The gene responsible is *LKB1*, which codes for a serine-threonine kinase
F. The gene responsible is the fibrillin-1 gene on chromosome 15.

Q22.27

A 39-year-old man presents with a painful, tender blistering eruption along one of the intercostal spaces. The rash was preceded by pain in the same area. With time the blisters have become pustular. The complications of this condition include

A. Myasthenia gravis
B. Motor neuropathy
C. Severe persistent pain
D. Ocular disease (when the ophthalmic nerve is involved)
E. Bell's palsy

Q22.28

A 28-year-old woman presents with a widespread subepidermal blistering and sloughing of most of the skin. There is an itch which has burning quality. She is febrile and there is involvement of the oral mucosa. The following drugs have been implicated in the causation of this condition

A. Steroids
B. Penicillin
C. Co-trimoxazole
D. Carbamazepine
E. NSAIDs

Q22.29

A 28-year-old man presents with separation of the distal nail plate. The following have been implicated in the causation of this condition

A. Iron deficiency anaemia
B. Psoriasis
C. Hyperthyroidism
D. Trauma
E. Photosensitive reaction to tetracycline

Q22.30

A 55-year-old man presents with itchy pinkish-red scaly plaques on the knees and elbows. On examination he has similar lesions on the lower back, ears and scalp. The nail changes in this condition include

A. Pitting of nail plate
B. Distal separation of the nail plate
C. Yellow-brown discoloration
D. Subungual keratosis
E. Damaged nail matrix and lost nail plate

Q22.31

A 57-year-old woman presents with itchy pinkish-red scaly plaques on the knees and elbows. On examination she has similar plaques on the lower back, ears and scalp. The patterns of joint involvement seen in this condition include

A. Distal interphalangeal arthritis
B. Peripheral mono- or oligoarthritis
C. Symmetrical rheumatoid arthritis pattern but seronegative
D. Spondylitis or sacroiliitis (especially if HLA-B27 positive)
E. Arthritis mutilans causing destruction and resorption of bone leading to 'telescoping' digits

Skin disease

Q22.32

An 18-year-old girl presents with skin swellings or weals that develop acutely over a few minutes. The lesions are intensly itchy but show no surface change or scaling. The patient should avoid the following medications

A. H_1 receptor blockers
B. Salicylates
C. Opiates
D. H_2 receptor blockers
E. Steroids

Q22.33

The following statements regarding phototherapy of skin conditions are correct

A. UVB is more likely to burn but it is less carcinogenic than UVA
B. Narrow-band UVB (311 nanometer) is superseding broad-band UVB because it is much more effective in the treatment of eczema and psoriasis
C. UVA is relatively ineffective on its own so is used in conjunction with a photosensitizer (psoralen)
D. Sunbeds are very effective in treating skin disease
E. PUVA is more effective than UVB but is limited by its carcinogenic potential

Q22.34

A 22-year-old woman presents with fever, malaise, joint pains and a painful rash on the shins. On examination she has tender dusky blue-red nodules on the shins. The following are known to cause this condition

A. Oral contraceptives
B. Streptococcal infection
C. Sarcoidosis
D. Inflammatory bowel disease
E. Aspirin

Q22.35

A middle-aged man presents with malaise, fever and erythematous nodules on the skin. Some of them have ulcerated and the ulcers have a typical bluish-black undermined edge and purulent surface. Biopsy shows an intense neutrophilic infiltrate. The following conditions can cause this clinical picture

A. Inflammatory bowel disease
B. Multiple myeloma
C. Rheumatoid arthritis
D. Primary biliary cirrhosis
E. Dermatomyositis

Q22.36

A 39-year-old woman presents with a thickened, hyperpigmented velvety skin in the axilla. This condition is associated with

A. Insulin resistance
B. Tuberculosis
C. Hyperandrogenism
D. Lupus
E. Gastrointestinal malignancy

Q22.37

An 18-year-old boy has a history of mental retardation and epilepsy. The history confirms that it has an autosomal dominant inheritance pattern. This condition has several cutaneous abnormalities including hamartomatous growths. The following cutaneous abnormalities are seen in this condition

A. Reddish papules/fibromas around the nose
B. Nodules arising from the nail bed
C. Firm, flesh-coloured plaques on the trunk
D. Pale macules best seen with UV light
E. Indurated flesh-coloured patch on the forehead

Q22.38

A 36-year-old man presents with weight loss, thirst and polyuria. Investigations show that his glycosylated haemoglobin is elevated. Skin changes described in this condition include

A. Spreading erythema over the shin which becomes yellowish and atrophic in the center with ulceration
B. Granuloma annulare
C. Red-brown flat-topped papules
D. Tight waxy skin over the fingers with limitation of joint movement due to increased collagen
E. Granuloma inguinale

Skin disease

A22.1

E

Dermatomyositis is a rare disease affecting skin and muscle with an associated vasculitis. The rash is distinctive. Facial erythema and a magenta-coloured rash around the eyes with associated oedema are often present. Bluish-red nodules or plaques may be present over the knuckles and extensor surfaces. The nail folds are frequently ragged with dilated capillaries.

A22.2

C

In venous ulcers high-compression bandaging (e.g. Unna boot or four-layer bandaging) and leg elevation are used to try to decrease the venous hypertension.

A22.3

C

The diagnosis of dermatomyositis is made from the clinical appearance, muscle biopsy, EMG and a serum creatine phosphokinase. Skin biopsy is not diagnostic.

A22.4

C

Chronic discoid lupus erythematosus presents with fixed erythematous, scaly, atrophic plaques with telangiectasia, especially on the face or other sun-exposed site. Hypopigmentation is common and follicular plugging may be apparent. Scalp involvement may lead to a scarring alopecia. Oral involvement (erythematous patches or ulceration) occurs in 25% of cases. Skin biopsy shows a dense patchy, dermal lymphohistiocytic infiltrate which often is centred around appendages.

Epidermal basal layer damage, follicular plugging and hyperkeratosis may be present.

A22.5

D

Herpes simplex virus is the most common identifiable cause of erythema multiforme.

A22.6

C

Hereditary angio-oedema is an extremely rare autosomal dominant condition due to an inherited deficiency of C1 esterase inhibitor, a component of the complement system. In the acute setting, treatment is with C1 esterase inhibitor concentrates and fresh frozen plasma. Adrenaline (epinephrine) and steroids are often ineffective. Maintenance treatment with the anabolic steroid stanozolol (or danazol) stimulates an increase in hepatic synthesis of C1 esterase inhibitor but this should not be used in children.

A22.7

E

Pityriasis rosea is a self-limiting rash seen in adolescents and young adults. The rash consists of circular or oval pink macules with a collarette of scale and is more prominent on the trunk than the limbs. The long axis of the oval lesions tends to run along dermatomal lines giving a 'Christmas tree' pattern on the back. The rash may be preceded by a large solitary patch with peripheral scaling ('herald patch') and this is most commonly found on the trunk. The rash is usually asymptomatic and spontaneously resolves over 4–8 weeks.

A22.8

C

In lichen planus the rash is characterized by small, purple flat-topped, polygonal papules that are intensely pruritic. It is common on the flexors of the wrists and the lower legs but can occur anywhere. There may be a fine lacy white pattern on the surface of lesions (Wickham's striae).

A22.9

D

Acne may occur secondary to corticosteroid therapy or Cushing's syndrome. Comedones and cysts are rare in this variant but involvement of the back and shoulders (rather than the face) is common. Clinically the rash often appears as a pustular folliculitis.

A22.10

B

In rosacea treatment is suppressive rather than curative. Long-term use of topical 0.075% metronidazole may help. Avoid topical steroids as they can exacerbate or trigger the condition. A 3-month course of oral tetracycline (500 mg twice daily) is also helpful. Oral metronidazole (400 mg twice daily) or oral isotretinoin (0.5–1 mg/kg/day) is occasionally given in resistant cases.

A22.11

D

Sézary syndrome is cutaneous T cell lymphoma and may present as erythroderma. Biopsy is diagnostic.

A22.12

D

Molluscum contagiosum is a common cutaneous infection of childhood caused by a pox virus. Clinically, lesions are multiple, small (1–3 mm) translucent papules which often look like fluid-filled vesicles but are in fact solid. Individual lesions may have a central depression called a punctum.

A22.13

C

Pityriasis versicolor is a relatively common condition of young adults caused by infection with *Pityrosporum*. In Caucasians it presents most commonly on the trunk with reddish-brown scaly macules which are asymptomatic. In black-skinned individuals (or in whites who are sun-tanned) it more commonly presents as macular areas of hypopigmentation. Inappropriate use of topical steroids tends to spread the rash.

A22.14

C

Head lice (pediculosis capitis) is a common infection world-wide, affecting predominantly children and being commoner in females. Spread is by direct contact and encouraged by overcrowding. It usually presents with itch or scalp excoriations. Occasionally, erythematous papules on the neck may be seen. Diagnosis can be confirmed by the presence of eggs ('nits') seen tightly bound to the hair shaft. Adult lice may be seen rarely in heavy infection.

Skin disease

A22.15

C

This patient has scabies. All other organisms listed are fungi and there are no mites and eggs in fungal infections.

A22.16

D

Atopic eczema can present as a number of distinct morphological variants. The commonest presentation is of itchy erythematous scaly patches, especially in the flexures such as in front of the elbows and ankles, behind the knees and around the neck. In infants, eczema often starts on the face before spreading to the body. Very acute lesions may weep or exude and can show small vesicles. Scratching can produce excoriations, and repeated rubbing produces skin thickening (lichenification) with exaggerated skin markings.

A22.17

B

Overgrowth of *Pityrosporum ovale* (also called *Malassezia furfur* in its hyphal form) together with a strong cutaneous immune response to this yeast produces the characteristic inflammation and scaling of seborrhoeic eczema. The condition is more common in parkinsonism as well as in HIV disease.

A22.18

D

Yellow-nail syndrome is a rare disorder of lymphatic drainage. It presents with thickened, slow-growing, yellow nails which may be associated with pleural effusions, bronchiectasis and lymphoedema of the legs.

A22.19

E

Lepromatous leprosy presents with multiple inflammatory papules, plaques and nodules. Loss of the eyebrows ('madarosis') and nasal stuffiness are common. Skin thickening and severe disfigurement may follow. Anaesthesia is much less prominent. Biopsy shows numerous acid-fast bacilli.

A22.20

D

Tuberculoid leprosy presents with a few hypopigmented or erythematous plaques with an active erythematous, raised rim. Lesions are usually markedly anaesthetic, dry and hairless reflecting the nerve damage. Nerves may be enlarged and palpable. Biopsy shows a granulomatous infiltrate centred on nerves, but scant acid-fast bacilli.

A22.21

1) B   2) C   3) E   4) A   5) D

The epidermis is a stratified epithelium of ectodermal origin that arises from dividing basal keratinocytes. The basement membrane zone is a complex proteinaceous structure consisting of type IV and VII collagen, hemidesmosomal proteins, integrins and laminin. Inherited or autoimmune-induced deficiencies of these proteins can cause skin fragility and a variety of blistering diseases. The dermis is of mesodermal origin and contains blood and lymphatic vessels, nerves, muscle, appendages (e.g. sweat glands, sebaceous glands and hair follicles) and a variety of immune cells such as mast cells and lymphocytes. It is a matrix of collagen and elastin in a ground substance. Hairs arise from a downgrowth of epidermal keratinocytes into the dermis. The hair shaft has an inner and outer root sheath, a cortex and sometimes a medulla. The lower portion of the hair follicle consists of an expanded bulb (which also contains melanocytes) surrounding a richly innervated and vascularized dermal papilla. The subcutaneous layer consists predominantly of adipose tissue as well as blood vessels and nerves. This layer provides insulation and acts as a lipid store.

A22.22

1) F   2) C   3) E   4) B   5) H

Impetigo presents as weeping, exudative areas with a typical honey-coloured crust on the surface. Cellulitis presents as a hot, sometimes tender area of confluent erythema of the skin owing to infection of the deep subcutaneous layer. It often affects the lower leg, causing an upwards-spreading, hot erythema. Ecthyma presents as chronic well-demarcated, deeply ulcerative lesions sometimes with an exudative crust. It is commoner in developing countries, being associated with poor nutrition and hygiene. It is rare in the UK but is seen more commonly in intravenous drug abusers and people with HIV. Boils or furuncles are a rather more deep-seated infection of the skin, often caused by *Staphylococcus*. They can cause painful red swellings. They are commoner in teenagers and often recurrent. Recurrent boils may rarely occur in diabetes mellitus or in immunosuppression. Hidradenitis suppurativa is a rare condition

characterized by a painful, discharging, chronic inflammation of the skin at sites rich in apocrine glands (axillae, groins, natal cleft). The cause is unknown but it is commoner in females, and within some families it appears to be inherited in an autosomal dominant fashion.

A22.23

1) B   2) C   3) A   4) D   5) E

Pemphigus vulgaris is a potentially fatal blistering disease. Skin biopsy shows a superficial intraepidermal split just above the basal layer with acantholysis (separation of individual cells). Both direct immunofluorescence (IMF) of skin (perilesional) and indirect IMF using patients' serum show intercellular staining of IgG within the epidermis. Bullous pemphigoid is more common than pemphigus. It presents in later life (usually over 60 years old) and mucosal involvement is rarer. Skin biopsy shows a deeper blister (than in pemphigus) owing to a subepidermal split through the basement membrane. Direct and indirect IMF studies show linear staining of IgG along the basement membrane. Dermatitis herpetiformis is a rare blistering disorder associated with gluten-sensitive enteropathy. Skin biopsy shows a subepidermal blister with neutrophil microabscesses in the dermal papillae. Direct IMF studies of uninvolved skin show IgA in the dermal papillae and patchy granular IgA along the basement membrane. Linear IgA disease is a further subepidermal blistering disorder of adults and children. Pathogenic autoantibodies can bind to a variety of basement membrane proteins including ladinin, BP 180 antigen and laminin 5. Direct IMF studies of skin show linear IgA deposition along the basement membrane.

Skin disease

Epidermolysis bullosa (EB) simplex is a group of autosomal dominant genodermatoses characterized by 'superficial' blistering owing to mutations of cytoskeleton proteins within the basal layer of the epidermis, e.g. keratin 5 (chromosome 12q) or keratin 14 (chromosome 17q). Most forms of EB simplex show mild disease with intermittent blistering of the hands and feet, especially in hot weather. The teeth and nails are normal and scarring is absent.

A22.24

1) A   2) B   3) C   4) D   5) E

Treatment of advanced Kaposi's sarcoma is with radiotherapy, immunotherapy or chemotherapy. More advanced disease of the skin, in cutaneous T cell lymphoma, may require radiotherapy, chemotherapy, immunotherapy or electron beam therapy. The treatment in malignant melanoma consists of urgent wide excision of the lesion. In squamous cell carcinoma treatment consists of excision or radiotherapy. Curettage should be avoided. In basal cell carcinoma treatment consists of surgical excision although radiotherapy can be useful for large superficial forms. Curettage may occasionally be used in older patients, although not for central facial lesions as they often recur.

A22.25

1) C   2) B   3) A   4) D   5) G

Ehlers–Danlos syndrome can be subdivided into at least 10 variants. They are all inherited disorders causing abnormalities in collagen of the skin, joints and blood vessels. Clinically this causes increased elasticity of the skin, hypermobile joints and fragile blood vessels causing easy bruising. The skin is hyperextensible but recoils normally after stretching. Pseudoxanthoma elasticum is a rare group of disorders characterized by abnormalities in collagen and elastic tissue affecting the skin, eye and blood vessels. The skin may be loose, lax and wrinkled. It can look yellowish and papular ('plucked chicken skin') and tends to lose its elastic recoil when stretched. Marfan's syndrome is an autosomal dominant disorder of connective tissue. The basic genetic defect is a mutation in the extracellular matrix glycoprotein fibrillin 1 (chromosome 15q). Vitiligo presents in childhood or early adult life with well-demarcated macules of complete pigment loss. There is no history of preceding inflammation. Patients are very susceptible to sunburn. Lesions are often symmetrical and frequently involve the face, hands and genitalia. Idiopathic guttate hypomelanosis occurs most commonly in black African people and is of unknown aetiology. It presents with small (2–4 mm) asymptomatic porcelain-white macules, often on skin exposed to sunlight. The borders are often sharply defined and angular.

A22.26

1) D   2) B   3) A   4) E   5) C

Freckles appear in childhood as small brown macules after sun exposure. They fade in the winter months. Lentigos are a more permanent macule of pigmentation similar to freckles but they tend to persist in the winter. Peutz–Jegher syndrome is an autosomal dominant genetic condition. The gene responsible is *LKB1*, which codes for a serine-threonine kinase. It presents with brown macules of the lips and perioral region. It is associated with gastrointestinal polyposis which almost never becomes malignant. Chloasma are brown macules often seen symmetrically over the cheeks and forehead and are most common in women. They can occur spontaneously but are also associated with pregnancy and the oral contraceptive pill. Urticaria pigmentosa presents most commonly with multiple pigmented macules in children. These lesions tend to become red, itchy and urticated if they are rubbed (Darier's sign). Skin biopsy shows an excess of mast cells in the skin.

A22.27

A) F B) T C) T D) T E) F

Complications of shingles include severe, persistent pain (post-herpetic neuralgia), ocular disease (if ophthalmic nerve involved) and, rarely, motor neuropathy.

A22.28

A) F B) T C) T D) T E) T

This patient has toxic epidermal necrolysis which is associated with penicillin, co-trimoxazole, carbamazepine and NSAIDs. Steroids and ciclosporin have been used to treat severe cases.

A22.29

A) F B) T C) T D) T E) T

Onycholysis (distal nail plate separation) is caused by psoriasis, hyperthyroidism, following trauma and, rarely, a photosensitive reaction to drugs such as tetracyclines.

A22.30

A) T B) T C) T D) T E) T

There are five types of nail change in psoriasis: a) pitting of the nail plate; b) distal separation of the nail plate (onycholysis); c) yellow-brown discoloration; d) subungual hyperkeratosis; e) rarely, a damaged nail matrix and lost nail plate.

A22.31

A) T B) T C) T D) T E) T

Up to 5% of individuals with psoriasis develop psoriatic arthritis and most of these will have nail changes. Five patterns are recognized: a) distal interphalangeal arthritis; b) peripheral mono- or oligoarthritis; c) symmetrical 'rheumatoid arthritis pattern' but seronegative; d) spondylitis or sacroiliitis (especially if HLA-B27 positive); e) rarely, arthritis mutilans causing destruction and resorption of bone leading to telescoping of affected digits.

A22.32

A) F B) T C) T D) F E) F

Patients with urticaria should avoid salicylates and opiates as they can degranulate mast cells. Oral antihistamines (H_1 blockers) are the most important part of treating idiopathic cases. If control proves difficult, addition of a sedating antihistamine or an H_2 blocker may be helpful. Angio-oedema of the mouth and throat may require urgent treatment with intravenous steroids and subcutaneous adrenaline (epinephrine).

A22.33

A) T B) T C) T D) F E) T

UVB and UVA are both used in the treatment of inflammatory dermatoses. UVB is more likely to burn but it is less carcinogenic than UVA. It is used in the treatment of eczema and psoriasis (especially in children) and is usually given

Skin disease

three times per week for 6–10 weeks. Narrow-band UVB (311 nanometer) is superseding broad-band UVB because it is much more effective in the treatment of eczema and psoriasis. Animal and in vitro studies show it to be less carcinogenic than PUVA but long-term data in humans are not yet available. UVA is relatively ineffective on its own so is used in conjunction with a photosensitizer (psoralen); hence the term 'PUVA'. It is more effective than UVB but is limited by its carcinogenic potential. It is used for many conditions including psoriasis, eczema, cutaneous T-cell lymphoma, some photosensitive dermatoses and vitiligo. Sunbeds are used for tanning and consist of predominantly UVA light; they are therefore rarely effective in treating skin disease. If used frequently there may be an increased risk of skin cancer.

A22.34

A) T   B) T   C) T   D) T   E) T

Causes of erythema nodosum include:
a) streptococcal infection; b) drugs
(e.g. sulphonamides, oral contraceptive, aspirin, NSAIDs); c) sarcoidosis; d) idiopathic; e) *Yersinia* infection; f) fungal infection (histoplasmosis, blastomycosis); g) tuberculosis; h) leprosy; i) inflammatory bowel disease; j) *Chlamydia* infection. Of these, the common causes in the UK are: streptococcal infection; drugs; sarcoidosis; and idiopathic.

A22.35

A) T   B) T   C) T   D) T   E) F

The main causes of pyoderma gangrenosum are: a) inflammatory bowel disease; b) rheumatoid arthritis;

c) myeloma, monoclonal gammopathy, leukaemia, lymphoma; d) liver disease (primary biliary cirrhosis); e) idiopathic (>20% in some series).

A22.36

A) T   B) F   C) T   D) F   E) T

Acanthosis nigricans presents as thickened, hyperpigmented skin predominantly of the flexures. It can appear warty or velvety when advanced. In early life it is seen in obese individuals who have very high levels of insulin owing to insulin resistance. In older people it normally reflects an underlying malignancy (especially gastrointestinal tumours). Rarely it is associated with hyperandrogenism in females

A22.37

A) T   B) T   C) T   D) T   E) T

Tuberous sclerosis is an autosomal dominant condition of variable severity which may not present until later childhood. It is characterized by a variety of hamartomatous growths. The three cardinal features are: a) mental retardation; b) epilepsy; c) cutaneous abnormalities – but not all have to be present. The skin signs include: a) adenoma sebaceum (reddish papules/fibromas around the nose); b) periungual fibroma (nodules arising from the nail bed); c) shagreen patches (firm, flesh-coloured plaques on the trunk); d) ash-leaf hypopigmentation (pale macules best seen with UV light); e) forehead plaque (indurated flesh-coloured patch); f) *café au lait* patches; g) pitting of dental enamel.

A22.38

A) T **B)** T **C)** T **D)** T **E)** F

Specific dermatoses of diabetes include:
a) necrobiosis lipoidica (a patch of
spreading erythema over the shin which
becomes yellowish and atrophic in the
centre and may ulcerate); b) diffuse
granuloma annulare; c) diabetic
dermopathy (red-brown flat-topped
papules); d) blisters (usually on the feet or
hands); e) diabetic stiff skin (tight waxy
skin over the fingers with limitation of
joint movement owing to thickened
collagen – also called cheiroarthropathy).

Index